Eye Care for Infants and Young Children

Eye Care for Infants and Young Children

Bruce D. Moore, O.D., F.A.A.O.

The Marcus Professor of Pediatric Studies, New England College of Optometry,
Boston; Clincal Assistant in Ophthalmology, Harvard Medical School, Boston;
Former Director of Pediatric Contact Lens Service, Former Staff Optometrist,
Active Medical Staff, The Children's Hospital, Boston

Butterworth–Heinemann
Boston   Oxford   Auckland   Johannesburg   Melbourne   New Delhi

Butterworth–Heinemann supports the efforts of American Forests and the Global ReLeaf program in its campaign for the betterment of trees, forests, and our environment.

Library of Congress Cataloging-in-Publication Data
Moore, Bruce D.
    Eye care for infants and young children / Bruce D. Moore.
      p.   cm.
    Includes bibliographical references and index.
    ISBN 0-7506-9646-X
    1. Pediatric ophthalmology.   I. Title.
    [DNLM: 1. Eye Diseases--in infancy and childhood. 2. Eye Diseases-
-therapy. 3. Eye Diseases--prevention & control.   WW 600 M821e
1997]
    RE48.2.C5M66   1997
    618.92'0977--dc21
    DNLM/DLC
    for Library of Congress   96-2666
                                          CIP

British Library Cataloguing-in-Publication Data
A catalogue record for this book is available from the British Library.

The publisher offers special discounts on bulk orders of this book.
For information, please contact:

Manager of Special Sales
Butterworth–Heinemann
225 Wildwood Avenue
Woburn, MA 01801–2041
Tel: 781-904-2500
Fax: 781-904-2620

For information on all Butterworth–Heinemann publications available, contact our World Wide Web home page at: http://www.bh.com

10 9 8 7 6 5 4 3

Printed in the United States of America

Contents

Contributing Authors

Sandra S. Block, O.D., M.Ed., F.A.A.O.
Associate Professor, Department of Clinical Education, Pediatrics
and Binocular Vision Service, Illinois College of Optometry, Chicago

Elise B. Ciner, O.D., F.A.A.O.
Associate Clinical Professor of Pediatrics and Binocular Vision and Director,
Infant Vision Service, Pennsylvania College of Optometry, Philadelphia

Susan A. Cotter, O.D., F.A.A.O.
Professor of Optometry, Vision Therapy Service, Optometric Center
of Fullerton, Southern California College of Optometry

Ellen Richter Ettinger, O.D., M.S., F.A.A.O.
Associate Professor of Optometry, Department of Clinical Sciences,
State University of New York State College of Optometry, New York

Kelly A. Frantz, O.D., F.A.A.O.
Associate Professor, Department of Clinical Education, Pediatrics
and Binocular Vision Service, Illinois College of Optometry, Chicago

Paul Kohl, O.D.
Professor of Optometry, Pacific University College of Optometry,
Forest Grove, Oregon

Richard C. Laudon, O.D., F.A.A.O.
Associate Professor of Optometry, New England College of Optometry, Boston;
Staff, Pediatric Binocular Vision Service, New England Eye Institute

Dominick M. Maino, O.D., M.Ed., F.A.A.O.
Professor of Pediatrics and Binocular Vision, Illinois Eye Institute and the
Illinois College of Optometry, Chicago; Adjunct Professor of Pediatrics,
Centro Boston de Optometria, Madrid, Spain; Chief, Optometric Services,
Illinois Eye Institute at the Gilchrist-Marchman Rehabilitation Center, Easter
Seal Society of Metropolitan Chicago

Ruth E. Manny, O.D., Ph.D., F.A.A.O.
Associate Professor and Chair of Clinical Sciences, College
of Optometry, University of Houston

Bruce D. Moore, O.D., F.A.A.O.
The Marcus Professor of Pediatric Studies, New England College of Optometry,
Boston; Clincal Assistant in Ophthalmology, Harvard Medical School, Boston;
Former Director of Pediatric Contact Lens Service, Former Staff Optometrist,
Active Medical Staff, The Children's Hospital, Boston

Donald O. Mutti, O.D., Ph.D., F.A.A.O.
Specialist and Assistant Clinical Professor of Optometry, School
of Optometry, University of California at Berkeley

Deborah Orel-Bixler, Ph.D., O.D., F.A.A.O.
Assistant Clinical Professor and Residency Director, School of Optometry,
University of California at Berkeley

Leonard J. Press, O.D., F.C.O.V.D., F.A.A.O.
Associate Professor, State University of New York, State College of Optometry,
New York; Associate Medical Staff, Department of Rehabilitative Medicine,
St. Lawrence Rehabilitation Hospital, Lawrenceville, New Jersey

Jack E. Richman, O.D., F.C.O.V.D., F.A.A.O.
Professor of Optometry, New England College of Optometry, Boston;
Chief of Pediatric Optometry and Binocular Vision Services,
New England Eye Institute

Janice Emigh Scharre, O.D., M.A., F.C.O.V.D., F.A.A.O.
Professor of Optometry and Associate Dean of Clinical Affairs,
Illinois College of Optometry, Chicago

Paulette P. Schmidt, O.D., M.S., F.A.A.O.
Associate Professor of Optometry and Physiological Optics,
The Ohio State University College of Optometry, Columbus

Karla Zadnik, O.D., Ph.D., F.A.A.O.
Assistant Professor of Optometry, The Ohio State University College of Optometry,
Columbus; Associate Clinical Professor of Optometry, University of California,
Berkeley School of Optometry, Berkeley

Preface

Optometry has continued its expansion into many new and exciting areas. Optometrists now routinely treat the full spectrum of eye disease, something unthinkable when I was a student 25 years ago. I believe that one of the next frontiers in optometric practice will be age related. Today, elderly patients are routinely seen in optometric clinical practice. This is due partly to their very considerable visual needs, partly to their rapidly growing numbers, and partly to their generally good health insurance coverage, along with the considerable interest of the optometric community in their care.

Young children, the opposite end of the age spectrum, are currently seen in significant numbers in only a relatively few optometric practices. This is due to the perceptions that young children cannot be examined and do not need vision care, and when some problem is suspected, the referral patterns historically bypass optometry. I believe that these perceptions will change for a number of reasons. As our profession's mode of practice continues to evolve, optometry's position as the entry point into the vision care delivery system will be solidified for infants and young children, as it is for the adult population today. The perception that young children cannot be examined and treated as well as older patients is being put to rest, as this text illustrates.

The standard of care as exemplified by the *Clinical Practice Guidelines on the Pediatric Eye and Vision Examination* issued by the American Optometric Association recommends for the routine vision care assessment of all 6-month-old children. As these guidelines are implemented, practicing optometrists will more routinely be providing care to young children. Students and practicing optometrists will need to develop skills in the care of these patients. The purpose of this text is to provide a theoretical and clinical basis for the optometric care of young children by current and future optometrists.

Historically, optometry has emphasized not only the care and treatment of vision disorders but also functional aspects of vision that have fallen outside the interest of ophthalmology. Indeed, this is what separates us from that profession. This is nowhere more true than within the realm of the child, where function is so critical in the relationship between vision and learning. A goal of this text is to stimulate optometric thought and research into these areas of visual function in the young child. It is hoped that this first optometric text on the young child will help to crystallize thinking on this developing area of optometric practice.

This text is the product of the combined efforts of a group of experts in pediatric optometry in the United States. Although all of the authors are active faculty at various colleges of optometry, this text is not intended solely for the student or faculty member. Indeed, practicing clinicians, those experienced or inexperienced in the care of children, will find the material of particular clinical value on a day-to-day basis. Because the care of infants and young children was relatively rare during their professional training, the established practitioner will be less experienced in the care of this population than with others. Clinicians will now have a centralized source of information about the optometric care of the young child.

Students will have available a comprehensive text that emphasizes the optometric care of young children. This includes both a theoretical framework and the clinical diagnosis and treatment of the full spectrum of vision care abnormalities in young children. With only minor additions, this text is inclusive enough to be used as a general pediatric optometry text for students. The emphasis on young children brings attention to the most important subject areas that differ from that of adult patients.

This text is highly clinical in nature. Each chapter is designed to be useful and accessible to the clinician. The background material included is also meant to be clinical in orientation. There are many excellent texts available that take a more didactic approach to the various aspects of pediatric eye and vision care. The reader is strongly encouraged to pursue his or her interest in particular topic areas in other sources.

The text begins with a discussion of clinical decision making. Ellen Ettinger sets forth the specific issues that the pediatric optometrist faces in obtaining information from young patients and their families. The obvious inability to inquire directly of the patient makes the process of examination and diagnosis more complex than for older patients, but the general considerations of the examination process are actually not so different, just more complex, and, I think, more interesting. The ability of the clinician to be a consummate detective in the quest for clues as to the child's visual status is critical. Likewise, the process of communication with parents and the child is more complex, necessitating skill and patience beyond that required for typical patients. Clinical decision making is a process that the experienced clinician probably rarely, if ever, considers as a didactic exercise but is the basis of good clinical care. The student, as well as the experienced clinician, is encouraged to give thought to this process.

Jan Scharre and Sandy Block describe the important subject of visual development in young children. This is a subject area that has changed enormously in the past few decades as our knowledge and appreciation of the developing child has grown. It was not very long ago that most authorities believed that infants had only rudimentary levels of vision. We now know this is untrue. Many visual functions reach excellent, even virtually adult levels, by 4–6 months of age. It is therefore critical that we identify abnormal visual development as early as possible to initiate treatment when it is most likely to prove effective. We now understand that abnormalities in visual development lead directly to many of the most common vision disorders, such as amblyopia and strabismus. Thus knowledge of visual development is essential for the student and clinician to understand the basis of optometric care of the child.

An awareness of the prevalence of vision disorders in young children is essential to provide a framework for their clinical care. With optometry's expansion into the realm of the treatment of eye disease, it is natural to place almost inordinate attention on this subject matter. This text does spend considerable effort to make the diagnosis and treatment of eye disease accessible to the reader, but it must be emphasized that pediatric eye disease is for the most part, uncommon, if not rare. Compare this with the prevalence of what might be thought of as the "bread and butter" of pediatric optometry—namely, the diagnosis and management of refractive error, amblyopia, strabismus, and vision-related learning problems. A review of the epidemiology and the clinical significance of vision problems in young children provides a foundation for making the clinician aware of those conditions most likely to be seen in actual clinical practice.

Refraction is perhaps the cornerstone of optometry. All of my generation of optometrists fondly remember the massive (and magnificent) work by Dr. Irving Borish, *Clinical Refraction*, as the centerpiece of our education. Optometry has always been viewed as the vision care profession most closely associated with refraction and the treatment of refractive error. I firmly believe that this is just as true today. The recent exciting work on the process of emmetropization and the early development of refractive error provides new importance to the old topic of refraction. Without question, refractive error is by far the most prevalent ocular disorder affecting all age groups and populations. A critical understanding of the topic is fundamental to understanding pediatric optometry.

Refraction is approached from two perspectives in this text. Don Mutti and Karla Zadnik share their views of refractive error in young children from a somewhat structural viewpoint. They have identified the role that the various ocular components play in determining refractive error, how those components are related to each other and the whole, and how these components evolve over time in the developing child. This information provides a basis of understanding the natural history of refractive error in young children. Elise Ciner takes a more classic approach, emphasizing the functional aspects of refractive error in young children, with a comprehensive approach to the management of those refractive errors. The clinician must have a clear knowledge of the natural history of refractive error in young children, so as not to prescribe inappropriately.

Elise Ciner and Deb Orel-Bixler next provide information on the actual clinical techniques of examination of the young child. Elise concentrates on the more general aspects of examination procedures in a practical manner especially useful to the student. Deb discusses more advanced procedures, those that are more useful in specialized clinical settings. These are the tools that are used in the diagnosis of less common pediatric ocular disorders. Although these tools may not be readily available to the general practitioner, it is important to understand when they are useful or even essential to the proper diagnosis. The general practitioner must understand how to interpret their results when patients are referred for special testing.

Two essential subject areas in pediatric optometry concern the diagnosis and treatment of strabismus and amblyopia. The relationship of these topics to refractive error is important. Together, these three (along with their relationship to learning related issues) make up the vast bulk of clinical patients seen by pediatric optometrists. Therefore, great emphasis is placed on these topics. The proper diagnosis and treatment of amblyopia (discussed in Chapter 9 by Lennie Press and Paul Kohl) and strabismus (discussed in Chapter 8 by Sue Cotter and Kelly Frantz) requires all of the knowledge base of our profession. The clinician must understand the underlying anatomic and physiologic basis of these disorders in order to treat them effectively. The clinician must use all of his or her management skills to oversee the long-term and difficult treatment entailed. And perhaps most important, the clinician must not forget that although most amblyopia and strabismus are due to what may be considered functional causes, organic causes such as those derived from ocular and systemic disease should always be suspected until they can be completely ruled out during the early and late decision-making phases.

The ideal situation for all children would be to follow the American Optometric Association guidelines on the frequency and timing of eye examinations. These guidelines state that all 6-month-old infants and 3-year-old children should have complete eye and vision evaluations. This is unfortunately neither the case today, nor even feasible, for logistic, financial, and geographic reasons. Therefore, the best approach that we should be following today would be a universal vision screening program. Paulette Schmidt discusses both the theoretical and practical aspects of such a vision screening program, including its rationale and a description of appropriate methods and implementation.

An extensive section on ocular disease, including congenital and acquired eye disease, its diagnosis and treatment, and ocular pharmacology as it relates to the young child follows. This is a relatively new area for optometry, as this was formerly almost entirely within the purview of ophthalmology. This change is indicative of the expansion in scope of our profession. Although the treatment of many of these disorders is currently beyond the scope of optometry, the detection and diagnosis are integral to pediatric clinical practice.

Dominick Maino discusses the important ocular and systemic issues related to children born with developmental disabilities. These children are more likely to have vision and eye abnormalities requiring early care and treatment by optometrists. They make up a significant component of the practice of pediatric optometry.

Contact lenses are a useful modality in the treatment of many ocular disorders affecting young children. The pediatric optometrist should be aware of their potential benefit to the patient.

Child abuse and neglect are difficult subjects for anyone to consider, but as health care providers, optometrists must confront these unpleasant issues. Ruth Manny provides an extensive evaluation of this issue and includes practical guidelines for the practitioner who suspects this in a patient. Our ability to identify this difficult problem is indicative of our coming of age as a health care profession.

Learning disabilities and the relationship of vision to learning problems have been an integral aspect of pediatric optometry. Extending these issues to younger children, in particular to preschoolers and even infants, may be difficult for some of our colleagues to accept. Nonetheless, I believe that Jack Richman and Rich Laudon have addressed an important issue. Clearly, "at-risk" infants and young children are at increased risk for the development of both eye and vision problems and learning related problems. Addressing these issues through early intervention programs, occupational and physical therapy, speech and language therapy, and early optometric vision therapy, and providing necessary medical and psychosocial support may improve the child's ability to learn and perform in school. Therefore, a broad definition of the role of optometry in the identification and treatment of potential learning disabilities in young children is, I think, quite appropriate.

I reiterate that this text is meant to be clinical in orientation. The reader should pursue background information elsewhere.

BDM

Acknowledgments

This text is based on my 21 years of personal experience while a member of the Department of Ophthalmology at Boston's Children's Hospital. I am very deeply indebted to my former Chief, Richard Robb, M.D., and to my former colleagues, Drs. Robert Petersen, Anne Fulton, and Lois Smith, for their enormous experience, guidance, and encouragement over the years. I would like to acknowledge all I have learned, in so many ways, from my patients and their families. I would like to thank the good people at Butterworth–Heinemann Publishers, especially my friends Barbara Murphy and Jana Friedman, for their encouragement and especially their patience during this long endeavor. Most important, I would like to thank my loving wife, Marcia, and my children, Rachel, Eric, and Kate, for their support and forbearance during this long effort.

Chapter 1
Clinical Decision Making

Ellen Richter Ettinger

Clinical decision making has been compared to detective's work [1]. The clinician must uncover clues and evidence (the case history and examination findings) that lead to the solution of a problem (the diagnosis and treatment plan). Just as a detective performs an investigation to search for evidence and clues, the doctor performs a clinical examination, with his or her clinical findings serving as the hints and clues that provide insight into the patient's diagnosis and the proper management plan. The clinical findings, therefore, are the input needed for decision making.

This chapter reviews how the optometrist gathers information for decision making, how the clinical clues and evidence are used in models of clinical decision making, and how epidemiology guides the development of rules for decision making.

GATHERING CLUES AND EVIDENCE

The untrained detective, like many parents, would be uncertain how to tell if an infant or toddler sees well or needs glasses. Clinicians who are intimidated by working with children identify many challenges in treating the pediatric population. Nonverbal infants and young children are not able to respond to many traditional clinical tests. Those who are old enough to respond are sometimes not cooperative or fully attentive for long periods of time. Therefore, results are often ambiguous, unreliable, or unobtainable.

These problems highlight two of the main difficulties in collecting data in pediatric patients: limited quantity and limited quality of information [2, 3]. The primary challenge in working with infants and young children is to collect "evidence" when the indicators and clues sometimes appear to be hidden or unobtainable.

Fortunately, many ocular testing techniques have been developed for use in infants and children. Preferential looking [4, 5], the Broken Wheel test [6], and Lighthouse acuity cards [7] are some of the many options available for testing pediatric patients. Clinicians should be comfortable with performing these tests and know with what age groups the tests are most effective. Expertise in using specific tests and procedures is important not only for collecting clinical data, but also for acquiring information that serves as a basis for making decisions.

Like a detective, the expert clinician working with pediatric patients knows how to maximize the input for the decision-making process. Table 1.1 outlines some of the strategies that enable the clinician to acquire maximum information from the patient.

The clinician should learn to communicate effectively with pediatric patients to maximize the amount of information that can be obtained. Successful communication and interaction with children requires good verbal and nonverbal communication skills [8]. Even children who do not speak or understand words are able to recognize communication. Infants do not always understand the content of verbal communications, but they appear to respond to sensitive, caring vocal intonations. Nonverbal communications such as facial expressions and eye con-

Table 1.1. Tips for Gathering Input for the Decision-Making Process

- Work quickly and efficiently to keep the child from fatiguing.
- If a child fatigues during one part of the examination, try to regain attention and cooperation by moving to another procedure.
- Use brightly colored, interesting visual targets to hold the child's attention.
- Become an expert in using special testing procedures that are effective in gathering clinical findings in children (e.g., preferential looking, the Broken Wheel test, Lighthouse acuity cards).
- Remember that separation anxiety occurs because the infant or child wants to be close to the parent or caregiver. Consider having the child sit on the parent's lap during the examination. If the child is old enough to sit in a chair alone, make sure the parent is within the child's view.
- Develop a caring, trusting relationship with the child and parents or caregivers.
- Do not schedule the examination during the child's normal nap or meal time.
- Use both verbal and nonverbal communication appropriately to build rapport and trust and to continue to reassure the patient.
- If you are not able to get all of the information that you want, consider having the patient return to complete the examination.

tact are also important. Infants also often respond well to gentle, therapeutic touch.

Doctors must also develop trust with young patients. This process is more of an art than a science. Building trust improves the quantity and quality of information acquired.

Clinicians who work with children are usually quick, attentive, and astute at making observations in patients (e.g., head tilt, eye turn) and in encouraging parents and caregivers to become good observers and therefore good reporters. Observations by the parents, caregivers, and doctor are all useful in evaluating the child's status.

MODELS OF CLINICAL DECISION MAKING

Pattern recognition, algorithmic reasoning, and hypothetico-deductive reasoning are three models of

clinical decision making that illustrate the different ways in which clinicians can use clinical data to reach a diagnosis [9–12].

Algorithmic Reasoning

The process of algorithmic reasoning is usually illustrated using a flow chart in which a sequence of questions are asked about the patient's problem. The answer to each question determines the path for the next step and the pathway leads to a final decision (or diagnosis).

A nonclinical example [13] frequently used to illustrate algorithmic reasoning is the path of questioning followed when a light does not work. First, you make sure the light fixture is plugged into the outlet. If that is not the problem, you check to make sure the light bulb is not burned out. If that is not the problem, you check to make sure the switch on the light fixture is working properly. If that is not the problem, you check to make sure the outlet is working properly or that there is not a power failure. If you still cannot solve the problem, you may refer the problem to an expert (in this case, an electrician).

A similar type of sequential inquiry can be made in a clinical situation to determine the cause of a red eye [9]. The optometrist can observe whether a yellow, purulent discharge is present (suggesting a bacterial cause); whether preauricular nodes are present (suggesting a viral cause); whether the redness is located at the episcleral vessels (suggesting episcleritis); whether the eyelids are red (suggesting blepharitis); whether there are cells in the anterior chamber (suggesting iritis); or whether there is corneal and pupillary involvement (suggesting a narrow-angle glaucoma attack). The optometrist may also ask if there is any history of allergy (suggesting an allergic cause) or any recent history of an upper respiratory infection (suggesting a viral cause).

Pattern Recognition

In pattern recognition, the doctor matches a set of signs and symptoms in the patient (referred to as the *sign-symptom complex*) with a previously learned picture or pattern of disease known as the *template*.

When the patient's sign-symptom complex matches the template of a known disease, a diagnosis can be made. Conditions that have very obvious and distinctive visual presentations such as subconjunctival hemorrhages, exophthalmos in Graves' disease [10], café au lait spots in neurofibromatosis [10], and albinism may be identified in this manner. Patients with a constant large-angle strabismus are often identified instantly by the experienced optometrist because the patient's appearance is easily matched to the clinician's template of a large-scale strabismic individual. Similarly, it is often easy to detect Down syndrome in a patient by the presence of characteristic features such as prominent epicanthal folds, oblique palpebral fissures, and flat nasal bridges [14]. Problems that have less prominent or less distinctive identifying features may be more difficult to diagnose using this model.

Hypothetico-Deductive Method

The clinician using the hypothetico-deductive method generates a list of possible diagnoses, referred to as the *working hypotheses* early in the clinical encounter. These potential hypotheses correspond to the patient's presenting symptoms. As data are gathered and analyzed, some hypotheses are reinforced, or ruled in; some are eliminated or ruled out; and other new ones are generated to correspond to the evolving group of known signs and symptoms. A cyclic process of data collection and hypothesis testing occurs until a final diagnosis is made.

The hypothetico-deductive method is the process used by clinicians to perform a differential diagnosis. The most likely conditions are identified and clinical testing is done to determine which diagnosis is most likely.

The hypothetico-deductive method is the form of decision making used most frequently by clinicians [10], although pattern recognition may help elicit diagnoses in conditions with highly recognizable cues. Algorithmic reasoning may also help explain the types of questions clinicians ask as they rule in and rule out hypotheses. In each of these three models, the clinician looks at the patient's signs and symptoms (the evidence) to make a diagnostic decision. The visual cues and other features observed by the clinician and the symptoms reported by the patient

are used to make a match in pattern recognition. In algorithmic reasoning, they are used to determine the pathway of inquiry. In the hypothetico-deductive method, the continuing collection of clinical signs and features facilitates the doctor's ability to rule in and rule out conditions until a final diagnosis is established. In all three models, it is the evidence that leads to the diagnosis.

EPIDEMIOLOGY

In addition to identifying signs and symptoms found in individual patients, the clinician working with pediatric patients must be aware of problems commonly found in infancy and childhood. Epidemiologic knowledge helps clinicians plan an appropriate testing sequence and identify management plans that work effectively in a pediatric population. Good clinical diagnostic and management skills require a clear understanding of the epidemiology and clinical and scientific knowledge of a patient population.

Clinical studies have found that refractive errors, nonstrabismic binocular disorders, strabismus, amblyopia, and accommodative disorders are the most prevalent visual anomalies in children [15]. Studies have also shown that early diagnosis and intervention is essential in treating vision problems in children [16–24]. Failure to detect and manage visual problems in a timely manner can result in amblyopia. For this reason and others, clinicians strongly encourage the eye examination of children by 6 months of age.

Studies have also shown that rapid changes in the visual system within the first 6 months of life affect visual acuity, accommodation, and binocular vision; interference with vision during this critical time can result in permanent and irreversible visual limitations [16–23]. Also, the prognosis is often worse if treatment is delayed, and additional cost and time burdens accrue if these problems must be treated later in life [24–27].

The clinical knowledge gained from these studies affects the optometrist's decision making. For example, current professional recommendations state that a child should have an eye examination by age 6 months. If anisometropia, strabismus, congenital cataracts, or any other amblyogenic risk factors are identified, rapid intervention is key. Studies have shown that it is best to actively treat patients with these conditions and not to just monitor patients with these conditions and have them back over the next few years of life to see if anything changes on its own.

Clinical research has also provided insights into treatment and therapeutic decisions. When using patching routines for amblyopia in infants, for example, it has been shown that it is best not to patch for extended periods of time or the patch itself can result in interference in vision. It is therefore recommended that patching be done for only short periods of time and for no more than 2 hours per day to reduce the risk of occlusion amblyopia [28].

Although there is a much lower incidence of ocular pathology compared with the incidence of the visual problems discussed previously, clinicians must also perform proper testing to identify the presence of any ocular diseases or conditions.

Optometrists should also remember that visual information processing and learning problems can affect visual performance. Optometrists should inquire about developmental milestones (e.g., when did the child first walk, talk, sit, crawl,) and pre-, peri-, and postnatal health (e.g., difficulties during pregnancy and birth, low birth weight, prematurity). Signs of perceptual and developmental lags require additional testing and intervention.

The information supplied by clinical and scientific studies provides tremendous guidance for decision making in the treatment of pediatric patients. The clinician who provides care to infants and young children must be familiar with new information relevant to the care of pediatric patients.

DECISION RULES

Clinicians constantly use decision rules to guide their care of patients. A decision rule may be as simple as the fact that distance vision in nearsighted patients is corrected with minus power lenses [29]. Decision rules are often more complex and cover a wide variety of factors, including testing patients, making a correct diagnosis, and choosing a proper management plan.

Not all clinicians use the same set of decision rules. Different clinicians may adopt different rules based on their own philosophies of clinical care and practice. It is important, however, for clinicians to be certain that their decision rules accurately reflect current clinical and scientific knowledge.

Clinical Testing

The following statements are examples of decision rules that involve choosing appropriate methods of clinical testing:

> To assess visual acuity in infants up to 12 months age of age, use preferential looking [30].
> To assess visual acuity in preschoolers, use the Broken Wheel test or Lighthouse cards [30].

Decision rules are general guidelines. When used for decisions regarding diagnostic testing, they provide the clinician with a suggested method of testing that may need to be adjusted to meet the individual patient's needs. For example, preferential looking generally works well with infants, but some older infants are too active to maintain attention and respond definitively. If this is the case, the clinician would likely not use preferential looking for testing or would attempt it at another time with the patient. Similarly, clinicians would anticipate that some children over a year would respond well to preferential looking testing.

Diagnosis

Decision rules that include analysis of clinical findings help to guide diagnosis. The following decision rules assist clinicians in making diagnoses:

> Patients with decreased visual acuity in one eye with at least a two-line difference in acuity between the eyes are amblyopic in the absence of pathology [31].
> Patients with a receded near point of convergence, greater exophoria at near than at distance, decreased positive fusional vergence, and a low accommodative convergence to accommodation ratio have convergence insufficiency [31].
> Patients with esophoria at near, orthophoria or low-to-moderate esophoria at distance, reduced negative fusional vergence, and a high accommodative convergence to accommodation ratio have convergence excess [31].
> Patients with opacified lenses have cataracts [32].

Patient Management

Many decision rules direct patient management and therapy, including rules about when to prescribe refractive corrections in children and young infants. These decisions are usually based on our understanding of the risks of amblyopia, the child's binocular status and age, and the developing eye and visual system. The following are examples of decision rules that affect patient management:

Myopia of greater than 5.00 D should be corrected in infants or children of any age [33].

Myopia of greater than 3.00 D should be corrected at 1 year of age [33].

Myopia of greater than 1.00 D should be corrected at 3 years of age [33].

Consider undercorrecting myopia with esodeviations to optimize binocular functioning [33].

If the refractive error is greater than 5.00 D, correction with contact lenses is preferable [33].

Prescribe the full prescription for full-time wear as expeditiously as possible for patients with refractive amblyopia [30].

Decision rules provide general diagnostic and therapeutic strategies to help guide treatment. It is important to realize that these guidelines are general rules that usually apply. There will always be cases that are exceptions to theses rules. For example, it may be best optically to prescribe a contact lens for a child with significant anisometropia, but if the child and parent are resistant to such treatment, a rigid rule requiring contact lens wear would not be satisfactory. Similarly, the general rule is to provide the full prescription for patients with refractive amblyopia, but if binocularity is compromised, the clinician would modify the prescription.

When clinical care becomes automatic and ingrained in the mind of the clinician, decision rules often become intuitive, and clinicians may not even be conscious or aware that they use them. It is important, however, for clinicians to be aware of the rules that they use so they can be sure to review and update their decision rules as new information becomes available. For example, when research showed that a spray administration of cyclopentolate was a good alternative to conventional eyedrops for cycloplegic examinations in pediatric patients [34], some clinicians chose

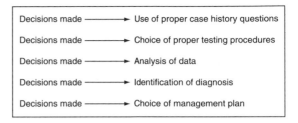

Figure 1.1. This figures illustrates that the process of clinical decision making occurs throughout the examination, not just at the end with the determination of the diagnosis and management plan. Making the proper decisions throughout case history, clinical testing, and case analysis enables the clinician to make correct diagnostic and therapeutic decisions.

to use this procedure since it eliminated the need to hold the child's eyelid open for eyedrop administration and therefore produced less avoidance response.

Special clinical procedures such as preferential looking [4, 5] and photorefraction [35] have been developed to help assess vision in infants and children. Other scientific and clinical findings relevant to the care of children should be evaluated by clinicians as they are reported. When warranted, new decision rules may be adopted by clinicians as a result of new testing techniques or treatment modalities and philosophies. Advances in scientific knowledge and appropriate implementation of this new knowledge by clinicians can improve the quality of care provided to our patients.

THE CLINICAL DECISION-MAKING PROCESS

Decision making often focuses on identifying the patient's diagnosis and determining a management plan. The discussion of pediatric care in this chapter demonstrates, however, that decision making is an ongoing process that starts at the first meeting with the patient and continues throughout the examination (Figure 1.1).

Excellent clinicians are adept at "putting the pieces of the puzzle together" and analyzing the patient's entire situation because they are thinking throughout the examination. Throughout all the processes discussed in this chapter—from communicating with the patient, to testing, to choosing decision rules—the clinician is constantly thinking

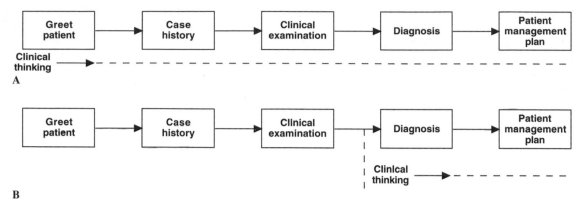

Figure 1.2. Two models of clinical decision making. A. The clinician uses clinical thinking throughout the encounter, beginning when he or she greets the patient. B. The clinician does not begin the process of clinical thinking and analysis until all data have been gathered. In B, the clinician would miss many cues (e.g., patient's head tilt, signs of discomfort) that the clinician in A would notice. In B, the clinician is essentially acting as a technician until all the data are collected. Clearly, the method illustrated in A is the optimal method for data collection and decision making.

(Figure 1.2A). The clinician is not a technician who collects data and analyzes it at the end when all clinical findings have been collected (Figure 1.2B). Like the detective, the optometrist gathers clues and evidence (case history and examination findings) during the investigation (examination), and these lead to the final answer (diagnosis and management plan). It is unlikely the investigator will reach an optimal final conclusion if he or she has not been alert throughout the process.

Incomplete Data Sets

Data are limited in pediatric patients for a number of reasons. Children are sometimes inattentive, anxious, or uncooperative. Standard procedures are difficult to perform with infants and children who are nonverbal. Even in children who can be tested, responses are sometimes questionable or unreliable. Clinicians learn very quickly that one of the primary challenges of working with young patients is making decisions with an incomplete set of data. Clearly, working with a pediatric patient is not like performing an examination on a highly responsive adult. When working with children, the clinician often has a set of tests and a list of the data that optimally would be obtained, but recognizes that for each individual patient pieces of the puzzle will probably be missing.

Many students and clinicians who begin working with young patients experience a feeling of insecurity when they realize that parts of the clinical data set are unobtainable. The first step in addressing this fear is recognizing that this is a problem inherent in work with pediatric patients. Instead of agonizing over unobtainable data, the experienced pediatric clinician understands that data are usually limited in this population. By becoming proficient in special testing techniques and procedures for children and strategies for maintaining a child's attention and cooperation, the clinician can become an expert in the art of acquiring as full a set of data as possible.

It is also important to realize that a clinician can still make excellent clinical decisions even in the absence of abundant data. When little information is available and the clinician is not confident about the data obtained, he or she may have to rely on alternate strategies to strengthen the patient's understanding. These include bringing a child back to finish an examination, asking parents or caregivers for additional input, or monitoring a child closely over time to reevaluate decisions.

Finally, it is important to remember that by staying alert throughout the examination for cues and clues, the doctor can gather maximum information about the child. It is the ability to make keen observations, the insights into choosing the proper testing procedures for a particular child, and the skill in interacting with the pediatric patient that enables the clinician to obtain an optimal—but not necessarily complete—set of data.

CONCLUSION

Good clinical decision making in infants and children involves the following:

1. Proper testing to gather the "clues and evidence"
2. Sound epidemiologic understanding of the problems found in the pediatric population and the options for correction and treatment in these patients
3. Use of updated decision rules that reflect current knowledge of testing and management in infants and young children
4. Skillful interactive abilities with pediatric patients and a sincere interest in infants, children, their parents, and caregivers
5. Dedication to keeping current in the research and advances on vision care and assessment in children and maintaining an open attitude toward changing clinical procedures and treatment decisions when new information warrants change
6. Dedication to thinking throughout the clinical encounter in order to avoid missing any cues or clinical insights during the examination

REFERENCES

1. Albert DA, Munson R, Resnik MD. Reasoning in Medicine—An Introduction to Clinical Inference. Baltimore: Johns Hopkins University, 1988.
2. Ettinger ER. Clinical Decision Making in Special Populations: Dealing with Incomplete Data. In M Maino (ed), Problems in Optometry: Diagnosis and Management of Special Populations. St. Louis: Year Book, 1995;207–226.
3. Weinstein MC, Fineberg HV. Clinical Decision Analysis. Philadelphia: Saunders, 1980.
4. Dobson V, McDonald MS, Kohl P, et al. Visual acuity screening of infants and children with the acuity card procedure. J Am Optom Assoc 1986;57:284–289.
5. Stebbins A. Clinical assessment of the PL 20/20 infant vision tester. J Am Optom Assoc 1986;57:465–469.
6. Richman JE, Petito GT, Cron M. Broken wheel acuity test: a new and valid test for preschool and exceptional children. J Am Optom Assoc 1984;55:561–565.
7. Hyvarinen L. The Lighthouse Symbol Tests. Long Island City, NY: Lighthouse Low Vision Products, 1992.
8. Ettinger ER. Communicating with Pediatric Patients. In ER Ettinger (ed), Professional Communications in Eye Care. Boston: Butterworth–Heinemann, 1994.
9. Ettinger ER. Clinical Decision Making Skills. In ER Ettinger, MW Rouse (eds), Clinical Decision Making in Optometry. Boston: Butterworth–Heinemann, 1996.
10. Sackett DL, Haynes RB, Guyatt GH, Tugwell P. Clinical Epidemiology: A Basic Science for Clinical Medicine. Boston: Little, Brown, 1991.
11. Kurtz D. Teaching clinical reasoning. J Optom Educ 1990;15:119–122.
12. Sox HC, Blatt MA, Higgins MC, Marton KI. Medical Decision Making. Boston: Butterworth, 1988.
13. Madsen EM, Kaminski MS, Yolton RL. Automated decision making: the role of expert computer systems in the future of optometry. J Am Optom Assoc 1993; 64:478–489.
14. Wesson MD, Maino DM. Oculovisual Findings in Children with Down Syndrome, Cerebral Palsy, and Mental Retardation without Specific Etiology. In M Maino, RL London (eds), Problems in Optometry: Diagnosis and Management of Special Populations. St. Louis: Year Book, 1995.
15. Scheiman M, Gallaway M, Coulter R, et al. Prevalence of vision and ocular disorders in a clinical pediatric population. Optom Vis Sci 1992;69(Suppl):108.
16. American Optometric Association. Pediatric Eye and Vision Examination (Clinical Practice Guideline). St. Louis: American Optometric Association, 1994.
17. Dobson V, Teller DY. Visual acuity in human infants: a review and comparison of behavioral and electrophysiological studies. Vision Res 1978;17:1469–1483.
18. Gwiazda J, Brill S, Mohindra I, et al. Preferential looking acuity in infants from two to fifty-eight weeks of age. Am J Optom Physiol Opt 1980;57:428–32.
19. Banks MS. The development of visual accommodation during early infancy. Child Dev 1980;51:646–66.
20. Brookman KE. Ocular accommodation in human infants. Am J Optom Physiol Opt 1982;60:91–99.
21. Banks MS, Aslin RN, Letson RD. Sensitive period for the development of human binocular vision. Science 1975;190:675–677.
22. Hohman A, Creutzfeldt OD. Squint and the development of binocularity in humans. Nature 1975;254: 613–614.
23. Ciner EB, Scheiman MM, Schanel-Klitsch E, et al. Stereopsis testing in 18 to 35 month old children using operant preferential looking. Optom Vis Sci 1989;66:782–787.
24. Epelbaum M, Milleret C, Buisseret P, Dufier JL. The sensitive period for strabismic amblyopia in humans. Ophthalmology 1993;100:323–327.
25. Angi MR, Pucci V, Forattini F, Formentin PA. Results of photorefractometric screening for amblyogenic defects in children age 20 months. Behav Brain Res 1992;49(1):91–97.

26. Neumann E, Friedman Z, Abel-Peleg B. Prevention of strabismic amblyopia of early onset with special reference to the optimal age for screening. J Pediatr Ophthalmol Strabismus 1987;24:106–110.

27. Franz KA. Children's vision: where primary optometric care begins. J Am Optom Assoc 1994;65:685–686.

28. Garzia RP. Management of Amblyopia in Infants, Toddlers, and Preschool Children. In M Scheiman (ed), Problems in Optometry: Pediatric Optometry. Philadelphia: Lippincott, 1990;438–458.

29. Madsen EM, Reinke AR, Fehrs MH, Yolton RL. Applications of expert computer systems. J Am Optom Assoc 1990;61:116–122.

30. Press LJ, Moore BM. Clinical Pediatric Optometry. Boston: Butterworth–Heinemann, 1993.

31. Scheiman M, Wick B. Clinical Management of Binocular Vision. Philadelphia: Lippincott, 1994.

32. Eskridge JB, Amos JF, Bartlett JD. Clinical Procedures in Optometry. Philadelphia: Lippincott, 1991.

33. Ciner EB. Management of Refractive Error in Infants, Toddlers, and Preschool Children. In M Scheiman (ed), Problems in Optometry: Pediatric Optometry. Philadelphia: Lippincott, 1990;394–419.

34. Bartlett JD, Wesson MD, Swiatocha J, Wooley T. Efficacy of a pediatric cycloplegic administered as a spray. J Am Optom Assoc 1993;64:617–620.

35. Duckman R. Using Photorefraction to Evaluate Refractive Error, Ocular Alignment, and Accommodation in Infants, Toddlers, and Multiply Handicapped Children. In M Scheiman (ed), Problems in Optometry: Pediatric Optometry. Philadelphia: Lippincott, 1990;333–354.

Chapter 2
Visual System Development

Janice Emigh Scharre and Sandra S. Block

Clinicians rely on a thorough understanding of normal visual development to guide the clinical decision-making process. To determine if an abnormality exists, developmental and behavioral norms are compared with the data collected on an individual patient, and a clinical decision-making model [1] is used to explore the patient's problem.

An understanding of the normal visual development process of the infant helps the clinician to accurately determine if the visual development observed deviates from normal, allowing for early identification of and intervention for infants at risk for vision problems. The earlier a visual impairment occurs, the greater the impact the impairment has on the child's motor and sensory development. The integrity of the visual system is essential for an infant's normal overall development [2].

Understanding of human visual development is rapidly expanding, and many of our previous conceptions of the visual capabilities of infants are obsolete. Significant advances in research on vision development in the infant have been made in the past 40 years. Research has traditionally concentrated on either the role of neural mechanisms in the development of vision [3] or on behavioral aspects of vision development in infants [4, 5]. Recently, knowledge of these two areas has been considered together [6], allowing for consideration of both the anatomic and functional aspects of the developing visual system. It has been shown that infants possess more visual capability than previously thought. Our ability to evaluate visual development has become more reliable. Instruments have been de-

signed and techniques modified to aid in improved evaluation of the young child. This allows more thorough assessment of preschool children and earlier intervention for significant visual disorders that are detected.

Visual development is not complete at birth. There are significant individual variations in visual developmental landmarks as there are in the areas of language and motor skill development [7].

VISUAL ACUITY

Visual acuity development has been studied using both behavioral and electrophysiologic methods. The behavioral methods are based on Fantz's [4, 8] early work on preferential looking in infants. This work demonstrated that infants did, in fact, have a preference for certain patterns that were shown to them. Electrophysiologic methods for evaluating visual acuity include the noninvasive visual evoked potential (VEP) test. VEP testing evaluates the integrity of the visual pathway from the retina to the visual cortex by recording brain wave activity synchronized with a visual stimulus. The VEP technique can be used to generate an acuity estimate under certain conditions.

Although it was once thought that infants had limited visual ability at birth, the use of preferential-looking VEP tests has shown that newborns are capable of seeing at birth and that their visual acuity significantly improves over the first 6 months. These techniques are also used to monitor treat-

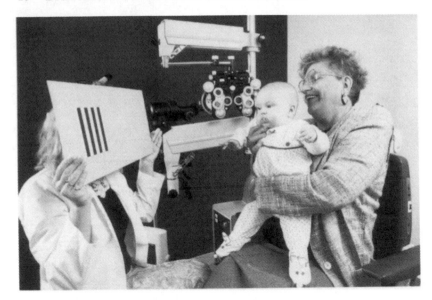

Figure 2.1. The acuity card procedure is an effective technique to measure visual acuity in young children.

ment outcome, specifically for amblyopia, in young children [9].

These test strategies provide reliable yet somewhat different information on visual acuity development. Behavioral methods rely on looking preferences to assess visual acuity. Fantz initially sought to determine whether infants could discriminate between two patterns. He determined that the infant will tend to fixate on the most novel or complex stimuli. Fantz's technique determined fixation preference by counting the number and duration of the fixations made on each pattern. This early work laid the foundation for the development of the use of the forced-choice preferential-looking technique (FPL). Teller and colleagues [10] developed FPL by modifying Fantz's technique to incorporate psychophysical methods. In FPL, a striped grating pattern and a uniformly illuminated area are displayed on opposing sides of panel. An observer who does not know the location of the grating pattern watches the infant and attempts to judge the pattern's location based on cues provided by the infant. The infant will have no fixation preference when the gray field and the grating pattern appear identical to them. The observer's responses will fall to chance level. The infant is tested with several different trials of grating patterns and the data are plotted with the observer's percentage of correct responses. Typ-

ically, threshold is defined as a 75% correct response level.

FPL techniques are most effective with infants 0–6 months old. In older infants, the technique is modified to allow for greater response compliance by incorporating behavior modification techniques into the operant preferential-looking (OPL) procedure. When rewards such as cereal, cartoons, or music were offered, older infants were more responsive to the procedure. In a study by Mayer and Dobson [11], OPL was effective in children from 5 months to 5 years of age. The evolution of FPL and OPL procedures has allowed many researchers to more fully explore visual acuity development in infants [11–13].

The acuity card procedure is a modified FPL technique [14–16] that allows clinicians to routinely assess a young child's visual acuity (Figure 2.1). This technique has also provided significant insights into the natural history of delayed visual maturation and has helped to quantify the severity of a visual defect in the infant and monitor the improvement of vision [17].

Just as no two infants attain motor and sensory skills at the same time [7], infants show marked individual variations [18] in visual acuity development in the early months of life. Development is rapid in the first few months. Studies using the FPL

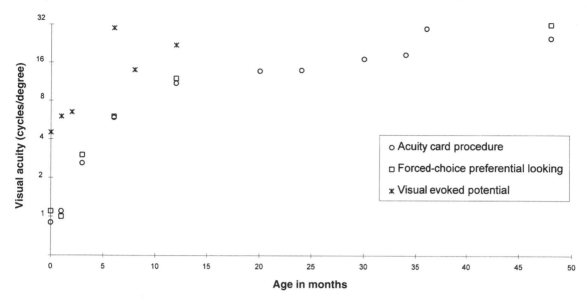

Figure 2.2. Binocular visual acuity as a function of age in normal children.

technique have shown that infants' visual acuity improves steadily with age and reaches adult levels (30 cyc/deg [20/20]) by 3–5 years old [12, 19]. Visual acuity is 1 cyc/deg (20/600) at birth, 3 cyc/deg at 3 months, 6 cyc/deg at 6 months, and 12 cyc/deg at 12 months [20].

Monocular and binocular visual acuity development has also been studied extensively with several studies, yielding similar results [11, 21–23]. Monocular and binocular visual acuity in infants improves rapidly from approximately 2.0 cyc/deg to 9.6 cyc/deg during the first year. For the first 6 months of life, monocular and binocular visual acuity develop at approximately the same rate. During the sixth to eleventh month of life, an infant's binocular visual acuity is superior to monocular visual acuity [23].

Normative information for the Teller Acuity Cards revealed results similar to those of FPL studies. Mayer et al. [24] found that the mean visual acuity of an infant improves rapidly from 1–6 months of age and more slowly after 6 months. They found that at 1 month, the infants' mean visual acuity was 1 cyc/deg and at 6 months, 6 cyc/deg. The infants' acuity did not change appreciably between 6 and 12 months of age. Salomao and Ventura [25] also tested children from low-income families ages 0–36 months using the Teller

Acuity Cards. Their findings were very similar to the results of Mayer et al. [24].

Studies using electrophysiologic methods have also provided valuable information on the infant's visual acuity development. A longitudinal study by Barnet et al. [26] followed children from 2 weeks until 3 years of age to determine if the VEP response is stable during a child's development. They found that the VEP undergoes rapid developmental changes during infancy.

VEP has been used to assess visual acuity in infancy (Figure 2.2). Sokol [27] used a pattern-reversal checkerboard stimulus to measure visual acuity in 2- and 6-month-old infants and found that visual acuity increased rapidly in the first 6 months of life from 20/150 at 2 months to 20/20 at 6 months. Marg et al. [28] used a transient VEP, a square-wave grating that alternated with a gray field, to test infants from 1 to 6 months old. Results were similar to Sokol's.

The sweep VEP technique has also been used to determine visual acuity in infants. The sweep VEP technique records the steady-state response continually while rapidly presenting a large range of stimuli. Norcia and Tyler [29] tested 197 infants from 1 week to 53 weeks old. They found a gradual increase in visual acuity from 4.5 cyc/deg at 2.5 weeks to 22.0 cyc/deg at 50.5 weeks of age. Hamer et al. [30] studied infants 2–52 weeks of age. They deter-

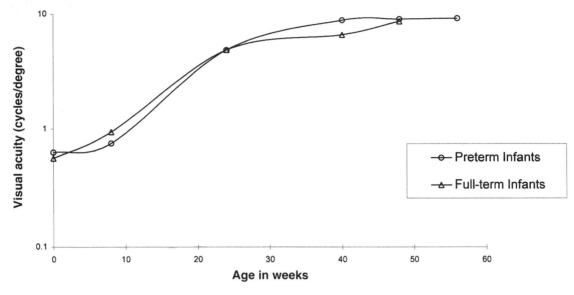

Figure 2.3. Acuity development in full-term and preterm infants; by preferential-looking methods.

mined that the mean acuity develops from about 6 cyc/deg at 1 month to 14 cyc/deg at 8 months. The monocular and binocular visual acuity in infants followed a similar growth curve and binocular visual acuity was only slightly better than monocular visual acuity until about 6 months of age. They also determined there was little difference between the eyes in visual acuity development.

Sokol and Moskowitz [31] used a pattern VEP to measure visual acuity in infants between 11–13 weeks old and compared these results to FPL data. They found similarity between results obtained using VEP latency (but not amplitude) and those using FPL data. Pattern VEP results and acuity card results yielded similar measures of visual acuity [32].

Visual acuity development in preterm infants has also been studied using preferential looking and electrophysiologic methods. van Hof-van Duin and Mohn [33] used FPL techniques to compare visual acuity of full-term and preterm infants. When postnatal age was used in comparing the two groups, visual acuity in the preterm infants lagged behind that of the full-term infants up to approximately 6–7 months of age. By 8 months, the mean visual acuity of preterm infants was equal to that of full-term in-

fants. In fact, 63% of the preterm infants had better visual acuities than the full-term infants. This would suggest a slightly faster rate of development in the preterm infants. When corrected age was used, the rate of acuity development between preterm and full-term infants was identical. The mean visual acuity of the preterm infants was slightly higher at all ages (Figure 2.3).

Sweep VEP in preterm infants found that mean visual acuity in healthy preterm infants was above that of full-term infants of equivalent corrected age [34]. The study also suggested that sweep VEP acuity begins developing at birth.

Hermans et al. [35] studied low-birth-weight full-term and preterm infants using the Acuity Card Procedure. They did not find a difference in mean visual acuity between healthy and high-risk or full-term and preterm infants.

The visual acuity of infants increases significantly from birth to 6 months of age regardless of the method used to measure it. The rate of improvement varies, however. When VEP is used, it demonstrates a higher rate of change in acuity between 2 and 4 months of age than between 4 and 6 months of age. In comparing VEP studies to preferential looking, VEP studies show a more significant increase in visual acuity than that seen with preferential-looking and acuity card procedures. This may be due to either the more rigorous scoring criteria used in preferential-looking methods or to the fact that the different methods are assessing information available at different levels of the neurologic system.

OCULOMOTOR CONTROL

Eye movement is often used as an indicator of how well an infant sees. Normal eye movements do not develop in visually impaired infants; abnormal eye movements are often the first symptom of a significant visual impairment [2]. Information on the development of oculomotor control in human infants has been limited because interpretation and methodology problems have occurred in studies on this subject [36, 37]. Studies are now using carefully calibrated eye movement recordings rather than relying primarily on qualitative descriptions of eye movements [37]. Variations in major calibration parameters among infants have still been found using these techniques, however [38].

Infants are capable of a variety of eye movements; however, these movements are not as sophisticated as an adult's. They are able to fixate on a stationary object, track moving stimuli, and move their eyes toward stimuli in the periphery of the visual field. All of these responses are dependent on the infant's interest and attention level. Interest in novel things is a typical feature of infants. If an infant is shown the same object or picture several times, he or she loses interest and becomes habituated to the target [39]. A new target needs to be introduced to attract the infant's visual attention.

Saccades

Although infants will look at a target that suddenly appears, the infant's eye movements are not mature at birth. The two primary voluntary eye movements of the infant, saccades and pursuits, are similar but not yet identical to an adult's under all conditions. Newborns are able to direct their attention toward an object using a saccadic eye movement. The newborn's individual saccade is basically similar to the adult's in dynamics; however, the programming of these saccades is different. Roucoux et al. [40] identified two types of saccades in infant: a hypometric foveate-like saccade associated with a small head movement and an afoveate-like coordinated eye-head movement that is often hypermetric. The former are primarily used to view an object whose image projects centrally on the fovea.

The infant's initial saccade is normally in the correct direction of the target but generally only covers a fraction of the distance. An adult is able to initiate a long saccadic movement that will bring the eye to the desired position with an error of only 5–10% of the distance. The infant tends to use a series of small saccades very similar in amplitude to the initial saccade to reach the target. These smaller, hypometric saccades are of a standard amplitude, rather than being matched to the target distance. They generally cover only 50% of the distance to the target. Thus, the infant takes longer than an adult to reach the target and in some cases does not reach the target for over a second [40–42]. The infant also takes longer to initiate the saccadic eye movement. In an adult, a saccade will start the eye moving toward the target within 200–250 milliseconds. The infant will often take as long as 500–800 milliseconds to initiate the saccadic eye movement. Therefore, the infant demonstrates both a longer latency of initial movement toward the target and longer target acquisition times [41].

A study by Harris et al. of saccadic accuracy in infants found that the hypometric saccades are part of normal development [43]. The saccadic hypometria was less conspicuous by 7 months of age, but the infant's accuracy was still not at an adult level. They found that infantile saccadic hypometria was a robust phenomenon readily detected with a large target.

Harris et al. [43] also found that a secondary saccade in the opposite direction from the primary saccade (saccadic hypermetria) is relatively rare. They indicated that a persistent hypermetria should be considered abnormal. Leigh and Zee [44] found that hypermetria is often associated with cerebellar disease.

Infants rely more heavily than adults on coordinated head and eye movements when viewing objects in their peripheral visual field. When infants attempt to fixate on a target in their periphery, the head will generally move toward the target with a compensatory saccadic movement to place the eyes on the target. The ability to change fixation onto a target in the periphery with one saccadic movement is evident by 1 year of age [40].

When presented with a target outside of their direct line of sight, newborns are able to move their eyes to bring visual targets onto or close to their fovea. Thus, if suddenly presented with a target 20 degrees from the fovea, a 2-week-old infant will slowly turn his or her eyes toward the target [42]. By 3 months, infants are able to identify targets in the periphery of their visual field well enough to guide their eyes to a preferred target. Bronson [45] also found that as infants grow older, their scanning ability improves. By 14 weeks, infants more consistently and accurately direct their saccades toward the contours of a stimulus.

Infants respond differently to different targets. McKenzie [46] did a longitudinal study of oculomotor responses of 101 infants to a variety of stimuli. Infants were found to be capable of fixation to faces at birth but were not as responsive to lights and visual and auditory targets until 3 months of age. Horizontal saccades showed a similar pattern; newborns showed a fixation to faces but responses to a penlight and other visual targets were not as evident until 3 months of age. It is important to use appropriate stimuli for clinical assessment of oculomotor skills in infants. The most effective stimulus for newborns is the examiner's face [47].

Horizontal saccadic eye movements develop before vertical movements. Vertical gaze movements are generally not seen until 4–6 weeks of age. By 3 months, response frequencies of horizontal and vertical saccadic fixation are very similar. The infant's horizontal and vertical saccadic abilities appear to develop independently of one another [46].

Pursuits

It was previously thought that infants used a series of hypometric saccades to track a steadily moving target [42] and that the ability to elicit smooth tracking did not develop until 3 months. Studies have now demonstrated that newborns are capable of smooth eye and head movements if certain conditions are met [40, 48]. First, the target velocity must be low for the pursuit of a moving visual target to be accomplished by a smooth eye and head movement. If the target velocity is increased, the infant will begin to demonstrate an afoveate type of saccadic tracking. As the child becomes older, the maximum speed of pursuit of a moving target increases.

The newborn's smooth pursuit movements are short in duration—about 300–400 milliseconds—and depend on target size. The target size must be 12 degrees or larger for the smooth pursuit movements to be maintained by the infant [49].

Aslin found that infants older than 6 weeks showed brief series of smooth pursuit movements interspersed among saccades [49]. The ratio of smooth pursuits to saccades increased with age. Although smooth pursuit movements are evident by 6–8 weeks of age, the accuracy of movements is poor because the velocity of the eye movements does not match the velocity of the target [40]. Roucoux suggests that smooth pursuit movements have improved considerably by 4 months of age [40]. McKenzie's [46] longitudinal study found that pursuit movement development follows a pattern similar to that in saccadic development.

Smooth pursuit eye movements are possible in newborns but are more often seen after 6–8 weeks of life. Even at this time, the child's eye movements depend on the size of the target and its velocity. A larger, highly stimulating, slow-moving target is most likely to elicit smooth pursuit movement in an infant (Table 2.1).

OPTOKINETIC NYSTAGMUS

Slow and fast phases of the optokinetic nystagmus (OKN) response can be elicited from infants from birth [50]. The monocular OKN response in infants is immature compared with the adult's, however. Visually normal infants have an asymmetric OKN response. They show a poor pursuit of targets, moving in a nasal to temporal direction before the fixating eye under monocular conditions. The temporal to nasal movement is easier to elicit. The OKN response becomes symmetric after 3–6 months of age [51–54].

The persistence of an asymmetric response in infants beyond 3–6 months of age indicates a problem in visual development. This asymmetric response frequently occurs in children and adults with poor binocular vision resulting from infant-onset strabismus [55], amblyopia, or unilateral congenital cataracts [56, 57].

HEAD AND EYE MOVEMENTS

Infants as young as 1–5 months of age actively use coordinated eye and head movements to locate visual targets. The velocity and duration of individual eye and head movements are very similar to those of an adult. The most noticeable difference is that infants use multiple eye and head movement components and that the latency before initial movement and the time to reach the target are longer in infants [41].

When a target is unexpectedly presented, saccadic eye movement aligns the eyes with the target, and the head then rotates toward the target. While the head is moving, the vestibulo-ocular reflex (VOR) maintains fixation on the target. Goodkin [58] studied the initiation of coordinated head and eye movements and the VOR in infants. In the first experiment, infants were shown a central target, and then stationary, visual targets were presented in the periphery of the infants' visual field. The infants either responded with an eye movement (saccade) alone or with an eye movement followed by a head movement. There was a clear difference in patterns of looking between 2- and 3-month-old infants. In general, 2-month-old infants moved their eyes toward the targets with no apparent head movements. By 3 months of age, infants showed the same pattern of coordinated movements as an adult: They moved their eyes and then their head toward the light stimulus within less than 1 second. Both 2-month-old and 3-month-old age groups tended to look more frequently at targets that were closer to the midline position and to use eye movements alone for targets nearer the midline.

The VOR is present from birth. It allows clear fixation during head movement. In a second experiment, Goodkin [58] found that the gain of VOR (velocity of eye movement to velocity of rotation) was the same for adults and 2- and 3-month-old infants, allowing infants to maintain clear vision of a target as they are moved or as they move their head.

Table 2.1. Development of Oculomotor Abilities

Skill	Age
Fixation to	
Lights	3 mons
Faces	Birth
Visual objects	3 mons
Auditory objects	3 mons
Optokinetic nystagmus	Birth
Saccadic movement	
Horizontal	Birth
Vertical upgaze	4–6 wks
Vertical downgaze	3 mons
Stimulus	
Faces	Birth
Penlight	3 mons
Pursuits	6–8 wks
Vestibulo-ocular reflex	Birth
Coordinated head-eye movements	3 mons

Newborns are capable of producing head and eye movements and by 4 weeks produce several forms of looking patterns with their head and eyes.

Some apparently abnormal eye movements may in fact be appropriate for a certain age. The development of eye movements therefore needs to be taken into account. Other abnormalities, such as asymmetries in binocular OKN and smooth pursuits and nystagmus, are abnormal at any age.

Binocular Fixation and Convergence

A newborn can binocularly fixate on an object but prefers to fixate on a face [46]. As infants become older, toys and lights also become popular targets. Slater and Findlay [59] found that infants were capable of bifoveal fixation on lights at a distance of 10 and 20 in. in 90% of the test sessions. Newborns are capable of reliable convergence if the target is visually stimulating and the distance from the infant's eyes to the target is 10 inches or greater [59].

Aslin and Jackson [60] found that by 3–4 months of age, infants showed accurate convergence. This finding was supported by the work of Hainline et al. [61], who found that infants younger than 1 year old showed appropriate convergence for the target distance. Infants older than 2 months old showed adult-like convergence ability. Thorn et al.

[62] found that by 11.9 weeks of age, 50% of infants demonstrated full convergence. By 18 weeks, 90% of the infants showed full convergence.

Vergence Movements

Aslin [42] studied the infant's ability to make reliable convergence and divergence eye movements. The frequency of reliable convergent and divergent movements increased considerably from 1 to 3 months of age. By 3 months of age, 70% of infants were capable of accurate convergent and divergent movements.

The ability of infants to respond to rapid changes in vergence demand has also been studied. Fusional vergence movements toward monocularly placed prisms were studied in 3- and 6-month-old infants. Prisms of the magnitudes of 5, 10, and 20 were placed base out in front of the infants [42, 46]. A distinctive fusional vergence movement was seen in 6-month-old infants in 70% of the trials [42]. McKenzie [46] found similar results with 10 and 20^Δ. By 6 months of age, the majority of the infants showed a fusion reflex response.

These studies collectively show that infants' ability to move their eyes depends on the infant's age, the type of target, and the speed of the target. Infants are generally able to demonstrate consistent convergence ability and fusional vergence movements by 4–6 months of age.

ACCOMMODATION

Infants' accommodative ability has not been studied as extensively as the development of visual acuity in infants. One of the first studies of accommodation in infants [63] found that infants from birth to 1 month do not adjust to the changes of the target distance. Results of a study by White [64] were similar with the exception of findings indicating a greater accuracy of the accommodative system during the first 2 months of life than previously thought.

Banks [65] studied the accommodative ability of 1- to 3-month-old infants. He found that accommodative responses in infants become more accurate with age and that variability of responses decreases with age. Banks found that the infant re-

sponses were adult-like by 3–4 months. Braddick et al. [66] studied the accommodative function of infants using photorefraction. They found that infants from birth to 6 months of age could accommodate accurately to targets at 75 and 150 cm. They concluded that the errors of accommodative ability in infants younger than 6 months old were not significant enough to account for the relatively low acuity demonstrated in preferential-looking studies. Banks [65] reached the same conclusion in retinoscopic studies.

A longitudinal study on infant accommodation proficiency by Brookman [67] found that 2-week-old infants were reasonably accurate in adjusting their accommodative response to low accommodative demands. As the accommodative stimulus demand increased, however, the infant's ability to adequately respond to the higher demands decreased. This study also supported Banks' conclusion that the accommodative ability of infants reached adult-like levels by 16–20 weeks [65].

A more recent study using paraxial photorefraction [61] assessed the development of accommodation and convergence in infants younger than 1 year old. Infants younger than 2 months of age tend to have a fixed accommodative response to a target at a distance of approximately 30 cm. When attempting to look at a distant object, they did not relax the accommodative system adequately. Most significant was the finding that the majority of emmetropic infants older than 2 months had accommodative responses that changed appropriately with the target distance. Hyperopic and myopic infants, however, displayed a variety of accommodative styles.

BINOCULARITY

Disparity Detection

Disparity detection is necessary for accurate binocular function and is poorly developed at birth. The cortical neurones that detect small disparities are probably absent or deficient [68]. It is generally agreed that infants are capable of detecting changes in disparity by 3–4 months of age. Held et al. [69] and Birch et al. [70] suggest that 50–60% of normal infants are sensitive to binocular disparity by 4 months of age. By 5 months, 80–90% of infants are sensitive to disparity.

Granrud [71] found that 4-month-old infants sensitive to binocular disparity were more consistent and accurate when reaching for objects than infants not sensitive to disparity.

Stereopsis

Preferential-looking techniques have also been used to assess sensory fusion and stereopsis. Birch et al. [72] found that sensory fusion was not present at birth but rapidly developed over the first 6 months of life. In their longitudinal study of nine infants, they found that the development of stereopsis and sensory fusion follow a similar time frame. Thorn et al. [62] also investigated the development of sensory binocular fusion in young infants using a fusion versus rivalry preferential-looking technique. Infants demonstrated binocular fusion at a mean age of 12.8 weeks.

Stereopsis was first demonstrated by infants at 16 weeks using a two-choice preference method [69]. By 21 weeks, infants were able to achieve 1 minute or more of arc. Held et al. [69] and Birch et al. [72] found that 5- to 6-month-old infants could respond to stereoacuity of less than 1 minute of arc using a preferential-looking paradigm. The average age of development of stereoscopic vision development is 3.5 months [72, 73]. A major developmental spurt occurs between 4 and 6 months of age.

Random dot stereopsis is not present at birth but has been demonstrated as early as 3–4 months. Infants have a binocular visual-evoked response to random dot stereograms at the median age of 11.4 weeks [73]. The youngest infant showing a binocular VEP response was 7–8 weeks [73]. Gwiazda et al. [74] also found responses to similar stimuli at 3 months of age.

During the first 3–5 months of life binocular function, and specifically stereopsis, is affected by interocular acuity differences. Birch et al. [75] found that infants who demonstrated a stereopsis response did not have significant interocular differences. Infants not responding to the stereopsis target did show a significant amount of acuity difference between eyes.

Random dot stereoacuity continues to develop throughout the first year. Ciner et al. [76] found that stereoacuity thresholds increased from a mean of 301.7 seconds of arc at 6–11 months to 28.8 seconds of arc by 60 months of age. Their study used a preferential-looking paradigm with a "happy face" target. A previous study by Ciner et al. [77] using random dot targets also found an improvement of stereopsis with age. Steady improvement in stereoacuity in children should occur if the visual system is normal (Figure 2.4).

Contrast Sensitivity

Contrast sensitivity (CS) is the minimum contrast needed to detect sine wave gratings of varying spatial frequencies. It also has not been studied as extensively as visual acuity development. The assessment of CS may be a significant component in the detection of visual system anomalies.

Studies suggest that contrast sensitivity function (CSF) in infants is not adult-like. Atkinson and Braddick [78] used preferential-looking and electrophysiologic methods to evaluate CS development in infants and found that there is a rapid improvement in visual capacities over the first 1–3 months of life. The infant shows an increased sensitivity to all spatial frequencies and the first appearance of the low spatial frequency cutoff by 2–3 months. Banks and Salapatek [79] also used a preferential-looking technique to measure CSF in infants. They found an increase in overall CS with age. The shape and height of the CSF at 2 and 3 months of age were similar in both studies. Other studies have shown that infants 6 months of age still exhibit a deficit in high-frequency sensitivity relative to adults. Evoked potential measurements and preferential-looking procedures show that the contrast threshold at 1 cyc/deg was very near to the adult level; however, sensitivity is still lower than over the range of 2–5 cyc/deg [80–82].

Adams and Courage [83] used the psychophysical card procedure to evaluate the monocular CS of 3- to 36-month-old infants. They found that binocular CS was significantly greater than monocular CS at 12 months of age. They conclude that this may be an indication that monocular and binocular CS follow a different developmental course at least until the end of the first year. This study and a previous one [84] of 2- to 3-year-old children showed that spatial vision is not yet adult-like at 3 years of age.

Studies by Richman and Lyons [85] and Scharre et al. [86] determined that monocular and binocular

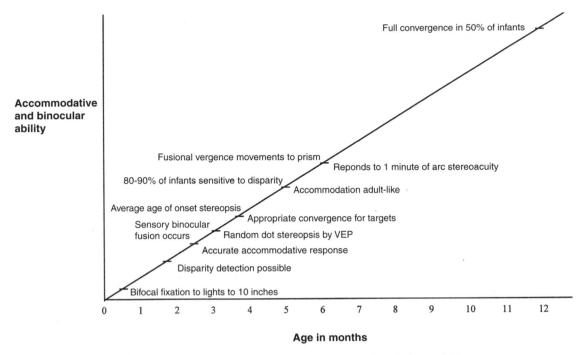

Figure 2.4. Development of accommodative and binocular skills. (VEP = visual evoked potential.)

CSF are not at adult-like levels in preschool children. Richman and Lyons used a forced-choice procedure to measure CS in preschoolers and found that with age the child's ability to detect lower contrast levels increased. Scharre et al. [86] used the Vistech Contrast Sensitivity distance chart to show that children's CS was significantly less than adults' and that adult-like levels were not yet reached at 7 years of age. When assessing CS in children appropriate normative information should be taken into consideration.

CONCLUSION

The infant's visual capabilities are more advanced than previously thought but still fall short of adult-like levels in many areas. The rapid development of visual skills in the first year of life slows in subsequent years. Individual variations do occur, and different visual skills are attained at different ages. Understanding of normal visual development allows the clinician to develop an appropriate test strategy for a young child and to decide if the observed behavior deviates from normal.

REFERENCES

1. Scharre JE, Marciniak MM. Pediatric clinical decision making. J Am Optom Assoc 1994;65:305–310.
2. Hyvarinen L. Assessment of visually impaired infants. Ophth Clin North Am 1994;7:2.
3. Hubel DH, Wiesel TN. Functional architecture of macaque monkey visual cortex. Proc R Soc Lond B Biol Sci 1977;198:1–59.
4. Fantz RL. The origins of form perception. Sci Am 1961;204:66–72.
5. Dobson V, Teller DY. Visual acuity in human infants: a review and comparison of behavioral and electrophysiological studies. Vision Res 1978;18:1469–1483.
6. Hung LF, Smith III EL. Extended-wear, soft contact lenses produce hyperopia in young monkeys. Optom Vis Sci 1996;73:579–584.
7. Illingworth RS. The Development of the Infant and Young Child (7th ed). London: Churchill Livingstone, 1980.
8. Fantz RL. Pattern vision in young infant. Psychol Rec 1958;8:43–47.
9. Lennerstrand G, Andersson G, Axelsson A. Clinical assessment of visual functions in infants and young children. Acta Ophthalmol Scand Suppl 1982;157:63–67.
10. Teller DY, Morse R, Barton R, Regal D. Visual acuity for vertical and horizontal gratings in human infants. Vision Res 1974;14:1433–1439.

11. Mayer DL, Dobson V. Visual acuity development in infants and young children, as assessed by operant preferential looking. Vision Res 1982;22:1141–1151.

12. Birch EE, Gwiazda J, Bauer JA Jr, et al. Visual acuity and its meridional variations in children aged 7–60 months. Vision Res 1983;23:1019–1024.

13. Dobson V, Salem D, Mayer DL, et al. Visual acuity screening of children 6 months to 3 years of age. Invest Ophthalmol Vis Sci 1985;26:1057–1063.

14. Teller DY, McDonald MA, Preston K, et al. Assessment of visual acuity in infants and children: the acuity card procedure. Dev Med Child Neurol 1986;28:779–789.

15. McDonald MA, Sebris SL, Mohn G, et al. Monocular acuity in normal infants: the acuity card procedure. Am J Optom Physiol Optics 1986;63:127–134.

16. McDonald MA, Dobson V, Sebris SL, et al. The acuity card procedure: a rapid test of infant acuity. Invest Ophthalmol Vis Sci 1985;26:1158–1162.

17. Fielder AR, Mayer DL. Delayed visual maturation. Semin Ophthalmol 1991;6:182–193.

18. Atkinson J, Braddick O. Assessment of visual acuity in infancy and early childhood. Acta Ophthalmol Scand Suppl 1982;157:18–26.

19. Teller DY. Measurement of visual acuity in human and monkey infants: the interface between laboratory and clinic. Behav Brain Res 1983;10:15–23.

20. Banks MS, Salapatcik P. Acuity and contrast sensitivity in 1-, 2-, and 3-month old infants. Invest Ophthalmol Vis Sci 1978;17:361–365.

21. Atkinson J, Braddick O, Pimm-Smith E. Preferential looking for monocular and binocular acuity testing of infants. Br J Ophthalmol 1982;66:264–268.

22. Dobson V. Clinical application of preferential-looking measures of visual acuity. Behav Brain Res 1983;10:25–38.

23. Birch EE. Infant interocular acuity differences and binocular vision. Vision Res 1985;25:571–576.

24. Mayer DL, Beiser AS, Warner AF, et al. Monocular acuity norms for the teller acuity cards between ages one month and four years. Invest Ophthalmol Vis Sci 1995;36:671–685.

25. Salomao SR, Ventura DF. Large sample population age norms for visual acuities obtained with Vistech-Teller Acuity Cards. Invest Ophthalmol Vis Sci 1995;36:657–670.

26. Barnet AB, Friedman IP, Weiss ES, et al. VEP development in infancy and early childhood. A longitudinal study. Electroencephalogr Clin Neurophysiol 1980;49:476–489.

27. Sokol S. Measurement of infant visual acuity from pattern reversal evoked potentials. Vision Res 1978;18:33–39.

28. Marg E, Freeman DN, Peltzman P, Goldstein PJ. Visual acuity development in human infants: evoked potential measurements. Invest Ophthalmol 1976;15:150–153.

29. Norcia AM, Tyler CW. Spatial frequency sweep VEP: visual acuity during the first year of life. Vision Res 1985;25:1399–1408.

30. Hamer RD, Norcia AM, Tyler CW, Hsu-Winges C. The development of monocular and binocular VEP acuity. Vision Res 1989;29:397–408.

31. Sokol S, Moskowitz A. A comparison of pattern VEPs and preferential-looking behavior in 3-month-old infants. Invest Ophthalmol Vis Sci 1985;26:359–365.

32. Moskowitz A, Sokol S, Hansen V. Rapid assessment of visual function in pediatric patients using pattern VEPs and acuity cards. Clin Vis Sci 1987;2:11–20.

33. Van Hof-van Duin J, Mohn G. The development of visual acuity in normal fullterm and preterm infants. Vision Res 1986;26:909–916.

34. Norcia AM, Tyler CW, Piecuch R, et al. Visual acuity development in normal and abnormal preterm human infants. J Pediatr Ophthalmol Strabismus 1987;24:70–74.

35. Hermans AJM, Van Hof-van Duin J, Oudesluys-Murphy AM. Visual acuity in low birth weight [1500–2500 g] neonates. Early Hum Dev 1992;28:155–167.

36. Jacobs M, Harris C, Shawkat F, Taylor D. The objective assessment of abnormal eye movements in infants and young children. Aust N Z J Ophthalmol 1992;20:185–196.

37. Shupert C, Fuchs AF. Development of conjugate human eye movements. Vision Res 1988;28:585–596.

38. Bronson GW. The accurate calibration of infants' scanning records. J Exp Child Psychol 1990;49:79–100.

39. Berg CA, Sternberg RJ. Response to novelty: continuity versus discontinuity in the developmental course of intelligence. Adv Child Dev Behav 1985;19:1–47.

40. Roucoux A, Culee C, Roucoux M. Development of fixation and pursuit eye movements in human infants. Behav Brain Res 1983;10:133–139.

41. Regal DM, Ashmead DH, Salapatek P. The coordination of eye and head movements during early infancy: a selective review. Behav Brain Res 1983;10:125–132.

42. Aslin RN. Normative Ocular Motor Development in Human Infants. In G Lennerstrand, GK von Noorden, EC Campos (eds), Strabismus and Amblyopia. New York: Plenum, 1988;133–142.

43. Harris CM, Jacobs M, Shawkat F, Taylor D. The development of saccadic accuracy in the first seven months. Clin Vis Sci 1993;8:85–96.

44. Leigh RJ, Zee DS. The Neurology of Eye Movements (2nd ed). Philadelphia: Davis, 1991.

45. Bronson GW. Infants' transitions toward adult-like scanning. Child Dev 1994;65:1243–1261.

46. McKenzie L. The ocular motor development of infants. Aust Orthopt J 1991;27:19–23.

47. Hainline L, Turkel J, Abramov I, et al. Characteristics of saccades in human infants. Vision Res 1984;24:1771–1780.

48. Kremenitzer JP, Vaughan HG Jr, Kurtzberg D, et al. Smooth-pursuit eye movements in the newborn infant. Child Dev 1979;50:442–448.

49. Aslin RN. Development of Smooth Pursuit in Human Infants. In DF Fisher, RA Monty, JW Senders (eds), Eye Movements: Cognition and Visual Perception. Hillsdale, NJ: Lawrence Erlbaum, 1981.

50. Fielder A. Neonatal eye movements: normal and abnormal. Br Orthopt J 1985;42:10–15.

51. Atkinson J, Braddick O. Development of Optokinetic Nystagmus in Infants: An Indicator of Cortical Binocularity? In DF Fisher, RA Monty, JW Senders (eds), Eye Movements: Cognition and Visual Perception. Hillsdale, NJ: Lawrence Erlbaum, 1981;53–64.

52. Naegele JR, Held R. The postnatal development of monocular optokinetic nystagmus in infants. Vision Res 1982;22:341–346.

53. Van Hof-van Duin J, Mohn G. Vision in the Preterm Infant. In HFR Prechtl (ed), Continuity of Neural Functions from Prenatal to Postnatal Life. Philadelphia: Lippincott, 1984;93–114.

54. Roy MS, Lachapelle P, Leporé F. Maturation of optokinetic nystagmus and the role of visual experience in normal and preterm infants. Invest Ophthalmol Vis Sci 1987;28(Suppl):313.

55. Aiello A, Wright K, Borchert M. Independence of optokinetic nystagmus asymmetry and binocularity in infantile esotropia. Arch Ophthalmol 1994;112:1580–1583.

56. Schor CM, Levi DM. Disturbances of small-field horizontal and vertical optokinetic nystagmus in amblyopia. Invest Ophthalmol Vis Sci 1980;19:668–683.

57. Maurer D, Lewis TL, Brent HP. Peripheral vision and optokinetic nystagmus in children with unilateral congenital cataract. Behav Brain Res 1983;10:151–161.

58. Goodkin F. The development of mature patterns of head-eye coordination in the human infant. Early Hum Dev 1980;4(4):373–386.

59. Slater AM, Findlay JM. Binocular fixation in the newborn baby. J Exp Child Psychol 1975;20:248–273.

60. Aslin RN, Jackson RW. Accommodative-convergence in young infants: development of a synergistic sensory-motor system. Can J Psychol 1977;33:222–231.

61. Hainline L, Riddell P, Grose-Fifer J, Abramov I. Development of accommodation and convergence in infancy. Behav Brain Res 1992;49:33–50.

62. Thorn F, Gwiazda J, Cruz AAV, et al. The development of eye alignment, convergence, and sensory binocularity in young infants. Invest Ophthalmol Vis Sci 1994;35:544–553.

63. Haynes H, White BL, Held R. Visual accommodation in human infants. Science 1965;148:528–530.

64. White BL. Human Infants: Experience and Psychological Development. Englewood Cliffs, NJ: Prentice Hall, 1971;69.

65. Banks MS. The development of visual accommodation during early infancy. Child Dev 1980;51:646–666.

66. Braddick O, Atkinson J, French J, Howland HC. A photorefractive study of infant accommodation. Vision Res 1979;19:1319–1330.

67. Brookman KE. Ocular accommodation in human infants. Am J Optom Physiol Optics 1983;60:91–99.

68. Atkinson J, Braddick O. Stereoscopic discrimination in infants. Perception 1976;5:29–38.

69. Held R, Birch E, Gwiazda J. Stereoacuity of human infants. Proc Natl Acad Sci U S A 1980;77:5572–5574.

70. Birch EE, Gwiazda J, Held R. Stereoacuity development for crossed and uncrossed disparities in human infants. Vision Res 1982;22:507–513.

71. Granrud CE. Binocular vision and spatial perception in 4- and 5-month old infants. J Exp Psychol Hum Percept Perform 1986;12:36–49.

72. Birch EE, Shimojo S, Held R. Preferential-looking assessment of fusion and stereopsis in infants 1–6 months. Invest Ophthalmol Vis Sci 1985;26:366–370.

73. Braddick OJ, Atkinson J. Some recent findings on the development of human binocularity: a review. Behav Brain Res 1983;10:141–150.

74. Gwiazda J, Bauer J, Held R. Binocular function in human infants: correlation of stereoptic and fusion-rivalry discriminations. J Pediatr Ophthalmol Strabismus 1989;26:128–132.

75. Birch EE, Stager DR. Monocular acuity and stereopsis in infantile esotropia. Invest Ophthalmol Vis Sci 1985;26:1624–1630.

76. Ciner EB, Schanel-Klitsch E, Scheiman M. Stereoacuity development in young children. Optom Vis Sci 1991;68:533–536.

77. Ciner EB, Schanel-Klitsch E, Herzberg C. Stereoacuity development: 6 months to 5 years. A new tool for testing and screening. Optom Vis Sci 1996;73:43–48.

78. Atkinson J, Braddick O. New techniques for assessing vision in infants and young children. Child Care Health Dev 1979;5:389–398.

79. Banks MS, Salapatek P. Acuity and contrast sensitivity in 1-, 2-, and 3-month old human infants. Invest Ophthalmol Vis Sci 1975;17:361–365.

80. Harris L, Atkinson J, Braddick O. Visual contrast sensitivity of a 6-month-old infant measured by the evoked potential. Nature 1976;264:570–571.

81. Norcia AM, Tyler CW, Allen D. Electrophysiological assessment of contrast sensitivity in human infants. Am J Optom Physiol Optics 1986;63:12–15.

82. Norcia AM, Tyler CW, Hamer RD. Development of contrast sensitivity in the human infant. Vision Res 1990;30:1475–1486.

83. Adams RJ, Courage ML. Monocular contrast sensitivity in 3- to 36-month old human infants. Optom Vis Sci 1996;73:546–551.

84. Adams RJ, Courage ML. Contrast sensitivity in 24- and 36-month olds as assessed with the contrast sensitivity card procedure. Optom Vis Sci 1993;70:97–101.

85. Richman JE, Lyons S. A forced choice procedure for evaluation of contrast sensitivity function in preschool children. J Am Optom Assoc 1994;64:859–864.

86. Scharre JE, Cotter SA, Block SS, Kelly SA. Normative contrast sensitivity data for young children. Optom Vis Sci 1990;67:826–832.

Chapter 3

The Epidemiology of Ocular Disorders in Young Children

Bruce D. Moore

This chapter provides an overview of the epidemiology of the most common clinically important eye and vision problems of young children. It is obviously useful for the clinician to have some sense of the frequency of abnormalities that are likely to be encountered on a day-to-day basis in the office.

REFRACTIVE ERROR

Significant refractive error is the most common cause of decreased vision in both children and adults. Much is known about refractive error. There are considerable data on refractive errors at different ages and how to optically correct the refractive error when required. We know less about the etiology of refractive error and its natural history.

Premature infants and low-birth-weight infants tend to be more myopic than full-term, normal-birth-weight infants. Banks [1] reported that premature infants tend to be myopic or less hyperopic than full-term neonates; the mean spherical equivalent of full-term neonates was +1.8 D, with a range of +0.6 to +2.6 D, and premature infants had a mean spherical equivalent of +0.24 D, with a range of −1.3 to +1.1 D. The prevalence of myopia among premature infants is said to be 15–20% [2]. Because 6–7% of births occur prematurely, prematurity accounts for approximately 1% of all cases of myopia. Fledelius [3] reported that myopia of prematurity results from small-sized eyes and highly curved corneas.

Goldschmidt [4] reported the results of other studies on the refractive error of newborns and found that myopia was relatively uncommon in full-term infants (mean refractions varied from +2.3 to +4.8 D). In his own study of 356 infants 2–10 days of age (all weighing more than 2,500 g), there was a much greater prevalence of myopia (24.2%), with a mean refraction of +0.55 D and standard deviation (SD) of 2.26.

Cook and Glascock [5] determined the average refractive state of 1,000 infants (625 black and 375 white). The data for whites indicated a mean spherical refractive error of +2.07 ± 0.14 D, SD was 2.73 ± 0.10 D, g1 (skewness) was −0.19 ± 0.13 D, and g2 (kurtosis) was +0.41 ± 0.25 D (note: ± is the standard error). Black infants in the study had a lower mean birth weight and accounted for 44 of the 56 cases of myopia of more than −4 D. Compared with other studies, the average refraction of +2.07 D is similar, and the standard deviation is greater than that reported earlier by Wibaut [6]. Hirsch and Weymouth [7] found this surprising, in part because this SD is much greater than for adults as reported by Stenstrom [8–13] (2.2 ± 0.05) and Kronfeld and Devney [14] (1.66 ± 0.03). Wibaut, whose study included only three myopes, determined that the SD for children should be the same as for adults. Cook and Glascock's data indicated decreased variability as children grow, instead of a lack of change of variability as previously thought. The skewness found by Cook and Glascock agreed with Wibaut's findings. The distribution was leptokurtic, as with adult data, but this finding by Cook and Glascock differed from Wibaut's data. Cook and Glascock's data showed that approximately 19% of eyes in their study were myopic. Atkinson [15] noted that only 0.5% of infants ages 6–9 months in their study exhibited more than –3.00 D of myopia.

It is well known that there are racial and ethnic variations in the type and degree of refractive error. Sperduto et al. [16] noted a significantly higher rate of high congenital myopia in blacks but a lower overall prevalence of low and moderate myopia generally in black children.

External factors may affect the refractive error of preschool-age children. Hirsch [17] noted a possible relationship between high fevers caused by measles in children and the sudden onset and rapid progression of myopia. A positive relationship with sudden onset and rapid progression of myopia may be seen in other febrile illnesses as well.

Sorsby [18] linked hyperopia to congenital and possibly hereditary factors but not to environmental factors. Nathan [19] pointed out that various ocular abnormalities affecting foveal vision lead to hyperopia. Robb and Rodier [20] showed that 90% of patients in their study with congenital esotropia were at least mildly hyperopic. Bilateral hyperopia of more than +2.50 D in young children is associated with future onset of strabismus [21]. Atkinson [15] found that 4.6% of infants 6–9 months of age in her study had more than +3.50 D.

Ingram and Barr [22] reported the refractive error of 148 children at 1 and 3.5 years of age. The prevalence of myopia and astigmatism decreased, and the prevalence of emmetropia increased over this period of time. Children with refractive error of +2.50 D or more at 1 year of age were equally likely to shift to more or less hyperopia at 3.5 years. This study showed that refractive error, especially hyperopia, is quite volatile and its progression uncertain at this young age. Children that are significantly hyperopic at 2 years old may be emmetropic later, and those that are emmetropic at 2 years may become hyperopic later.

Astigmatism is variable, even over short periods of time in the same young children. Many studies have shown a high incidence of against-the-rule astigmatism in infants, ranging up to 90% of premature infants in a study by Abrahamsson et al. [23] and 83% by London and Wick [24]. Howland [25]

noted that 63% of infants had astigmatism of 0.75 D or greater, whereas Fulton et al. [26] found 19% had 1.00 D or more. This astigmatism tended to regress to adult levels by about 4 years of age. Gwiazda et al. [27] found greater amounts of astigmatism by noncycloplegic techniques—56% against-the-rule with a mean magnitude of 2.00 D.

Many authors have noted high degrees of astigmatism in Native Americans (especially with-the-rule astigmatism) and in several other racial and ethnic groups. There is a suggestion that uncorrected astigmatism before 3 years of age, especially at an oblique axis of astigmatism, may stimulate the development of myopia [28]. Dobson et al. [29] found that in premature infants, the shorter the gestation the more likely the infants were to be myopic and astigmatic. Almost 80% of patients with astigmatism had against-the-rule. Fetal alcohol syndrome has been found to cause high degrees of congenital against-the-rule astigmatism [30].

In premature infants, Fulton et al. [31] found a 32% prevalence of anisometropia, decreasing to 18% of full-term infants. Other studies have noted a prevalence of 1.0–8.8% in children 1–6 years of age, depending on the definition (from 0.50 to 2.00 D) of anisometropia. Anisomyopia is much more common than anisohyperopia [32, 33]. Ingram and Barr found that anisometropia can increase or decrease during childhood [22]. Abrahamsson et al. [34, 35] also noted the changeability of anisometropia in the first 4 years of life. Some children who were anisometropic early became isometropic later; in others, the reverse occurred. They also noted that children who experienced increasing degrees of anisometropic astigmatism were most likely to develop amblyopia. Their conclusion was that a failure of emmetropization played an important role in visual development. Friedman et al. [36] reported that, in a large-scale screening program, anisometropia of 2.00 D or more was found in 9.4% of the 360 cases of esotropia. It was especially prevalent in those cases with constant unilateral esotropia. Atkinson [15] noted a prevalence of anisometropia of more than 1.00 D in 1.3% of children between 6 and 9 months of age. Goldschmidt [4] found myopic anisometropia in 2.5% of boys and 2.9% of girls.

Perhaps of greatest importance is the recognized association between anisometropia and amblyopia and strabismus. Ingram and Walker [37] have noted that 1.00 D of anisometropia is associated with strabismus, amblyopia, or both. Ingram [38] also noted the association of anisohyperopia, strabismus, and amblyopia. Significant unilateral myopia can also be induced by visual deprivation during the critical period of visual development. Miller-Meeks [39] reported on a series of six infants with traumatic vitreous hemorrhages who developed significant myopia in the affected eye. Hoyt [40] reported a heterogeneous group of patients with neonatal eyelid closure who developed unilateral myopia.

Modest, symmetric, refractive errors in the youngest age groups do not generally require refractive correction and do not lead to vision loss. High refractive errors, particularly when unequal, cause both temporary (correctable soon after application of spectacles) and more permanent, difficult-to-treat loss of vision (i.e., amblyopia). Anisometropia is the leading cause of amblyopia, with studies indicating that up to 60% of all amblyopia is due to anisometropia. High refractive errors are also more often associated with both structural and functional abnormalities of the eye and visual system. The prevalence of high refractive error is uncertain but may be 5–10% of the pediatric population.

AMBLYOPIA

The prevalence of amblyopia in the general population is estimated at 2–3%. The annual incidence is estimated to be approximately 0.4% in the preschool years [41]. Approximately six million Americans are amblyopic in one or both eyes. Based on findings that amblyopia develops only during the first 6–8 years of life [42], it has been estimated that each year in the United States a cohort of approximately 75,000 3-year-olds will develop amblyopia. Fulton [43], giving a prevalence of amblyopia at approximately 2% of children, estimated that, including only today's preschool population, amblyopia will cause 20 million people years (20 million children × 2% amblyopes × 50 years) of preventable vision loss. This is a surprising and widely underappreciated statistic. The amount of public health effort expended on amblyopia education and prevention pales in comparison to that dedicated to cataracts and glaucoma in the adult population.

Epidemiologic Studies of Amblyopia

As seen in the following sections, there is an extensive amount of literature on the epidemiology of amblyopia. Many of these studies are flawed, however. Some of the larger population-based studies did not actually measure a reduced level of visual acuity but inferred that unilateral constant strabismus equated with amblyopia. These studies probably underidentified cases of amblyopia with microtropia and mistakenly included cases in which there was no amblyopia in spite of the strabismus. Studies of military recruits were based only on a selected population of men instead of the entire population of all men in any age cohort. Studies based on clinic populations suffer from the obvious fact that the subjects who attended for examination presumably either had or were suspected of having eye problems, including amblyopia. Therefore, as Hillis et al. [42] pointed out, the true epidemiology of amblyopia, and indirectly, the sensitivity and specificity of amblyopia screening programs are unknown.

Population-Based Studies

Population-based studies have estimated a prevalence of amblyopia as being between 0.5 and 1%. Most consider this to be an underassessment of the actual prevalence. Friedman et al. [36] and Nawratzki et al. [44], in large population-based studies in Israel, found 0.5% of toddlers were amblyopic. These studies were based on a presumption of amblyopia by the presence of unilateral strabismus only, being insensitive to the presence of a microtropia. They did not actually measure visual acuity. Studies derived from extensive screening programs sponsored by the National Society For the Prevention of Blindness and commented on by Ehrlich et al. [45] reported a prevalence of almost 1% in 3- to 6-year-olds. These screenings suffered from a procedure using volunteers of various skill levels and from a very high number of untestable patients. This screening procedure also used a single "E" optotype, which underidentifies amblyopia because it does not invoke the crowding phenomenon.

Studies Based on Military Recruits

Studies of military recruits estimated amblyopia prevalence at 1–5% [46, 47]. Although they imply a broadly based sampling of young men, they may not fully represent those having more severe known vision problems that were automatically exempt from draft physicals. In addition, they are open to the criticism of potential malingerers not being accurately identified. The quality of the screening or examination is also somewhat suspect.

Clinic-Based Population Studies

Clinic population studies have generally elicited higher amblyopia prevalence levels. This is not surprising, given that patients with reduced vision may be more likely to attend for clinical care than those with normal vision. Because these patients are receiving full eye examinations instead of merely a screening battery, the accuracy of the results is greater than in many other studies. For example, microtropic patients with true amblyopia will likely be identified, whereas those same patients would be more likely to be missed in other study designs, particularly those depending only on the presence of constant unilateral strabismus. Cole [48], in a study of 10,000 consecutive clinic patients in England, noted a prevalence of amblyopia of 5.3%. Cholst et al. [49] found a prevalence of 4.7% in 3,000 clinic patients in New York City. A study in the United Kingdom by Thompson et al. [50] arrived at a prevalence of amblyopia of 3% of children. An interesting study [51] of elderly people in Denmark who were not previously screened or treated for amblyopia arrived at a prevalence of 2.9% overall: 2.3% due to strabismus and 0.6% from anisometropia.

Risk Factors Associated with Amblyopia

A number of important risk factors are related to the development of amblyopia. Sjostrand and Abrahamsson [52] determined the relative risk factors in their study of 310 children. The greatest risk factors were oblique astigmatism and strabismus, followed by increasing levels of with-the-rule and against-the-rule astigmatism, anisometropia, and hyperopia of more than +3.50 D. They and others have also made clear the association of premature birth and low birth weight, birth defects, mental retardation, hereditary factors, and eye diseases with amblyopia. Ingram and Walker [37] noted that children whose siblings

had strabismus or amblyopia were four times more likely to have vision disorders if the siblings had refractive errors. These and other data indicate that siblings of children with strabismus, amblyopia, and high refractive errors (especially hyperopia) are at increased risk for similar problems.

The percentage of amblyopic patients having strabismus has been estimated at 25–55% in various studies involving large numbers of military draftees [53, 54]. Schapero [32] pointed out that esotropia leads to more strabismic amblyopia than exotropia, due in part to the fact that esotropia is more common than exotropia [55]. Strabismic amblyopic patients are more likely to be identified earlier than those with apparently straight eyes [56].

High symmetric refractive error may cause bilateral refractive amblyopia. There is relatively little literature on this cause of amblyopia [57], but anecdotally it is well recognized. Astigmatism seems to play a significant role in many of these patients. High refractive errors may cause strabismus, as in the case of accommodative esotropia. Agaston [58], in a large population of military recruits, found that only a minute percentage of amblyopic patients had symmetric bilateral high refractive error, but Ingram and Barr [22] noted an association between high hyperopia and strabismus (primarily due to accommodative esotropia).

Anisometropic amblyopia is more common than strabismic amblyopia. Although the majority of anisometropic patients are myopic [33] as opposed to hyperopic, most patients with anisometropic amblyopia are hyperopic [59, 60]. Phillips [59] found that 71% of 131 amblyopic patients had hyperopic anisometropia (more than half were strabismic), 14% had myopic anisometropia (only one was strabismic), and 15% had antimetropic anisometropia (seven were strabismic). Horwith [60] found that 66% of 51 strabismic anisometropic patients had hyperopic anisometropia, and 33% had astigmatic anisometropia. Townshend et al. [61] noted that the depth of anisometropic amblyopia is related closely to the degree of anisometropia. Interestingly, they found a greater correlation in myopic patients than hyperopic patients, the reverse of what is usually assumed. It is possible that the myopic anisometropic patients in their study may have had reduced vision not only from amblyopia, but from organic causes as well, such as foveal abnormalities or severe myelinated nerve fibers.

Astigmatism may directly cause amblyopia. Meridional amblyopia has been described by Mitchell et al. [62], Mitchell [63], and Gwiazda et al. [64]. It is well known that there is great variability in the magnitude and orientation of astigmatism in the first 2½–3 years of life. Gwiazda et al. [64] suggest that astigmatism present before 1 year of age does not result in meridional amblyopia, but astigmatism present in the second year of life may be detected as meridional amblyopia later. The duration of the critical period for the development of this type of amblyopia is not yet known. Sjostrand and Abrahamsson [52] noted the significance of oblique astigmatism and any increasing degree of astigmatism at any axis as risk factors in the development of amblyopia.

Individuals with unilateral (anisometropic) astigmatism clinically are recognized as having a high risk for the development of amblyopia, but the prevalence is not reported. One relatively uncommon group of patients with unilateral astigmatism caused by large eyelid hemangiomas has been reported by Robb [65]. The timing of onset and the natural history of these patients is well known and studied. These patients invariably develop dense and persistent amblyopia, but their clinical course is sufficiently different than the more typical cases of unilateral astigmatism in which the depth of amblyopia is not as great.

STRABISMUS

There is both a less extensive literature on the prevalence of strabismus than of amblyopia and also less disagreement on those prevalence levels. The prevalence of esotropia in the general population is estimated at approximately 3% and that of exotropia at approximately 1.5%. There is little mention in the literature of the prevalence of vertical deviations, which is likely due to its low prevalence. There is even less mention of the prevalence of strabismus syndromes such as Duane's, Brown's, and Möbius' syndromes because of their low prevalence in the general population.

Convergence and the control of oculomotor function occurs rather abruptly at 3–4 months of age [66]. Esotropia present at birth is said to be rare. Nixon et al. [67] was unable to find a single case among 1,219 neonates. The definition of congenital esotropia is often broadened to include infants with demonstrable esotropia by 6 months of age. Using this definition, von Norden [68] and others have estimated the prevalence of congenital (or infantile as it is sometimes called) esotropia at 1–2%. This includes about one-fourth to one-half of all cases of strabismus [69, 70]. Some of these cases appear to be hereditary in nature, with various patterns observed. Other cases may be due to neurologic events that occur before, during, or after birth, such as cerebral palsy, meningitis, hydrocephalus, and head trauma. Other causes include trisomy 21, the strabismus syndromes (Duane's, Brown's, Möbius', and congenital fibrosis), and a myriad of unilateral and bilateral eye diseases and malformations. Many of these patients may also have refractive errors that are great enough to require optical correction. Refractive error may play some role in the onset of infantile esotropia. Robb and Rodier [71] found that 75% of patients with infantile esotropia had significant refractive error, primarily hyperopia.

Accommodative esotropia is an important cause of acquired strabismus. Onset is usually around 2–3 years of age but in a few cases may be as early as 4–6 months of age. Ingram [38] has shown that infants with more than +2.50 D of hyperopia are 20 times more likely to develop strabismus than those with emmetropia. Ingram et al. [71] noted that almost 50% of children with +3.50 D or greater at 1 year of age eventually developed strabismus. Atkinson [15] found that 4.6% of infants 6–9 months of age had more than +3.50 D. When both Atkinson's prevalence of hyperopia in the infant population and Ingram et al.'s estimate that up to 50% of infants with hyperopia of more than +3.50 D develop strabismus are combined, approximately 2.0–2.5% of infants may develop strabismus of an accommodative nature.

It is difficult to arrive at prevalence estimates for other acquired forms of esotropia because there are many possible etiologies. Several large population-based studies have estimated the total prevalence of strabismus in pediatric populations, but they have problems in the method of actual diagnosis of the strabismus. The largest is a multicenter study by Chew et al. [72] involving more than 50,000 patients who were followed from pregnancy until 7 years of age. Strabismus was diagnosed by pediatricians or neurologists from the Hirschberg light reflexes, with statistical validation by ophthalmologists. The study found a prevalence of esotropia of 3% and exotropia of 1.2%. This is likely an underestimation of the actual prevalence of strabismus because of insensitivity of testing to the presence of microtropia and small-angle strabismus. As clinicians are all too aware, cases of strabismus may be easily missed by Hirschberg reflex alone. Chew et al. also noted that esotropia was more prevalent in whites (3.9%) than in blacks (2.2%). The prevalence of strabismus increased in low-birth-weight infants by 3.26 times for esotropia and 4.01 times for exotropia compared with normal infants. There was also an increased risk for infants whose mothers smoked during pregnancy, and for those with increasing maternal age. The prevalence of strabismus in the general population in several other studies was also estimated at approximately 3–4% [73, 74].

OCULAR DISEASE

Severe structural abnormalities and various disease processes may cause marked vision loss in children. Deprivation amblyopia is the most severe form of amblyopia. It occurs in neonates prevented from obtaining form vision before the end of the critical period of visual development. Deprivation amblyopia is usually caused by congenital cataracts, but it also may be due to corneal opacities or severe ptosis. All of these causes together are rare, occurring in approximately 1 per 10,000 births [75].

It is often difficult to differentiate the amblyopic and anatomic components of vision loss in young children. Among the specific causes of vision loss in this category are cataracts and other media opacities, congenital glaucoma, albinism, aniridia, retinopathy of prematurity, metabolic diseases, neurologic disorders, and many others. Treatment is directed at remediation of the structural defects to the degree possible, correcting any refractive error, and patching for amblyopia. Early detection is critical for any chance of success in arriving at useful levels of vision, even after aggressive treatment. Abnormalities such as these are far more common in high-risk populations, such as those of low birth weight and those with a history of prenatal exposure to drugs such as cocaine. Although there is uncertainty over the maximum age when these conditions may be treated, there is no disagreement over the best time to detect these conditions—as early as possible. All high-risk infants should be screened in the first year of life.

OTHER OCULAR CONDITIONS AFFECTING CHILDREN

Other categories of ocular conditions affect vision in children and are considered screenable. Color vision defects are common and identifiable in children. These occur primarily in boys and are believed to be a significant functional issue by many optometrists and educators. Although it might be argued that they are not of great importance in children, color vision defects can place the child at a disadvantage in certain situations. For example, the child may experience difficulty identifying colors when drawing in preschool and school environments.

Visual perceptual problems, visual motor integration, eye-hand coordination, and learning disabilities all have important implications for affected children. These conditions are covered in greater depth in Chapter 19.

SIGNIFICANCE AND TREATABILITY OF OCULAR DISORDERS IN YOUNG CHILDREN

The epidemiologic evidence presented above provides a framework for understanding which vision disorders affect children. Clinical experience helps in estimating the depth of the vision loss and the likelihood of remediation. This is useful on a clinical basis, but there are no definitive answers based on careful studies of the short- and long-term effects on vision and functioning for most of these disorders. We are uncertain how treatable many of these conditions are, and we do not necessarily know the best ways to treat them. There are, however, widely shared clinical impressions of the natural history of these disorders, both treated and untreated.

There is certainty that high refractive error causes reduced visual acuity. Providing appropriate optical correction to these patients usually improves vision, often immediately. Certain types of refractive errors respond better than others. For example, myopic patients corrected for the first time show immediate improvements in acuity. Patients with refractive amblyopia, however, show little if any improvement in visual acuity immediately after initial optical correction. Acuity may improve spontaneously over a period of days or weeks, or the patient may require active forms of amblyopia treatment to expedite improvements in acuity. If treatment is instituted too late, there may be no possibility of improvement in acuity. There is little question that correcting refractive error in children is both useful and cost effective when the uncorrected refractive error impairs visual acuity sufficiently to cause functional problems, especially in the context of education.

The treatment of amblyopia is more complicated. There are few large-scale, controlled studies that have focused on the treatment of amblyopia. Clinically, amblyopia is treated primarily by patching, but the details of the treatment are very much determined by the practitioner, the patient, and the family, and there is no standardization in technique or duration. There is also little agreement on the efficacy of the treatment, with various studies showing anywhere from a 30% to a 90% success rate (there is not even agreement on what the definition of successful treatment is). The variability is due to the specifics of the cause of amblyopia, temporal issues such as onset of the amblyopia, when treatment was initiated, and the treatment chosen and how consistently it was carried out. These factors make careful study of amblyopia treatment difficult. This is just as true for the patient—the practitioner essentially must depend on the parents and child for accurate reporting of all phases of the treatment. We never really know if our recommendations are being followed as directed.

It is easier to ascertain the extent of vision loss in patients with amblyopia. We are able to accurately measure patients' visual acuity, but there is disagreement as to how closely vision at a young age compares to that later. Well-treated amblyopic patients may not hold their improvements in visual acuity into adulthood for a number of reasons. It has even been argued that the benefits of good binocular vision may not be worth the efforts of intensive amblyopia treatment during childhood, unless of course the amblyopic patient later loses vision in the nonamblyopic eye due to trauma or disease.

The effectiveness of treating strabismus is also uncertain. There is a large body of literature that has looked at the issues of whether to treat strabismus [76] and compared the efficacy of optometric with ophthalmologic treatment of strabismus [77, 78]. The restoration of binocularity and the elimination or at least minimization of amblyopia is the usual goal, but one that is at best only occasionally achieved. The ophthalmologic criteria of cosmetically straight eyes seems an unacceptable goal for the efforts of early detection and treatment of strabismus.

There is no disagreement on the necessity of treating ocular disease when found. Conditions such as anterior segment inflammatory or infectious disease are often obvious on casual inspection and will likely be identified by parents or others in close contact with the child. Treatment will then be instituted by conventional systems of care.

In summary, the conditions that most frequently have adverse effects on children's vision include refractive error, amblyopia, and strabismus. These meet the criteria of significant prevalence; likelihood for successful treatment, at least under suitable conditions; and likelihood of causing significant vision loss if not adequately corrected.

REFERENCES

1. Banks MS. Infant refraction and accommodation. Int Ophthalmol Clin 1980;20:205–232.
2. Quinn GE, Dobson V, Repka MX, et al. Development of myopia in infants with birth weights less than 1251 grams. Ophthalmology 1992;99:329–340.
3. Fledelius H. Prematurity and the eye—ophthalmic 10-year follow-up of children of low and normal birth weight. Acta Ophthalmol 1976;54(Suppl 128): 1–245.
4. Goldschmidt E. Refraction in the newborn. Acta Ophthalmol (Copenh) 1969;47:570–578.
5. Cook RC, Glascock RE. Refractive and ocular findings in the newborn. Am J Ophthalmol 1951;34:1407–1413.
6. Wibaut JF. Uber die Emmetropisation und den Ursprung der spharischen Refrakionsanomalien. Albrecht von Graefes Arch fur Ophthalmol 1926; 116:596–612.
7. Grosvenor T, Flom MC (eds). Refractive Anomalies. Boston: Butterworth–Heinemann, 1991;20.
8. Stenstrom S. Investigation of the variation and the covariation of the optical elements of human eyes. D Woolf (trans). Am J Optom and Arch Am Acad Optom 1948;25(5):218–232.
9. Stenstrom S. Investigation of the variation and the covariation of the optical elements of human eyes. D

Woolf (trans). Am J Optom and Arch Am Acad Optom 1948;25(6):286–299.

10. Stenstrom S. Investigation of the variation and the co-variation of the optical elements of human eyes. D Woolf (trans). Am J Optom and Arch Am Acad Optom 1948;25(7):340–350.

11. Stenstrom S. Investigation of the variation and the co-variation of the optical elements of human eyes. D Woolf (trans). Am J Optom and Arch Am Acad Optom 1948;25(8):388–397.

12. Stenstrom S. Investigation of the variation and the co-variation of the optical elements of human eyes. D Woolf (trans). Am J Optom and Arch Am Acad Optom 1948;25(9):438–449.

13. Stenstrom S. Investigation of the variation and the co-variation of the optical elements of human eyes. D Woolf (trans). Am J Optom and Arch Am Acad Optom 1948;25(10):496–504.

14. Kronfeld PD, Devney C. Ein Beitragzur Kenntnis der Refractions Kurve. Graefes Arch Ophthalmol 1931; 126:487.

15. Atkinson J, Braddick O, Durden K, et al. Screening for refractive errors in 6–9 month old infants by photorefraction. Br J Ophthalmol 1984;68:105.

16. Sperduto RD, Seigel D, Roberts J, et al. Prevalence of myopia in the United States. Arch Opthalmol 1983;101: 405–407.

17. Hirsch MJ. The relationship between measles and myopia. Am J Optom Arch Am Acad Optom 1957;34: 289–297.

18. Sorsby A, Benjamin B, Davey JB, et al. Emmetropia and its aberrations. Medical Research Council Special Report Series, No. 293, 1957.

19. Nathan J, Kiely PM, Crewther SG, et al. Disease associated visual image degradation and spherical refractive errors in children. Am J Optom Physiol Opt 1985; 62:680–698.

20. Robb RM, Rodier DW. The broad clinical spectrum of early infantile esotropia. Trans Am Ophthalmol Soc 1986;84:103–116.

21. Ingram RM, Traynar MJ, Walker C, et al. Screening for refractive errors at age 1 year: a pilot study. Br J Ophthalmol 1979;63:243–250.

22. Ingram RM, Barr A. Changes in refraction between the ages of 1 and 3 1/2 years. Br J Ophthalmol 1979;63: 339–342.

23. Abrahamsson M, Fabian G, Sjostrand J. Changes in astigmatism between the ages of 1 and 4 years: a longitudinal study. Br J Ophthalmol 1988;72:145–149.

24. London R, Wick BC. Changes in angle lambda during growth: theory and clinical implications. Am J Optom Physiol Opt 1982;59:568–572.

25. Howland HC, Atkinson J, Braddick D, et al. Infant astigmatism measured by photorefraction. Science 1978;202:331–333.

26. Fulton AB, Dobson V, Salem D, et al. Cycloplegic re-

fractions in infants and young children. Am J Ophthalmol 1980;90:239–247.

27. Gwiazda J, Mohindra I, Brill S, et al. Infant astigmatism and meridional amblyopia. Vision Res 1985; 25:1269–1276.

28. Fulton AB, Hansen RM, Petersen RA. The relation of myopia and astigmatism in developing eyes. Ophthalmology 1982;89:298–302.

29. Dobson V, Fulton AB, Manning K, et al. Cycloplegic refractions of premature infants. Am J Ophthalmol 1981;91:490–495.

30. Stromland K. Ocular abnormalities in the fetal alcohol syndrome. Surv Ophthalmol 1987;31:277–293.

31. Fulton AB, Manning K, Salem D, et al. Cycloplegic refractions of premature infants. Am J Ophthalmol 1981; 91:490–495.

32. Schapero M. Amblyopia. Philadelphia: Chilton, 1971; 63–64.

33. Jampolsky A, Flom BC, Weymouth FW, et al. Unequal corrected visual acuity as related to anisometropia. Arch Ophthalmol 1955;54:893–905.

34. Abrahamsson M, Fabian G, Andersson AK, Sjostrand J. A longitudinal study of a population based sample of astigmatic children. I. Refraction and amblyopia. Acta Ophthalmol (Copenh) 1990;68:428–434.

35. Abrahamsson M, Fabian G, Sjostrand J. A longitudinal study of a population based sample of astigmatic children. II. The changeability of anisometropia. Acta Ophthalmol (Copenh) 1990;68:435–440.

36. Friedman Z, Neumann E, Hyams SW, et al. Ophthalmic screening of 38,000 children, age 1 to 2 1/2 years, in child welfare clinics. J Pediatr Ophthalmol Strabismus 1976;17:261–267.

37. Ingram RM, Walker C. Refraction as a means of predicting squint or amblyopia in preschool siblings of children known to have these defects. Br J Ophthalmol 1979;63:238–242.

38. Ingram RM. Refraction of 1 year old children after atropine cycloplegia. Br J Ophthalmol 1979;63:343–347.

39. Miller-Meeks MT, Bennett SR, Keech RV, Blodi CF. Myopia induced by vitreous hemorrhages. Am J Ophthalmol 1990;109:199–207.

40. Hoyt CS, Stone RD, Fromer C, et al. Monocular axial myopia associated with neonatal eyelid closure in human infants. Am J Ophthalmol 1981;91:197–200.

41. Hillis A. Amblyopia: prevalent, curable, neglected. Public Health Rev 1986;14(3–4):213–235.

42. Hillis A, Flynn JT, Hawkins BS. The evolving concept of amblyopia: a challenge to epidemiologists. Am J Epidemiol 1983;118:192–205.

43. Fulton AB. Editorial: screening preschool children to detect visual and ocular disorders. Arch Ophthalmol 1992;110:1553–1554.

44. Nawratzki I, Oliver M, Neumann E. Screening for amblyopia in children under three years of age in Israel. Isr J Med Sci 1972;8:1469–1471.

45. Ehrlich MI, Reinecke RD, Simons K. Preschool vision screening for amblyopia and strabismus: programs, methods, and guidelines, 1983. Surv Ophthalmol 1983; 28:145–163.

46. Theodore FH, Johnson RM, Miles NE, et al. Causes of impaired vision in recently inducted soldiers. Arch Ophthalmol 1946;31:399–402.

47. Helveston EM. The incidence of amblyopia ex anopsia in young adult males in Minnesota in 1962–1963. Am J Ophthalmol 1965;60:75–77.

48. Cole RBW. The problems of unilateral amblyopia: a preliminary study of 10,000 national health patients. Br Med J 1959;1:202–206.

49. Cholst MR, Cohen LJ, Losty MA. Evaluation of amblyopia problems in the child. N Y J Med 1962; 62:3927–3930.

50. Thompson JR, Woodruff G, Hiscox FA, et al. The incidence and prevalence of amblyopia detected in childhood. Br J Ophthalmol 1991;105:455–462.

51. Vinding T, Gregersen E, Jensen A, et al. Prevalence of amblyopia in old people without previous screening and treatment. An evaluation of the present prophylactic procedures among children in Denmark. Acta Ophthalmol (Copenh) 1991;69:796–798.

52. Sjostrand J, Abrahamsson M. Risk factors in amblyopia. Eye 1990;4:787–793.

53. Glover LP, Brewer WR. An ophthalmologic review of more than 20,000 men at the Altoona Induction Center. Am J Ophthalmol 1944;27:346–348.

54. Downing AH. Ocular defects in 60,000 selectees. Arch Ophthalmol 1945;33:137–143.

55. Flom MC, Neumaier RW. Prevalence of amblyopia. Public Health Rep 1966;81:329–331.

56. Shaw DE, Fielder AR, Minshull C, et al. Amblyopia— factors influencing age of presentation. Lancet 1988;2:207–209.

57. Abraham SV. Bilateral ametropic amblyopia. J Pediatr Ophthalmol Strabismus 1964;1:57–61.

58. Agaston H. Ocular malingering. Arch Ophthalmol 1944;31:223–231.

59. Phillips CI. Strabismus, anisometropia, and amblyopia. Br J Ophthalmol 1959;43:449–460.

60. Horwith H. Anisometropic amblyopia. Am Orthopt J 1964;14:99–104.

61. Townshend AM, Holmes JM, Evans LS. Depth of anisometropic amblyopia and difference in refraction. Am J Ophthalmol 1993;116:431–436.

62. Mitchell DE, Freeman RD, Millodot M, et al. Meridional amblyopia: evidence for modification of the human visual system by early visual experience. Vision Res 1973;13:535–558.

63. Mitchell DE. Astigmatism and neural development (editorial). Invest Ophthalmol Vis Sci 1979;18:8–10.

64. Gwiazda J, Bauer J, Thorn F, et al. Meridional amblyopia does result from astigmatism in early childhood. Clin Vis Sci 1986;1:145–152.

65. Robb RM. Refractive errors associated with hemangiomas of the eyelids and orbit in infancy. Am J Ophthalmol 1977;83:52–58.

66. Thorn F, Gwiazda J, Cruz AAV, et al. The development of eye alignment, convergence, and sensory binocularity in young infants. Invest Ophthalmol Vis Sci 1994;35:544–553.

67. Nixon RB, Helveston EM, Miller K, et al. Incidence of strabismus in neonates. Am J Ophthalmol 1985; 100:798–801.

68. von Norden GK. Infantile esotropia: a continuing riddle. Am Orthopt J 1984;34:52–62.

69. Nordlow W. Age distribution of onset of esotropia. Br J Ophthalmol 1953;37:593–600.

70. Robb RM, Rodier DW. The variable clinical characteristics and course of early infantile esotropia. J Pediatr Ophthalmol Strabismus 1987;24:276–281.

71. Ingram RM, Walker C, Wilson JM, et al. Prediction of amblyopia and squint by means of refraction at age 1 year. Br J Ophthalmol 1986;70:12–15.

72. Chew E, Remaley NA, Tamboli A, et al. Risk factors for esotropia and exotropia. Arch Ophthalmol 1994; 112:1349–1355.

73. Graham PA. Epidemiology of strabismus. Br J Ophthalmol 1974;58:224–231.

74. Woodruff ME. Vision and refractive status among grade 1 children in the Province of New Brunswick. Am J Optom Physiol Opt 1986;63:545–552.

75. Edmonds LD, James LM. Temporal trends in the prevalence of congenital malformation at birth based on the Birth Defects Monitoring Program, United States, 1979–1987. MMWR CDC Surveill Summ 1990; 39:SS4:19–23.

76. Flom MC. Issues in the Clinical Management of Binocular Anomalies. In E Rosenbloom, Morgan M (eds), Principles and Practice of Pediatric Optometry. Philadelphia: Lippincott, 1990;219–244.

77. Scheiman M, Ciner E. Surgical success rates in acquired, comitant, partially accommodative, and nonaccommodative esotropia. J Am Optom Assoc 1987; 58:556–561.

78. Scheiman M, Ciner E, Gallaway M. Surgical success rates in infantile esotropia. J Am Optom Assoc 1989; 60:22–30.

Chapter 4

Biometry of the Eye in Infancy and Childhood

Donald O. Mutti and Karla Zadnik

Refractive error is actually an unusual finding in a general population of young children, although it may seem to be a common occurrence in clinical practice. The prevalence of refractive error at the age of 6 is approximately 8%, with 2% of children being myopic ($\leq$–0.50 D) and 6% hyperopic ($\geq$+1.50 D) [1]. Yet, by the age of 15 years, nearly 15% of children are myopic, whereas the prevalence of hyperopia remains at about 6% [1]. Nearly 25% of the adult population of the United States is myopic [2].

If most myopia develops in childhood, why study ocular growth in infancy? Although juvenile myopia is classically associated with axial elongation, most eye growth and change in the power of the eye's refractive surfaces take place in infancy. The fact that most of this eye growth occurs without creating refractive error, in fact more often reducing neonatal refractive error (emmetropization), makes infant eye growth an important model for appropriate and normal ocular development.

Refractive error and ocular component development have fascinated clinicians and vision scientists alike for hundreds of years. Tools such as retinoscopy, cycloplegia, keratometry, and phakometry have been available since the last century for the evaluation of refractive error and the ocular components that contribute to it. Recent technologic developments and trends in the delivery of eye care have created special opportunities for assessing ocular dimensions. For example, the advent of refractive surgery has created a renaissance of interest in corneal topography. The availability of charge-coupled device (CCD), or "chip" cameras, interfaced with personal computers has allowed for the rapid capture and digitization of video-based information generated by these topographers. Increases in computer power and speed in the last decade have allowed for processing and storage of these large video image files. The increased demand for cataract surgery from our active aging population has stimulated continual improvement of modern ultrasonography units, resulting in the availability of more efficient, compact, and powerful machines.

BIOMETRIC TECHNIQUES

Keratometry and Corneal Topography

Obviously, the chief obstacle in obtaining biometric data in infants is their lack of cooperation. Two Laws of Infant Examination, attributed to Howard Howland of Cornell University, govern infant examination: (1) infants wiggle; and (2) a lot. Conventional keratometry is therefore difficult but has been successfully performed in newborns with the help of an eyelid speculum [3, 4]. Several photographic methods have been used successfully. Mandell [5] has used a 35-mm camera equipped with a tube extending from a lens that has clear rings at set intervals. When the tube is illuminated by the flash ring around it, these circles form mires that make concentric reflections on the cornea, serving as a small and portable corneoscope. Howland and Sayles [6] have used a 35-mm camera with a lens surrounded by eight optical fibers connected to the flash. This serves as a keratometer that works simultaneously in four meridians. The examiner can have the infant sit on the parent's lap and attract the baby's attention in the direction of the camera.

Ultrasonography

Measurement of the eye's axial dimensions presents special challenges in infants. Since the ultrasound probe must come into contact with the cornea or eyelid, infants tend to object more strongly to it than to other, less invasive procedures. The dimensions obtained from ultrasonography that are important in refractive development are anterior chamber depth (ACD), lens thickness, and vitreous chamber depth (VCD). The sum of all three is the axial length of the eye. Because of the difficulty in examining awake infants, much ultrasonography data have been obtained on sedated or anesthetized infants [7, 8], although cooperative infants and newborns may tolerate the procedure while awake [8, 9]. Recently, it has been shown that performing A-scan ultrasonography with the probe over the closed eyelid, similar to the procedure used for B-scan, is a feasible method for infant ultrasonography [10]. Measures on sleeping infants or cooperative toddlers may thus be accomplished without sedation or use of a lid speculum.

Phakometry

One of the least studied ocular components contributing to refraction in the infant eye is the crystalline lens. This is unfortunate, as the lens is critical to the refractive development of the eye, second only to axial length in importance. The lens undergoes a greater dioptric change (20 D), on average, than the cornea (5 D), and it continues to develop with respect to power and curvature from infancy through childhood. On the other hand, the cornea is nearly fully developed by the age of 2 years. Therefore, compensation for axial growth to maintain emmetropia is more likely to come from the crystalline lens. Technologic limitations have hampered previous investigators, limiting our cur-

rent knowledge. The first descriptions of crystalline lens radii in the newborn came in 1909, in which the estimates were made from frozen sections of seven cadaver eyes [11]. Up until the present, these were the only available data for use in creating schematic eyes and modeling of infant dioptrics. Phakometric techniques have been known, however, since the time of Tscherning [12]. He described how viewing a pair of Purkinje images could yield the equivalent radius of curvature of a lens surface, since the separation of the two images was proportional to the radius of curvature. Figure 4.1 depicts how incoming, parallel light forms images after reflection from the cornea and the anterior surface of the crystalline lens. These images form at the focal points of the respective mirror surfaces, or r/2. By similar triangles, the heights of the images will be proportional to the radius of curvature of the mirrors as viewed in air. By knowing the position of the mirror surfaces from ultrasound data, ray tracing equations can be applied to find the true radius for each lens surface within the eye.

Phakometry has been performed in several studies of children in conjunction with 35-mm photography. This format has several disadvantages, however. The number of images collected is small because of the time needed to take a picture, the camera flash may disturb or surprise photophobic children, and a child's motion during measurement may result in out-of-focus or poorly aligned images. Given that film development takes time, an examiner may not be aware of the poor data quality until long after the measurement session. Since phakometry generally requires pupillary dilation, repeating the measurement to obtain complete data becomes an added burden to the child. Advances in video and computer technology address many of these issues. Using a video format means that no flash is required and the camera may change focus to follow the patient's movement more easily. More important, the clinician can know that acceptable images are being recorded at the time of data collection without delays for processing. Computer hardware can grab multiple frames of video, increasing the number of samples obtained from each subject and improving the repeatability of the video technique [13].

We have recently built a video-based phakometer suitable for use in infants (Figure 4.2). The unit consists of a CCD camera equipped with a fixed-focus lens mounted on an extension tube. The working distance from the infant is set at 25 cm, close enough to obtain adequate magnification and precision, but far enough away to be out of the baby's reach or to have the baby taking a bottle without blocking the phakometer. The light sources for the Purkinje images are infrared light-emitting diodes (LEDs). The room lights can therefore be dim, without dazzling the baby with bright lights. CCD cameras have excellent sensitivity in the infrared once the infrared filter is removed. The phakometry LEDs are arranged in two pairs, one to measure the vertical meridian and one for the horizontal meridian. Additionally, three rings of eight dimmer keratometry lights are mounted on the faceplate of the unit in order to measure infant corneal toricity and topography.

REFRACTIVE ERROR IN INFANCY

The typical newborn is hyperopic under cycloplegia (Table 4.1). Cycloplegia is a valuable tool in refracting the newborn to reveal any latent hyperopia. Many infants who are myopic by noncycloplegic retinoscopy can be hyperopic after instillation of a cycloplegic, such as atropine [14]. Mean refractive error is also less hyperopic when near retinoscopy is used compared with cycloplegic retinoscopy [15]. The distribution of newborn refractive error also lacks the sharply peaked, leptokurtic distribution typical in children and adults. On the other hand, myopia is not uncommon in newborns, with prevalences ranging from 0 to 25% (see Table 4.1) [16]. Figure 4.3 shows the normal distribution skewed toward hyperopia, which is typical of neonatal refractive error. During ocular growth, the process of emmetropization results in a reduction in the average amount of hyperopia in infancy, as well as a reduction in the variance of refractive errors. This process is responsible for transforming the distribution of refractive errors from normal to narrow. Recent evidence suggests that the highest rates of emmetropization seen during the first 12–17 months of life occur in infants with the highest initial ametropia, whether hyperopic [17, 18] or myopic [19]. The mechanism underlying emmetropization is unknown. Based on considerable work in animal models of refractive error, it has been hypothesized that the eye senses the sign and magnitude of its refractive error, then modulates its rate of growth

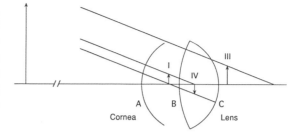

Figure 4.1. Parallel rays from a distant object are reflected from three reflecting surfaces of the eye: Purkinje image I from the cornea, III from the anterior surface of the crystalline lens, and IV from the posterior surface of the lens. Reflected images are formed at the focal points of the three equivalent mirrors when observed in air by the examiner. Their heights are determined by the nodal ray through the center of curvature of each equivalent surface. Their relative heights are therefore proportional to the radius of curvature of each surface.

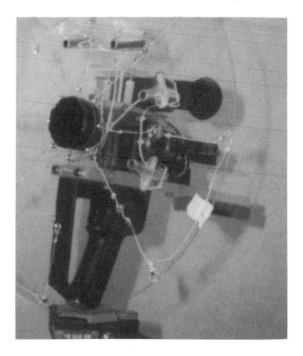

Figure 4.2. Photograph of a keratophakometer. A plastic faceplate is mounted on the camera lens. Purkinje images III and IV are generated by two pairs of brighter infrared light-emitting diodes (LEDs) mounted horizontally and vertically, and the corneal reflections by three concentric rings of dimmer infrared LEDs mounted on the faceplate in four meridians. Images are recorded on a VHS-format videocassette recorder separate from the camera and faceplate.

Table 4.1. Newborn Refractive Errors as Measured by Retinoscopy

Author	Number	Age	Method	Mean Refraction (D)	% Myopic
Goldschmidt [65]	356 infants	2–10 days	Atropine 0.5%	+0.62 ± 2.24	24.2
Santonastaso [14]	34 infants	0–3 mons	Atropine	+1.67 ± 2.54	8
Luyckx [7]	104 eyes	0–1 wk	Cyclopentolate 1%	+2.4 ± 1.2	0
Cook and Glasscock [16]	1,000 eyes	After post-delivery care	Atropine 1% ointment	+1.54	25.1
Zonis and Miller [66]	600 eyes	48–72 hrs	Mydriaticum	+1.1 ± 1.6	14.5
Mohindra and Held [15]	48 infants	0–4 wks	Noncycloplegic near retinoscopy	−0.70 ± 3.20	Not given
	27 infants	5–8 wks		−0.35 ± 2.30	
	78 infants	9–16 wks		−0.52 ± 2.25	
	70 infants	17–32 wks		+0.13 ± 1.39	
	50 infants	33–64 wks		+0.78 ± 0.97	

Source: Reprinted with permission from DO Mutti, K Zadnik. Refractive Error. In K Zadnik (ed), The Ocular Examination. Philadelphia: Saunders, 1997;55.

through an active, visual feedback mechanism in order to reduce that error [20]. Eyes myopic at birth would reduce their refractive error by growing slowly while the cornea and lens lost power during development, and neonatal hyperopic eyes would reduce that error by growing more rapidly.

An interesting feature of infant refractive error is the high prevalence of against-the-rule astigmatism (Table 4.2). Anywhere from 17% [21] to 63% [22] of infants may have astigmatism of more than 1.00 DC. Most reports place the orientation as against-the-rule in 40–100% of cases. There are several potential sources for this astigmatism, such as a large-angle lambda [23], off-axis peripheral refractive astigmatism, or a change in accommodation between measurement of the two principal meridians during noncycloplegic retinoscopy [24]. From photokeratometric measures, Howland and Sayles [6] showed that this astigmatism is primarily corneal, especially in infants younger than 1 year old. This astigmatism is also transient. The prevalence of refractive astigmatism ≥1.00 DC decreases rapidly during the first year of life, reaching levels found in childhood by the age of 18 months [25] to 2 years [26]. Interestingly, this is similar to the time when the corneal radius of curvature has stabilized.

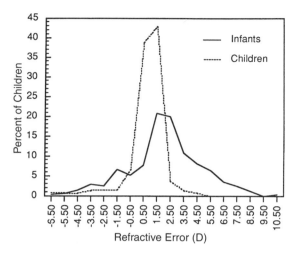

Figure 4.3. Comparison of refractive error distribution from newborns [16] to that from children (Orinda Longitudinal Study of Myopia, vertical meridian cycloplegic autorefraction, unpublished data, 1993). Note the reduced standard deviation and higher peak near emmetropia in the data for children, indicating the process of emmetropization. (Reprinted with permission from DO Mutti, K Zadnik. Refractive Error. In K Zadnik [ed], The Ocular Examination. Philadelphia: Saunders, 1997;55.)

OCULAR COMPONENT DEVELOPMENT IN INFANCY

The infant eye presents an interesting puzzle in ocular development. The average eye of a newborn is about 17 mm in length [7–9, 27–29], with a corneal power of about 49 D (Tables 4.3 and 4.4) [3–5, 30]. During the first 5 years of life, the eye grows another 4 mm in length on average. If uncompensated by changes in the other ocular components, this increase in length would result in a refractive error of –18 D. Obviously, other optical components must change so that myopia can be avoided. The cornea loses only approximately 5 D of power during those years. The crystalline lens is the component that undergoes the greatest dioptric change to create and preserve emmetropia. During the first 5 years of life, it loses an average of 20 D of power. The surprising feature of this phase of ocular development is that despite this substantial rate of growth, the prevalence of myopia is low by age 6 years (about 2%), lower perhaps even than at birth. These

changes in ocular dimensions occur rapidly. Both axial length and corneal curvature undergo the majority of their development in the first 2 years of life (Figure 4.4). Although the overall power of the eye decreases from 90 D at birth to 75 D at age 12 months [7, 31], studies have shown little residual spherical equivalent refractive error by age 12 months, averaging approximately +1.00 D, with standard deviations of less than ±2.00 D [14, 32–35].

Ocular growth is much slower in childhood, in contrast to the rapid changes occurring during the first 2 years of life. During the age period of 6–14 years, the eye grows only about 1 mm, the lens loses another 3.00 D of power, and the cornea remains virtually unchanged (flattening by 0.10 D per year) [36]. It is puzzling that during this period of slow growth when the increases in axial length should present little challenge to the compensating mechanisms of the eye, the prevalence of myopia increases from 2% at age 6 to 15% by age 15 years [1]. Is the eye growing more rapidly than it was during infancy? Inspection of Figure 4.4 shows that this is probably not the case, but clearly the eye is growing more rapidly than is appropriate—that is, more

Table 4.2. Estimates of the Prevalence and Orientation of Astigmatism ≥1.00 DC in Infancy (Younger Than 1 Year)

Author	Number	Method	Age	Prevalence of Astigmatism % (≥1.00 DC)	Orientation
Ingram and Barr [32]	296 eyes	Atropine 1% retinoscopy	1 yr	29.7	Not given
Fulton et al. [33]	133 infants	Cyclopentolate 1% retinoscopy	0–1 yr	19	71% ATR 21% WTR 8% Oblique
Dobson et al. [21]	46 infants 187 infants	Cyclopentolate 1% retinoscopy	0–6 mons 6–18 mons	17 19	100% ATR 70% ATR 18% WTR 2% Oblique
Santonastaso [14]	63 infants	Atropine retinoscopy	0–12 mons	52.4	15% ATR 85% WTR
Howland et al. [67]	93 infants	Noncycloplegic photorefraction	0–12 mons	47	70% "horizontal and vertical"
Gwiazda et al. [68]	521 infants	Noncycloplegic near retinoscopy	0–11 mons	53	44% ATR 39% WTR 16% Oblique
Howland and Sayles [22]	117 infants	Noncycloplegic photorefraction	0–12 mons	63	55% ATR 3% WTR 42% Oblique
Mohindra et al. [26]	276 right eyes	Noncycloplegic near retinoscopy	<1–50 wks	45	40% ATR 40% WTR 20% Oblique

ATR = against-the-rule (astigmatism); WTR = with-the-rule (astigmatism).
Source: Reprinted with permission from DO Mutti, K Zadnik. Refractive Error. In K Zadnik (ed), The Ocular Examination. Philadelphia: Saunders, 1997;56.

Table 4.3. A Summary of Previous Literature on the Keratometer Power (K) of the Infant Eye

Author	Number	Age	K (D)
York and Mandell [30]	8	0–3 mons	47.75
Mandell [5]	5	4–15 days	48.80
Blomdahl [39]	28	1–4 days	48.21
Inagaki [3]	11 (22 eyes)	14 days	47.00
Insler et al. [4]	19 (38 eyes)	39 wks (gestational age)	46.98

Source: Reprinted with permission from ICJ Wood, DO Mutti, K Zadnik. Crystalline lens parameters in infancy, © 1996;16:310–317, with kind permission from Elsevier Science Ltd, The Boulevard, Langford Lane, Kidlington, 0X5 1GB, UK.

Table 4.4. Summary of Previous Literature on the Axial Dimensions of the Infant Eye

Author	Number	Age	Anterior Chamber Depth (mm)	Lens Thickness (mm)	Axial Length (mm)
Gernet [27]	36 (70 eyes)	1–5 days	2.9	3.4	17.1
Luyckx [7]	52 (104 eyes)	4–7 days	2.6	3.7	17.6
Larsen [8, 28, 29]	80 (160 eyes)	1–5 days	2.4	4.0	16.6
Blomdahl [39]	28	1–4 days	2.6	3.6	16.6
Fledelius [9]	25	37–43 wks (gestational age)	2.6	3.8	17.3

Source: Reprinted with permission from ICJ Wood, DO Mutti, K Zadnik. Crystalline lens parameters in infancy, © 1996;16:310–317, with kind permission from Elsevier Science Ltd, The Boulevard, Langford Lane, Kidlington, 0X5 1GB, UK.

rapidly than the ability of the other components to compensate. An alternate possibility is that some mechanism that keeps the axial length coordinated with the focal length of the eye breaks down.

PREMATURITY AND REFRACTIVE ERROR

Several factors may interfere with normal refractive and ocular component development, such as low birth weight or pathology that deprives the eye of normal, high-contrast form vision (e.g., cataract). Lorenz et al. [37] studied the impact of unilateral and bilateral congenital cataract surgery followed by contact lens correction in the first year of life. Refraction was measured by retinoscopy; corneal radius was inferred from the base curve of contact lenses worn by the infants; and the axial length was measured by A-scan ultrasound. Eyes with a unilateral cataract were longer at the time of surgery, then appeared to grow at a normal rate compared with unaffected children. Corneal radius also flattened at

a rate similar to that for normal infants. Bilateral cataract patients tended to have initially shorter eyes than expected for their age, accompanied by a higher initial aphakic refractive error (approximately +35 D, compared with approximately +29 D for the unilateral cataract group). The bilateral cataract patients continued to display slow rates of growth, ending up with shorter eyes than expected at age 5–8 years. Their corneas did not appear to flatten during eye growth. The net impact on refractive error of these two trends was that both groups decreased in hyperopia by about 13 D during the first 3 years of life in a nearly linear manner. The bilateral group was always more hyperopic than the unilateral group. These rates are similar to those found by Moore [38] for infants with unilateral cataracts operated on in the first 6 months of life and corrected with contact lenses. Moore found that a polynomial provided a better fit to the rate of decrease than a line—refractive error = 31.897 − (0.753 · age in months) + (0.013 · [age in months]^2) − (0.00005556 · [age in months]^3).

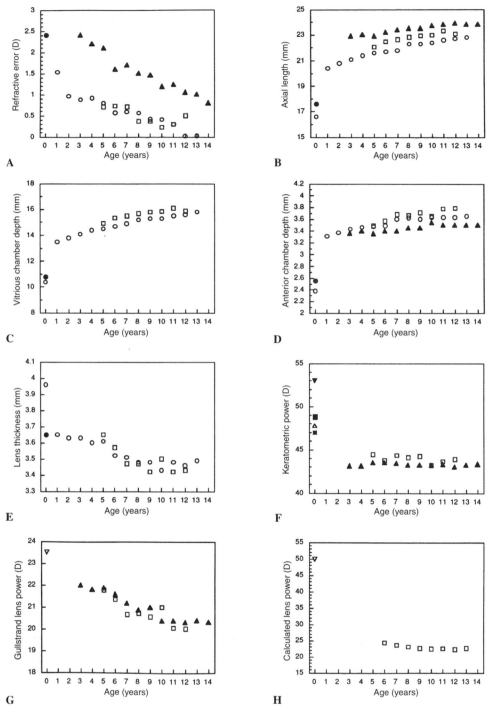

Figure 4.4. Growth curves for the various ocular components from birth through the age of 14 years. A. Refractive error: ● Luyckx [7]; ○ Larsen [28]; ▲ Sorsby et al. [71]; □ Zadnik et al. [69]. B. Axial length: same with ○ Larsen [8]. C. Vitreous chamber depth: same with ○ Larsen [51]. D. Anterior chamber depth: same as A. E. Lens thickness: same with ○ Larsen [29]. F. Keratometer power: same with ▼ Grignolo and Rivara [31]; △ York and Mandell [30]; ■ Mandell [5]; × Inagaki [3]; + Insler et al. [4]. G. Gullstrand lens power. H. Calculated lens power: same with ▽ Wood et al. [49]. (Reprinted with permission from DO Mutti, K Zadnik. Refractive Error. In K Zadnik [ed], The Ocular Examination. Philadelphia: Saunders, 1997;54.)

The finding that changes in both axial length and corneal radius of curvature occur slowly in infants who have undergone surgery for bilateral cataracts is consistent with the strong relationship that exists between these two components in infancy. The correlation between corneal radius and axial length in infants is 0.69, indicating that flatter radii are typically associated with longer eyes [39]. This correlation also continues into childhood and beyond but at a reduced level of correlation of 0.29–0.31 [40, 41]. The correlation between birth weight and axial length is also very significant at 0.66, consistent with the eyes of premature babies being smaller than those born at term [9, 31]. Tucker et al. [42] also found high correlations between birth weight and axial length ($r = 0.866$), as well as axial length and postconceptual age ($r = 0.906$). Strangely, the correlation between axial length and refractive error, which is so significant in childhood and adulthood ($r = -0.76$) [40], is either not seen in infancy ($r = -0.132$) [39], or is somewhat reduced ($r = -0.49$) [9]. This may be due to the higher degree of correlation between axial length and corneal radius described above.

Despite the shorter axial length of the premature infant eye, it is typically less hyperopic than that of an infant born at term. Dobson et al. [43] found that the average refraction of 146 premature infants was –0.55 D, which is much more myopic than expected for full-term newborns. In a study of 380 children between the ages of 6 months and 3.5 years who had birth weights of less than 2,000 g and no retinopathy of prematurity (ROP), Shapiro et al. [44] found that 5% displayed myopia. The correlation between cycloplegic (cyclopentolate) refractive error and birth weight was low ($r < 0.28$). Scharf et al. [45] found that 43% of babies weighing less than 2,500 g were myopic. Refractions fell into a bimodal distribution, with peaks centered on low hyperopia and moderate myopia. The use of a milder cycloplegic agent in this study, mydriaticum, may explain the greater prevalence of myopia. Again, no association was found between the prevalence of myopia and birth weight.

Grignolo and Rivara [31] studied both refractive error and ocular components in 58 full-term and 57 premature infants. Premature newborns had a mean refractive error of +0.50 D, and were about –1.00 D less hyperopic on average than full-term infants. The source of this relative myopia was the greater refractive power of the cornea and crystalline lens in the premature infants. The axial length of the eye in premature infants was actually 0.75 mm shorter (equivalent to about +4.5 D in an infant eye) than in full-term babies. In addition to less hyperopia and shorter axial lengths, Fledelius [9] found that premature infants had thicker crystalline lenses (3.99 versus 3.76 mm) and shallower ACDs (2.38 versus 2.65 mm) compared with full-term infants. These differences are greatly diminished during the first 6 months of life [31]. Fledelius [46] has found that some differences may persist into childhood, however. At age 10 years, children who were premature infants still had shorter axial lengths, thicker crystalline lenses, steeper corneas, and a greater prevalence of myopia (13.2% compared with 9.2%) than children who were born at term. Myopia is a more common and a more severe consequence of prematurity in the presence of retinopathy. Quinn et al. [47] found that myopia occurs in 18.1% of eyes of infants at 3 months whose birth weights were less than 1,251 g, with high myopia ($\leq$–5.00 D) occurring in 2%. At 24 months, the prevalence of myopia was virtually the same (19.9%), but high myopia was more common (4.6%). The severity of myopia was closely associated with that of the ROP and with birth weight.

CRYSTALLINE LENS DEVELOPMENT—PHAKOMETRIC RESULTS

The crystalline lens appears to be more important than the cornea for offsetting the potential for myopia posed by axial elongation. The lens undergoes a greater amount of dioptric change than the cornea by a factor of 4–5, and its development continues during the period when the majority of juvenile myopia has its onset. The cornea appears to have its adult radius of curvature by the age of 2. Despite the importance of the crystalline lens, relatively little is known about its development. Because phakometry has not been applied to the developing crystalline lens in vivo, knowledge of the infant lens comes from data taken nearly 90 years ago on a small series of frozen cadaver eyes [11]. The infant schematic eye of Lotmar is based on these limited data [48]. We measured the crystalline lens radii of curvature of 27 infants ranging in age from 3 months to 18 months using the video-phakometric technique [49].

Fifteen of the infants were boys, and 12 were girls. There were 25 white and two black infants.

Measurements were taken using cyclopentolate 1% cycloplegia (1 drop) following 1 drop of 0.5% proparacaine. The infants were refracted by spot retinoscopy 20 minutes after drop instillation, with each meridian neutralized separately for an estimate of refractive astigmatism. Corneal and lens curvatures were measured using a portable, hand-held video-based keratophakometer similar to the one described above. This unit consists of a series of infrared LEDs mounted on a clear, plastic faceplate. Two pairs of bright phakometric LEDs are mounted on the right side and at the top of the faceplate. The angle between the phakometric LEDs and the center of the disc was 40 degrees at the infant's eye, with 17-degree separation between each member of the pair. Dimmer infrared LEDs are arranged in three concentric circles to measure corneal radius of curvature in eight meridians. Results are reported for the horizontal meridian only.

The infrared LEDs in the instrument must have a margin of safety with respect to cataract formation. The infrared radiance of the keratometric and phakometric LEDs was determined using a Photodyne 44XL radiometer. The radiance of a single keratometric LED was 0.01 W/cm^{2}sr, and that of a single phakometric LED was 0.166 W/cm^{2}sr. The irradiance of the 880-nm infrared sources at the cornea was calculated at 0.34 mW/cm^2 for the 24 keratometric LEDs and 0.47 mW/cm^2 for the two phakometer LEDs. The maximum permissible exposure is less than 10 mW/cm^2 using the 1988 American Conference of Government Industrial Hygienists' standard for infrared radiation beyond 770 nm [50]. This is also below British Standard 7192 of less than 200 mW/cm^2 for exposures more than 10 seconds. The margin of safety was therefore at least a factor of 20 compared with published standards.

As previously mentioned, ultrasonography is difficult to perform on awake infants. At the time of this study, we had not yet used the technique of performing ultrasonography with the probe over the closed lid. In this analysis, we used age- and sex-appropriate values for ACD, lens thickness (LT), and VCD from Larsen [28, 29, 51] to obtain lens radii and refractive index from the phakometric data.

The median cycloplegic refractive error in the horizontal meridian was +1.50 D—in good agreement with expected values for infants in this age range [15, 32–35]. There is a significant trend toward reduction of this hyperopia with age (Figure 4.5A, $r = -0.47$, $p = .043$).

The median radius of corneal curvature in the horizontal meridian of the infants in this study was 7.76 mm (43.5 D), ranging from 7.35 to 8.46 mm (45.9–39.9 D). Interestingly, this was somewhat flatter than expected considering previously reported values (see Table 4.3), yet there was also no correlation between the corneal radius of curvature and age (Figure 4.5B, $r = 0.00$, $p = .99$).

The infant lens is 3.4–4.0 mm thick at birth (see Table 4.4). Examination of changes in lens wet weight indicates that the lens grows most rapidly during the first 2 years of life, doubling in wet weight during the first 8–10 years of life. Lens growth in later childhood through adulthood is much slower, with a further doubling in weight again during the course of adult life (Figure 4.6) [52]. Interestingly, despite this rapid increase in lens substance in infancy, the thickness of the lens is fairly stable throughout this time, remaining at an average of 3.6 mm at the age of 6 years. From 6 to 10 years of age, the lens actually thins by about 0.2 mm [29, 53]. After age 10, lens thickness is again constant on average in childhood and may begin to increase in the early teens. Although it is a textbook truism that the lens grows throughout life, it appears that it does not always increase in axial thickness. The lens may lay down new fibers throughout life, but forces discussed below must be at work to distribute these new fibers into a thinner profile.

In our study, the median anterior and posterior lens radii of curvature in the horizontal meridian were 8.7 and 5.6 mm, respectively, much flatter than the 5.0- and 3.7-mm values given by Lotmar for the infant schematic eye [48]. No age-related trends were observed for either anterior or posterior lens radius over the range of ages tested in this study at this sample size (see Figure 4.5C, $r = 0.25$, $p = .30$; see Figure 4.5D, $r = 0.00$, $p = .99$).

If the infant lens had the equivalent refractive index of 1.43 provided by Lotmar but had the surface curvatures found in this study, it would

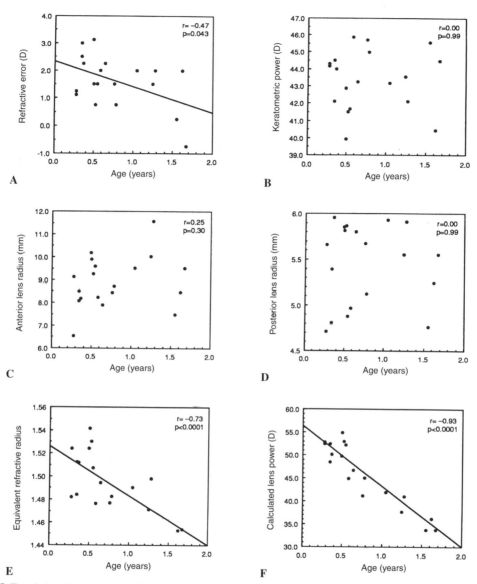

Figure 4.5. Trends in refractive error and the ocular components with age. A significant negative correlation was found for refractive error (A), but no correlations with age are apparent for central keratometric power (B), or anterior (C) or posterior (D) lens radius of curvature. Both equivalent refractive index of the crystalline lens (E) and lens power (F) show substantial age-related decreases. (Reprinted with permission from ICJ Wood, DO Mutti, K Zadnik. Crystalline lens parameters in infancy, © 1996;16:310–317, with kind permission from Elsevier Science Ltd, The Boulevard, Langford Lane, Kidlington, 0X5 1GB, UK.)

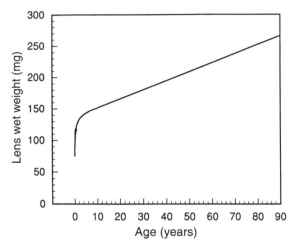

Figure 4.6. Growth in lens wet weight as a function of age. Note the rapid increase in the first 2 years of life with a more gradual increase in later childhood and adulthood. (Data from J Bours, HJ Födisch. Human fetal lens: wet and dry weight with increasing gestational age. Ophthalmic Res 1986;18:363–368.)

clearly have too little power and would result in more than the +1.50 D of hyperopia seen in these infants. To obtain the correct match of lens dimensions and measured refractive error, the equivalent index must be higher, namely 1.49. This index of refraction has a significant negative correlation with increasing age (see Figure 4.5E, $r = -0.73$, $p < .0001$). Lens power also decreases with age (see Figure 4.5F, $r = -0.93$, $p < .0001$). Since curvatures are changing substantially with age, the major contributor to this decrease in lens power must be the decrease in equivalent index. The lens power calculated from the median curvatures and equivalent index in Table 4.5 is 44.8 D in infancy and 25.0 D at age 6 years. If the equivalent refractive index remained at 1.49 throughout infancy, the decrease in lens power due to curvature changes alone would be 4.9 D, or only 25% of the 19.7 D of power loss over those years. The decrease in equivalent index from 1.49 to 1.431 accounts for the remaining 14.8 D, or 75% of the power change.

The flatness of crystalline lens curvatures indicates a degree of maturity in infant lens shape resembling that of a child. Gwiazda et al. [54] have shown that refractive error in later childhood may

be associated with the noncycloplegic retinoscopic result at the age of 1 year. Perhaps this maturity of lens shape in infancy may provide some basis for the similarity in refractive error between infancy and childhood.

POSSIBLE ROLE FOR THE CRYSTALLINE LENS IN EMMETROPIZATION AND MYOPIA

Since refractive error is in some sense a structural error—that is, the eye is either too long or too short for its focal length—understanding the development of the eye as a structural entity is useful. At best, it may provide some insight into the etiology of refractive error itself. In the previous section, we saw how the radii of the infant crystalline lens are much closer to those found in childhood than previously thought, how critical lens power is to compensation for axial growth, how equivalent index plays a major role in these power reductions, and how the crystalline lens maintains a nearly constant thickness in infancy despite rapid growth, then thins in childhood. Reductions in lens equivalent index most likely indicate changes in the equatorial gradient index profile, rather than a decrease in core or increase in superficial cortical indices. The responsiveness of the equatorial gradient profile may be an important characteristic of the process in which lens power keeps pace with axial elongation throughout childhood to maintain emmetropia and to avoid myopia.

If one tries to envision how the eye might grow to produce reductions in lens power through both flattening of lens radii of curvature and changes in the equatorial gradient index, as well as crystalline lens thinning, it could be pictured as overall growth in both the axial and equatorial directions of the eye. Equatorial ocular growth might result in crystalline lens stretching in the equatorial plane, which in turn flattens lens radii, changes the equatorial gradient index, and thins the lens. The matching of axial and focal lengths to produce emmetropia across species [55, 56] and evidence of increased frequency of myopia and higher refractive error variability when normal visual input is disrupted [57, 58] have prompted others to assume that eye growth and the process of emmetropiza-

Table 4.5. Median, Maximum, and Minimum Refractive, Keratometric, and Phakometric Values for 19 Infants

	Refractive Error (D)	Keratometer Power (D)	Anterior Lens Radius of Curvature (mm)	Posterior Lens Radius of Curvature (mm)	Number	Lens Power (D)
Median	+1.50	43.5	8.7	5.6	1.49	46.7
Maximum	+3.12	45.9	11.6	6.0	1.54	54.9
Minimum	−0.75	39.9	6.5	4.7	1.43	33.7
Lotmar [46]	+2.8	48.9	5.0	3.7	1.43	43.4
Average for age 6 yrs [69]	+0.73	43.75	10.7	6.0	1.431 [70]	25.0*

Note: All measures were made in the horizontal meridian.
*Calculated assuming lens radii of 10.7 and 6.0 mm, lens equivalent refractive index of 1.431, aqueous refractive index of 4/3, and lens thickness of 3.6 mm.
Source: Reprinted with permission from ICJ Wood, DO Mutti, K Zadnik. Crystalline lens parameters in infancy, © 1996;16:310–317, with kind permission from Elsevier Science Ltd, The Boulevard, Langford Lane, Kidlington, 0X5 1GB, UK.

tion are controlled by visually guided feedback loops [40, 59]. Compensation by the chick eye for the defocus imposed by spectacle lenses is consistent with refractive error arising from visually mediated processes [60, 61]. Although clear visual input free from deprivation is obviously required for normal refractive development, we propose that mechanical effects from the connection between globe axis, equator, and crystalline lens may create an additional simple, mechanical feedback loop. If rapid rates of ocular growth are accompanied by similarly rapid rates of lens flattening or changes in the distribution of the gradient of the refractive index of the crystalline lens due to lens stretch, the focal length of the eye may keep pace with the physical length of the eye. This type of physically and optically coordinated growth has been proposed by several previous investigators [40, 62–64].

This model may also have implications for the etiology of myopia. In contrast to the traditional view that eye growth only occurs in the axial dimension, the eye probably grows in three dimensions, displaying equatorial as well as axial expansion. In infancy, the growth of the lens is well matched to the growth of the eye, allowing for the proportional growth that maintains emmetropia at any eye size. In childhood years, this pattern is maintained in emmetropic patients, in whom reduc-

tion in crystalline lens power still occurs in concert with the eye's increasing axial length. In myopic patients, the lens may no longer be able to meet the challenge of the continued growth of the eye, perhaps because it has reached some physical limit, such as an inability to thin further. Figure 4.7 shows the thickness of the lens as a function of refractive error status and age. In all ages above 7, myopic patients have thinner lenses than emmetropic patients, and emmetropic patients have thinner lenses than hyperopic patients [53]. In myopia, the crystalline lens may not be able to make compensating power changes in the larger eye sizes of myopic eyes. It may have reached some intrinsic physical limit or be constrained by anatomic limits on equatorial expansion. As the eye at risk for myopia continues to grow and the axial length starts to exceed the focal length, the crystalline lens may be unable to further thin or to further decrease its power in order to increase the eye's focal length. The result is the excessive, uncompensated axial length characteristic of myopia.

It is hoped that improved biometric techniques will be used in the future to study infant refractive and ocular development in longitudinal studies. Such studies will document the course of eye growth that maintains emmetropia, thereby providing a contrast with the patterns of eye growth that produce myopia in children.

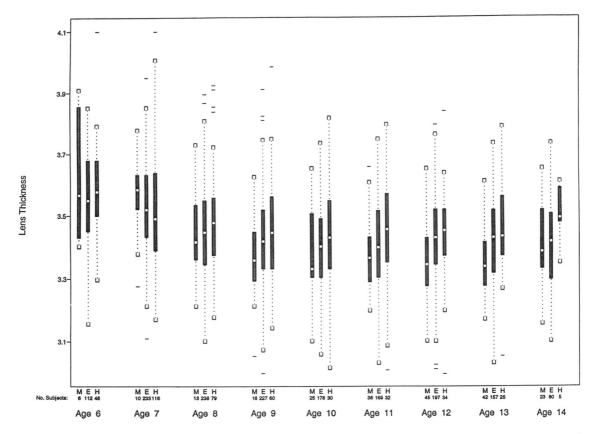

Figure 4.7. Age-specific sets of boxplots for lens thickness categorized by current refractive error status. For each group of subjects, the shaded bar represents the interquartile range (connecting the twenty-fifth and seventy-fifth percentiles), whereas the white box within the bar represents the median. The dotted lines reach out for 1.5 times the length of the interquartile range or to the most extreme observation, if closer. Any points beyond this range are represented by horizontal dashes. (M = myopia [at least –0.75 D]; E = emmetropia [between –0.75 D and +1.00 D]; H = hyperopia [at least +1.00 D]). (Reprinted from Zadnik K, Mutti DO, Fusaro RE, AJ Adams. Longitudinal evidence of crystalline lens thinning in children. Invest Ophthalmol Vis Sci 1995;36:1581–1587. Copyright Association for Research in Vision and Ophthalmology, published by Lippincott–Raven Publishers.)

REFERENCES

1. Blum HL, Peters HB, Bettman JW. Vision Screening for Elementary Schools: The Orinda Study. Berkeley: University of California, 1959.
2. Sperduto RD, Siegel D, Roberts J, et al. Prevalence of myopia in the United States. Arch Ophthalmol 1983; 101:405.
3. Inagaki Y. The rapid change of corneal curvature in the neonatal period and infancy. Arch Ophthalmol 1986;104:1026–1027.
4. Insler MS, Cooper HD, May SE, et al. Analysis of corneal thickness and corneal curvature in infants. CLAO J 1987;13:182–184.
5. Mandell RB. Corneal contour of the human infant. Arch Ophthalmol 1967;77:345–348.
6. Howland HC, Sayles N. Photokeratometric and photorefractive measurements of astigmatism in infants and young children. Vision Res 1985;25:73–81.
7. Luyckx J. Mesure des composantes optiques de l'oeil du nouveau-né par échographie ultrasonique. Arch Ophtalmol (Paris) 1966;26:159–170.
8. Larsen JS. The sagittal growth of the eye. IV. Ultrasonic measurement of the axial length of the eye from birth to puberty. Acta Ophthalmol 1971;49:873–886.
9. Fledelius HC. Pre-term delivery and the growth of the eye. An oculometric study of eye size around term-time. Acta Ophthalmol Suppl 1992;204:10–15.
10. Twelker JD, Kirschbaum S, Zadnik K, et al. Compari-

son of corneal vs. through-the-lid A-scan ultrasound biometry. Optom Vis Sci (in press).

11. von Pflugk A. Die Fixierung der Wirbeltierlinsen, insbesondere der Linse des neugeborenen Menschen. Klin Monatsbl Augenheilkd 1909;47:1–14.

12. Tscherning M. Physiologic Optics (4th ed). Philadelphia: Keystone, 1924;84–85.

13. Mutti DO, Zadnik K, Adams AJ. A video technique for phakometry of the human crystalline lens. Invest Ophthalmol Vis Sci 1992;33:1771–1782.

14. Santonastaso A. La rifrazione oculare nei primi anni di vita. Ann Ottalmol Clin Oculist 1930;58:852–884.

15. Mohindra I, Held R. Refraction in humans from birth to five years. Doc Ophthalmol Proc Series 1981; 28:19–27.

16. Cook RC, Glasscock RE. Refractive and ocular findings in the newborn. Am J Ophthalmol 1951;34: 1407–1413.

17. Atkinson J. Infant Vision Screening: Prediction and Prevention of Strabismus and Amblyopia from Refractive Screening in the Cambridge Photorefraction Program. In K Simons (ed), Early Visual Development: Normal and Abnormal. New York: Oxford University, 1993;342.

18. Saunders KJ, Woodhouse M, Westall CA. Emmetropisation in human infancy: rate of change is related to initial refractive error. Vision Res 1995;35:1325–1328.

19. Ehrlich DL, Atkinson J, Braddick O, et al. Reduction of infant myopia: a longitudinal cycloplegic study. Vision Res 1995;35:1313–1324.

20. Norton TT, Siegwart JT. Animal models of emmetropization: matching axial length to the focal plane. J Am Optom Assoc 1995;66:405–414.

21. Dobson V, Fulton A, Sebris S. Cycloplegic refractions of infants and young children: the axis of astigmatism. Invest Ophthalmol Vis Sci 1984;25:83–87.

22. Howland HC, Sayles N. Photorefractive measurements of astigmatism in infants and young children. Invest Ophthalmol Vis Sci 1984;25:93–102.

23. London R, Wick BC. Changes in angle lambda during growth: theory and clinical applications. Am J Optom Physiol Opt 1982;59:568–572.

24. Banks MS. Infant refraction and accommodation. Int Ophthalmol Clin 1980;20:205–232.

25. Atkinson J, Braddick O, French J. Infant astigmatism: its disappearance with age. Vision Res 1980;20: 891–893.

26. Mohindra I, Held R, Gwiazda J, et al. Astigmatism in infants. Science 1978;202:329–330.

27. Gernet H. Achsenlänge und refraktion lebender augen von neugeborenen. Graefes Arch Ophthalmol 1964; 166:530–536.

28. Larsen JS. The sagittal growth of the eye. I. Ultrasound measurement of the depth of the anterior chamber from birth to puberty. Acta Ophthalmol 1971;49:239–262.

29. Larsen JS. The sagittal growth of the eye. II. Ultrasonic measurement of the axial diameter of the lens and the anterior segment from birth to puberty. Acta Ophthalmol 1971;49:427–440.

30. York MA, Mandell RB. A new calibration system for photokeratoscopy. Part II—corneal curvature measurements. Am J Optom Arch Am Acad Optom 1969; 46:818–825.

31. Grignolo A, Rivara A. Observations biométriques sur l'œil des enfants nés à terme et des prématurés au cours de la première année. Ann Oculist 1968;201:817–826.

32. Ingram RM, Barr A. Changes in refraction between the ages of 1 and 3 1/2 years. Br J Ophthalmol 1979; 63:339–342.

33. Fulton AB, Dobson V, Salem D, et al. Cycloplegic refractions in infants and young children. Am J Ophthalmol 1980;90:239–247.

34. Howland HC, Sayles N. A photorefractive characterization of focusing ability of infants and young children. Invest Ophthalmol Vis Sci 1987;28:1005–1015.

35. Wood ICJ, Hodi S. Longitudinal changes in refractive error in infants during the first year of life. Eye 1995;9:551–557.

36. Friedman NE, Mutti DO, Zadnik K. Corneal changes in schoolchildren. Optom Vis Sci 1996;73:552–557.

37. Lorenz B, Wörle J, Friedl N, et al. Ocular growth in infant aphakia. Bilateral versus unilateral congenital cataracts. Ophthalmol Paedtr Gen 1993;14: 177–188.

38. Moore BD. Changes in the aphakic refraction of children with unilateral congenital cataracts. J Pediatr Ophthalmol Strabismus 1989;26:290–295.

39. Blomdahl S. Ultrasonic measurements of the eye of the newborn infant. Acta Ophthalmol 1979;57:1048–1056.

40. van Alphen GWHM. On emmetropia and ametropia. Ophthalmol Suppl 1961;142:1–92.

41. Sorsby A, Benjamin B, Davey JB, et al. Emmetropia and Its Aberrations. London: Her Majesty's Stationery Office, 1957. Medical Research Council, Special Report Series.

42. Tucker SM, Enzenauer RW, Levin AV, et al. Corneal diameter, axial length, and intraocular pressure in premature infants. Ophthalmology 1992;99:1296–1300.

43. Dobson V, Fulton AB, Manning K, et al. Cycloplegic refractions of premature infants. Am J Ophthalmol 1981;91:490–495.

44. Shapiro A, Yanko L, Nawratzki I, et al. Refractive power of premature children at infancy and early childhood. Am J Ophthalmol 1980;90:234–238.

45. Scharf J, Zonis S, Zeltzer M. Refraction in Israeli premature babies. J Pediatr Ophthalmol 1975;12:193–196.

46. Fledelius H. Prematurity and the eye. Acta Ophthalmol Suppl 1976;128:1–245.

47. Quinn GE, Dobson V, Repka MX, et al. Development of myopia in infants with birth weights less than 1251 grams. Ophthalmology 1992;99:329–340.

48. Lotmar W. A theoretical model for the eye of new-born infants. Graefes Arch Klin Exp Ophthalmol 1976;198: 179–185.

49. Wood ICJ, Mutti DO, Zadnik K. Crystalline lens parameters in infancy. Ophthal Physiol Opt 1996;16: 310–317.

50. Committee on Threshold Limit Values. ACGIH Transactions 1985. Cincinnati: American Conference of Government Industrial Hygienists, 1986;13:84.

51. Larsen JS. The sagittal growth of the eye. III. Ultrasonic measurement of the posterior segment (axial length of the vitreous) from birth to puberty. Acta Ophthalmol 1971;49:441–453.

52. Bours J, Födisch HJ. Human fetal lens: wet and dry weight with increasing gestational age. Ophthalmic Res 1986;18:363–368.

53. Zadnik K, Mutti DO, Fusaro RE, AJ Adams. Longitudinal evidence of crystalline lens thinning in children. Invest Ophthalmol Vis Sci 1995;36:1581–1587.

54. Gwiazda J, Thorn F, Bauer J, et al. Emmetropization and the progression of manifest refraction in children followed from infancy to puberty. Clin Vis Sci 1993; 8:337–344.

55. Norton TT, McBrien NA. Normal development of refractive state and ocular component dimensions in the tree shrew *(Tupaia belangeri)*. Vision Res 1992; 32:833–842.

56. Wallman J, Adams JI, Trachtman JN. The eyes of young chickens grow toward emmetropia. Invest Ophthalmol Vis Sci 1981;20:557–561.

57. Rabin J, Van Sluyters RC, Malach R. Emmetropization: a vision-dependent phenomenon? Invest Ophthalmol Vis Sci 1981;20:561–564.

58. Nathan J, Kiely PM, Crewther SG, et al. Disease-associated visual image degradation and spherical refractive errors in children. Am J Optom Physiol Opt 1985; 62:680–688.

59. Schaeffel F, Howland HC. Mathematical model of emmetropization in the chicken. J Opt Soc Am A 1988; 5:2080–2086.

60. Schaeffel F, Glasser A, Howland HC. Accommodation, refractive error, and eye growth in chickens. Vision Res 1988;28:639–657.

61. Wildsoet C, Wallman J. Choroidal and scleral mechanisms of compensation for spectacle lenses in chicks. Vision Res 1995;35:1175–1194.

62. Gernet H, Olbrich E. Excess of the Human Refractive Curve and Its Cause. In KA Gitter, AH Keeney, LK Sarin, D Meyer (eds), Ophthalmic Ultrasound. An International Symposium. St. Louis: Mosby; 1969; 142–148.

63. Mark HH. Emmetropization. Physical aspects of a statistical phenomenon. Ann Ophthalmol 1972;4: 393–401.

64. Sorsby A. The Functional Anomalies of the Eye. Section I. In A Sorsby (ed), Refraction and Accommodation. Modern Ophthalmology (2nd ed). Philadelphia: Lippincott, 1972;9–29.

65. Goldschmidt E. Refraction in the newborn. Acta Ophthalmol 1969;47:570–578.

66. Zonis S, Miller B. Refractions in the Israeli newborn. J Pediatr Ophthalmol 1974;11:77–81.

67. Howland HC, Braddick O, Atkinson J, et al. Infant astigmatism measured by photorefraction. Science 1978;202:331–333.

68. Gwiazda J, Scheiman M, Mohindra I, et al. Astigmatism in children: changes in axis and amount from birth to six years. Invest Ophthalmol Vis Sci 1984;25: 88–92.

69. Zadnik K, Mutti DO, Friedman NE, et al. Initial cross-sectional results from the Orinda Longitudinal Study of Myopia. Optom Vis Sci 1993;70:750–758.

70. Mutti DO, Zadnik K, Fusaro RE, et al. Longitudinal changes in the equivalent refractive index of the crystalline lens in childhood. Invest Ophthalmol Vis Sci 1995;36:S939.

71. Sorsby A, Benjamin B, Sheridan M. Refraction and Its Components During the Growth of the Eye from the Age of Three. London: Her Majesty's Stationery Office, 1961. Medical Research Council, Special Report Series No. 301.

Chapter 5
Refractive Error in Young Children

Elise B. Ciner

The ability to appropriately detect, evaluate, and manage refractive error in young children is rapidly becoming an essential skill for primary care optometrists. This trend toward earlier optometric intervention has been sparked by significant research in infant visual development. This research has changed our views of both how and when the visual system develops. We now know, for example, that there is a period of rapid growth and significant changes in vision during the first few years of life. It has been shown that infants are normally born with very poor visual resolution capabilities, yet approach adult levels of visual acuity by approximately 1 year of age [1–3]. Research on infant vision has also resulted in the development of both objective and behavioral methods of evaluating young children in the laboratories. These methods have subsequently been introduced into clinical practice [4–6]. Using new and different tools, clinicians are now able to perform a complete clinical evaluation of the visual system in preverbal children. Each of these advances toward a more complete understanding of infant visual development provides compelling support for the early clinical assessment of the visual system by as early as 6 months of age [7, 8].

The profession of optometry is at the forefront of this trend toward early vision assessment and intervention by recognizing the need for assessment of infants and young children [8–10]. The evaluation and management of refractive error is a basic and integral component of optometric practice, including the visual evaluation of infants and preschool children.

IMPORTANCE OF EARLY DETECTION AND MANAGEMENT OF REFRACTIVE ERROR

Although it is widely accepted that a thorough assessment of refractive error should be completed in adult vision examinations, it is of even greater importance to detect, monitor, evaluate, and manage refractive error in young children. The following list highlights the importance of performing a careful and accurate refractive examination on young children. Table 5.1 summarizes the more common signs and symptoms of uncorrected refractive error in young children.

1. Refractive error development undergoes a more complex and dynamic process of changes during the first 5 years of life than at any other period of human development [11–15]. It is imperative for clinicians to be familiar with these changes and understand when refractive correction should be provided and when an error is a normal part of development and needs only monitoring.

2. The impact of refractive error on other aspects of visual development, specifically visual acuity and binocularity, is also significant. Providing appropriate corrective lenses in young children can significantly reduce the prevalence of amblyopia. This in turn reduces accompanying vision rehabilitation and health care costs.

3. A child who is not seeing comfortably or clearly will be less likely to develop normal fine and gross motor, language, and social skills during the

Table 5.1. Signs and Symptoms of Uncorrected Refractive Error in Young Children

Experiences difficulties with depth perception
Experiences eye-hand and coordination difficulties
Confuses likeness and minor differences (i.e., the child sees
    things as identical when there are minor differences)
Frequently rubs eyes
Blinks excessively
Complains of double vision
Cannot maintain fixation on a task
Frequently closes or covers one eye
Displays lack of interest in outdoor activities
Positions self close to television or books
Squints
Displays lack of interest in near tasks
In some cases, displays no signs or symptoms

Source: Reprinted from EB Ciner. Refractive error in young children: evaluation and prescription. Pract Optom 1992;3:4.

first years of life. Prescriptive lenses that help a child attain visual comfort for near tasks can be the difference between success and failure in a preschool setting.

4. It is important to consider that young children are often unaware of what it means to have 20/20 vision. A child with uncorrected 20/80 visual acuity often does not know that this level of vision is not typical for his or her age. Even if a child senses that something is not right with his or her vision, he or she may be unable to verbally express that something is wrong.

TECHNIQUES FOR DETECTING AND MEASURING REFRACTIVE ERROR

There are several clinical techniques for detecting or measuring refractive error in young children. Some are primarily used to screen for the presence of refractive error, whereas others can be used to measure refractive error and prescribe appropriate correction. There are techniques that are considered secondary measures of refractive error and are useful in confirming the presence of a refractive error. Each requires varying levels of technical knowledge, clinical understanding, and cost. These techniques are each designed to be performed in just a few minutes. Because young children cannot communicate as well as adults, it is important for the

optometrist to carefully assess refractive error by using one or more of these measures to make as accurate an assessment as possible.

Near Retinoscopy

Near retinoscopy, a technique developed by Mohindra, is useful in evaluating children from birth to 3 years of age and also in older children as necessary [16]. The advantage of the Mohindra technique is that the retinoscopy is performed in a very dark room with no extraneous sources of light other than the retinoscope. The child's attention is therefore directed toward the plane of the retinoscope beam, which should be set at a minimum light level. A blackened lens rack or loose lenses are used to measure the refractive error (Figure 5.1). A working distance of 50 cm is maintained throughout the test. Sound effects, singing, or songs from a tape recorder placed near the examiner are very useful in maintaining the child's attention on the retinoscope. Mohindra originally recommended calculating the net refractive error by subtracting a correction factor of 1.25 D from the gross finding, thus compensating for both the working distance and residual accommodation. There is no change in the cylinder power or axis. Saunders and Westall have proposed a correction factor of 0.75 D for children younger than 2 years old [17].

Distance Retinoscopy

Distance retinoscopy as normally performed in adults is useful in children who are approximately 3 years of age and older. Children younger than 3 years old are often unable to maintain attention on a distance task for any prolonged period of time. Therefore, accommodation is difficult to control. To determine if distance retinoscopy may be helpful, ask the parent if the child watches television. Children who easily focus on a television set across the room are also easy to perform distance retinoscopy on. Appropriate distance fixation targets are the key to maintaining attention. The ideal fixation targets are television programs that the child enjoys, such as cartoons, "Sesame Street," or sing-along programs. A television and videocassette player allow the optometrist to individualize the target to the child's interests and

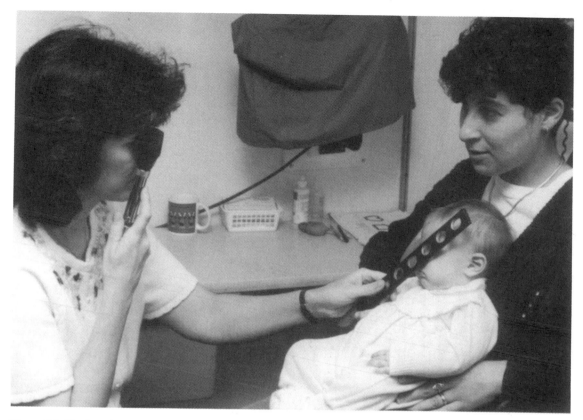

Figure 5.1. Blackened lens rack used for near point retinoscopy on an infant. (Reprinted with permission from EB Ciner. Refractive error in young children: Evaluation and prescription. Pract Optom 1992;3:4. Photo by Ron Davidoff.)

provide a visual and auditory stimulus that is constantly changing to keep the child's attention. Less expensive alternatives include a slide projector with cartoons or eye-catching pictures; blinking lights across the room; a commercially available "barking dog" or talking Big Bird toy; or any toy with sound, lights, or music that can be controlled by the optometrist from across the room [18].

Accommodation should be further controlled by performing the refraction using a lens rack instead of using a phoropter. Children often lose attention and fixation behind the phoropter. The examiner is able to maintain good eye contact with the child during a lens rack refraction. Refracting glasses that fog the child's vision and control accommodation should be used whenever possible. This is especially important when latent hyperopia, strabismus, or pseudomyopia is present. A hand-held mirror should be used to show children how they look in glasses and encourages them to keep the

glasses on during the examination. These glasses should be in attractive frames with flexible hinges. The examiner's working distance should correspond to the lens correction (e.g., +1.50 D lenses). This simplifies the interpretation of the results because the child's refractive error is simply whatever the examiner scopes in each meridian (Figure 5.2). The modifications made in distance retinoscopy when evaluating young children are summarized in Table 5.2.

Cycloplegic Retinoscopy

It is usually not necessary to perform cycloplegic retinoscopy on most children if good results are obtained with either near or distance retinoscopy. Cycloplegic retinoscopy can be helpful in confirming a refractive error, diagnosing an accompanying condition, and deciding on a final prescription. It should

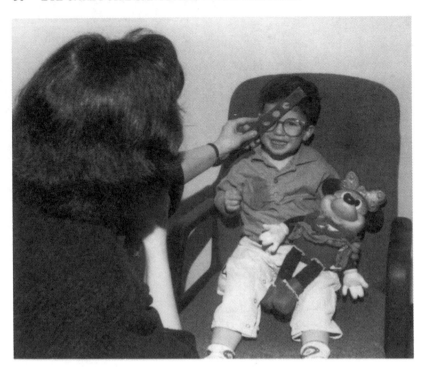

Figure 5.2. Fogging lenses used during distance refraction in a toddler. (Photo by Ron Davidoff.)

be used when there is a fluctuating reflex and an endpoint is difficult to obtain, the child cannot maintain attention at distance or near long enough to scope both meridians, a significant esodeviation or amblyopia is present, latent hyperopia is suspected, or large amounts of astigmatism or anisometropia are present on near or distance retinoscopy.

Cycloplegic agents include homatropine, atropine, cyclopentolate, and tropicamide. Homatropine is an unpredictable cycloplegic agent and is therefore falling into disfavor. Atropine is useful in certain circumstances and provides the best overall cycloplegic refraction. It has a prolonged action time (several days to weeks), however, and a significant number of side effects in young children. It also must be prescribed for several days before examination due to its delayed onset of action, making its use impractical on a routine basis. Cyclopentolate is generally the drug of choice because of its rapid action and minimal side effects [19, 20]. The use of 2% cyclopentolate, however, is strongly discouraged because of its side effects [21]. Cyclopentolate 1% is usually recommended for routine cycloplegic refractions. Table 5.3 lists commonly used cycloplegic agents, and Table 5.4 outlines a recommended regimen for cycloplegic refractions in young children. Cycloplegic refraction should be completed approximately 30–40 minutes after installation of the cycloplegic agent. Mydriasis is not necessarily a good indicator of when full cycloplegia has taken place; therefore, it is best to check for cycloplegia by looking at the reflex with a retinoscope. Variability or a change in appearance or brightness of the reflex should be watched for. If variability is present, there are three options: (1) Use another drop of cyclopentolate, (2) wait a few more minutes, or (3) consider use of atropine at home. No more than three drops of cyclopentolate should be used in each eye due to the risk of toxic central nervous system reactions. It is also wise to use refracting glasses when the cycloplegic retinoscopy is performed. This further helps to ensure that the child is relaxing his or her accommodation and that residual efforts at accommodation will be controlled. It will also make calculation of the net refractive error quicker and easier.

The use of a cycloplegic spray can be particularly helpful in young, uncooperative children [21], particularly those with light irides (Figure 5.3). It consists of (1) 3.75 ml of 2% cyclopentolate, (2) 7.5

Table 5.2. Modifications for Retinoscopy for Young Children

Modification	Purpose
Trial lens/lens rack refraction	This method allows continual observation of behavioral responses. A phoropter should never be used in young children.
Occlusion of one eye	Occluding one eye is sometimes helpful and necessary when a constant or intermittent strabismus is present. The nonoccluded eye maintains fixation and retinoscopy is performed on-axis with less chance of error.
Placement of prism in front of eye not being scoped	This technique is useful when a strabismus is present. This allows on-axis fixation of the eye that is being scoped.
Use of refracting glasses	Colorful, comfortable frames with the examiner's "working distance" (i.e., +1.50 D or +2.00 D) controls accommodation. With refracting glasses, it is not necessary to subtract the examiner's working distance when determining the refractive error.
Use of age-appropriate distance targets	These targets can help maintain the child's attention at distance and controls accommodation using video tapes, talking toys, or a parent's voice.
Use of trial frame to check retinoscopy	It may be useful to trial frame the retinoscopy and recheck the retinoscopy and visual acuities with corrective lenses in place when prescribing. This requires extra time and good cooperation from the child.

Table 5.3. Use of Cycloplegic Agents in Young Children

Cycloplegic Agent	Side Effects	Dosage	Comments
Cyclopentolate	Drowsiness, incoherent speech, ataxia, disorientation, restlessness, and visual hallucinations	0.5% gtts* (infants) 1% gtts* (children >1 yr)	Cycloplegic agent of choice Onset of action = 15–30 mins Duration of action = 8 hrs
Tropicamide	Minimal	Same as cyclopentolate dosage*	Minimally effective cycloplegic agent Onset of action = 15–30 mins Duration of action = 4–6 hrs Consider use in cases of hypersensitivity to cholinergic agents (e.g., in Down syndrome patients).
Atropine	Same as those of cyclopentolate	0.5% ointment in lightly pigmented irises; 1% ointment in darkly pigmented irises at bedtime every night for 3 nights before examination	Most effective cycloplegic agent Onset of action = 3–6 hrs Duration of action = 1–2 wks
Cyclomydril	Same as those of cyclopentolate	1 gtt; repeat if necessary	Combination drug consisting of 0.2% cyclopentolate and 1% phenylephrine; not as effective with dark irides

gtt = drop.
*Drops can be preceded by application of a local anesthetic to promote action.

Table 5.4. Guidelines for Selection of Age-Appropriate Cycloplegic Agents

Age	Recommended Agent
Premature or low-birth-weight neonate	1 gtt Cyclomydril[a, b]
Neonates–3 mons	1 gtt Cyclomydril or 0.5% cyclopentolate[a] (repeat in 5–10 mins if necessary)
4 mons–1 yr	1 gtt Cyclomydril or 0.5% cyclopentolate[a] (repeat in 5–10 mins if necessary)
1–5 yrs	1 gtt 1% cyclopentolate or 1 gtt 1% tropicamide[a] (Mydriacyl) (repeat in 5 mins)

gtt = drop.
[a]Drops can be preceded by application of a local anesthetic to promote action.
[b]Cyclomydril = 0.2% cyclopentolate and 1% phenylephrine in combination.
Source: Adapted from E Ciner, ML Parisi, H Herzberg. Pediatric Optometry. In K Alexander (ed), The Lippincott Manual of Primary Eye Care. Philadelphia: Lippincott, 1995;438.

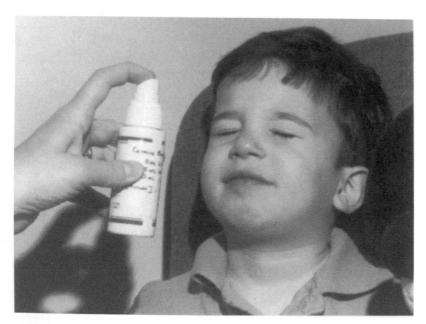

Figure 5.3. Application of a cycloplegic spray in a young child. (Photo by Ron Davidoff.)

ml of 1% tropicamide, and (3) 3.75 ml of 10% phenylephrine. When combined in an atomizer, the actual spray applied to the child's closed eyelids consists of 0.5% cyclopentolate, 0.5% tropicamide, and 2.5% phenylephrine [22].

Photorefraction

Photorefraction is the newest retinoscopy technique. It is particularly good for use in young children because it is noninvasive, nonthreatening, requires very little time or expertise to administer, produces a permanent record of the child's refractive status, and can detect as little as 0.50 D of ametropia. Photorefraction uses a camera, special lens, and strobe to simultaneously evaluate the refractive status of both eyes [23–25]. When a picture is taken, the strobe light enters the child's eye, is refracted by the media, strikes the retina, becomes focused or forms a blur circle on the retina, reflects off the retina, and is refracted by the media as it leaves the eye [26]. This light is then captured on the film. While the pupil of an emmetropic eye appears as a homogeneous red reflex on the developed film, any ametropia appears as a whitish crescent. The larger the crescent, the higher the magnitude of ametropia. When the ametropia is greater than approximately 6.00 D, the pupil is entirely filled by the white crescent. The crescents of myopia, hyperopia, and astigmatism are distinguished by their positioning in the pupil relative to strobe placement on the camera. Photorefraction is also useful in detecting other visual abnormalities including strabismus, anisocoria, and media opacities [27, 28].

Photorefraction is potentially valuable for use in large screenings and in pediatrician's offices; however, there are still several drawbacks to its use in routine diagnosis and prescribing. For example, it may take days to develop the film. Other computerized techniques [23] that provide instant results are still too costly to be practical for use in routine clinical care. Although photorefraction can detect refractive errors of more than 6.00 D, some techniques are unable to obtain an actual measurement necessary for prescribing corrective lenses for these high-magnitude refractive errors. The sensitivity and specificity of photorefraction as a screening device precludes its use in isolation in detecting refractive error and other vision anomalies in a screening setting [29, 30]. The development of Polaroid camera photorefraction units such as the Medical Technology and Innovations (MTI) photorefractor, which produces photographs of the blur circles within minutes, offers the most promise for the expanded use of this technique in the future [31, 32] (see Chapter 7 for more information on photorefraction).

Keratometry

Keratometry can be performed on cooperative children who are approximately 3 years of age or older. Maintaining fixation is the key to achieving good results. Keratometry should be considered a secondary test for refractive error and should be attempted if retinoscopy shows a significant degree of astigmatism that the optometrist wants to confirm. The test can be administered as a game in which the child is asked to look at his or her eye through the tube [33].

Autorefraction

Autorefraction has been advocated for use in measuring refractive error in children. Although some

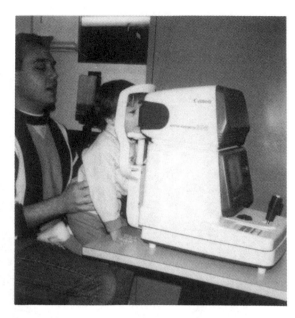

Figure 5.4. Autorefraction of a young child. (Photo by Ron Davidoff.)

studies have shown autorefraction is more useful in children ages 3–5 than cycloplegic refractions [34, 35], there is little research to support its efficacy in children younger than 3 years old. Adequate positioning and steady fixation for several seconds are necessary to obtain an accurate reading, making this technique very difficult to perform on young children. Autorefractors manufacturers have begun to address these problems by making instruments more portable (e.g., the Nikon hand-held autorefractor, Retinomax) and using colorful fixation targets (Canon autorefractors). Autorefraction can be useful for confirming retinoscopy findings when prescribing for high refractive error in children 3 years of age and older [35, 36]. As a screening tool, autorefraction has questionable reliability in young children, particularly those younger than 3 years of age. Therefore, most practitioners still rely primarily on other methods of refraction in these very young children (Figure 5.4).

Keratoscopy

The keratoscope is useful for confirming the presence of large amounts of astigmatism in young chil-

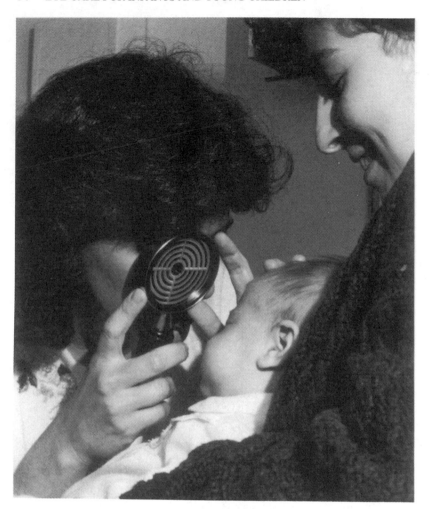

Figure 5.5. Use of a keratoscope for detection of astigmatism in an infant. (Reprinted with permission from EB Ciner. Refractive error in young children: evaluation and prescription. Pract Optom 1992;3:4. Photo by Ron Davidoff.)

dren [20]. It is portable, easy to use, and noninvasive. The examiner simply holds the instrument close to the child's eye so that the internally illuminated Placido's disk is reflected off the child's cornea. When a significant degree of corneal astigmatism is present (>1.50 D) the pattern of the Placido's disk becomes elongated along the cylinder axis. This instrument is a useful adjunct to other methods of retinoscopy, since large amounts of astigmatism are common in young children (Figure 5.5).

Summary

Depending on the associated ocular findings and symptoms, the method of choice for evaluating refractive error in children younger than age 2 is ei-

ther near retinoscopy or a cycloplegic refraction. In 2- to 5-year-old children, either distance retinoscopy or a cycloplegic refraction can be performed. The other methods, including keratometry, autorefraction, keratoscopy, and photorefraction, should be considered screening or secondary methods to confirm the presence or absence of significant refractive error. Table 5.5 provides guidelines for difficult refractions in young children. The advantages and disadvantages of each method are outlined in Table 5.6.

NATURAL HISTORY AND EPIDEMIOLOGY

Refractive error occurs in approximately 15–30% of young children [37–51]. The amount of error

Table 5.5. Guidelines for Difficult Refractions

Observation	Solution
Reflex is difficult to interpret (e.g., scissors motion is present).	Try to focus on the central portion of the reflex as the peripheral portion can be confusing and distorted due to spherical aberration and coma.
	WR motion is easier to interpret than AR motion. Add minus lenses until WR motion is easily seen, reduce until definite AR motion is seen, and then bracket inwards until neutrality can be determined.
	Move toward or away from the child to verify changes in reflex.
No reflex is seen with retinoscopy.	Check for media opacity with the ophthalmoscope. If red reflex is present, note amount of plus or minus in ophthalmoscope to clear retina.
	Scope with high amounts of plus and minus in 5 D increments (to 20 D if necessary) until red reflex is seen.
Adequate fixation of child is difficult to achieve.	Ask parent to sit across room and attempt to keep child's interest.
	Attempt cycloplegic refraction.
Reflex appears to change.	Accommodative fluctuations or off-axis scoping may be occurring.
	Cycloplegic refraction may be indicated.

AR = against-the-rule; WR = with-the-rule.

Table 5.6. Methods of Refraction

Method	Primary Use	Equipment Needed	Advantages	Disadvantages
Near retinoscopy	Testing	Retinoscope	Useful in very young children; fixation more accurate	May not give same results as cycloplegic refraction
Distance retinoscopy	Testing	Retinoscope and distance fixation target	Similar to refractions performed with adults	May be difficult to perform in children younger than age 2
Cycloplegic refraction	Testing	Retinoscope and cycloplegic agent	Increases accuracy of refraction; controls accommodation	Requires use of drops, which can be stressful for the child; increases examination time
Keratometry	Confirmation of cylinder	Keratometer	Allows for assessment of cornea and confirmation of astigmatism	May be difficult to perform in children younger than age 3
Autorefraction	Confirmation of refractive error; screening	Autorefractor	Can be performed by a technician	May be difficult in children younger than age 3; results may not be reliable
Photorefraction	Screening	Photorefractor	May be used to confirm refractive error	Results may not be reliable; may only provide estimate of refractive error
Keratoscopy	Confirmation of cylinder	Keratoscope	May be used to confirm astigmatism	Useful only for higher magnitudes of astigmatism

often fluctuates considerably during the first 5 years of life. Although the evaluation of refractive error in young children is relatively easy, optometrists must also be familiar with the appropriate management of refractive errors and know what types of error are considered normal, how refractive error changes with time, and when refractive error interferes with normal visual development.

Changes in Refractive Error

Infants

Most full-term infants are born with a mild to moderate degree of hyperopia. The amount of refractive error varies widely and averages 2.00 D of hyperopia [52, 53]. The prevalence of myopia detected with cycloplegic refractions is approximately 25% [52, 53]. There is also a high prevalence of both astigmatism (approximately 50%) [11, 12, 45, 54–58] and anisometropia (11–22%) [42, 45, 46] in young infants. In white infants, much of this astigmatism is the against-the-rule (AR) type. As the child approaches his or her first birthday, the distribution of refractive error narrows and there is less variability in the population [13, 38, 40, 42]. The average refractive error remains mild to moderately hyperopic. Astigmatism also changes during this time with generally lower magnitudes and a lower overall prevalence of astigmatism [12, 42, 54, 55, 59–62]. AR astigmatism shows the most volatility, whereas oblique astigmatisms show the most stability with regard to changes in magnitude [59, 61, 63].

Toddlers and Preschool Children

Significant changes in refractive error continue to occur from 1–5 years of age, including a continual process toward emmetropization [11, 64]. By 5 years of age, the distribution of refractive error is a peaked or leptokurtic distribution that is skewed toward mild hyperopia [53, 65, 66]. The prevalence of significant astigmatism also drops dramatically to approximately 10% by 5 years of age [60, 67], a level equal to that of adult populations. There is a further shift away from AR astigmatism and toward with-the-rule (WR) astigmatism [55, 68].

Knowing the magnitude and type of refractive error present during the early years helps the clinician to predict how a child's refractive error might change during the school years. Children who have transient myopia during the first few years of life and then go through emmetropization are more likely to have their myopia reappear during the school years [69]. The child's refraction when beginning school is also a predictor of what can be expected later on. Children with greater than 1.50 D of hyperopia at 5 years of age tend to remain hyperopic. Children with 0.50–1.25 D of hyperopia

tend to become emmetropic. Children with 0.50 D of hyperopia or less or those with myopia tend to become more myopic during the school years [70]. Changes in the degree of anisometropia are also significant during these years. The high prevalence of anisometropia present at birth decreases rapidly so that the prevalence is relatively low by the time a child enters school [71–73].

Astigmatism

Mohindra and colleagues used near retinoscopy to study astigmatism in infants and young children. They found that large amounts of astigmatism are common in children younger than 3 years of age. The magnitude of this astigmatism appears to decline over the first few years of life until adult levels are reached at approximately 2½–5 years of age. These findings have been confirmed in several other studies [12, 42, 54, 55, 59–62]. There is general agreement that astigmatism is more prevalent in infants, ranging from 20% to 60%. In comparison, the prevalence of astigmatism in adults is 10% [11, 12, 54, 58, 60–63, 68, 74, 75]. Mohindra found the prevalence of astigmatism (≥1.00 D) to be approximately 30% at birth. The prevalence peaks at 51% between 9 and 32 weeks and then gradually declines [11]. Gwiazda and colleagues found that the prevalence and magnitude of astigmatism are highest in the first 2 years of life and are greatly reduced or eliminated by 4 years of age (Figure 5.6) [55].

This trend toward a decrease in the magnitude of the astigmatism with age is especially common when AR astigmatism is present [55, 68]. The transition from these high levels to those seen in adult populations appears to occur somewhere between 18 months and 3–5 years of age [55, 59]. Investigators have also found no increase in the amount of astigmatism over time. Children who have little or no astigmatism in the first year of life did not develop significant astigmatism over the next 4 years. This implies that if the magnitude of astigmatism decreases during early childhood, astigmatism will rarely reappear. Astigmatic errors of high magnitude (>3.00 D), however, may not completely disappear with age [59]. An overall shift in axis toward WR astigmatism also occurs during development [55, 68]. From birth until 3 years of age, there is a higher prevalence of AR astigmatism than that seen

Figure 5.6. Total astigmatism in young children. (Reprinted with permission from WM Lyle. Astigmatism. In T Grosvenor, MC Flom [eds], Refractive Anomalies. Boston: Butterworth–Heinemann, 1991;154.)

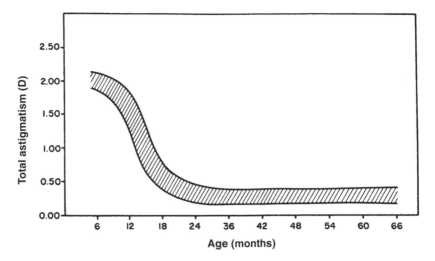

Figure 5.7. Relative proportions of against-the-rule (AR) and with-the-rule (WR) astigmatism in young children. (Reprinted with permission from WM Lyle. Astigmatism. In T Grosvenor, MC Flom [eds], Refractive Anomalies. Boston: Butterworth–Heinemann, 1991;154.)

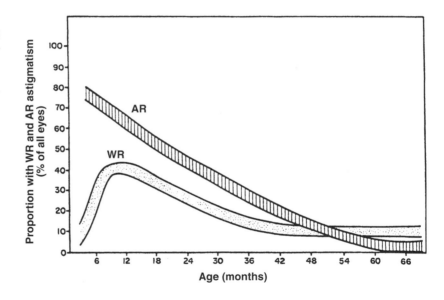

in a normal adult population. By 5 years of age, there is a higher prevalence of WR astigmatism (Figure 5.7). Increases in the magnitude of WR astigmatism with age have also been reported [61]. Only a small percentage of children have been found to have oblique axis astigmatism, which generally remains more stable or can increase in magnitude during the early years of life [54, 55, 59, 61, 68]. Oblique astigmatism is more difficult to manage and may be associated with other visual disorders in young children [59]. Follow-up is therefore

recommended for children found to have oblique astigmatism at 1 year of age.

The age of 3½ years generally is seen as a significant milestone with respect to astigmatism. The prevalence of astigmatism has dropped significantly by this age, approaching that of adult populations. The prevalence of AR versus WR astigmatism also appears to shift at this time. AR is more prevalent before the age of 3½. The period from 3½ years to 5½ years is one of transition. In children older than 5½ years, WR astigmatism is more common [76].

The mechanism by which the developmental changes in astigmatism occur is not yet well understood. Howland and Sayles determined that the amounts of corneal and total astigmatism in infants are approximately equal, decrease during the first 3 years of life, and are significantly and positively correlated with each other. They suggest that astigmatism arises from unequal tension on the pairs of vertical and horizontal rectus muscles, with the tension on the horizontal rectus muscles exceeding that on the vertical rectus muscles. This bends the cornea more in the horizontal meridian, causing an increase in myopia [60].

Dobson suggested that the amount of pressure exerted on the eye by the horizontal rectus muscles may be a possible cause of astigmatism. It has also been speculated that changes in eyelid pressure during the early years may cause the developmental changes in astigmatism [60, 68, 77].

Banks summarized other research that concluded that changes in astigmatism were due to measurement error [13]. London and Wick postulated that the high prevalence of AR astigmatism that occurs early in life is an artifact caused by the presence of a large angle lambda in infancy. They proposed that the measurement of refractive error using retinoscopy along the line of sight results in off-axis retinoscopy and the measurement of a false degree of astigmatism. As angle lambda is greatest in the horizontal meridian, a higher percentage of AR astigmatism could be predicted from this model. They concluded that astigmatic errors should not be corrected until angle lambda approaches adult levels at approximately 2 years of age [78].

Anisometropia

The prevalence of anisometropia is negatively correlated with age. Anisometropia of at least 1.00 D is a common vision anomaly in premature infants, with a prevalence of 32% [74]. A significant number of full-term infants also demonstrate anisometropia, although the prevalence is somewhat lower (11–22%) [11, 45, 79]. By 1 year of age, the prevalence of anisometropia has dropped significantly (4–7%) [11, 12, 58] and continues at this low level through 2½ years. By 5 years of age, the prevalence of anisometropia is reported to be even lower (1–4%) [71–73, 80].

Anisometropia has the additional unusual developmental feature of "flip-flopping" in its presentation. Children who had little anisometropia at 1 year of age were found to have significant amounts by 4 years of age, and those with significant amounts of anisometropia at 1 year of age were often found to have little anisometropia at 4 years [12, 81, 82]. Abrahamsson emphasized the need to consider the stability of the anisometropia before prescribing glasses for very young children. Likewise, a vision examination that is normal at 1 year of age still necessitates reevaluation at 3 and 5 years of age.

The presence of aniseikonia and the possibility of inducing strabismus as a result of full correction for anisometropia in young children has been addressed in the literature [83–85]. Nordlow provided full optical correction with conventional or iseikonic lenses for 4-year-old children with more than 2.00 D of anisometropia. In this study, two-thirds of the children with conventional lenses continued to demonstrate reduced visual acuity, whereas only one in 15 of the children with iseikonic lenses did. The children with iseikonic lenses also demonstrated better foveal fixation. Nordlow recommends providing full optical correction when 2.00 D or more of anisometropia is present with an iseikonic correction of 0.75–1.25% per diopter [84]. Additional studies have demonstrated improved visual acuity and functioning with application of full correction for anisometropia [86, 87].

Myopia

The prevalence and magnitude of myopia in premature infants is higher than in full-term infants [88–91]. In summarizing the work of several researchers, Banks found the mean refractive error of premature infants to be less hyperopic than that of full-term neonates and within 1.00 D of emmetropia [13]. Premature infants who deviate from this pattern have been shown to do so at the myopic end of the spectrum with the degree of myopia higher in premature infants [92]. The gestational age of infants is also correlated with refractive error, with the more premature infants demonstrating higher degrees of myopia [74]. The prevalence of myopia in premature infants is reported to be as high as 45%, with almost half of these children becoming emmetropic by 7 years of age. Overall, myopia in pre-

Figure 5.8. Refractive states of 375 eyes of newborn infants and 333 children between the ages of 6–8 years. (Reprinted with permission from MJ Hirsch, FW Weymouth. Prevalence of Refractive Anomalies. In T Grosvenor, MC Flom [eds], Refractive Anomalies. Boston: Butterworth–Heinemann, 1991;22.)

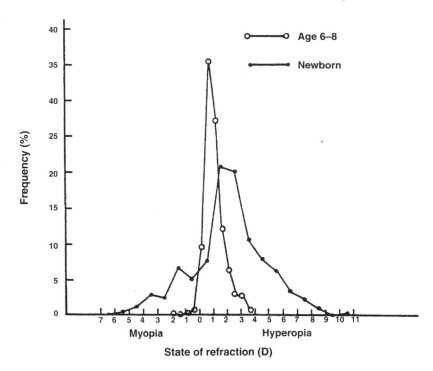

mature infants tends to decrease over time [88, 93], and children who remain myopic show a lower degree of myopia than at birth. Premature infants who were born hyperopic show the same changes in refraction as full-term neonates [94].

Infants are typically born with a spherical refractive error of +2.00 D with a standard deviation of ±2.00 D using cycloplegic refraction [3]. Other studies using near retinoscopy show newborns to be slightly myopic (mean = –0.69, SD = 3.21) [11]. Mohindra has attributed these differences to the loss of ciliary muscle tone when cycloplegic refractions are performed. When this is taken into account, the results of these studies do not differ significantly.

There is a bell-shaped distribution of refractive error with wide variability during infancy [95]. A subsequent change in distribution of spherical refractive error from the bell-shaped curve to a leptokurtic (peaked) curve takes place between the first and second years of life, with only small changes occurring after this time [1, 11–13]. Children with myopia generally become less myopic or slightly hyperopic, and children with hyperopia generally became less hyperopic [12]. The mean refractive error changes from mildly myopic at birth to mildly hyperopic by age 5 (+0.59 D) [11]. This change re-

flects the wide range of maturity of the eye at birth [52, 96] and also supports Fabian's concept that emmetropization is taking place during visual development (Figure 5.8) [64].

DEVELOPMENTAL IMPACT

Understanding the impact of uncorrected ametropia on a child's developing visual system is important for the proper management of refractive error. Ametropia can result in amblyopia or binocular anomalies and can prevent a child from developing the appropriate visual, perceptual, and eye-hand coordination skills, which are necessary prerequisites to learning. The benefits of providing full optical correction include normal binocular vision, enhanced stereopsis, clear peripheral images, equal accommodative stimulus, and the prevention of amblyopia.

Relationship to Amblyopia

High magnitudes of myopia can result in amblyopia when the magnitude of the myopia exceeds 8.00 D, although there is little documentation of this occurring [97]. Loss of vision can also result from lesser degrees of myopia. For example, the presence of pathologic myopia is usually considered in myopia of greater than 6.00 D and is based on ophthalmoscopic appearance rather than retinoscopy. Pathologic myopia may be a sign of the presence of ocular health problems that could result in degenerative changes in the posterior segment of the eye and a subsequent loss of vision. These changes are primarily due to an increased axial length and cause stretching and thinning of the retina, choroid, and sclera. Both the magnitude of the myopia and its associated complications increase with age, making it a leading cause of blindness in the United States. Pathologies associated with high-magnitude myopia include posterior staphyloma and the resultant spreading of cones, macular damage, retinal tears, chorioretinal degenerations, and associated reduced visual function. Approximately 31% of cases of pathologic myopia are present at birth, with 61% occurring from 6 to 12 years of age and 8% after age 12 [98].

Although hyperopia does not pose any significant ocular health risks in a young child, there is an association between amblyopia and uncorrected hyperopia of more than 2.00 D [97, 99]. Hyperopia is particularly troublesome when the magnitude of the hyperopia is unequal between the two eyes. Amblyopia can also develop when as little as 1.50 D of astigmatism is present.

Martin first provided evidence that orientation differences in visual acuity were present in those whose astigmatism had been totally corrected [100]. This was later elaborated on and confirmed by Mitchell, who demonstrated a relationship between the amount of astigmatism and degree of amblyopia and the meridian of amblyopia and axis of astigmatism [101]. These two studies demonstrated the connection between the optical defect of astigmatism and the neural defect of amblyopia, although the time sequence for the occurrence of this meridional amblyopia was not determined until several years later.

Several other studies have clarified the relationship between early astigmatism and amblyopia. Dobson and colleagues found that early astigmatism had little effect on the vision of young infants in their studies [68, 102]. This is attributed to the poor visual acuity and large depth of focus of infants. In very young infants, this large depth

of focus results from miotic pupils and poorly developed dilator muscles. Teller and colleagues found variations in grating acuity with stimulus orientation in an infant with astigmatism [63]. These same variations were not present when the infant was retested with correction, indicating that neural-based meridional amblyopia emerges after approximately 6 months of age. Others found no meridional amblyopia during the first year of life or found decreased vision in infants with astigmatism [103–106]. The latter condition was correctable with lenses. Meridional amblyopia has been reported before the end of the third year of life [54]. Even at this age, the amblyopia disappeared within a couple of months after optical correction was provided. The chronologically late onset for this type of amblyopia is thought to involve the high lability of the astigmatism, the poor resolution capabilities of the neonate, and the relative neural insensitivity of the very young child to blur [11]. Clinically, this means that much of the transient astigmatism seen during infancy does not have a long-term effect on the developing visual system and may not need to be optically corrected unless it persists past the age of 2 years.

Generally, uncorrected astigmatism can cause meridional amblyopia when the magnitude exceeds 1.25 D. Meridional hyperopia of 2.50 D or more has also been associated with the eventual identification of squint or amblyopia. A child with meridional hyperopia is more at risk for the development of amblyopia than a child with bilateral hyperopia, anisometropia, or astigmatism [99, 107, 108]. With this in mind, the presence of +2.50 D or more of hyperopia in any one meridian should be monitored carefully.

Amblyopia can also develop when as little as 1.00 D of anisometropia is present. This is particularly true when there is bilateral anisometropic hyperopia present [97, 99, 102, 109, 110]. The presence of anisometropia increases the likelihood that a significant degree of amblyopia or astigmatism (1.50 D or greater) will be present. Children who have a significant degree of anisometropia at 4 years of age also maintained their astigmatic refractive error [81]. Jampolsky et al. suggest that when anisometropia is present, the visual acuity of the more ametropic eye often decreases [111]. Ingram and Walker found that children with 1.00 D or more of anisometropia were likely to develop strabismus or amblyopia 2 or more years later [112]. Studies have also shown that visual acuity tends to be better when a low degree of anisometropia is present [99, 109]. The final degree of amblyopia has been attributed to the age at which the anisometropia first appears. Abrahamsson found a marked increase in the prevalence of amblyopia in children whose anisometropia was unchanged or increased in magnitude during a 3-year period [81]. The association between anisometropia and amblyopia may be partially due to the significant association between anisometropia and hyperopic refractive error of more than 2.00 D. The referral criteria for the Orinda study has addressed these concerns and recommends referral for further vision care when 1.00 D or more of anisometropia is detected during a vision screening program [113]. More specifically, anisometropia is considered an amblyogenic risk factor when astigmatism is greater than 1.50 D, hyperopic anisometropia is greater than 1.00 D, or myopic anisometropia is greater than 3.00 D.

Because amblyopia is a cause for concern when deciding when to correct refractive error, it is extremely important to measure and monitor its presence using age-appropriate visual acuity tests. The clinical methods of choice for monitoring visual acuity are listed in Table 5.7 and discussed in more detail in Chapter 6.

Relationship to Binocularity

Significant uncorrected hyperopia can require a child to make excessive accommodative responses, resulting in a large esophoria or esotropia; reduced stereopsis; and the development of abnormal sensory findings, including diplopia, suppression, or anomalous retinal correspondence. The diagnosis of accommodative esotropia secondary to moderate bilateral hyperopia is common in children 1–3 years of age [114]. Uncorrected anisometropia can also compromise a child's binocularity by reducing stereopsis and causing suppression [114, 115]. Correction of significant refractive error throughout infancy may reduce the likelihood of strabismus [116]. Hyperopic children who receive optical correction are less likely to develop strabismus by age 4 than are those who do not (6.3% versus 21%) [117].

Table 5.7. Visual Acuity Tests for Refractive Amblyopia

Age	Visual Acuity Test
Birth–2 yrs	Forced-choice preferential looking
2–3 yrs	Forced-choice preferential looking or LEA symbols
3–5 yrs	LEA Symbols, Broken Wheel, HOTV, Allen Pictures

Correction of hyperopia would typically be contraindicated when an exodeviation is present. In these cases, application of plus lenses would theoretically reduce the child's accommodative effort and, based on the accommodative convergence-to-accommodation (AC/A) ratio, reduce the accommodative convergence. This would normally result in a higher exodeviation. There are reports, however, of cases of exotropia in which application of plus lenses resulted in a paradoxical response [118]. The application of plus lenses actually reduced the exodeviation and resulted in better alignment. Although the reasons for this response are unclear, the most likely explanation is that the visual system of the child with significant hyperopia ultimately has two choices when responding to this uncorrected refractive error. The child can make an attempt to compensate for the refractive error by exerting greater accommodative effort. This frequently results in an accommodative esotropia. If the hyperopia is too much to overcome or the child's accommodative skills are insufficient, the child may cease accommodating altogether. Relaxation of accommodation followed by relaxation of accommodative convergence could result in the child exhibiting an exodeviation if the AC/A ratio is large enough. Application of plus lenses in these cases could result in greater visual comfort for the child. If part of the accommodation is provided optically, the accommodative system could provide the remaining accommodative and accommodative convergence effort. This would in turn result in better ocular alignment.

When a binocular vision problem is present along with a refractive error, it is important to monitor the child's motor and sensory binocular ability. Application of lenses can often be helpful in developing and maintaining binocularity in cases such as

Table 5.8. Tests for Binocular Assessment of Young Children

Age	Motor Assessment	Sensory Assessment
Birth–2 yrs	Cover test Bruchner test Hirschberg test Krimsky test Four base-out test Convergence near point test	Stereo smile test
3–5 yrs	All of the above tests Prism bar vergences	Randot Stereo Smile Test Randot Stereo Test Lang-Stereotest Randot Preschool Stereoacuity Test Three-figure flashlight Stereo Fly Stereo Butterfly Goggle-Free stereo test

accommodative esotropia. There are conditions, however, in which the prescription of lenses can actually create a binocular vision problem. Children with moderate to high hyperopia, fragile binocularity, a receded near point of convergence, amblyopia, more than 4.00 D of hyperopia, or a high AC/A ratio are especially at risk for developing optically induced consecutive exotropia [119].

A child's ocular alignment should always be measured with a unilateral and alternating cover test. Any significant deviation should be measured with loose prisms or a prism bar. Other useful adjuncts to the cover test and clinical techniques to evaluate a child's sensory binocular status are listed in Table 5.8 and described in more detail in Chapter 6.

Relationship to Learning

Any uncorrected refractive error that results in decreased visual acuity or fragile binocularity can contribute to a learning-related vision problem. In preschool children, this can result in a lack of interest in close work, poor development of eye-hand coordination and perceptual skills, or an inability to sit still for long periods of time. Moderate degrees of uncorrected hyperopia have been associated with diminished academic performance in school-age children [120–123] and delays in visual perceptual skills in preschool children [124, 125]. Asthenopia and decreased reading performance in adults have also been linked to uncorrected hyperopia [126, 127]. It is therefore important to note signs and symptoms of these problems in preschool children before they interfere with the acquisition of reading readiness skills (see Table 5.1).

Although AR astigmatism in children younger than 2 years of age is common, transient, and often of little concern, its presence in older preschool children, who are beginning to engage in sustained near tasks, should be addressed. There is an association between the presence of AR astigmatism, reduced accommodative skills, and the impending onset of myopia. Hirsch has demonstrated that small amounts of AR astigmatism can result in asthenopia or visual discomfort and often precede the development of myopia [108]. Birnbaum has hypothesized that AR astigmatism is a functional adaptation made to reduce near-point stress by permitting reduced accommodative output while maintaining a sufficient resolution for the primarily vertically oriented characters of the English alphabet [128]. Although most preschool children are not required to complete lengthy, detailed near tasks, some preschools today place strong emphasis on reading readiness skills through computer learning or sustained near-point tasks. It is therefore possible that some children might develop a small degree of AR astigmatism in response to these environmental demands.

Table 5.9. Types of Refractive Error Associated with Developmental Disabilities

Condition	Myopia	Hyperopia	Astigmatism	Anisometropia
Aarskog syndrome		X		
Albinism	X	X	X	
Aphakia				
Bardet-Biedl syndrome			X	
Blepharoptosis				X
Cohen's syndrome	X			
Congenital glaucoma	X			X
Congenital pendular nystagmus			X	
Cornea plana		X		
Down syndrome	X			
Duane's syndrome				X
Ehlers-Danlos syndrome	X			
Fetal alcohol syndrome	X			
Homocystinuria syndrome	X		X	
Kennedy's syndrome		X		
Keratoglobus			X	
Kniest syndrome	X			
Leber's congenital amaurosis		X		
Marcus Gunn's syndrome				X
Marfan syndrome	X		X	
Marshall syndrome	X			
Microcornea	X			
Noonan's syndrome	X			
Retinopathy of prematurity	X	X		
Rubinstein-Taybi syndrome		X		
Stickler's syndrome	X			
Treacher Collins syndrome			X	
Weill-Marchesani syndrome	X			

Relationship to Developmental Disabilities

It is not uncommon for refractive error to be associated with various syndromes, systemic conditions, or developmental disabilities [129–131]. In some cases, the condition is specific as to the type of refractive error present. For example, there is an association between Leber's congenital amaurosis and the presence of moderate to high hyperopia [132]. Other types of disabilities are known to be associated with refractive error in general, but are not associated with any specific condition. For example, Down syndrome is associated with significant refractive error, including high myopia, hyperopia, or astigmatism. Table 5.9 lists some of the more common systemic conditions and their associated refractive conditions. Because the prevalence of refractive error in special-needs populations is higher than in the general population, careful evaluation, prescription, and management is imperative when evaluating these children [133–135].

PRESCRIBING FOR REFRACTIVE ERROR

Myopia

Low myopia (<1.00 D) has little significance in infants and preschool children and is not usually corrected. Findings of low degrees of myopia in a young child may often be an artifact resulting from excessive accommodation during retinoscopy procedures and would not be detected with cycloplegic refraction. Correction of myopia of less than 1.00 D should be considered only in older preschool children (4–5 years of age) who are showing signs of myopia (squinting, difficulty with distance vision) or at any age when an exodeviation is present and the resultant accommodative effort is useful in helping maintain binocular alignment [76, 136].

Moderately low degrees of myopia (1.00–3.00 D) should be corrected in children who are 3 years of age or older. At this age, most children are in a nursery school, preschool, or day care setting and need reasonably good distance visual acuity in order to sit in a classroom, watch a movie, or observe distance objects (e.g., people, signs, airplanes).

By the time children approach their first birthday, they are just beginning to walk and explore their environment. They are also beginning to become interested in such distance tasks as television or watching other children at play and should be able to sight small objects across a room or a person entering a doorway at a distance. For these reasons, moderately high degrees of myopia in infants (3.00–5.00 D) should be corrected by 1 year of age [15].

High myopia presents a particular risk for the development of amblyopia in children of all ages. Infants naturally have a close working distance and lower degrees of myopia would still allow for good visual acuity at near. When the myopia exceeds 5.00 D, the child no longer has any point in space beyond 8 in. at which he or she can obtain a clear retinal image. These children are therefore at a significant risk for amblyopia development and need to be corrected regardless of age. The visual acuity in these children should be monitored by the use of appropriate visual acuity tests both before and after prescribing [76].

Hyperopia

Hyperopic refractive errors should be corrected when the magnitude of the hyperopia exceeds 2.50 D and there is no binocular dysfunction; this provides maximum visual acuity, minimizes the risk of amblyopia, and reduces the demand placed on the accommodative system. This will provide the child with clear, comfortable vision at near and allow for the normal acquisition of visual perceptual and reading readiness skills. In children younger than 3 years of age, it is acceptable to monitor low to moderate degrees of hyperopia for a period of time before prescribing, providing that the child's visual acuity and binocularity are normal.

Hyperopic refractive errors in young children should always be corrected if they facilitate ocular alignment and enhance binocularity when an eso-deviation is present. The actual amount of the prescription should be dependent on the child's AC/A ratio. Although there is a tendency to provide maximum plus whenever esotropia is present with hyperopia, care must be taken not to overprescribe, which may result in an optically induced consecutive exotropia [119, 137]. Risk factors for the development of this condition include hyperopia of more than 4.50 D, a receded near point of convergence, amblyopia, fragile binocularity (e.g., reduced stereopsis), and a high AC/C ratio [119].

Astigmatism

Astigmatism is often transient in early childhood and has little effect on visual acuity development. Most astigmatic refractive errors that are present before 2 years of age do not need immediate correction, provided that the child's visual acuity is normal and assessed periodically. The type of astigmatism present plays a significant role in how closely the astigmatism is monitored. Since oblique and WR astigmatism usually remain stable, these types should be monitored carefully every 3–4 months, even during the first years of life. AR astigmatism, which is very common in young children, has a tendency to decrease significantly in the early years and may need less frequent monitoring (every 6–9 months) [76].

During the period between 1 and 3 years of age, the prevalence and magnitude of astigmatism decreases significantly. Most of the notable astigmatism present during infancy is no longer detectable. A small number of children will continue to have residual astigmatism and are at risk for developing meridional amblyopia. This astigmatism should be corrected once the child reaches 2 years of age and the refractive error is more than 1.25 D and is stable over a 3- to 6-month period. These guidelines apply regardless of the type of astigmatism present. Full correction should be provided in order to minimize the risk for amblyopia. Once glasses are prescribed, visual acuity as well as changes in the refractive error should be checked at least every 6 months [15, 76].

Meridional hyperopia of +2.50 D or more has also been associated with the eventual identification of strabismus (squint) or amblyopia [58]. Children with significant meridional hyperopia need to be monitored closely every 3 months. Full prescription is given when the refractive error is stable, reduced visual acuity is present, or both [15, 76].

Anisometropia

Anisometropia contributes to vision loss and is easily detectable and treatable at an early age. Unfortunately, many vision screenings do not adequately detect this problem. Parents who are otherwise fastidious about their child's health may be lulled into security when no visible eye problem is present and their child passes a vision screening. Michaels explains the functional vision problems associated with anisometropia: "Since accommodation is always binocular, the uncorrected anisometropic hyperope flounders between unequal acuity, aniseikonia, amblyopia, induced heterophorias and potential strabismus" [138].

When more than 1.00 D of anisometropia is present, the child's visual acuity as well as motor and sensory binocularity should be carefully evaluated. If these are normal, the anisometropia can be reevaluated approximately every 6 months. When the anisometropia exceeds 1.00 D and the visual acuity or the binocular findings are abnormal, it is important to provide optical correction to prevent abnormal sensory development. Thal and Grisham emphasize the importance of correcting anisometropia despite the lack of patient symptoms [86]. Benefits include improved binocularity and stereopsis, a clearer central and peripheral image in the more ametropic eye, equal stimulus to accommodation, and the prevention of amblyopia. Direct, minimal occlusion therapy to prevent amblyopia from developing in the more ametropic eye is beneficial while changes in refractive error are being monitored. Care must be taken, however, because occlusion may add another dissociative factor to the anisometropia and precipitate or aggravate a squint, especially in young children. It is important to consider the type of anisometropia present when managing refractive error.

When low to moderate myopia is present in both eyes (myopic anisometropia), each eye will receive a clear retinal image at some point in space, preventing the development of amblyopia [111]. Typically, the less myopic eye will be used for distance

viewing, whereas the more myopic eye will be used at near. Once the anisometropia stabilizes, a full correction for the myopia can be provided to enhance binocularity [139].

Hyperopic anisometropia should raise more serious concerns and is more difficult to manage because (1) hyperopic anisometropia is not a predictable or stable condition in children younger than the age of 4 years and (2) the more hyperopic eye is not used at any distance due to the excessive accommodative demand required. The risk of amblyopia development is significant, even with as little as 1.00 D of anisometropia [99]. Careful, periodic visual acuity assessment is important in these cases. Correction should be provided if the refraction stabilizes or the visual acuity measurements are asymmetric. When bilateral hyperopic anisometropia of more than 5.00 D is present, there is a far greater risk for the development of amblyopia. These refractive errors should be corrected as soon as they are identified [15, 76].

When antimetropia is present (one eye myopic, the other hyperopic), amblyopia is less likely because the myopic eye is used for near and the hyperopic eye for distance vision. Antimetropia can affect the development of normal binocularity and stereopsis. In these cases, a full correction is indicated once the refractive error has stabilized in order to provide equal accommodative demand to the eyes.

In cylindrical anisometropia the type of astigmatism must be considered. WR and oblique astigmatism tend to be more permanent and should be monitored closely and treated more aggressively than AR astigmatism. Mohindra demonstrated the advantages of full correction for anisometropia in her successful treatment of a 4-year-old child with anisometropia, astigmatism, and strabismus [87]. Correction of the anisometropia and subsequent patching for amblyopia not only resulted in a change in visual acuity from 20/60 to 20/20 but also dramatically improved binocular functioning and stereopsis.

Unequal image size (aniseikonia) in the preschool population does not commonly raise concern but should not be ignored. The routine use of aniseikonic lenses may be contraindicated in this population due to lack of patient symptoms, high costs, and difficulty assessing their effectiveness. The optometrist should be aware of this problem and con-

Table 5.10. Summary of Prescribing Guidelines

Refractive Error	Level at Which Amblyopia Concern is Indicated	Binocularity Considerations	Interference with Learning	Refractive Error at Which Prescription Should be Considered
Myopia	>5.00 D	Undercorrect esodeviation; fully correct exodeviation to maximize binocularity	Dependent on child's age	>5.00 D (any age) >3.00 D (>1 yr) >1.00 D (>3 yrs)
Hyperopia	>2.00 D	Undercorrect exodeviation; fully correct esodeviation to maximize binocularity	>2.50 D	>2.00 D
Astigmatism	>1.25 D	No specific considerations	Depends on visual acuity	>1.25 D
Anisometropia	>1.00 D	Monitor binocularity and stereopsis	>1.00 D	>1.00 D

sider it when the child shows signs or symptoms of aniseikonia, including refusal to wear glasses, complaints of discomfort, decreased visual acuity, and reduced binocularity with correction.

Table 5.10 presents a summary of guidelines for prescribing lenses for correction of significant refractive error in infants and young children.

GENERAL MANAGEMENT RECOMMENDATIONS

Evaluating and managing refractive error in young children is a challenging part of any primary care optometric practice. There are several general guidelines to consider when managing refractive error.

Initial and Subsequent Evaluation

Although most refractive error decreases during the early years, some, such as astigmatism, may remain stable, and others, such as anisometropia, can increase. Periodic evaluations are therefore a key element in good management. All children should initially be examined for refractive error by approximately 6 months of age [7, 8]. Evaluation at this time allows for early detection and management of the higher magnitude refractive errors and also allows identification of lower degrees of refractive error, which may need to be monitored on a regular basis before prescribing.

Children who initially present with a refractive error that does not need correction should be evaluated again between 2 and 3 years of age. This allows for identification of early astigmatism that has not resolved and that now places the child at risk for amblyopia and also allows for the detection of moderate degrees of hyperopia that may begin to affect binocularity due to excessive accommodative efforts at near or a high AC/A ratio [8].

A final routine evaluation during the preschool years should be done just before the child enters kindergarten (approximately 5 years of age). This evaluation will ensure that the child has no significant refractive error that might interfere with learning and will also help the optometrist to predict how that child's refractive error might change during the school years [8].

When a significant refractive error is found during the early years, it should be periodically monitored regardless of whether a prescription is given. These evaluations should take place every 3–6 months to determine if a prescription is needed and to evaluate compliance, wearing schedules, frame fit, visual acuity, binocularity, and behavioral and refractive changes.

Case Example

A 2-year-old child comes in for a routine vision examination. There are no parental concerns other than a family history of myopia. A refraction indicates –1.00 D of myopia, orthophoria on cover testing, and normal visual acuities with preferential looking (a near visual acuity test). No glasses are prescribed, but a follow-up visit is recommended in 6 months. As this child approaches 3 years of age, visual acuities using optotypes such as the LEA symbols will be possible and a more accurate assessment of distance visual acuity can be done. A return visit at 3 years of age indicates reduced distance visual acuities and a slight increase in myopia. Glasses to correct the myopia are now indicated.

Amount of Prescription

A full prescription is generally recommended for young children, unless this compromises some other aspect of the child's visual system (e.g., binocularity). When the combination of significant myopia with an esodeviation or hyperopia with an exodeviation is present, management can be particularly problematic. In these cases, it may be advisable to modify the prescription to provide maximum visual acuity along with minimal binocular dysfunction. These children may also benefit from vision therapy in order to prevent secondary strabismic deviations from occurring [119].

Case Example

Two 3-year-old children present for vision examinations. They both have 2.50 D of hyperopia. The first child has 14^Δ of esophoria at distance and near, with reduced stereopsis and normal visual acuities in each eye. Application of +2.50 spheres results in orthophoria and increased stereopsis. The second child is orthophoric at distance and near, with normal stereopsis and normal visual acuities. The first child should be given the full hyperopic prescription. The second child's refractive error can be monitored periodically without prescribing.

Wearing Schedule

Another issue when prescribing for refractive error is wearing time. In general, prescriptions to correct refractive error are intended to prevent amblyopia, improve visual acuity, increase learning efficiency, or enhance binocularity. For this reason, it is usually advisable to recommend full-time wear. Modifications to this wearing schedule can then be implemented when necessary on an individual basis.

Although most children will actually appreciate their new or improved visual skills and reach for their glasses every morning, some children will be resistant to wearing glasses. In these cases, the optometrist should always check first to make sure the glasses are not too tight or loose and fit properly on the child's face and behind his or her ears. These are some of the main reasons for noncompliance. Next, a modified wearing schedule and behavioral modification should be considered if necessary. The keys to obtaining maximum compliance are flexibility and willingness to work with the parent and child in establishing a reasonable wearing schedule. For example, a child with 3.00 D of hyperopia and 15^Δ esophoria present at near could remove his or her glasses for distance viewing or active outdoor play if necessary without severe consequences. Likewise, a child with 3.00 D of myopia could remove his or her glasses for near activities.

LENSES AND EYE WEAR FOR YOUNG CHILDREN

Bifocals

A bifocal prescription should be considered in certain cases of convergence excess or accommodative esotropia in which the esodeviation is significantly greater at near than at distance. Bifocals are generally not recommended until the child is well into his or her second year of life and is walking comfortably. It is preferable to "over-plus" an infant who is in need of additional plus at near rather than to provide a bifocal. For example, full correction would allow a 10-month-old child with bilateral aphakia and a refraction of +20.00 D to see at a distance but not at near, where most activity and learning is taking place for a child. In this case, it would be appropriate to "over-plus" the child and provide corrective lenses of +22.50 D in order to allow for clear vision at near. When the child learns to walk and run comfortably without stumbling (approximately 1½ to 2 years of age), it would be appropriate to change to a bifocal prescription of +20.00 D with a +2.50 D add.

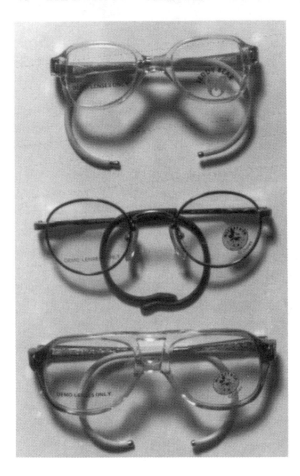

Figure 5.9. Infant and toddler frames with riding cables. (Photo by Ron Davidoff.)

Bifocals are most frequently considered for use in cases of accommodative esotropia, which has an onset at approximately 2–3 years of age. When full application of plus does not result in ocular alignment at distance and near (due to a high AC/A ratio) a bifocal prescription is recommended to improve binocularity. The bifocal segment preferred for use in young children is a flat-top (either 25 mm or 28 mm) with the segment set to split the pupil when the child is looking straight ahead. Application of other types of bifocals or a lower segment height will require larger eye movements by the child and is more likely to result in lack of use of the bifocal with the child looking through the carrier for both distance and near. Blended or progressive bifocals are most appropriate for school-age children and adults. An ex-

ecutive segment provides a wide reading area and high optical center, but is cosmetically unacceptable for most children.

Contact Lenses

Contact lenses should be considered when the magnitude of the ametropia or anisometropia is greater than 5.00 D and is strongly recommended when it exceeds 10.00 D [15, 76]. Since most astigmatic corrections are in the low to moderate range and contact lenses require more expertise for fitting, they are generally not recommended for young children. Contact lenses have several benefits, including improved cosmesis, reduced prismatic effect, enhanced peripheral field, decreased peripheral distortion, and improved binocularity. There are also several disadvantages, including increased cost of lenses, need for more frequent follow-up visits, careful hygiene, and optimum child and parent compliance. Each of these factors should be carefully discussed with parents when contact lenses are considered [139].

Case Example

A 4-year-old boy born with retinopathy of prematurity now has a refraction of +1.00 OD and –8.00 OS. Wearing glasses presents a cosmetic problem, and the child is resistant to wearing glasses because they are "weightier" on one side. The child's peripheral vision is reduced on the left side due to the distortion from the lenses. The hyperopia in the right eye is considered normal for his age, since there is no accompanying strabismus. The child is provided with a single contact lens for his left eye. This allows him to achieve better visual acuity and he is able to demonstrate a higher level of binocular vision.

Appropriate Eye Wear for Young Children

It is important to provide appropriately sized frames for young children. A frame that is too large will be uncomfortable, unsightly, and increase peripheral distortions. For infants, a frame with a riding cable is strongly recommended (Figure 5.9). Most of these frames have flexible cables that young chil-

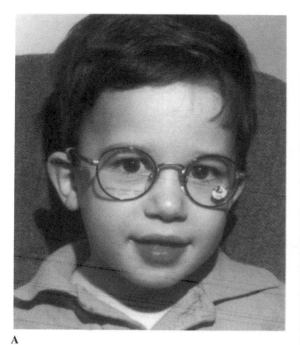
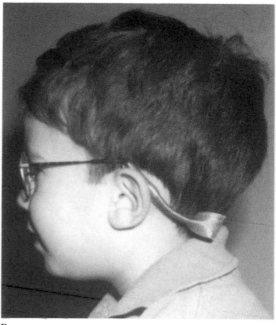

A   B

Figure 5.10. A. Appropriately fitting toddler frame. B. Side view of same toddler showing use of Croakie strap to keep frames on. (Photos by Ron Davidoff.)

dren tolerate better. For children older than 1 or 2 years of age, a regular ear piece may be sufficient, although a strap—for example, a Croakie—or other type of holding device will help prevent the glasses from slipping (Figure 5.10) In all cases, the frame should have spring hinges. These allow the frames to withstand rough handling. They also maintain their alignment for a longer period of time and provide increased comfort and overall better compliance.

Polycarbonate is the recommended lens material for young children because it is the material that is least likely to break. An alternative is a CR 39 or plastic lens. If polycarbonate is recommended, this must be specified on the prescription because it is typically more costly than standard plastic for lenses. Optometrists should inform parents that CR-39 and glass lenses provide limited impact resistance [140] and should never be prescribed or dispensed to young children due to the danger of breakage and resultant eye injury.

The actual fit of glasses is critical for ensuring maximum patient compliance. A tight nose pad or pinched ears can make a young child unwilling to wear the prescribed glasses, regardless of the visual benefits. It is also important to inform the parents

that frame adjustments should be performed periodically, especially if the child becomes more resistant to wearing the glasses.

Sun sensitivity has become an increasing concern. It is recommended that children wear protective sun lenses when outdoors. It is important to help parents select the most appropriate sun lenses, which should also allow the child to wear his or her refractive correction. Fortunately, there are many options available, including separate tinted corrective lenses for outdoors, clip-on sun lenses, and slip-behind lenses designed for children. When severe photophobia is present, it is important to provide the child with sun lenses that shield the eyes from extraneous light and glare. Any type of tinted lens should have ultraviolet protection. Polycarbonate lenses always provide protection against ultraviolet light even if there is no tint.

ACHIEVING SUCCESS AFTER PRESCRIBING TREATMENT

Prescribing accurate and useful refractions is only the first step in achieving successful refractive error management. Compliance can be ensured only if the optometrist, parents, and child work together as a team.

Frequency of Follow-Up

When glasses are prescribed, it is important to continue to monitor a child's adaptation to the glasses, their effect on the other aspects of the child's vision, and changes in refraction, which will occur during the preschool years.

Parent Education

The most important aspect of managing refractive error in young children is parent education. Parents who understand why their child needs to wear glasses, how the glasses will improve their child's visual skills, and when the glasses should be worn will be motivated to ensure compliance from their children and work with the optometrist to achieve optimum results.

The initial step in parent education is demonstration of how the child is seeing without lenses and how lenses will improve the child's vision.

Case Example

The parents of an 18-month-old boy with a refractive error of +7.50 OU, no strabismus, and a subnormal visual acuity are told that their child will need to wear strong corrective lenses on a full-time basis. They are given −7.50 trial lenses to hold in front of their eyes to demonstrate their child's refractive error. They attempt to read through these lenses, and the optometrist explains that these lenses simulate how their child sees without any glasses. While the parents are holding these lenses to their eyes, +7.50 trial lenses are placed over the minus lenses. The optometrist explains that the +7.50 lenses are the same prescription as their child's glasses and will provide them with a clearer and more comfortable image.

Parents should also be made aware of the possibility that periodic lens changes may need to be made due to changes in the child's visual system in response to the initial application of lenses, increased accuracy of refraction with increased cooperation from the child during subsequent visits, and changes in the actual refractive state of the eye.

Parents need to understand that periodic monitoring of their child's refractive error is essential to provide their child with optimal visual acuity, binocularity, and visual comfort during their early developmental years.

Child Motivation

In most cases, children gladly welcome the opportunity to see clearly and comfortably with their new glasses. When the child is able to talk, it is important for both the optometrist and parents to discuss the child's need for glasses with him or her at an age-appropriate level. Allowing the child to be involved in frame and case selection at an early age is also helpful in achieving compliance. Developing a structured wearing schedule along with a safe, easily located place to store the glasses when they are not being worn will help decrease uncertainty and anxiety associated with their wear.

CONCLUSION

The evaluation and management of refractive error in young children is easily accomplished using tools that are often available in most optometric offices. The management of refractive error in young children, however, differs from that of adults. This is due to the continual changes that are occurring in the visual system of children during their early years. Uncorrected refractive error can have serious consequences on the visual development of children as well as their ability to interact with and learn from their environment. Optometrists who consider these issues and prudently monitor and correct these refractive errors will find working with young children a rewarding and beneficial part of their practice.

REFERENCES

1. Boothe RG, Dobson V, Teller DY. Postnatal development of vision in human and nonhuman primates. Ann Rev Neurosci 1985;8:495–545.

2. Mayer DL, Beiser AS, Warner AF, et al. Monocular acuity norms for the Teller Acuity Cards between one month and four years. Invest Ophthalmol Vis Sci 1995;36(3):671–685.

3. Teller DY. The Development of Visual Function in Infants. In B Cohen, I Bodis-Wollner (eds), Vision and the Brain. New York: Raven, 1990;109–118.

4. Ciner EB, Schanel-Klitsch E, Herzberg H. Stereoacuity development: 6 months to 5 years: a new tool for testing and screening. Optom Vis Sci 1996;73(1):43–48.

5. Pease PL, Allen J. A new test for screening color vision: concurrent validity and utility. Am J Optom Physiol Opt 1988;65:729–738.

6. Dobson V, McDonald MA, Kohl P, et al. Visual acuity screening of infants and young children with the acuity card procedure. J Am Optom Assoc 1986;57(4):284–289.

7. Committee on Practice and Ambulatory Medicine. Vision screening and eye examination in children. Pediatrics 1986;77:918–919.

8. Scheiman MM, Amos CS, Ciner EB, et al. Pediatric Eye and Vision Examination. Optometric Clinical Practice Guideline. St. Louis: American Optometric Association, 1994.

9. Zolot M. Infant Vision Examination. In Curriculum II Continuing Education Courses. Optometric Extension Program, 1979;Series 1, No. 1:1–70.

10. Lewerenz DC. Visual acuity and the developing visual system. J Am Optom Assoc 1978;10:1155–1160.

11. Mohindra I, Held R. Refraction in humans from birth to five years. Doc Ophthalmol Proc 1981;28:19–27.

12. Ingram RM, Barr A. Changes in refraction between the ages of 1 and 3 1/2. Br J Ophthalmol 1979;63:339–342.

13. Banks MS. Infant refraction and accommodation. Int Ophthalmol Clin 1979;19:205–232.

14. Cron MT, Garzia R, Richman J. Infant visual development. J Optom Vis Dev 1986;17:6–18.

15. Ciner EB. Refractive error in young children: evaluation and prescription. Practical Optom 1992;3(4):182–190.

16. Mohindra I. A non-cycloplegic refraction technique for infants and young children. J Am Optom Assoc 1977;48:518–523.

17. Saunders KJ, Westall CA. A comparison between near and cycloplegic retinoscopy in the refraction of infants and young children. Optom Vis Sci 1992;69:615–622.

18. Ciner EB. Examination procedures for infants and young children. J Optom Vis Dev 1996;27:54–67.

19. Moore BD. Pediatric Ocular Pharmacology. In LJ Press, BD Moore (eds), Clinical Pediatric Optometry. Boston: Butterworth, 1993;347.

20. Ciner EB, Parisi M, Herzberg H. Examination of Children. In K Alexander (ed), Clinical Optometry. Philadelphia: Lippincott, 1995;422–498.

21. Jaanus SD, Pagano VT, Bartlett JD. Drugs Affecting the Autonomic Nervous System. In JD Bartlett, SD Jaanus (eds), Clinical Ocular Pharmacology. Boston: Butterworth, 1984;113.

22. Bartlett JD, Wesson MD, Swiatocha J, Woolley T. Efficacy of a pediatric cycloplegic administered as a spray. J Am Optom Assoc 1993;64:617–621.

23. Duckman RH. Photorefraction: an update. J Optom Vis Dev 1996;27:68–79.

24. Braddick OJ, Atkinson J, Wattam-Bell J, et al. Video-refractive screening of accommodative performance in infants. Invest Ophthalmol Vis Sci 1988;29(Suppl):60.

25. Atkinson J, Braddick O. The use of isotropic photore-fraction for vision screening in infants. Acta Ophthalmol 1983;157:36–45.

26. Duckman R. Using Photorefraction to Evaluate Refractive Error, Ocular Alignment and Accommodation in Infants, Toddlers and Multiply Handicapped Children. In M Scheiman (ed), Problems in Optometry—Pediatric Optometry. Philadelphia: Lippincott, 1990;333–353.

27. Kaakinen K, Ranta-Kemppainen L. Screening of infants for strabismus and refractive errors with two flash photorefraction with and without cycloplegia. Acta Ophthalmol (Copenh) 1986;64:578–582.

28. Cogan MS, Ottemiller DE. Photorefractor for detection of treatable eye disorders in preverbal children. Ala Med 1992;62:16–20.

29. Lewis RC, Marsh-Tootle WL. The reliability of interpretation of photoscreening results with the MTI PS-100 in Head Start preschool children. J Am Optom Assoc 1995;66(7):429.

30. Schmidt PP, Orel-Bixler D, et al. Analytical comparisons of photorefraction in screenings. Optom Vis Sci 1995;72(12S):209.

31. Freedman HL, Preston KL. Polaroid photoscreening for amblyogenic factors: an improved methodology. Ophthalmology 1992;99(12):1785–1795.

32. Ottar WL, Scott WE, Holgado SI. Photoscreening for amblyogenic factors. J Pediatr Ophthalmol Strabismus 1995;32:289–295.

33. Press L. Examination of the Preschool Child. In LJ Press, BD Moore (eds), Clinical Pediatric Optometry. Boston: Butterworth, 1993;47–62.

34. Aslin RN, Shea SL, Metz HS. Use of the Canon R-1 autorefractor to measure refractive errors and accommodative responses in infants. Clin Vis Sci 1990;5:61–70.

35. Evans E. Refraction in children using the Rx1 auto-refractor. Br Orthop J 1984;41:46–52.

36. Helveston EM, Pachtman MA, Cadera W, et al. Clinical evaluation of the Nidek AR Auto Refractor. J Pediatr Ophthalmol Strabismus 1984;21:227–230.

37. Friedman Z, Neumann E, Hyams SW, et al. Ophthalmic screening of 38,000 children, age 1 to 2 years, in child welfare clinics. J Pediatr Ophthalmol Strabismus 1976;17:261.

38. Shapero M, Yanko L, Nawratzki I, et al. Refractive power of premature children at infancy and early childhood. Am J Ophthalmol 1980;90:234.

39. Garner L, Grosvenor T, McKellor M, et al. Refraction

and its components in Melanesian school children in Vanuatu. Am J Optom Physiol Opt 1988;65:182.

40. Wibaut F. Uber die Emmetropisation und den Ursprung der spharischen Refracktionsanomalien. Graefes Arch Klin Exp Ophthalmol 1926;116:596.

41. Lyle WM. Changes in corneal astigmatism with age. Am J Optom Arch Am Acad Optom 1971;48:467.

42. Atkinson J, Braddick OJ, Durden K, et al. Screening for refractive errors in 6–9 month old infants by photorefraction. Br J Ophthalmol 1984;68:105.

43. Fulton AB, Hanson R, Peterson R. The relation of myopia and astigmatism in developing eyes. J Ophthalmol 1982;89:298.

44. Ingram R, Barr A. Refraction of 1 year old children after cycloplegia with 1% cyclopentolate: comparison with finding after atropinization. Br J Ophthalmol 1979;63:348.

45. Fulton A, Dobson V, Salem D, et al. Cycloplegic refractions in infants and young children. Am J Ophthalmol 1980;90:239–247.

46. Santanastaso A. La refraziene oculare nei primi anni de vita. Ann Ottal Clin Ocul 1930;58:852.

47. Angle J, Wissmann DA. The epidemiology of myopia. Am J Epidemiol 1980;3:220.

48. Woodruff ME. Cross-sectional studies of corneal and astigmatic characteristics of children between the twenty-fourth and seventy-second months of life. Am J Optom Physiol Opt 1971;48:650.

49. Hodi S. Screening of infants for significant refractive error using video refraction. Ophthalmic Physiol Opt 1994;14(7):310.

50. Brown EVL, Kronfeld P. Net average yearly changes in refraction of atropinized eyes from birth to beyond middle life. Arch Ophthalmol 1938;19:719.

51. Abrahamsson M, Fabian G, Sjostrand J. Changes in astigmatism between the ages of 1 and 4 years: a longitudinal study. Br J Ophthalmol 1988;72:145.

52. Goldschmidt E. Refraction in the newborn. Acta Ophthalmol (Copenh) 1969;47:570.

53. Cook RC, Glasscock RE. Refractive and ocular findings in the newborn. Am J Ophthalmol 1951;34:1407–1413.

54. Mohindra I, Held R, Gwiazda J, Brill S. Astigmatism in infants. Science 1978;202:329–330.

55. Gwiazda JE, Scheiman MM, Mohindra I, et al. Astigmatism in children: changes in axis and amount from birth to six years. Invest Ophthalmol Vis Sci 1984;25:88–92.

56. Howland HC, Sayles N. Photokeratometric and photorefractive measurements of astigmatism in infants and young children. Vision Res 1985;25(1):73–81.

57. Saunders KJ. Visual function in infants and young children with and without a family history of strabismus and/or amblyopia. Ph.D. thesis, University of Wales, College of Cardiff, 1993.

58. Ingram R, Traynar M, Walker C, Wilson J. Screening for refractive errors at age 1 year. A pilot study. Br J Ophthalmol 1979;63:243.

59. Atkinson J, Braddick O, French J. Infant astigmatism: its disappearance with age. Vision Res 1980;20:891.

60. Howland HC, Sayles N. Photorefractive measurement of astigmatism in infants and young children. Invest Ophthalmol Vis Sci 1984;25:93–102.

61. Abrahamsson M, Fabian G, Sjostrand J. Changes in astigmatism between the ages of 1 and 4 years: a longitudinal study. Br J Ophthalmol 1988;72:145–149.

62. Howland HC, Atkinson J, Braddick O, et al. Infant astigmatism measured by photorefraction. Science 1978;202:331–333.

63. Teller DY, Allen JL, Regal DM, Mayer DL. Astigmatism and acuity in two primate infants. Invest Ophthalmol Vis Sci 1978;17:344–349.

64. Van Alphen GWHM. On emmetropia and ametropia. Ophthalmologica 1961;142(Suppl):1–92.

65. Kempf GA, Collins SD, Jarman EL. Refractive Errors in the Eyes of Children as Determined by Retinoscopic Examination with a Cycloplegic. In Public Health Bulletin No 182. Washington DC: Government Printing Office, 1928.

66. Hirsch MJ, Weymouth FW. Prevalence of Refractive Anomalies. In T Grosvenor, M Flom (eds), Refractive Anomalies—Research and Clinical Applications. Boston: Butterworth, 1991;15–38.

67. Nathan J, Kiely PM, Crewther SG, Crewther DP. Astigmatism occurring in association with pediatric eye disease. Am J Optom Physiol Opt 1986;63:497–504.

68. Dobson V, Fulton A, Sebris SL. Cycloplegic refractions of infants and young children: the axis of astigmatism. Invest Ophthalmol Vis Sci 1984;25:83–87.

69. Gwiazda J, Thorn F, Bauer J, et al. Prediction of school age myopia from infant refractive errors. Invest Ophthalmol Vis Sci 1990;31:233.

70. Hirsch MJ. Anisometropia: a preliminary report of the Ojai longitudinal study. Am J Optom Arch Am Acad Optom 1967;44:581–585.

71. Hirsch MJ. Vision anomalies among children of grammar school age. J Am Optom Assoc 1952;23:663–671.

72. Flom MD, Bedell HE. Identifying amblyopia using associated conditions, acuity and nonacuity features. Am J Optom Physiol Opt 1985;62:153–160.

73. Blum H, Bettman J, Peters HB. Vision Screening for Elementary Schools: The Orinda Study. Berkeley: University of California Press, 1959.

74. Dobson V, Fulton AB, Manning K, et al. Cycloplegic refractions of premature infants. Am J Ophthalmol 1981;91:490–495.

75. Ingram RM. Refraction of 1-year-old children after atropine cycloplegia. Br J Ophthalmol 1979;63:343–347.

76. Ciner EB. Management of Refractive Error in Infants, Toddlers and Preschool Children. In MM Scheiman (ed), Problems in Optometry—Pediatric Optometry. Philadelphia: Lippincott, 1990;394–419.

77. Anstice J. Astigmatism—its components and their changes with age. Am J Optom Physiol Opt 1971;48:1001.

78. London R, Wick B. Changes in angle lambda during growth: theory and clinical applications. Am J Optom Physiol Opt 1982;59:568.

79. Zonis S, Miller B. Refraction in the Israeli newborn. J Pediatr Ophthalmol Strabismus 1974;2:77.

80. Almeder LM, Peck LB, Howland HC. Prevalence of anisometropia in volunteer laboratory and school screening populations. Invest Ophthalmol Vis Sci 1990;31:2448–2455.

81. Abrahamsson M,Sjostrom A,Sjostrand J. A longitudinal study of changes in infantile anisometropia (abstract 83). Assoc Res Vis Ophthalmol 1989;30 (Suppl):141.

82. Abrahamsson M, Fabian G, Sjostrand J. A longitudinal study of a population based sample of astigmatic children. II. The changeability of anisometropia. Acta Ophthalmol (Copenh) 1990;68:435.

83. Rubin L. The clinical handling of anisometropia. Optical J Rev 1950;15:34–36.

84. Nordlow W. Anisometropia, amblyopia, induced aniseikonia and estimated correction with iseikonic lenses in 4 year olds. Acta Ophthalmol 1970;48:959–970.

85. Davis RJ. Empirical corrections for aniseikonia in preschool anisometropes. Am J Optom Arch Am Acad Optom 1959;36:351–364.

86. Thal LS, Grisham JD. Correcting high anisometropia: two case reports. Am J Optom Physiol Opt 1976;53:85–87.

87. Mohindra I. Early treatment of anisometropic astigmatism and strabismus. Am J Optom Physiol Opt 1977;54:479–484.

88. Fletcher MC, Brandom S. Myopia of prematurity. Am J Ophthalmol 1955;40:474–480.

89. Scharf J, Zonis S, Zeltzer M. Refraction in Israeli premature babies. J Pediatr Ophthalmol 1975;12:193.

90. Yamamoto M, Tatsugami H, Bun J. A follow-up study of refractive error in premature infants. Jpn J Ophthalmol 1979;23:435–443.

91. Fledelius H. Prematurity and the eye. Acta Ophthalmol 1976;128(Suppl):78–98.

92. Lomichkova H. Notes on myopia in premature infants. Cs Oftalmologov 1964;20:195–201.

93. Graham MV, Gray OP. Refraction of premature babies' eyes. Br Med J 1963;1:1452–1453.

94. Scharf J, Zonis S, Zeltzer M. Refraction in premature babies: a prospective study. J Pediatr Ophthalmol Strabismus 1978;15:48–50.

95. Wibaut F. Biologisch-statistische Refraktionsuntersuchungen. Master's thesis, Amsterdam, 1932.

96. Goss DA. Childhood Myopia. In T Grosvenor, M Flom (eds),Refractive Anomalies:Research and Clinical Applications. Boston: Butterworth, 1991;82.

97. Rouse MW, Cooper JS, Cotter SA, et al. Optometric Clinical Practice Guideline. St. Louis:American Optometric Association, 1994.

98. Goss DA, Eskridge JB. Myopia. In J Amos (ed), Diagnosis and Management in Vision Care. Boston: Butterworth, 1987;122.

99. Ingram RM. Refraction as a basis for screening children for squint and amblyopia. Br J Ophthalmol 1977;61:8–12.

100. Martin G. Amblyopie astigmatique. Condition du developpement parfait de la vision. Bull Soc Ophtalmol Fr 1890;8:217.

101. Mitchell DE, Freeman RD, Millodot M, Haegerstrom G. Meridional amblyopia: evidence for modification of the human visual system by early visual experience. Vision Res 1973;13:535–558.

102. Dobson V, Howland HC, Moss C, et al. Photorefraction of normal and astigmatic infants during viewing of patterned stimuli. Vision Res 1983;10:1043.

103. Gwiazda J, Mohindra I, Brill S, et al. Infant astigmatism and meridional amblyopia. Vision Res 1985; 25:1269.

104. Gwiazda J, Mohindra I, Brill S, Held R. The development of visual acuity in infant astigmats. Invest Ophthalmol Vis Sci 1985;26:1717–1723.

105. Held R. Development of Visual Acuity in Normal and Astigmatic Infants. In SJ Cool, EL Smith (eds), Frontier in Visual Science. Berlin:Springer, 1978;712–719.

106. Mohindra I, Jacobson SG, Thomas J, Held R. Development of amblyopia in infants. Trans Ophthalmol Soc U K 1979;99:344–346.

107. Ingram RM, Walker C. Refraction as a means of predicting squint or amblyopia in preschool siblings of children known to have these defects. Br J Ophthalmol 1979;63:238–242.

108. Hirsch MJ. Changes in astigmatism during the first eight years of school—an interim report from the Ojai longitudinal study. Am J Optom Arch Am Acad Optom 1963;40:127.

109. Malik SRK, Gupta AK, Choudhry S. Anisometropia: its relation to amblyopia and eccentric fixation. Br J Ophthalmol 1968;52:773–776.

110. Schapero M. Amblyopia. Philadelphia: Chilton, 1971;35–55.

111. Jampolsky A, Flom BC, Weymouth FW, et al. Unequal corrected visual acuity as related to anisometropia. Arch Ophthalmol 1955;54:893.

112. Ingram RM, Walker C. Refraction as a means of predicting squint or amblyopia in preschool siblings of children known to have these defects. Br J Ophthalmol 1979;63:238–242.

113. Peters HB, Blum HL, Bettman JW, et al. The Orinda Vision Study. Am J Optom Physiol Opt 1959; 36:455–469.

114. Von Noorden GK. Binocular Vision and Ocular Motility. Princeton:Mosby, 1985;280.

115. Calorosa EE, Rouse MW. Clinical Management of Strabismus. Boston: Butterworth,1993.

116. Smith EL, Fung L, Harwerth RS. Effects of optically induced blur on the refractive status of young monkeys. Vision Res 1994;34(3):293–301.

117. Atkinson J. Infant Vision Screening: Prediction and Prevention of Strabismus and Amblyopia from Refractive Screening in the Cambridge Photorefraction Program. In K Simons (ed), Early Visual Development: Normal and Abnormal. New York: Oxford, 1993;342.

118. Iacobucci IL, Archer SM, Giles CL. Children with exotropia responsive to spectacle correction of hyperopia. Am J Ophthalmol 1993;116:79–83.

119. Ciner EB, Herzberg H. Optometric management of optically induced consecutive exotropia. J Am Optom Assoc 1992;63:266–271.

120. Eames TH. Comparison of eye conditions among 1000 reading failures, 500 ophthalmic patients and 150 unselected children. Am J Optom Physiol Opt 1948;31:713–717.

121. Rosner J, Rosner J. Comparison of visual characteristics in children with and without learning difficulties. Am J Optom Physiol Opt 1987;64:531–533.

122. Young FA. Reading, measures of intelligence and refractive errors. Am J Optom Physiol Opt 1963;40:257–264.

123. Grosvenor T. Refractive state, intelligence test scores and academic ability. Am J Optom Physiol Opt 1970;47:355–361.

124. Rosner J, Rosner J. Some observations of the relationship between the visual perceptual skills development of young hyperopes and age of first lens correction. Clin Exp Optom 1986;69:166–168.

125. Rosner J, Gruber J. Differences in the perceptual skills development of young myopes and hyperopes. Am J Optom Physiol Opt 1985;62:501–504.

126. Walton HN, Schubert DG, Clark D, Burke W. Effects of induced hyperopia. Am J Optom Physiol Opt 1978;55:451.

127. Garzia RP, Nicholson SB, Gaines CS, et al. Effects of nearpoint visual stress on psycholinguistic processing in reading. J Am Optom Assoc 1989;60:38–44.

128. Birnbaum MH. Functional relationship between myopia, accommodative stress and against-the-rule astigmia: a hypothesis. J Am Optom Assoc 1978;49:911–914.

129. Laird K. Anisometropia. In T Grovenor, MC Flom (eds), Refractive Anomalies—Research and Clinical Applications. Boston: Butterworth,1991;174.

130. Ciner EB, Macks B, Schanel-Klitsch E. A cooperative demonstration project for early intervention vision service. Occup Ther Pract 1991;3(1):42–56.

131. Wesson MD, Maino DM. Oculovisual Findings in Children with Down Syndrome, Cerebral Palsy, and Mental Retardation without Specific Etiology. In DM Maino (ed), Diagnosis and Management of Special Populations. Philadelphia:Mosby, 1995;17–54.

132. Quinn G. Vitreous and Retina. In SJ Isenberg (ed), The Eye in Infancy. Chicago: Yearbook,1989;340–360.

133. Van der Pol BA. Causes of visual impairment in children. Doc Ophthalmol 1986;61:223–228.

134. Hill AE,McKendrick O, Poole JJ, et al. The Liverpool visual assessment team: 10 years' experience. Child Care Health Dev 1986;21:37–51.

135. Press LJ. Prescribing and Fitting of Children's Eyewear. In LJ Press, BD Moore (eds), Clinical Pediatric Optometry. Boston: Butterworth,1993;253.

136. Caltrider N, Jampolsky A. Overcorrecting minus lens therapy for treatment of intermittent exotropia. Ophthalmology 1983;90(10):1160–1165.

137. Beneish OC, Williams F, Polomeno RC, Little JM. Consecutive exotropia after correction of hyperopia. Can J Ophthalmol 1981;169(1):16–18.

138. Michaels DD. Indications for prescribing spectacles. Surv Ophthalmol 1981;25(2):55–74.

139. Moore BD. Contact Lens Problems and Management in Infants, Toddlers and Preschool Children. In MM Scheiman (ed), Problems in Optometry (Vol. 2). Philadelphia:Lippincott, 1990;365–393.

140. Cho MH, Wild BW. Spectacles for Children. In AA Rosebloom, MM Morgan (eds), Principles and Practices of Pediatric Optometry. New York:Lippincott, 1990;192–206.

Chapter 6

Examination Procedures for Infants and Young Children*

Elise B. Ciner

Professional organizations and practitioners generally agree that a child's first eye examination should take place at approximately 6 months of age [1, 2]. With the recent advancements in research and the development of new clinical tools, it is now possible to complete as comprehensive an examination on an infant as would be performed on an adult. Although the result is essentially the same in terms of obtaining an accurate diagnosis, the process by which a young child is examined is different in many ways.

The approach used and actual areas evaluated depend somewhat on the child's age and cognitive and language skills. This chapter presents a model for the evaluation of young children. Although there are many different tests available, those presented represent an optimal test battery. Because the prevalence of ocular disorders is higher in this age group than in older children or young adults [3], it is imperative that the evaluation be completed carefully and thoroughly. Table 6.1 lists the approximate age, developmental factors, and visual concerns for each of these groups.

GENERAL GUIDELINES FOR EXAMINING A YOUNG CHILD

- Schedule appointments when the child is usually awake and alert.

*Reprinted with permission with adaptations from EB Ciner. Examination procedures for infants and children. J Optom Vis Dev 1996;27(2):54–67.

- Learn to work quickly.
- Refrain from wearing a white lab jacket, which may frighten a child.
- Engage the child throughout the examination with eye contact, funny gestures, familiar songs, etc.
- Become knowledgeable about familiar children's characters, such as Elmo, Barney, Lambchop, Puzzle Place characters, and Thomas the Tank Engine.
- Have several of these familiar characters available as pictures, puppets, or toys.
- Use these and other age-appropriate fixation targets for testing.
- Use verbal praise, stickers, or prizes.
- Use an adhesive patch or colorful pirate patch— never have a child hold the occluder for testing.
- Allow the child to remain with a parent or on a parent's lap during testing.

HISTORY

Before examining a young child, it is essential to obtain a comprehensive visual, medical, and developmental history. Table 6.2 lists the components of a comprehensive history for young children. To obtain the information listed easily and quickly, develop a checklist or questionnaire that can be mailed to the parent before the examination. This will save examination time and help ensure that the child does not become fatigued or

Table 6.1. Visual Concerns for Young Children

	Approximate Age	Communication and Language Skills	Visual Concerns
Infants	Birth to 18 mons	Minimal	Congenital malformations Neurologic disorders Ocular pathologies Developmental delays Significant refractive error Strabismus and amblyopia
Toddlers	18 mons to 3 yrs	Beginning receptive and expressive	Moderate refractive error Ocular pathologies Neurologic disorders Developmental delays Accommodative esotropia Amblyopia
Preschoolers	3–5 yrs	Well-developed receptive and expressive	Mild to moderate refractive error Oculomotor dysfunction Significant phorias and tropias Visual perceptual deficiencies Learning difficulties Color vision anomalies

Table 6.2. Information to Obtain When Taking a History on a Young Child

Areas to Assess During History	Examples of Relevant Information
Chief complaint	Routine check; vision problems in family; eye turning; red eyes; rubs eyes; gets close to things
Family vision history	Refractive error; amblyopia; strabismus; blindness
Child's vision history	Previous glasses; patching; medication; surgery; therapy
Pregnancy	Length of pregnancy; illnesses or smoking during pregnancy; prescribed medications; nutrition; hygiene
Delivery	Length of labor; type and duration of delivery; complications during delivery
Postdelivery period	Birth weight; Apgar score; number of days in hospital; jaundice; infections; breathing or swallowing difficulties; birth defects
General health	Asthma; allergies; medications; injuries; illnesses; seizures; HIV; colic; name of pediatrician; date of last physical examination
Development	Normal or delayed; diagnosis of cerebral palsy, Down syndrome, mental retardation, developmental delay, etc.
Previous specialized testing	Neurologic, psychological, nutritional, lead levels, and developmental testing
Special information about the child	Favorite toys, games, and songs; fears child might have

HIV = human immunodeficiency virus.

inattentive because of lengthy discussions between doctor and parent.

EXAMINATION PROCEDURES

The following areas are important to assess in a routine visual evaluation of a young child: (1) visual acuity, (2) binocular status, (3) ocular motilities, (4) color vision, and (5) ocular health. Additional areas that can also be assessed, depending on the chief complaint, age of the child, and diagnosis, are visual fields and contrast sensitivity. These areas, however, are not typically part of the primary care examination of a young child.

Visual Acuity

Visual acuity must be assessed to ensure normal and equal development in each eye and to rule out amblyopia and associated ocular or systemic conditions that could cause reduced vision.

Infants and Toddlers

When examining a very young child who has not yet developed effective communication skills, the optometrist must rely on either objective tests (e.g., retinoscopy) or the behavioral responses of the child (e.g., objects to covering one eye). With the development of tools that quantify behavioral responses, such as preferential looking, it has become relatively easy to complete an accurate assessment of even the youngest infant.

There are many methods to evaluate visual acuity in young children. These include use of an optokinetic nystagmus (OKN) drum, Stycar balls, binocular fixation pattern, and visual evoked response. Each of these has significant limitations, however. For example, the OKN drum and Stycar balls are "motion-detecting" devices. A child with no central vision and greatly reduced visual acuity might still respond to these tests [4]. The binocular fixation pattern test is only useful in detecting a difference in responsiveness between the two eyes, is highly subjective, and requires a significant level of experience to properly interpret the results. Although the visual evoked response provides reliable results, it requires expensive equipment, is time consuming, and is not practical for a clinical setting. Each of these tests can be used as secondary measures to evaluate visual acuity, but they are not the methods of choice.

The clinical method of choice for evaluating visual acuity in young children is forced-choice preferential looking. One device, the Teller Acuity Cards (TACs), has been widely researched and has published, normative values for use in a clinical setting [5, 6]. In this technique, children are shown a gray card with a square grating of black and white stripes set off to one side of the card. If children are able to see the stripes, they will instinctively move their eyes or head toward the pattern. If children cannot see the stripes, both sides will appear to be unpatterned (gray), and no distinct eye or head movement will be observable. The TACs

have a peephole in the center of each card that allows the examiner to observe children's responses without being seen. To prevent bias, it is important for the examiner to be unaware of the side on which the stripes appear until a firm decision as to where the child is looking can be made.

Toddlers and Preschoolers

As with younger children, there are several methods available to examine visual acuity in children who are beginning to develop expressive and receptive language skills. The fact that these children can now communicate allows visual acuity testing to become more sophisticated and closer to the "gold-standard" Snellen charts used for adults. Among the tests available are the HOTV, the tumbling E chart, and the American Optical (AO) picture chart. Each of these has its limitations. For example, the HOTV test requires the child to say or match letters, depending on how the test is administered. In addition, the letters themselves do not blur out equally and thus can give clues to the child. The tumbling E test, in contrast, requires some development of laterality and directionality skills that are not well developed in most toddler and preschool children. The figures on the AO picture chart are often difficult for a child to interpret, do not blur out equally, and usually test only to the 20/30 level.

Both the Broken Wheel Test [7] and the LEA picture symbols [8] are appropriate clinical methods to evaluate visual acuity in toddlers and preschoolers. Each is calibrated for 10 feet and requires minimal development of language skills. The LEA symbols have a slight advantage because this test is based on a logarithmic Minimum Angle of Resolution (logMAR) scale as recommended by the National Research Council Committee on Vision in 1979. [9] Another advantage is the availability of a matching puzzle that children hold on their lap. This allows for motor involvement of the child and is often beneficial in maintaining the child's attention to the task for longer periods, thus allowing a more accurate assessment of visual acuity (Figure 6.1).

Although visual acuity can be evaluated effectively in children from infancy until the time they enter school using the sequence of tests above, it is important to remember that these tests differ in

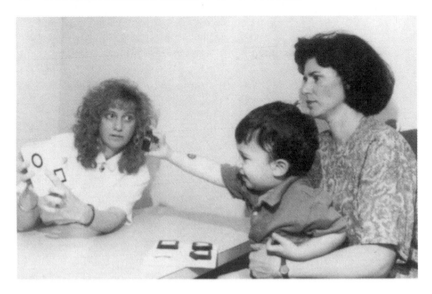

Figure 6.1. LEA symbol test with matching puzzle.

Table 6.3. Comparison of Visual Acuity Testing in Young Children

	Preferential-Looking Test or Teller Acuity Cards Test	LEA Symbol Test or Broken Wheel Test
Type of acuity task	Resolution	Recognition
Distance	Near (typically 55 cm)	Distance and near available
Field size	Large field of target	Small field of target
Communication needed	None	Child must have receptive language skills Child must complete a task
Advantage	Based on child's behavioral "looking" response—easy to accomplish on noncommunicative children	Most closely related to "gold standard" acuity tests for adults
Limitations	May miss strabismic amblyopes, foveal anomalies; valuable for deprivation amblyopia [9–12]	Only appropriate for children who are at a cognitive age of approximately 2–3 yrs

many ways (Table 6.3). These differences may result in an overestimation of visual acuity using preferential looking [10–13].

Refractive Error

See Chapter 5 for an in-depth discussion of the evaluation of refractive error.

Binocular Status

Excellent visual acuity in each eye does not ensure normal visual development in other areas. A child with a 40$^\Delta$ constant alternating esotropia may demonstrate 20/20 visual acuity with each eye, yet have no binocular vision. When evaluating binocular status it is necessary to evaluate both the motor component (how the eyes look) and sensory component (what the eyes see). The motor component is a cosmetic concern when there is a large, manifest strabismus. The sensory component is a functional concern, as amblyopia may be present or lack of depth perception may have an impact on a child's acquisition of normal gross, fine motor, and mobility skills.

Motor Evaluation

The motor evaluation of all young children can be accomplished with either the cover test, Hirschberg

Figure 6.2. Prism-bar assessment of cover test, with a sticker on the examiner's nose for fixation.

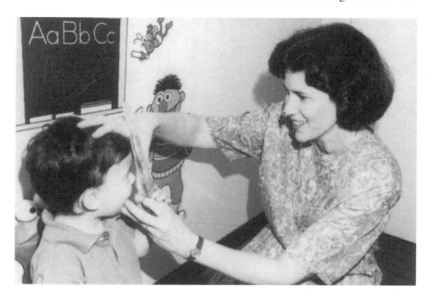

test, or Krimsky test. The Hirschberg and Krimsky tests use the corneal light reflex to evaluate and measure ocular alignment. They give only a rough estimate of alignment and therefore are not sensitive enough to detect large phorias or small tropias [14]. The cover test is more precise and easily administered using the examiner's hand as a cover along with an appropriate fixation target for distance and near. It is important to have an assortment of targets available. An example of appropriate fixation targets at near include illuminated finger puppets or penlights for infants. In older children, it is desirable to use an accommodative target such as a swing toy, a collapsible toy, or an attractive, detailed sticker. It is useful to actually place the sticker on the examiner's nose. This frees up both hands to hold the cover paddle and a prism bar for accurate measurement (Figure 6.2). At distance, a talking Big Bird, hand puppets, other engaging toys, or another person's face could adequately maintain the child's attention long enough to complete testing. The cover test is conducted by resting the examiner's hand on top of the child's head and using the examiner's thumb as a swinging occluder. It is important to have several targets available in case the child tires or becomes bored. To ensure adequate fixation, periodically move the target and watch for the child to change fixation appropriately. The cover test should be repeated in nine positions of gaze at either distance or near to ensure comitance. Table 6.4 lists useful variations on cover testing for young children. It is es-

Table 6.4. Modifications of Cover Testing for Young Children

Modification	Purpose
Use examiner's hand and thumb as occluder	Reduces distractibility in young children
Change target periodically during testing	Increases child's interest and attention
Use distance objects with sound (i.e., talking Big Bird doll)	Allows fixation for distance cover test
Cover test in nine positions of gaze	Tests for comitance
Turn finger-puppet light off periodically	Ensures that the child is fixating properly
Move target periodically during testing	Ensures that the child is fixating properly
Use prolonged occlusion during testing	Helps elicit a latent strabismus
Place colorful sticker on examiner's nose for fixation	Allows examiner to have both hands free to measure deviation with prism

sential to record the magnitude, type (eve, exo, hypo, hyper), comitance, frequency, and laterality of any deviation noted on a cover test.

Supplemental Motor Testing.   The near point of convergence is a supplemental motor test that is useful to perform when an exodeviation is present. The near point of convergence should be within 2–3 in. from the nose using an accommodative target at approximately 3–4 months of age. The break and recovery points are easily observed by the optometrist as a small-detailed, age-appropriate, high-interest target is slowly brought toward the child's nose. Fusional vergence ranges using a prism bar can also be measured in a toddler or preschool child. Children especially enjoy this technique if it is made into a game. For example, if a "bubblegum"-colored sticker is used as a target, the child can be asked to announce when they see the "double bubble" (after the optometrist demonstrates what "double" looks like by using a high amount of prism). Monitoring verbal responses along with careful observation of eye movements makes this an easy test to administer to young children.

It is useful to evaluate the centration point when a strabismus (esotropia) is present. An accommodative target is slowly brought toward the child's nose while the optometrist performs a cover test. The centration point is that point in space at which no movement is noted on a cover test. The centration point can be valuable information if the optometrist is considering a program of vision therapy to treat strabismus.

Sensory Evaluation

It is important to obtain a sensory assessment that evaluates the presence of suppression, diplopia, fusion, stereopsis, and anomalous and normal retinal correspondence.

Infants and Toddlers. Although some children are able to respond to tests such as the stereo fly or the random dot butterfly, these targets are often of little interest to the very young child. In addition, the stereo fly is a very rough measure of stereopsis. A child with amblyopia or strabismus could show a positive response to this test. The only test currently available to evaluate stereopsis in preverbal children is the Stereo Smile Test [15]. This test is similar to the TACs, except that the card consists of a random dot pattern with a disparate image in the shape of a face on one side. There is a nonstereo training card that is used to assess the child's ability to understand the task. This is a forced-choice test whereby the test plate is presented in front of the child and the examiner observes whether the child is looking at the stereo smile. This test has no monocular cues, and the child must have reasonable visual acuity (approximately 20/80) and no constant strabismus in order to pass (Figure 6.3).

Toddlers and Preschoolers. For children who are cognitively at a 2- or 3-year level, it is fairly easy to administer one of several tests. Although these children are still readily willing to play the Randot Stereo Smile Test, there are several alternatives available. The Three-Figure Flashlight test is similar to the Worth's four-dot test, except that the stimulus is three figures: a red girl, a green elephant, and a white ball. While wearing anaglyphic (red/green) glasses, children are shown the flashlight at distance, at near, or both, and are asked what pictures they see. The three-bear test is a simple test in which children are shown three small 1-in. bears while they are wearing anaglyphic glasses. They are asked what color each of the bears is [16] (Figure 6.4). Several stereopsis tests are also available, including the Random Dot Butterfly, Lang-Stereo Test, and Goggle-Free Random dot tests [17]. Table 6.5 lists each test of binocularity along with its associated features.

Ocular Motilities

An evaluation of pursuits, saccades, and position maintenance (ability to maintain fixation on a target) are all components of an ocular motility evaluation. It is important to use a high-interest, age-appropriate fixation target and to be ready to change that target periodically if the child begins to lose attention. For infants and young children, targets can range from collapsible toys, small swing toys, or illuminated finger puppets to flicker bulbs, bubbles, or a large hand mirror (Figure 6.5). For older toddlers and preschoolers, a detailed picture or sticker pasted on a tongue depressor is also appropriate. (Table 6.6 lists modifications of ocular motility testing for young children.)

Pursuits

The examiner should note the quality of movement, the presence of nystagmus, limitations in gaze, smoothness of movements, under- and overshoot-

Figure 6.3. Randot Stereo Smile Test: training card and children's polarized glasses (A), test plate (B), and reinforcement for preferential looking (C).

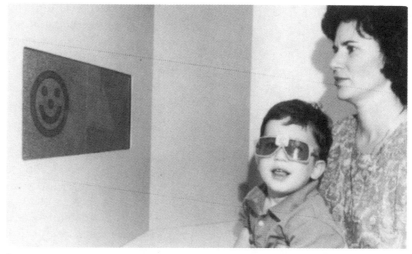

A

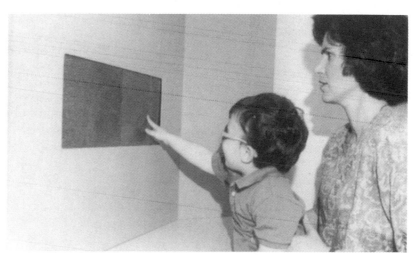

B

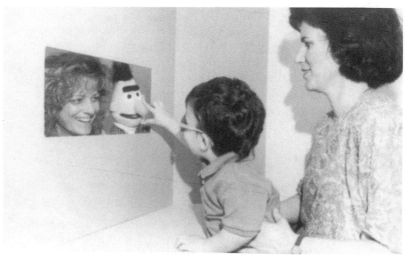

C

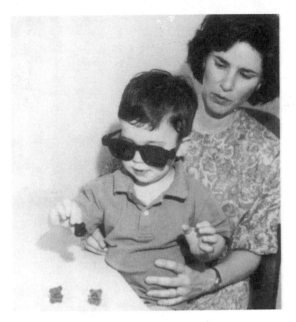

Figure 6.4. The three-bear test.

ing for saccades, the presence of associated head tracking, and the ability to cross the midline. Head tracking and inaccurate saccades could indicate a possible loss of visual field in addition to a motility

problem. Disorders of pursuits can include abnormalities of initiation, velocity, or asymmetries [17].

Saccades

When evaluating saccades, the child is asked to look back and forth between two targets. In young babies, this can easily be accomplished by using two finger puppets on penlights and alternately turning one, then the other, on or off. In older children, use swing or collapsible toys, alternately moving one, then the other, or ask the child to voluntarily look toward each target in succession. Disorders of saccades include abnormalities of speed, latency, and accuracy as well as inappropriate saccades [17].

Position Maintenance

Evaluation of nystagmus can easily be accomplished by careful observation at the time other testing is being completed, including pursuits, saccades, cover test, and retinoscopy. Detection of nystagmus is particularly easy during direct ophthalmoscopy in which the illumination, increases in magnification, and close working distance make it easier to detect

Table 6.5. Interpretation of Sensory Tests of Binocularity

Test	Cognitive Age	Task Required	Normal Retinal Correspondence	Suppression	Anomalous Retinal Correspondence	Diplopia
Worth 4-Dot	4 yrs +	Counts dots	4 dots and no strabismus	2 red or 3 green	4 and strabismus present	5 dots
Three-Figure Flashlight	2 yrs +	Names pictures	3 pictures and no strabismus	2 pictures	3 pictures and strabismus present	4 pictures
Randot Stereofly	1 yr +	Pinches wings	Pinches wings above page	Pinches wings on page	May pinch wings on or above page	Pinches wings on page
Randot Stereo-tests Goggle-Free Stereo Tests Lang-Stereotest Randot Preschool Stereoacuity Test	3 yrs +	Names or matches pictures	Names or matches pictures	No picture seen	No picture seen	No picture seen
Stereo smile	6 mons +	Forced choice	Child looks at face	No preference for face	No preference for face	No preference for face

Figure 6.5. Fixation targets for ocular motility testing.

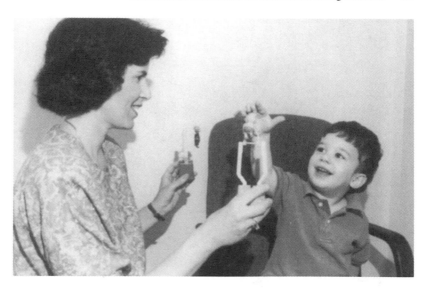

even a low-amplitude nystagmoid eye movement. The presence of a low-amplitude nystagmus is also more easily observable as direct retinoscopy is performed. Evaluation of nystagmus should include an assessment of amplitude, frequency, and type (pendular or jerky), presence of a "null" point, latent nystagmus, associated anomalous head positions or head nodding, and symmetry and conjugacy of the two eyes. Any nystagmus, especially one that is of recent onset and as yet undiagnosed, requires careful consideration of associated systemic and neurologic disorders and appropriate referral [17].

Color Vision

Color vision assessment of young children is typically not a concern until the child is 3–4 years old. At this age, children are often enrolled in a preschool or in day care where many of the reading readiness activities involve color discrimination or sorting. When assessing color vision, it is useful to differentiate an actual color deficiency from difficulty naming or labeling colors [16]. The latter two problems are language-based or perceptual in nature.

Color Naming

The ability to use language skills to name colors is directly related to a child's developmental level or

Table 6.6. Modifications of Ocular Motility Testing for Young Children

Modification	Purpose
Use age-appropriate targets	Increases attention and accuracy of test
Change target periodically during testing	Increases child's interest and attention
Gently hold child's head still while moving the target	Allows for isolation of eye movements from head movements
Test with an OKN drum or tape to look for asymmetries	Allows testing of slow phase of OKN (pursuit) or fast phase of OKN (saccade)
Turn finger-puppet light off periodically	Ensures that child is fixating properly
Observe movement of disc during ophthalmoscopy	May detect small nystagmus
Repeat monocularly	Detects latent nystagmus

OKN = optokinetic nystagmus.

cognitive abilities. When evaluating color naming, any type of identical objects with varying colors can be used. Examples include colored blocks, beads, balls, or bears. An assortment of colors in bright primary, pastel, and darker colors is most useful. It is important to provide good illumination for testing. The examiner points to or isolates one of the objects and asks the child to name the color. Always begin with the primary colors and proceed

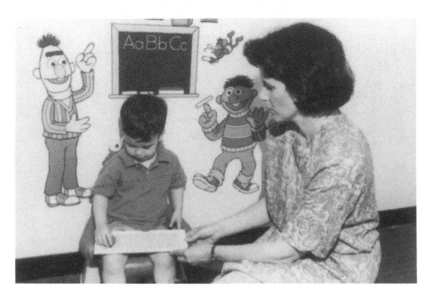

Figure 6.6. Preferential color vision testing with F2 plates.

to the pastel and darker colors. This skill usually develops by the time a child is at a cognitive age of 3–4 years.

Color Identification

This skill evaluates the child's ability to point to various colors without the need for expressive language skills. The same tools and illumination can be used as for color naming. Ask the child to point to each color. Begin with the primary colors and proceed to pastel and darker colors. Identify the colors or shades the child is having difficulty with. This skill is dependent on appropriate receptive language skills and usually develops by approximately age 3–4 years.

Detection of Color Vision Defects

Although color naming and pointing provide useful information for educational programs, it is important to remember that they are not considered acceptable indicators of true color vision deficits. A child with a color deficiency may learn to differentiate colors using other cues, such as brightness or position of objects. Because 1 of 12 boys and 1 of 200 girls have an actual color deficiency, a simple, easy-to-administer test would be ideal to alleviate parental concerns and provide useful educational information. The F2 test, or Pease-Allen Color Test

(PACT) preferential-looking plates test, is a forced-choice test of color vision that can be used beginning in infancy [18]. There is no understanding of the task required. These are pseudoisochromatic, rectangular plates with a square shape visible to color-normal individuals on one side. The examiner holds the plate in front of the child and either asks him or her to point to the square or uses preferential looking by observing eye movements. Alternatively, a matching task can be used in which the child is asked to "park the block" in its matching space (Figure 6.6). These plates are designed to detect mild, moderate, or severe red-green defects and moderate to severe blue-yellow defects [19]. The advantage of this test is that it is simple to understand, very quick to administer, and sensitive to color defects. A newer version uses a happy face as the target in place of the square target [20].

Supplemental Tests of Color Vision

There are several other clinically useful tools for evaluating color vision defects in children, although most are useful for children beginning at approximately 3 years of age because the tests require a higher level of verbal and cognitive skills than the F2 plates.

Portnoy Plates and Berson Plates. The Portnoy plates and Berson plates are similar forced-choice tests [21]. The Portnoy plates test differentiates mild from moderate and severe color defects as well as protan, deutan, and tritan anomalies, whereas the Berson plates test differentiates autosomal, recessive, complete rod monochromacy and sex-linked blue cone monochromasy. These tests use Munsell's colors similar to those used in the D-15 test for adults. The plates consist of four colored circles. The child must point to or identify which one of the four colored circles appears different.

Infant Color Vision Test and Color-Vision-Testing-Made-Easy Test.   The Infant Color vision test and the Color-Vision-Testing-Made-Easy test are pseudoisochromatic plates that present a picture instead of the traditional numbers used in adult color vision tests. The child must identify or point to the picture. These tests identify mild, moderate, or severe color vision defects as well as deutan versus protan anomalies.

PV-16 Quantitative Color Vision Test.   The PV-16 quantitative color vision test is modeled after the adult D-15 test with caps that are larger and easier to handle by young children. This test requires some time to administer but can be useful in older preschoolers when there is a desire to carefully confirm or quantify a color defect.

Ocular Health

A comprehensive ocular health assessment is performed at the completion of the evaluation. This should include assessment of pupils and anterior and posterior ocular health.

Anterior Segment Evaluation

The anterior segment can be evaluated initially by inspection with a penlight. An optimal assessment is performed in a slit-lamp if possible. It is important to check for the following [17]:

- Patent nasolacrimal system
- Pupillary anomalies
- Iris color and appearance
- Intact structures: lids, lashes, sclera, vasculature, cornea, anterior chamber, and lens
- Leukocoria

- Ptosis or lid anomalies
- Orbital anomalies
- Palpation of orbital region to detect masses

When the child's age and cooperation prevents the use of a standard slit-lamp, alternative tools include the use of a Burton lamp or, preferably, a portable, hand-held slit-lamp. Ocular pressures are ideally evaluated using a Goldmann tonometer, which is either mounted on a slit-lamp or hand-held. Other tools that are also useful include the portable noncontact (air-puff) tonometer and the Tono-Pen and Schiötz tonometers. Although each of these is fairly easy to administer, the Tono-Pen tonometer requires the least amount of physical contact or patient cooperation.

It is also important to monitor other signs of increased intraocular pressure, including the following [22]:

- Increased corneal diameter
- Corneal clouding
- Large or asymmetric cupping
- Optic atrophy
- Other associated systemic anomalies

Posterior Segment Evaluation

It is important to complete a dilated fundus evaluation using binocular, indirect ophthalmoscopy on all children at their first examination. (See Table 6.7 for suggested procedures.) When cooperation levels are poor, the practitioner may consider referral for evaluation under restraints or general anesthesia. Table 6.8 lists appropriate dilating drops for young children. In general, never use concentrations of phenylephrine of more than 2.5% in children.

When gathering information on the visual skills of a child, it is important for the optometrist to compare his or her findings with a table of expected findings in each area. A general summary of developmental data for each component of the vision evaluation is presented in Table 6.9.

CONCLUSION

This chapter presents a model for evaluating vision in young children. Although representative tests are listed for each of the seven areas evaluated,

Table 6.7. Procedures for Evaluating the Posterior Segment in Young Children

Procedure	Infants	Toddlers	Preschoolers
Stabilize child	√	√	—
Lay the child down in examination chair or on parent's lap	√	—	—
Positioning important	√	√	—
Attempt peripheral views	√	√	√
Often easier to obtain same view (i.e., superior retina) of each eye instead of examining one, then the other eye	√	√	√
Easy to examine infants if they are sound asleep or relaxed (i.e., drinking from a bottle)	√	—	—
Dim ophthalmoscope beam when possible	√	√	√
Use appropriate high-interest targets or lights to guide fixation	√	√	√
Refer for examination under sedation or general anesthesia when cooperation is poor, views unobtainable, or suspect pathology	√	√	√
Consider using dilating spray to increase cooperation and avoid drops [27]	—	√	√

Table 6.8. Dilating Agents for Young Children

Age	Dilating Agents[a]
Newborn to 6 mons	1 drop Cyclomydril[b] or 1 drop 0.5% or 1% tropicamide (Mydriacyl)
6 mons to 1 yr	1 drop Cyclomydril or 0.5% or 1% tropicamide and 2.5% phenylephrine
1–5 yrs	0.5% or 1% tropicamide and 2.5% phenylephrine

[a]All drops generally preceded by 1 drop of a local anesthetic to promote drug action.
[b]Cyclomydril = 0.2% cyclopentolate and 1% phenylephrine in combination.
Source: Adapted from EB Ciner, ML Parisi, H Herzberg. Pediatric Optometry. In K Alexander (ed), The Lippincott Manual of Primary Eye Care. Philadelphia: Lippincott, 1995;438.

there are other commercially available products that may provide similar results. Although a complete listing of all available products is beyond the scope of this chapter, this information can be found elsewhere in comprehensive chapters and texts devoted to pediatric vision care [17, 23–26]. Each optometrist should identify which equipment and special techniques provide the maximum information and ease of administration. With knowledge, patience, and caring, the evaluation of young children can be enjoyable and rewarding for both doctor and child.

Table 6.9. Early Visual Development

Area Tested	Level of Skill at Birth	Rapid Changes in Visual Skills
Visual acuity	20/600 grating with FPL at 1 mon [28]	20/20 grating acuity at 3 yrs
Binocularity		
Motor alignment	Strabismus may be present; vergence slower, less magnitude, no fusional vergence to prism present [29, 30]	Eyes should be straight by 6 mons; fusional vergence to prism present [31]
Stereopsis	No stereopsis present	Emerges at 3–4 mons; adult-like by 6 mons to 2 yrs [28, 29, 32–34]
Ocular motilities		
Pursuits	Brief and intermittent responses interspersed with saccades [35–37]	Normal by 6–8 wks of age [29, 36, 37]
Saccades	Present at birth. Until 2 mons, hypometric with a large latency [38–40]	2 mons of age, large single saccades to reach fixation target
Accommodation	Focusing errors for distance to 1 mon [41–44]	Adult-like by 3–4 mons [41–44]
Refractive error	Moderate hyperopia at birth, large amounts of astigmatism common [22, 41, 45–47]	Continues to change dramatically during first 5 yrs [22, 41, 45–47] Trends include the following: • Decrease in astigmatism • Decrease in anisometropia • Decrease in hyperopia and myopia • Shift from hyperopia to emmetropia
Color vision	Blue cones at 1 mon; dichromats at 2 mons [39, 48, 49]	Trichromats at 3 mons [28, 50]
Ocular health	Macula immature [39]	Fovea adult-like by 45 mons [51]

FPL = forced-choice preferential looking.

REFERENCES

1. Scheiman MM, Amos CS, Ciner EB, et al. Pediatric Eye and Vision Examination. Optometric Clinical Practice Guideline. St. Louis: American Optometric Association, 1994.
2. Committee on Practice and Ambulatory Medicine. Vision screening and eye examination in children. Pediatrics 1986;77:918–919.
3. Scheiman M, Gallaway M, Coulter H, et al. Prevalence of vision and ocular disease conditions in a clinical pediatric population. J Am Optom Assoc 1996;67:193–202.
4. Wang FM. Perinatal Ophthalmology. In PD Duane, EA Jaeger (eds), Clinical Ophthalmology (Vol 5). Philadelphia: Lippincott, 1984;14–16.
5. Salomao SR, Ventura DF. Large sample population age norms for visual acuities obtained with Vistech-Teller Acuity Cards. Invest Ophthalmol Vis Sci 1995;36:657–670.
6. Mayer DL, Beiser AS, Warner AF, et al. Monocular acuity norms for the Teller Acuity Cards between one month and four years. Invest Ophthalmol Vis Sci 1995;36:671–685.
7. Richman JE, Petito GT, Cron M. Broken Wheel Acuity Test: a new and valid test for preschool and exceptional children. J Am Optom Assoc 1984;55:561–565.
8. Orel-Bixler D, Moore B, Ciner E, et al. Validity of the LEA symbols visual acuity chart. Optom Vis Sci 1995;72:198.
9. National Research Council Committee on Vision. Recommended standard procedures for the clinical measurement and specification of visual acuity 1979. Adv Ophthalmol 1980;41:103.
10. Birch EE, Stager DR. Prevalence of good visual acuity following surgery for congenital unilateral cataract. Arch Ophthalmol 1988;106:40–43.
11. Birch EE, Stager DR. Monocular acuity and stereopsis in infantile esotropia. Invest Ophthalmol Vis Sci 1985;25:1624–1630.
12. Catalano RA, Simon JW, Perkins PL, Kandel GL. Preferential looking as a guide for amblyopia therapy in monocular infantile cataracts. J Pediatr Ophthalmol Strabismus 1987;24:56–63.
13. Stager DR. Preferential looking and recognition acuities in clinical amblyopia: discussion. J Pediatr Ophthalmol Strabismus 1991;28:326–327.
14. Griffin JR. Diagnosis of a Deviation of the Visual Axes. In JR Griffin (ed), Binocular Anomalies: Procedures for Vision Therapy. Chicago: Professional Press, 1982;3–4.

15. Ciner EB, Schanel-Klitsch E, Herzberg H. Stereoacuity development: 6 months to 5 years: a new tool for testing and screening. Optom Vis Sci 1996;73:43–48.

16. Ciner EB, Appel S, Graboyes M, Zambone AM. Assessment and rehabilitation of children with special needs. Optom Clin 1996;5:187–226.

17. Ciner EB, Parisi M, Herzberg H. Pediatric Optometry. In K Alexander (ed), The Lippincott Manual of Primary Eye Care. Philadelphia: Lippincott, 1995;442–498.

18. Pease PL, Allen J. A new test for screening color vision: concurrent validity and utility. Am J Optom Physiol Opt 1988;65:729–738.

19. Mohindra I. A non-cycloplegic refraction technique for infants and young children. J Am Optom Assoc 1977;48:518–523.

20. Ventocilla M, Orel-Bixler D, Haegerstrom-Portnoy G. Pediatric color vision screening: AO HRR vs. Mr. Color. Optom Vis Sci 1995;72(12S):203.

21. Haegerstrom-Portnoy G. Color Vision. In A Rosenbloom, M Morgan (eds), Principles and Practice of Pediatric Optometry. Philadelphia: Lippincott, 1990;449–466.

22. Mohindra I, Held R. Refraction in humans from birth to five years. Doc Ophthalmol 1981;28:19–27.

23. Press L, Moore B. Clinical Pediatric Optometry. Boston: Butterworth, 1993.

24. Rosner J, Rosner J. Pediatric Optometry (2nd ed). Boston: Butterworths, 1990.

25. Scheiman M. Problems in Optometry—Pediatric Optometry (Vol 2, No 3). Philadelphia: Lippincott, 1990.

26. Rosenbloom A, Morgan M. Principles and Practice of Pediatric Optometry. Philadelphia: Lippincott, 1990.

27. Bartlett JD, Wesson MD, Swiatocha J, Woolley T. Efficacy of a pediatric cycloplegic administered as a spray. J Am Optom Assoc 1993;64:617–621.

28. Teller DY. The Development of Visual Function in Infants. In B Cohen, L Bodis-Wollner (eds), Vision and the Brain. New York: Raven, 1990;109–118.

29. Cron MT, Garzia R, Richman J. Infant visual development. J Optom Vis Dev 1986;17:6–18.

30. Slater AM, Findlay JM. Binocular fixation in the newborn baby. J Exp Child Psychol 1975;20:248–273.

31. Aslin RN. Development of binocular fixation in human infants. J Exp Child Psychol 1977;23:133–150.

32. Fox R, Aslin RN, Shea SL, Dumais ST. Stereopsis in human infants. Science 1980;207:323–324.

33. Birch EE, Gwiazda J, Held R. Stereoacuity development for crossed and uncrossed disparities in human infants. Vision Res 1982;22:507–513.

34. Ciner EB, Schanel-Klitsch E, Herzberg H. Stereoacuity development: 6 months to 5 years. Optom Vis Sci 1996;73:44–48.

35. Kreminitzer JP, Vaughan HB, Kurtzberg D, Dowling K. Smooth-pursuit eye movements in the newborn infant. Child Dev 1979;50:442–448.

36. McGinnis JM. Eye movements and optic nystagmus in early infancy. Genet Psychol Monogr 1930;8:321–340.

37. Aslin RN. Development of Smooth Pursuit in Human Infants. In DF Fisher, RA Monty, JW Senders (eds), Eye Movements: Cognition and Visual Perception. Hillsdale, NJ: Lawrence Eribaum, 1981;31.

38. Tronick E, Clanton C. Infant looking patterns. Vision Res 1971;11:1479–1486.

39. Boothe RG, Dobson V, Teller DY. Postnatal development of vision in human and nonhuman primates. Annu Rev Neurosci 1985;8:495–545.

40. Aslin RN, Salapatek P. Saccadic localization of visual targets by the very young human infant. Percept Psychophys 1975;17:293–302.

41. Banks MS. Infant refraction and accommodation. Int Ophthalmol Clin 1979;20:205–232.

42. Braddick O, Atkinson J, French J, Howland HC. A photorefractive study of infant accommodation. Vision Res 1979;19:1319–1330.

43. Haynes H, White BL, Held R. Visual accommodation in human infants. Science 1965;148:528–530.

44. Banks MS. The development of visual accommodation during early infancy. Child Dev 1980;51:646–666.

45. Ingram RM, Barr A. Changes in refraction between the ages of 1 and 3 1/2. Br J Ophthalmol 1979;63:339–342.

46. Abrahamsson M, Fabian G, Sjostrand J. Changes in astigmatism between the ages of 1 and 4 years: a longitudinal study. Br J Ophthalmol 1988;72:145–149.

47. Ciner EB. Refractive error in young children. Evaluation and prescription. Pract Optom 1992;3:182–187.

48. Peeples DR, Teller DY. Color vision and brightness discrimination in two month old human infants. Science 1975;189:1102–1103.

49. Boynton RM. Human Color Vision. New York: Holt, Rinehart & Winston, 1979.

50. Teller DY, Bornstein MH. Color Vision. In P Salapatek, L Cohen (eds), Handbook of Infant Perception (Vol 1). New York: Academic Press, 1987;185–236.

51. Hendrickson AK, Youdelis C. The morphological development of the human fovea. Ophthalmology 1984;91:603–612.

Chapter 7

Electrodiagnostics, Ultrasound, Neuroimaging, and Photorefraction

Deborah Orel-Bixler

Technological advances have made noninvasive assessment of the human visual system possible through the use of electrodiagnostics, neuroimaging, ultrasound, and photorefraction. This chapter reviews these specialized techniques and their clinical application for the diagnosis of vision disorders and eye disease in the pediatric population. Electrodiagnostics includes the electroretinogram (ERG), electro-oculogram (EOG), and the visual evoked potential (VEP) to assess function of the retina, retinal pigment epithelium, and visual cortex, respectively. Neuroimaging provides in vivo depiction of normal and pathologic central nervous system (CNS) structures. Diagnostic tests in neuroimaging include computed tomography (CT), magnetic resonance imaging (MRI), and positron emission tomography (PET). A-scan and B-scan ultrasound provide imaging of the orbit and measurement of ocular structures. The chapter concludes with a review of photorefraction, a photographic technique that has received much interest as a means of vision screening for amblyogenic factors in infants and preverbal children.

ELECTRODIAGNOSTICS

Electrodiagnostics serve primarily as an adjunct to the clinical impression of an ocular or visual system disorder. The ERG and EOG can provide information that aids in the diagnosis of disturbance of retinal function. The VEP can provide information to aid in the diagnosis of disturbance of the visual pathway up to the level of the visual cortex. Often, electrodiagnostic test results are abnormal before ophthalmoscopic changes are noted. Furthermore, electrodiagnostics can be used to verify the patient's subjective account of a vision problem as well as to assess visual function in patients from whom a subjective account is not possible (e.g., infants, nonverbal children, and patients with multiple disabilities).

Electroretinogram

The ERG is a measure of the bioelectrical response generated in the retina in response to stimulation by light. The clinical ERG is recorded with a contact lens recording electrode under both light-adapted (photopic) and dark-adapted (scotopic) viewing conditions using single and multiple flash presentations. The amplitude (size of the response) and latency (time for the response to occur) of the ERG components are compared with normative data to establish the clinical diagnosis.

Clinical Paradigm for the Electroretinogram

The components needed for recording the ERG are a light source, recording electrodes, an amplification system, and a device for registering the amplified response. [For more information on international standards for ERG protocol and technical specifications, see references 1 and 2.]

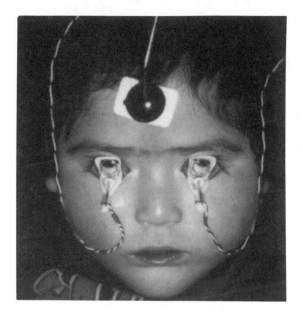

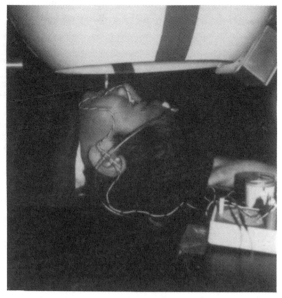

Figure 7.1. Pediatric Burian-Allen electroretinogram recording electrodes and their placement. (Courtesy of Wayne Verdon, O.D., Ph.D.)

Figure 7.2. An overhead mounted Ganzfeld allows the infant or child to recline during the electroretinogram testing session. (Courtesy of Wayne Verdon, O.D., Ph.D.)

The standard ERG recording electrode is the Burian-Allen corneal electrode, which is a ring of stainless steel (active electrode) surrounding a central polymethylmethacrylate core [3]. The attached lid speculum has a conductive coating of silver to serve as the reference electrode. An additional ground electrode is typically placed on the forehead or earlobe. The ERG recording electrodes and placement are illustrated in Figure 7.1. A topical ophthalmic anesthetic and a methylcellulose cushioning solution are needed with contact lens electrodes. The pupils are maximally dilated to control retinal illumination.

The Burian-Allen electrode is available in sizes appropriate for adults as well as premature infants [3]. The ERG can also be recorded using skin electrodes rather than a corneal electrode. This is an alternative when testing noncooperative patients such as infants and children. However, the amplitude of the ERG measured with skin electrodes is reduced 10–100× that measured with corneal electrodes [4] and therefore may not be comparable to established norms. In one study, ERGs measured with infraorbital electrodes were one-eighth the size of the flash ERG obtained with corneal electrodes; however, reliable ERGs could be obtained when signal averag-

ing was used [5]. Although corneal electrodes remain the preferred recording device, even in infants and children, recording from sedated or anesthetized young patients is not recommended as the first line of approach, since anesthesia or sedation may alter the electrophysiologic responses [6].

The typical light source used to elicit the ERG is a xenon-arc photo stimulator presented as a full field in a Ganzfeld dome (diffusing sphere) (Figure 7.2.) The ERG protocol states that the procedure should begin with a period of dark adaptation [1, 2]. The first response measured after dark adaptation is the rod response to either a dim white flash or blue light (equated to the white standard). Next, the maximal response elicited by a single white standard flash is recorded in the dark-adapted eye. After a 10-minute period of light adaptation to a background luminance that serves as a rod-suppressing background, the single-flash cone response is recorded. The cone-generated response to flicker concludes the testing.

Electroretinogram Components and Interpretation

The components of the ERG vary depending on the adaptation state, light level, and stimulus parame-

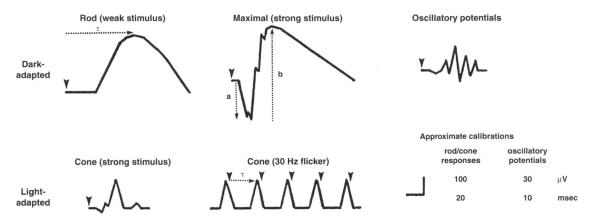

Figure 7.3. The five basic electroretinogram responses. These waveforms are for example only, and are not intended to indicate minimum, maximum, or even average values. Dotted arrows indicate the measurement of implicit time (time to peak) in a and b waves. (Reprinted with permission from MF Marmor, GB Arden, S Nilsson, E Zrenner. Standard for Clinical Electrophysiology. In JR Heckenlively and GB Arden [eds], Principles and Practice of Clinical Electrophysiology of Vision. St. Louis: Mosby–Year Book, 1991;283–288.)

ters used to elicit the ERG. These components include the early receptor potential, a-wave, b-wave, oscillatory potentials (OP), c-wave, d-wave, and flicker response.

The a-wave is a negative wave with a photopic or cone component (a1) and a scotopic or rod component (a2). It originates in the retinal photoreceptors. The b-wave is a positive wave with a photopic component (b1) ascribed to cone activity and a scotopic component (b2) ascribed to rod activity. It originates in the bipolar layer, mostly in the cells of Mueller. Under scotopic, high-intensity flash conditions, OPs appearing as 3–5 wavelets on the ascending limb of a b-wave may be recorded using a high-pass filter setting. The OP originates in the inner nuclear layer (bipolar/amacrine cells) and is thought to be sensitive to oxygen deprivation. It may have limited value since it is difficult to elicit in normals. The 30-Hz flicker response is mediated by cones since rods do not follow flicker past 20 Hz.

The five basic ERG responses include a maximal response in the dark-adapted eye, a response developed by rods (in the dark-adapted eye), oscillatory potentials, a response developed by cones, and responses obtained to flicker (Figure 7.3). Interpretation of the ERG and comparison with norms are based on the amplitude and implicit time of the ERG components. Amplitude of the a-wave is measured from the baseline voltage to the maximum

voltage of the a-wave. Amplitude of the b-wave is measured from the a-wave maximum to the b-wave maximum voltage. Implicit time is measured from stimulus onset to the corresponding waveform peak (see Figure 7.3).

Table 7.1 lists the "normal" range of ERG values for amplitude and implicit time under maximum-intensity stimuli conditions. Each electrodiagnostic laboratory needs to establish its own norms based on stimulus intensity [7].

Value of the Electroretinogram in the Infant

Developmental Changes in the Electroretinogram. An ERG can be recorded from infants within a few hours after birth. Implicit times are prolonged compared with adult values [8]. By 2 months of age, the photopic component is comparable to adult values, but the dark-adapted b-wave is about half the amplitude of an adult's [8]. The dark-adapted b-wave amplitude reaches adult values by 1 year of age [9]. The largest developmental changes in the ERG occur in the first year. In general, the interpretation of electrophysiologic responses depends upon comparisons to age-matched norms. It may be difficult to interpret the results when an infant has clinically abnormal vision yet a recordable ERG. Often serial testing will be necessary for a conclusive diagnosis [10].

Table 7.1. Normal Ranges for Electroretinogram Values with Maximum-Intensity Stimuli

		Amplitude (µV)	Implicit Time (ms)
A-wave	Photopic	20–50	14–20
	Scotopic	190–300	20–26
B-wave	Photopic	90–180	26–34
	Scotopic	400–700	40–56

Source: Reprinted with permission from GA Fishman. Measurements of the ERG Components in Electrophysiologic Testing in Disorders of the Retina, Optic Nerve, and Visual Pathway. In GA Fishman and S Sokol (eds), Ophthalmology Monographs 2. San Francisco: American Academy of Ophthalmology, 1990;9.

Clinical Value of the Electroretinogram in Infants. The ERG is particularly useful in the differential diagnosis of four disorders of the retina that produce vision impairment and nystagmus in an infant without producing obvious retinal or eyeground changes. These disorders include (1) achromatopsia, (2) albinism, (3) congenital stationary night blindness, and (4) Leber's congenital amaurosis.

ACHROMATOPSIA. Achromatopsia, or rod monochromacy, has an autosomal recessive inheritance pattern and an incidence of 0.003% [11, 12]. It is characterized by extremely reduced or absent cone function resulting in reduced visual acuity (20/160 on average) [13], very little if any color vision, nystagmus, and significant photophobia [12, 14]. The fundus appearance is normal.

The diagnosis of achromatopsia can be confirmed by an ERG that shows normal or near-normal dark-adapted (scotopic) responses but extremely reduced or absent light-adapted (photopic) responses (Figure 7.4) [15].

There is no medical treatment for achromatopsia per se. Appropriate refractive error correction and use of low vision aids [16] and adaptations to compensate for the photophobia, such as wearing sunglasses with very low transmission and squinting by partial closure of the eyelids, will help improve the person's ability to function [17]. Standard gray sunglass tints generally do not provide adequate relief from the photophobia since they are rarely made dark enough (<1% transmission). Individuals with achromatopsia are effectively light blind due to rod

saturation in bright lights. Since rods are very insensitive to long-wavelength radiation (red light), red-tinted lenses with side shields turn daylight into dusk and allow affected individuals to maintain optimal vision function even in bright daylight (Plate 7.1). Red lenses have anecdotally been reported to be an effective intervention for photophobia in adults [17]. In children with achromatopsia, early intervention with red lenses corresponded to a more rapid improvement in visual acuity and earlier attainment of adult-like levels [18].

Because cone function is virtually absent in achromatopsia, the condition is of particular interest in vision research since the rod visual system can be studied independent of cone intrusion. The development of visual acuity of the rod visual system has been studied by measuring visual acuity development in achromats. The rod-mediated visual acuity in achromats is not fully developed at birth and improves during the first three years of life. Rod-mediated visual acuity shows a similarly shaped developmental time course to cone-mediated visual acuity but it is delayed in time compared to cone acuity [19].

Blue cone monochromatism should be considered a possibility in males with nystagmus, poor vision, and photophobia that is less severe than that of rod monochromats. Blue cone monochromatism is an X-linked recessive disorder. Affected males have normal rod and blue (short-wavelength sensitive) cone function [14] but dichromat color vision at low photopic light levels, which can be revealed with the Berson test for color vision [20]. The ERG findings are identical to those in the rod monochromat. The differential diagnosis for blue-cone versus rod monochromacy is accomplished through mode of inheritance and psychophysical testing including measures of spectral sensitivity and the Berson test. Magenta-tinted lenses are recommended to protect the rods from saturation and provide relief from the photophobia but to also allow retention of dichromat color vision by permitting transmission of blue light [21].

ALBINISM. Albinism is a heterogeneous group of congenital hypomelanotic disorders with at least 10 distinct forms of oculocutaneous albinism and four types of ocular albinism [22]. Mild forms of albinism are inherited as an autosomal dominant trait, severe forms are inherited as autosomal recessive

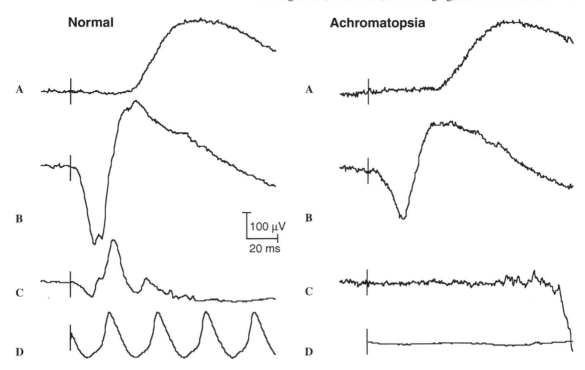

Figure 7.4. Electroretinogram recordings from an adult with normal vision and achromatopsia using the following stimuli: (A) dim flash to the dark-adapted eye, (B) bright flash to a dark-adapted eye, (C) single flash to a light-adapted eye, and (D) 30-Hz flicker to a light-adapted eye. The cone-mediated responses to a single flash under photopic conditions and 30-Hz flicker are absent in the adult with achromatopsia. (Courtesy of Wayne Verdon, O.D., Ph.D.)

traits, and ocular albinism is typically an X-linked recessive trait. In ocular albinism, the hypopigmentation of the iris and retinal pigment epithelium manifests clinically as iris transillumination, macular hypoplasia, and chorioretinal hypopigmentation. The extent of ocular involvement varies greatly but nystagmus, reduced vision, and photophobia are usually present. The reduced visual acuity in albinism (20/70 or worse) is due to foveal hypoplasia. Rods are present in the fovea and cones are distributed away from the fovea [23]. Mild ocular or oculocutaneous albinism have often been misdiagnosed as idiopathic congenital nystagmus [24].

Electrodiagnostic testing can aid in the differential diagnosis of albinism. The amplitude of the scotopic ERG exceeds the normal range in all forms of albinism. The most sensitive and specific test to diagnose albinism, however, is the VEP. There is an asymmetry in the amplitude of the VEP recorded from the cerebral hemispheres [25]. This asymmetry reflects the underlying anatomic miswiring in albinism. Axons from the temporal retina (within 20

degrees of the vertical midline) erroneously cross at the chiasm, resulting in an abnormal layering of the lateral geniculate nucleus and an abnormal visual pathway to the visual cortex.

The appropriate interventions for ocular albinism include tinted lenses for photophobia and low vision aids [23]. Since color vision is normal in albinism, red-tinted lenses are inappropriate, since this tint reduces color discrimination abilities.

CONGENITAL STATIONARY NIGHT BLINDNESS.   There are several forms of congenital stationary night blindness: autosomal recessive, autosomal dominant, and X-linked inheritance types. The X-linked disorder is the most difficult to diagnose due to the normal fundus appearance. Clinical manifestations of congenital stationary night blindness (CSNB) include poor night vision, myopia in the range of −4.00 to −8.00 D, nystagmus, and reduced visual acuity ranging from 20/40 to 20/200 [14]. Peripheral visual fields are normal, and the dark adaptation curve shows no abnormalities of the cone photoreceptors in children able to complete the task. The disorder is nonprogressive.

The major abnormality shown in the ERG, which is also diagnostic, is the absence of a positive response (b-wave) in the scotopic ERG [26, 27]. The initial negative response (a-wave) is normal. The presumed abnormality is one of neural transmission in the bipolar cell layer [28].

LEBER'S CONGENITAL AMAUROSIS.   Leber's congenital amaurosis [29] is an autosomal recessive disorder characterized by blindness at birth, the development of roving eye movements or nystagmus during the first few months after birth, sluggish or absent pupillary responses, high ametropia (more commonly high hyperopia) [30], and a relatively normal fundus during infancy. In one study of 45 children with Leber's congenital amaurosis, 75% had a normal fundus appearance during infancy [31]. By 8 years, diffuse pigmentary stippling may be seen, although up to 50% have a normal pigmentary pattern and some have macular dysplasia and pigmentary abnormalities of the peripheral retina. Pigmentary retinopathy with bony spicules, attenuated retinal arterioles, and optic atrophy may emerge gradually [32]. It is believed that the attenuated arterioles are present at birth but rarely detected.

The visual acuity of children with Leber's ranges from no light perception to 20/200. It is rare that it is as good as 20/200, however [31]. Persistent pressing on the eye with the finger or fist is known as the *oculodigital reflex* and is characteristic of children with Leber's and other severe retinal disorders [33]. It has been suggested by Jan et al. [34] that this pressure stimulates the visual cortex by mechanically triggering ganglion cell action potentials, thus producing phosphenes or entoptic flashes of light in the retina. This persistent eye pressing should be discouraged for eye health. Eye pressing disperses the surrounding orbital fat and causes the eyes to appear sunken with time as well.

It is estimated that Leber's accounts for 10–18% of childhood blindness [32] and may be isolated or associated with systemic conditions such as Joubert's syndrome, which is characterized by a specific malformation of the cerebellum, cerebral vermis hypoplasia, and oculomotor anomalies and respiratory problems in the neonatal period [35].

The ERG is the definitive test for establishing the diagnosis of Leber's congenital amaurosis in an infant with visual impairment and nystagmus but normal ocular findings. Both the light-adapted (photopic) and dark-adapted (scotopic) ERG components are markedly reduced or absent [33].

Differential Diagnosis for Vision Impairment in Infancy.   Congenital retinal disorders are usually accompanied by nystagmus, habitual pressing of the eyes, sluggish pupillary responses or pupillary constriction in darkness (CSNB), and highly myopic (CSNB) or hyperopic (Leber's) refractive errors. The ERG aids in the early differential diagnosis of these disorders.

An ERG is not necessary in other disorders that cause nystagmus and vision impairment in infants when abnormal ophthalmoscopy findings are present. Nystagmus and visual impairment in infancy may be associated with ocular abnormalities or media opacities such as bilateral congenital cataracts or corneal opacities, macular scarring, vitreous hemorrhage, retinopathy of prematurity, optic nerve hypoplasia, and optic nerve atrophy. With careful examination, the anomalies of the optic disc are detectable. Fundus signs and nystagmus are absent in infants with vision impairment due to cortical visual impairment and delayed visual maturation. In cases of suspected cortical visual impairment, delayed visual maturation, and optic nerve anomalies little information is gained from an ERG. Instead, a referral for VEP testing and neuroimaging would be recommended (for more information on these procedures, see the sections on neuroimaging and VEP).

Value of the Electroretinogram in Children

Most infantile retinal dystrophies display severe rod and cone involvement from onset. Retinal dystrophies with an onset in childhood involve predominantly the rods or the cones at presentation. The differential diagnosis for retinal dystrophies with an onset in childhood is obtained by comparison of the photopic and scotopic ERG. Fundus abnormalities are often not present early in the disease.

Retinitis Pigmentosa.   Retinitis pigmentosa (RP), a progressive rod-cone dystrophy, is a genetically heterogeneous group of disorders characterized by night blindness, visual field loss, and an abnormal or extinguished ERG [36]. RP inherited in the X-linked or autosomal recessive mode tends to have an earlier onset and more severe involvement than the autosomal dominant type. The dystrophic process primarily affects rods.

Although children with RP may initially present with night blindness or visual field loss, the appearance of the fundus in the early stages of RP is variable and abnormalities may be very subtle in young children. Mild pigment epithelial atrophy in the midperiphery appears early and is followed by pigment deposition in the equatorial retina with narrowing of the retinal arterioles and a waxy, pallid appearance of the optic disc. In more advanced disease, bone spicule pigmentation is seen with optic disc pallor and retinal arteriole attenuation. Visual acuity may decline due to associated posterior subcapsular opacities, macular edema, or macular involvement in the dystrophic process.

Children with RP often lack ophthalmoscopic findings early in the disease; however, the scotopic ERG is absent or reduced in amplitude at an early stage. The ERG photopic responses may be reduced in amplitude but the flicker response may be preserved [36].

Usher's Syndrome. Usher's syndrome is an autosomal recessive disorder characterized by RP and a severe, congenital neurosensory hearing loss [37]. In type I Usher's, the scotopic ERG is usually absent. Profound deafness and an absent or abnormal vestibular response may also be accompanied by mental retardation, ataxia, or psychosis. In type II Usher's, a scotopic ERG of reduced amplitude may be recorded. Hearing loss is variable. Some patients develop intelligible speech and normal vestibular responses. Other neurologic problems are rare [38]. Included in the differential diagnosis for Usher's is congenital rubella with its accompanying pigmentary retinopathy and profound deafness. The ERG is normal in congenital rubella syndrome [39], whereas the scotopic ERG is absent or reduced in amplitude early in Usher's syndrome.

Other Causes of Pigmentary Retinopathy. The differential diagnosis for pigmentary retinopathy may be aided by ERG testing. In congenital rubella syndrome, the most common ocular abnormality is pigmentary retinopathy, which is found in up to 40% of cases [40]. The ERG findings are normal [39], however, and no visual impairment accompanies the disorder. Pigmentary retinopathy may be associated with infectious retinopathy from congenital syphilis and in severe cases may result in extensive pigmentary changes resembling RP. This form of chorioretinitis is referred to as pseudoretinitis pigmentosa. In the chorioretinitis associated with congenital syphilis, diffuse chorioretinitis associated with virus inclusion, and Leber's congenital amaurosis, the ERG is abnormal and visual impairment accompanies the disorder. Attenuated retinal arterioles may be the sole finding in an infant with syphilis or Leber's congenital amaurosis. The ERG distinguishes between these two conditions. In Leber's, the ERG is severely reduced; in syphilis, the ERG is moderately reduced.

Cone-Rod Dystrophy. Cone-rod dystrophy is a hereditary, degenerative retinal disease that primarily affects cones. Unlike achromatopsia, which presents in infancy and is stationary, the progressive cone dystrophies are not usually symptomatic until late childhood or early adulthood and progressive vision loss accompanies the disorder [14]. Clinical signs of cone-rod dystrophy include a bull's eye maculopathy with symptoms of photophobia and progressive loss of central and color vision [41].

In cone-rod dystrophy, the photopic ERG is abnormal. The flicker and photopic b-wave are characteristically absent and the response to a bright flash is decreased. The scotopic b-wave amplitude may be normal.

Electroretinogram Versus Neuroimaging

Neuroimaging, such as an MRI or CT scan, is not usually indicated in children with retinal disorders unless other neurologic abnormalities or developmental delays are present [42]. The ERG is severely reduced in the retinal disorder Leber's congenital amaurosis, which may be accompanied by optic atrophy. Other causes of optic atrophy, without any retinal disorder, have normal ERG findings [43]. Therefore, neuroimaging studies are vital in all infants with optic atrophy or optic nerve hypoplasia [44, 45].

Summary

The ERG confirms the diagnosis in many retinal disorders associated with visual impairment or blindness and nystagmus during infancy. Leber's congenital amaurosis, achromatopsia, albinism, and CSNB have a similar clinical presentation characterized by reduced vision and nystagmus, but the ERG can differentially diagnose these disorders. In Leber's congenital amaurosis, the photopic and scotopic ERG is extinguished. In achromatopsia, the flicker and single flash photopic (cone) ERG is absent. In all forms of albinism, including oculocutaneous albinism, the scotopic ERG is supernormal. In CSNB, the scotopic b-wave is absent. In retinal dystrophies with an onset in childhood (RP and cone-rod dystrophy), abnormal ERG findings may precede the ophthalmoscopic appearance of ocular anomalies.

Electro-Oculogram

The EOG is a measure of the relative electrical potential of the eye. The clinical EOG uses a comparison of the voltage difference between the cornea and the posterior pole of the eye in the light-adapted and dark-adapted state. Physiologically, the EOG is a measure of the slow changes in potential that occur as a result of alterations in the metabolism of the pigment epithelium [46]. Clinically, the EOG is useful in the detection of ocular disorders, especially abnormalities of the retinal pigment epithelium.

Clinical Paradigm for Electro-Oculogram

The equipment required for recording the EOG includes skin electrodes, a direct current or alternating current amplifier for each eye, and a data storage device such as a strip chart recorder, storage oscilloscope, or computer. The recording electrodes are placed on the skin close to the medial and lateral canthus. An additional recording electrode serving as the common ground is typically placed on the forehead. The silver-silver chloride or gold-disc skin electrodes are attached to the skin with double adhesive tape and a small amount of conducting electrode paste after the skin is cleansed with isopropyl alcohol.

The EOG is recorded as the patient alternately fixates on two red light-emitting diodes (LEDs) which are typically presented in a Ganzfeld globe. The LEDs are horizontally separated so that the eyes rotate laterally through a constant angle of about 30 degrees. The EOG protocol requires the attention and cooperation of the patient, who must fixate on the alternately illuminated LEDs several times per minute, repeating these eye excursions at 1-minute intervals for up to 15 minutes in the dark followed by 12 minutes in the light [47]. The eye acts like an electrical dipole inducing an electrical field in the periocular tissue. The electrode in close proximity to the cornea of the eye registers a positive voltage while the electrode in close proximity to the fundus registers a negative voltage. The average amplitude of the EOG (maximum to minimum) during several eye excursions is calculated and plotted in microvolts as a function of time in the recording session.

In the EOG protocol, baseline recordings are obtained during a 5-minute adaptation period, with the background field of the Ganzfeld globe illuminated. The lights are extinguished and the saccadic eye movements producing the EOG are recorded at 1-minute intervals during 12–15 minutes of dark adaptation. The amplitude of the EOG reaches a minimum within 8–9 minutes in the dark. This minimum is referred to as the first dark trough. The background field is then illuminated and the EOG is recorded at 1-minute intervals during 12 minutes in the light. The EOG reaches a maximum amplitude after 8–9 minutes in the light. This maximum is referred to as the first light peak.

The EOG is interpreted by means of the Arden ratio [47], which is calculated using the ratio of the voltage for the light peak (LP) and the dark trough (DT):

$$\text{Arden ratio} = \text{LP/DT} \times 100\%$$

An Arden ratio of more than 180% is considered normal, a ratio of 165–180% is marginally subnormal, and a ratio of less than 165% indicates pathology of the retinal pigment epithelium [7, 47]. Figure 7.5 shows the amplitude of the standing potential of the eye (in microvolts) for the right eye (circles) and left eye (squares) plotted as a function of time (in minutes) for the pre-, dark, and light adaption periods in the EOG recording session. The dark trough

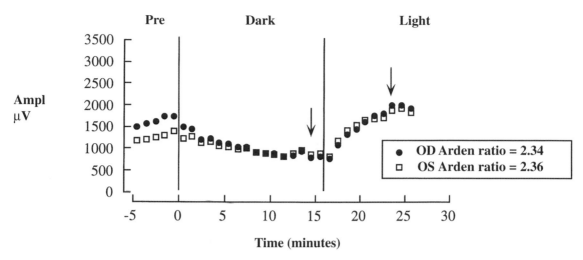

Figure 7.5. Standing potential of the eye as a function of time during the recording of the electro-oculogram (EOG). (Courtesy of Wayne Verdon, O.D., Ph.D.)

and light peak are indicated by arrows. The calculated Arden ratios are normal.

In general, interpretation of electrophysiologic responses depends on comparison to age-matched norms. No age-related changes in Arden ratios have been found [10]; however, due to variations in recording equipment and artifactual electrical noise, each laboratory needs to establish its own norms.

Children older than 5 years of age can generally cooperate sufficiently to complete the EOG protocol. Infants have been tested by inducing passive eye movements via vestibular reflexes [48]. Patients with less than 20/200 acuity may not be able to see the fixation lights but could be requested to make consistent, full excursion eye movements during testing.

Ocular Diseases Associated with an Abnormal Electro-Oculogram

To obtain a normal light peak in the EOG, rods and the retinal pigment epithelium must be functioning, the retina and the retinal pigment epithelium must be in contact, and an adequate choroidal blood supply must be present. An abnormal EOG is found in ocular disorders in which one of these conditions is not fulfilled [14]. These ocular disorders include rod-cone degenerations, cone degenerations, achromatopsia, CSNB, Leber's congenital amaurosis, albinism, toxic retinopathy, diabetic retinopathy, retinal detachment, and vitelliform macular degeneration (Best's disease).

Value of the Electro-Oculogram in Infants

The ERG is more useful than the EOG in the differential diagnosis of retinal disorders in infancy. The ERG findings in achromatopsia, albinism, CSNB, and Leber's congenital amaurosis may be supplemented by EOG findings, which may contribute supplemental information for the diagnosis. The EOG is usually abnormal in progressive cone degenerations and normal in nonprogressive cone disorders such as achromatopsia. The ERG is more diagnostic for achromatopsia due to an absent flicker and photopic ERG. Supernormal values are obtained when the EOG is recorded in albinism; these results are similar to those obtained with the ERG. The combination of ERG and EOG results is useful since the incomplete universal and ocular forms of albinism are often difficult to recognize clinically. In CSNB, the EOG is abnormal in the autosomal dominant condition but appears normal in the X-linked recessive and autosomal recessive variants. The absence of the ERG scotopic b-wave is most diagnostic for CSNB. The EOG may be predictive of the visual prognosis in Leber's congenital amaurosis. In this cone-rod disorder, the ERG is

Normal EOG

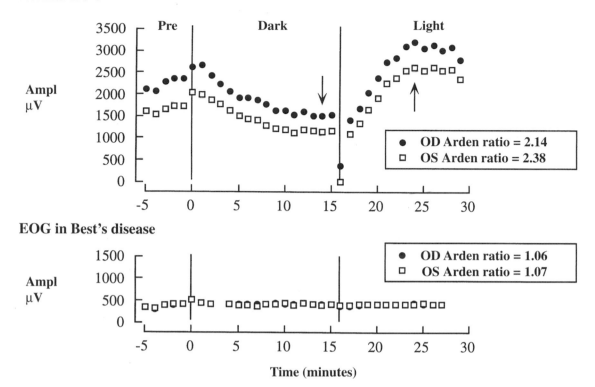

EOG in Best's disease

Time (minutes)

Figure 7.6. The electro-oculogram (EOG) findings in Best's disease indicated by bilateral abnormal Arden ratios. Findings from a nonaffected individual are shown for comparison. (Courtesy of Wayne Verdon, O.D., Ph.D.)

typically extinguished; however, the EOG is abnormal when the disorder is progressive and near normal in stationary forms of the disease.

Value of the Electro-Oculogram in Children

Vitelliform macular degeneration, or Best's disease, is an autosomal dominant, pleomorphic, progressive, retinal pigment epithelium disease usually manifesting in the second decade of life [49]. The classic ophthalmoscopic finding is a well-defined, egg yolk–like, yellow lesion beneath the pigment epithelium in the macular area. There is no loss of visual acuity during the early stages of the disease. The clinical presentation of the macular lesion is variable; it may include partially reabsorbed vitelliform cysts or appear normal. Best's can usually be diagnosed on the basis of the clinical evaluation and examination of family members and inheritance pattern. The EOG is particularly diagnostic,

since it always yields abnormal results regardless of the severity of Best's disease [50]. The light rise in the EOG is abnormal, whereas the ERG is usually normal. This dichotomy between the ERG and EOG is not typical and therefore is diagnostic for Best's disease (Figure 7.6) [28]. EOG can also confirm if a nonsymptomatic individual is a carrier of the disease [51].

Value of Electro-Oculogram in Retinal Disorders

The EOG is abnormal in diffuse rod-cone degenerations such as RP, diffuse choroidal sclerosis, and choroideremia [36]; however, the ERG is a more sensitive and reliable indicator of early disease. The EOG shows moderate to severe abnormalities in advanced stages of the following diseases, which are classified as the flecked retina syndromes: Stargardt's disease, fundus flavimaculatus, and fundus albipunctatus [52]. Both the EOG and ERG may be

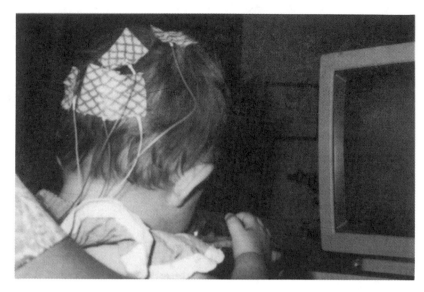

Figure 7.7. Placement of visual evoked potential recording electrodes over the occipital cortex. The fixation monitor on the right presents pattern stimuli during the visual evoked potential recording session.

abnormal in toxic retinopathy in patients after prolonged use of chloroquine for the treatment of rheumatoid arthritis or as an antimalarial drug. However, the tests are not predictive of early retinal toxicity [53]. Fortunately, the introduction of a less toxic drug, hydroxychloroquine, has reduced the occurrence of toxic retinopathy [54]. In a study of diabetes, the EOG was abnormal before the retinopathy was apparent clinically [55]. The degree of retinal detachment is reflected in a progressively abnormal EOG ratio as contact between the retina and retinal pigment epithelium is compromised [7].

Summary

The EOG is an important adjunct test for the diagnosis of abnormalities of the retinal pigment epithelium. It is particularly useful in the diagnosis of Best's disease, since the EOG is always abnormal in the presence of this condition. Its application to the infant or young child is limited, since consistent and repetitive eye movements are required for testing.

Visual Evoked Potential

Definition

The VEP is an electrical signal generated in the occipital region of the cortex in response to visual

stimulation [56]. Also referred to as the *visual evoked response* or the *visual evoked cortical potential*, the VEP is a specific occipital lobe response to visual stimuli. The VEP can be isolated from the background electroencephalogram (EEG) by recording the VEP in relation to a time-locked stimulus presentation. The VEP is elicited at a designated time after the presentation of the stimulus, whereas the EEG is random in its timing with respect to the visual stimulus. If the VEP to a specific number of stimuli is recorded, the VEP will be continuously added at equal and constant intervals in time, whereas the background EEG noise will average out to zero [56].

Clinical Paradigm for Recording the Visual Evoked Potential

The VEP is recorded with EEG-type electrodes and 1-cm gold cup disks, which are adhered to the scalp with an electroconductive paste or gel and gauze (Figure 7.7). Before electrode placement, small regions of the scalp are cleansed with a mild abrasive gel containing pumice to reduce electrical impedance. As in other electrodiagnostic recordings, a minimum of three electrodes are needed: the active, reference, and ground electrodes. Due to placement of the recording electrodes over the occipital cortex, underlying cortical anatomy, and cortical magnification, the VEP assesses primarily foveal

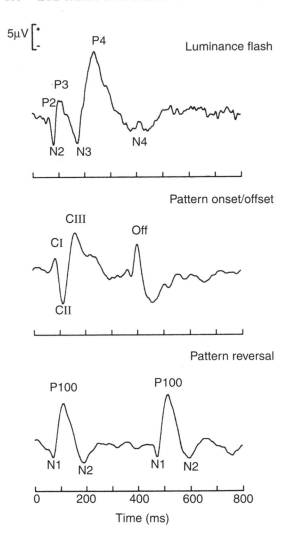

Figure 7.8. Transient visual evoked potential response waveforms to luminance, pattern onset/offset, and pattern-reversal stimuli. The different component structures and labeling conventions for each type of visual evoked potential response are shown. (Reprinted with permission from P Apkarian, H Spekreijse. In JE Desmedt [ed], Visual Evoked Potentials. New York: Elsevier, 1990.)

projections to the visual cortex. One millimeter of tissue in the cortex is devoted to 2 minutes of visual angle when the cortical projections originate from the fovea [57]. Amplification and computer averaging or analysis is required to isolate the VEP from the background EEG.

The VEP stimulus may be a flash from a xenon-arc photostimulator or patterned stimuli (checkerboards or gratings) generated on a video monitor. There are two presentation modes for patterned stimuli: pattern-reversal, in which the pattern is phase-reversed at a specific rate, and pattern onset-offset, in which the pattern appears briefly and then is replaced with a blank field of the same mean luminance as the pattern [58]. It is important to keep the overall mean luminance constant during either the pattern-reversal or onset-offset presentations in order to eliminate contamination of the pattern VEP by luminance components.

Temporal stimulation in VEP recordings is either transient or steady state. When recording the *transient* VEP, the stimulus is presented briefly at regular, slow intervals, usually with less than 6–10 presentations per second. Repeated stimulus presentations and signal averaging is required to isolate the VEP response from the background EEG noise. Since the noise is reduced by the square root of the number of stimulus presentations, typically up to 100 stimulus repetitions are presented to reduce the noise by a factor of 10 [59]. The transient VEP is a complex waveform consisting of a series of negative and positive components when plotted as amplitude versus time (Figure 7.8) [58, 60, 61]. The luminance flash VEP is recorded after very brief strobe flashes (see Figure 7.8, upper panel). The transient VEP recorded to pattern onset-offset stimuli (see Figure 7.8, middle panel) has three components, with positive, negative, and positive peaks called CI, CII, and CIII, respectively [60]. The transient VEP recorded to pattern-reversal stimuli (see Figure 7.8, lower panel) shows a positive peak at latency around 100 ms called P100, which is preceded and followed by negative peaks (N1 and N2, respectively) [58].

The steady-state VEP is recorded in response to a continuous, fast, temporal presentation, with the local changes in the pattern producing a response that is approximately sinusoidal [62]. The steady-state VEP is analyzed in the frequency domain and expressed as the amplitude of the VEP at the temporal frequency of the stimulus used to elicit the VEP. The primary advantage of the steady-state VEP is that stimuli can be more rapidly presented than in the transient paradigm and thus may be less affected by changes in patient cooperation [63]. The swept parameter VEP technique [63, 64] enables presentation of up to 20 different patterned stimuli during brief, 10-second recording trials. This allows for a better sampling of the relationship between VEP amplitude and changes in the visual stimulus. The improved speed in testing with sweep VEP techniques has increased clinical applicability.

VEP testing in pediatric patients is usually performed in a darkened room to decrease distraction. Attention to the video monitor is achieved by dangling small fixation toys on the video screen and speaking or singing to the infant or child being tested. A pause/resume remote control is used by the examiner to start and stop the VEP recording during fixation lapses. Electrical artifact caused by excessive movements of the subject can be eliminated with appropriate data analysis techniques. With skill of the examiner and rapid recording paradigms such as the sweep VEP technique, sedation or general anesthesia is unnecessary.

The latency and amplitude of the pattern VEP is sensitive to changes in contour and edges of the stimulus. The amplitude of the major positive component of the VEP decreases as the contrast or angular subtense of the visual stimulus is decreased. It is this consistent relationship between VEP amplitude and the visual stimulus that enables objective measurement of visual thresholds such as visual acuity and contrast sensitivity.

To measure visual acuity, the amplitude of the transient VEP is measured for a series of grating patterns. Grating patterns are defined in terms of spatial frequency or the number of cycles (light and dark bar pairs) of the grating per degree of visual angle (Figure 7.9). The amplitude of the P100 component is plotted versus the spatial frequency of the grating used to elicit the VEP. A straight line is fit from the peak of the amplitude versus spatial frequency function and is extrapolated to 0 µV to yield the acuity estimate in cycles/degree (see Figure 7.9).

Conversion of grating acuity (measured in cycles/degree) to Snellen notation is done using the following equivalency:

Grating with 30 cycles/degree = 1 minute of arc
of visual angle (or 20/20 visual acuity)

It is important to note that this mathematical translation of grating acuity into Snellen notation is not appropriate in some eye disorders with accompanying low vision.

Estimation of acuity by extrapolation techniques is dependent upon the number and range of pattern

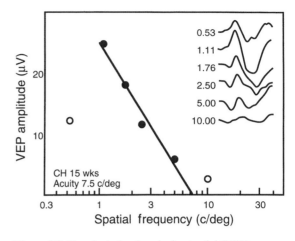

Figure 7.9. Transient visual evoked potential (VEP) responses to pattern-reversal grating stimuli in a 15-week-old infant. The amplitude of the major positive component is plotted (as circles) versus the spatial frequency of the grating used to elicit the visual evoked potential. The visual acuity threshold was determined from a linear extrapolation of the visual evoked potential amplitude to 0 µV. Solid circles indicate data points used in the extrapolation. The visual evoked potential acuity estimate is 7.5 cycles/degree (20/80 in Snellen notation).

sizes presented [64]. Maximal sampling of the amplitude versus spatial frequency function is ideal but time consuming; therefore, transient VEPs have limited clinical applicability for threshold measures of visual acuity. A more rapid technique for measuring visual acuity is the swept spatial frequency VEP paradigm [64]. To determine visual acuity with the sweep VEP, the spatial frequency of the reversing grating target is linearly incremented over a 20 to 1 range of spatial frequencies during a 10-second trial. The amplitude and phase of the steady-state VEP at the reversal frequency is determined using a discrete Fourier transform [65]. Acuity is determined by an extrapolation to 0 µV of the function relating VEP amplitude and linear spatial frequency (Figure 7.10).

The primary advantage of the sweep VEP is the increased sampling of the spatial frequency function, with 20 different spatial frequencies eliciting a VEP amplitude. In addition, the VEP trials are scored by a computer that uses phase information, local noise estimation, and signal-to-noise information in its scoring criteria. The time advantage of a 10-second trial for an acuity measure allows for re-

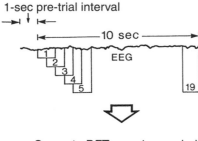

1-sec pre-trial interval

Compute DFT over 1-sec window
for signal and noise frequency

Slide window by 0.5 sec

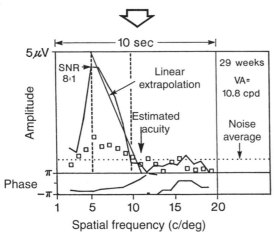

Figure 7.10. Estimate of visual acuity from the spatial frequency sweep visual evoked potential paradigm. Acuity is estimated by extrapolation to 0 μV of the declining portion of the visual evoked potential amplitude versus spatial frequency function. (EEG = electroencephalogram; VA = visual acuity; DFT = discrete Fourier transform; SNR = signal-to-noise ratio.) (Reprinted with permission from AM Norcia, CW Tyler. Spatial frequency sweep visual evoked potential: visual acuity during the first year of life. Vision Res 1985;25:1399.)

peated measures and monocular and binocular recordings within the clinical setting.

In normal adults, visual thresholds determined with extrapolation to 0 μV for VEP amplitude agree with psychophysical measures of contrast threshold [58, 66, 67], grating acuity [68, 69], stereoacuity [70], and vernier acuity [71]. Good correlations between psychophysical and VEP thresholds, with

changes in luminance, optical blur [68, 72] and retinal location [73] have also been reported.

Visual Evoked Potential Studies of Normal Visual Development

Maturation of the Visual Evoked Potential Waveform. The VEP shows maturational changes during the first 6 months of life. In young infants, the pattern VEP consists of a single positive peak [74, 75]. With age, the VEP waveform becomes more complex, the amplitude increases, and the latency of the main positive component decreases [75].

Assessment of Visual Function in Infancy. Within the past two decades, there has been considerable interest in the assessment of visual function in infancy [for a review, see reference 76]. The two methods effective in quantifying the visual capabilities of infants are assessment of the "looking" behavior of infants in response to visual stimuli with preferential looking (PL) techniques and the recording of the VEP.

VISUAL ACUITY. Use of VEP has shown that visual acuity develops rapidly during the first year of life [67, 74, 77, 78] and continues to develop into late childhood [69, 74]. Adult levels of grating acuity are reached as early as 6–8 months of age [67, 77–80]. VEP grating acuity develops rapidly until the age of 8 months and then develops more slowly until 5–11 years [69, 74].

VEP measurement of visual acuity development indicates much more rapid growth than behavioral measures with preferential looking (PL) techniques do. The development of grating acuity during the first few years of life has been investigated by several groups using forced-choice preferential looking (FPL) techniques [81, 82] operant FPL techniques [83], FPL acuity cards [84, 85], and the acuity card procedure [86]. Studies have generally agreed that PL grating acuity develops from approximately 1 cycle/degree at 1 month of age and improves to 6 cycles/degree by 6 months of age; however, PL grating acuity does not reach adult levels until approximately 3 years of age [85]. The 99% confidence limits for the mean acuity are on average a factor of ±2.4 octaves (an octave is a factor of two in MAR [minimum angle of resolution]) over the first year of life [82, 87].

Table 7.2. Mean Expected Monocular Grating Acuity Values

Age (Months)	VEP (Cycles/Degree)	PL (Cycles/Degree)	VEP (Snellen Notation)	PL (Snellen Notation)
1	5	0.94	20/120	20/638
2.5	7.8	2.16	20/77	20/278
4	12	2.68	20/50	20/224
6	18	5.65	20/33	20/106
9	23	6.79	20/26	20/88
12	25	6.42	20/24	20/93
18		8.59		20/70
24		9.57		20/62
30		11.52		20/52
36		21.81		20/28
48		24.81		20/24

VEP = visual evoked potential; PL = preferential looking.
Source: VEP grating acuity data from AM Norcia, CW Tyler. Spatial frequency sweep VEP: visual acuity during the first year of life. Vision Res 1985;25:1399–1408. Monocular grating acuity data from DL Mayer, AS Beiser, AF Warner, et al. Monocular acuity norms for the Teller acuity cards between ages one month and four years. Invest Ophthalmol Vis Sci 1995;36:671–685.

Additionally, the 99% confidence limits for interocular differences range from 0.5 octaves [86] to 3.2 octaves [85].

The sweep VEP technique [80] had relatively small test-retest variability and narrow confidence limits in comparison to previously reported data for PL techniques. The 99% confidence limits and interocular differences for the sweep VEP were 2–4 times smaller than PL measures. Likewise, monocular VEP grating acuities were higher than PL acuity by a factor ranging from 1 to 5 octaves. Therefore, the sweep VEP technique may have higher sensitivity than PL techniques and therefore would better detect amblyopia or visual acuity deficits in infants (Table 7.2).

The validity of the VEP measurement of visual acuity has been supported by two studies of normal populations. Optotype acuity measured with Landolt C targets was similar to VEP acuity (recorded to checkerboard stimuli) in subjects 3–71 years old [74]. Acuity determined by sweep VEP (recorded to grating stimuli) and letter acuity was in good agreement in normally sighted adults and in children 5–11 years old [69].

CONTRAST SENSITIVITY. The development of contrast sensitivity has been studied with the VEP [88, 89]. In a study using the sweep VEP, contrast sensitivity for low spatial frequency grating targets (1 cycle/degree) developed rapidly between birth and 10–12 weeks of age. The contrast sensitivity for coarse targets of a 10-week-old infant was only a factor of two lower than an adult's [89].

STEREOPSIS. Petrig et al. [90] measured VEPs elicited by dynamic random dot stereograms and correlograms in infants. Stereoscopically evoked potentials could be recorded at the age of 10–19 weeks, suggesting that the onset of cortical binocularity precedes stereopsis. Braddick et al. [91] recorded VEPs to the onset and offset of binocular correlation in a large-screen dynamic random dot display and reported that infants have a functional binocular visual cortex by 3 months of age, with some individuals showing cortical binocularity at an earlier age.

COLOR VISION. VEP studies indicate that infants as young as 2 weeks of age have functional medium- and long-wavelength–sensitive cones and postreceptoral circuits, which relay information to the visual cortex [92]. Infants as young as 5 weeks of age have functional short-wavelength–sensitive cones [93]. These findings do not imply, however, that neonates have mature color vision because behavioral measures of color discrimination indicate that development occurs later [94]. A complete spectral sensitivity function for infants has been recorded using the VEP to heterochromatic flicker photometry [95]. The infant heterochromatic flicker photometry functions had an elevation in sensitivity at short wavelengths.

Clinical Applications for the Visual Evoked Potential

Determination of Refractive Error. A small amount of optical blur can attenuate the amplitude of the VEP to centrally fixated fine checks [72]. Although it is possible to estimate refractive error based on the attenuation of VEP amplitude with increasing dioptric blur, it is impractical and less accurate than retinoscopy [96]. The dependence of VEP amplitude on optical blur underscores the importance of correcting the underlying refractive error when estimating visual acuity using VEP amplitudes.

Visual Evoked Potentials in Amblyopia: Contrast Sensitivity. Abnormal contrast responses across a wide range of spatial frequencies have been found using the pattern-reversal VEP in amblyopia [97]. These results were consistent with psychophysical measures of contrast sensitivity functions in individuals with strabismus and anisometropia [98]. Differences in the contrast sensitivity functions between strabismic and anisometropic amblyopia have also been measured with the pattern-reversal VEP [99]. Individuals with strabismic amblyopia showed an abnormal contrast sensitivity function only in the high spatial frequency range, whereas those with anisometropic amblyopia showed an abnormal contrast sensitivity function both in the low and high spatial frequency range.

Visual Evoked Potentials in Amblyopia: Visual Acuity. Several studies have reported an abnormal pattern VEP in patients with amblyopia [100–102]. The pattern-reversal VEP of the amblyopic eye has smaller amplitudes than the fellow eye [103] and smaller signal-to-noise ratios [97]. The determination of which eye is amblyopic could be made in 66% of the adults tested on the basis of the interocular VEP amplitude difference; however, no acuities were reported, so the magnitude of the acuity deficit could not be inferred from the interocular VEP amplitude difference [103].

A few studies have evaluated the usefulness of the VEP in the diagnosis of amblyopia in pediatric patients. Sokol et al. [104] calculated interocular

VEP amplitude differences for children with various ocular disorders, including strabismus and anisometropia, and compared these with normals. The interocular VEP amplitude ratios did not correlate with the magnitude of the interocular differences in Snellen acuity. Twenty-five of 26 children (96%) with a two-fold (three lines) or more interocular difference in Snellen visual acuity tests had abnormal VEP interocular ratios. The proportion of abnormals correctly identified dropped to 50% for an acuity difference of two lines and to 30% for an acuity difference of one line. Friendly et al. [105] assessed the clinical usefulness of pattern-reversal VEPs in the diagnosis of amblyopia in 27 children with anisometropia and 4 children without amblyopia. Measurements of visual acuity with letter charts were compared to normalized VEP amplitudes to reversing checks subtending 15 minutes of visual arc. Of the 31 children in their study, 25 (80%) were correctly identified with amblyopia by VEP testing only. Odom et al. [106] reported the usefulness of the VEP in monitoring acuity changes during patching therapy in preverbal amblyopes. Acuity was determined from an extrapolation to 0 μV of the transient VEP amplitude versus several checksizes; however, neither normative data nor validation of the VEP measures by comparison with subjective acuities were reported. A limitation of these VEP studies of amblyopia in children is that the VEP measures of acuity were not validated by comparison with optotype acuity [106] or a single VEP amplitude criterion was used to predict the amblyopic eye without yielding any information as to the magnitude of the amblyopia [104, 105]. Studies using the sweep VEP technique enable rapid and direct measures of visual acuity thresholds in a clinical setting.

Validation studies using the sweep VEP reported good correlations between VEP grating acuity and optotype acuity in adults and children with strabismus, anisometropia, or both and age-matched normals [69] and in children with various visual disorders [107]. Sweep VEP grating and optotype acuities were well correlated in amblyopia, in spite of substantial absolute differences between the two measures in patients with significant amblyopia [69]. There was substantial agreement between VEP and optotype acuity in observers with optotype acuity better than 20/60; however, an increasing discrepancy accompanied poorer acuity (Figure 7.11).

Figure 7.11. A comparison of sweep visual evoked potential (VEP) grating acuity and optotype acuity in 72 observers with strabismus, anisometropia, or both. Observers with a factor of three reduction in grating acuity from the norm are plotted as circles. These grating acuity values were converted into a predicted optotype acuity. The acuity measures plotted as squares represent the measured grating and optotype acuity scores without use of the conversion factor. (Reprinted with permission from DA Orel-Bixler. Subjective and visual evoked potential measures of acuity in normal and amblyopic adults and children. Ph.D. diss., University of California at Berkeley, 1989.)

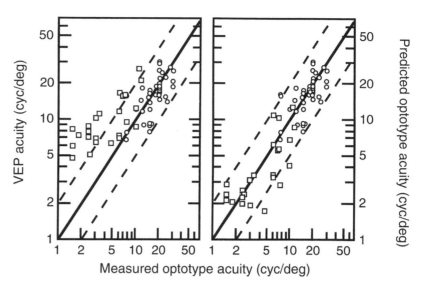

Tests using gratings overestimated acuity compared with optotypes by a discrepancy factor of 2.5 in MAR. Therefore, a measured grating acuity of 6 cycles/degree is expected to yield an optotype acuity of approximately 20/250. The more exact conversion factor [69] is determined using the following equation:

$$\{[(MAR_{grating} - 1)/0.4] \cdot 1.3\} + 1 = MAR_{predicted\ optotype}$$

This equation uses the loss of grating acuity (compared to normal) to predict optotype acuity by considering the limitations imposed by retinal or cortical magnification. Several other studies have indicated that visual acuities measured with grating targets are higher than those measured with optotypes in amblyopic observers [108, 109] and pediatric patients with significant ocular structural anomalies [110]. A better prediction of optotype acuity from the VEP grating acuity can be made by taking this systematic overestimation into account.

Visual Evoked Potentials in Clinical Populations.
The VEP has been shown to be a sensitive indicator of early acuity losses in studies of infants with strabismus. Measurements of monocular and binocular acuity of esotropic infants with the sweep VEP technique were significantly below the mean for age-matched normal infants. [111]. The acuity reductions, although small, were significant. The infants with esotropia and alternating fixation did not have significant interocular differences. The VEP has been used to monitor changes in the vision of the amblyopic and fellow eye during occlusion therapy [106, 112] and to record the postoperative acuity in infants with congenital cataract. Cataracts were removed from infants 7 hours to 41 days after birth with final acuity outcomes of 20/30 in five patients and 20/80 in three patients. No patients showed a major discrepancy between VEP recording and eye chart visual acuity measurements when the child was old enough to perform both tasks [113].

PATIENTS WITH VISUAL IMPAIRMENT AND MULTIPLE DISABILITIES. Several studies have reported that the VEP measurement of visual function can be useful in the clinical management of nonverbal patients including patients with multiple disabilities [114, 115], pediatric patients [107], and visually impaired children [116].

ALBINISM. The clinical findings in albinism include nystagmus, iris and fundus hypopigmentation, high refractive error, and strabismus. Not all albinos display every one of these clinical features, however. All forms of albinism involve foveal hypoplasia, reduced visual acuity, and a preponderance of ipsilateral retinal fiber decussation that disrupts retinotopic organization throughout the visual pathway [117]. Nerve fibers from the temporal retina erroneously decussate at the optic chiasm, resulting in a decreased proportion of uncrossed fibers and an abnormal visual pathway from the lateral geniculate nucleus to the occipital cortex [118]. The VEP correlate of misrouted optic pathway projections is indispensable for the detection and differential diagnosis of albinism [25]. With full-field stimulation to the right eye, the largest VEP amplitude is recorded over the left hemisphere (contralateral asymmetry). This VEP test is more difficult to interpret in children younger than 3 years old due to the immaturity of the pattern-onset response, but the luminance flash condition may still illustrate the asymmetry [119].

CORTICAL BLINDNESS.   Cortical blindness is a loss of vision secondary to damage to the geniculostriate pathways and is characterized by reduced vision and absence of optokinetic nystagmus with normal ocular examination findings and intact pupillary light responses [120]. Cortical blindness results from hypoxic insults, meningitis, encephalitis, metabolic disturbances, head trauma, or hydrocephalus. The recovery of vision is often protracted and only partial; however, in some cases, recovery may be complete and rapid. For this reason, *cortical visual impairment* (CVI) is the more appropriate term to describe this condition [121]. The most common causes are generalized cerebral hypoxia at the striate, parietal, and premotor regions and vascular lesions of the striate cortex [122].

Several studies have evaluated flash VEP responses in CVI. The large variations in waveform and amplitude of flash VEPs make them more difficult to interpret than pattern VEPs. The studies were often limited to single case reports or small population studies of patients with CVI. Both normal and abnormal flash VEP responses have been reported, as well as VEP responses that improved with time [122]. Frank and Torres [123] found no difference in the amplitude of the flash VEPs recorded from 30 children with CVI compared with age-matched children with neurologic disorders but no vision impairment. Conversely, Aldrich et al. [124] reported abnormal flash and pattern VEPs in 15 of 19 patients with CVI; however, the VEP was

not correlated with the degree of visual loss. Other studies have reported that the recovery of vision was paralleled by normalization of the VEP response. In one study, the VEP was used to determine visual prognosis following perinatal asphyxia [125]. In this study, flash VEPs were recorded from 25 asphyxiated infants. Sixteen infants had normal or only transient abnormalities of the VEP and with follow-up all of these infants developed normal vision. The remaining nine infants who had abnormal flash VEPs never developed normal vision. The VEP findings in CVI remain controversial since subjective measures of visual function cannot be determined for comparison to the VEP measures and the lesions that cause CVI are not often localized exclusively to the striate cortex [122].

DELAYED VISUAL MATURATION.   Infants with delayed visual maturation (DVM) appear to have CVI with poor or no fixation up to 5–6 months of age. At this time, visual responsiveness rapidly increases to normal levels [126–128]. Pupillary response, ocular examination, and neuroimaging studies are normal even though the infant appears visually nonresponsive before 6 months. Although DVM may be suspected, the diagnosis is confirmed only retrospectively after vision improvement. One study reported normal ERGs but absent or immature flash VEPs in infants suspected of having DVM. When the infants showed vision improvement, the flash VEPs were found to be normal; however, these VEP responses were not compared with age-matched norms [129]. A subsequent study compared the VEP of 9 infants with DVM with age-matched norms and reported normal pattern and flash VEPs [127]. The authors concluded that intact pattern VEPs indicate a good visual prognosis in visually unresponsive infants. At present, DVM is incompletely understood and the anatomic and molecular developments that underlie the visual recovery have not yet been identified [127].

Summary

There are several clinical applications of VEPs in the pediatric population. The VEP is noninvasive and can be used in a population that cannot communicate or cooperate for standard assessment of visual function. Taylor and McCulloch [130] state that the major application of VEPs in pediatric patients has been to quantify visual impairment by using measures of visual acuity or contrast sensitivity or by quantifying flash or pattern VEP abnormalities. The flash VEP may help establish the prognosis for visual recovery for specific pediatric disorders, including perinatal asphyxia in full-term neonates and acute-onset CVI. In some cases, flash VEP may contribute to the differential diagnosis. The VEP can help monitor patients who are at risk for visual complications either from diseases (e.g., hydrocephalus) or as a complication of therapeutic intervention (e.g., neurosurgery). VEPs have become an indispensable tool in pediatric ophthalmology and neurology and will probably play an increasingly important role in the future sensitivity of the VEP to subclinical damage [130].

A-SCAN AND B-SCAN ULTRASOUND

Background

A-scan and B-scan ultrasonography are diagnostic procedures for the detection and differentiation of ocular and orbital disorders [131, 132]. Thijssen [133] provides an excellent review of the 50-year history of the application of ultrasound in ophthalmology and optometry.

Definition

Ultrasound uses focused, short-wavelength, acoustic waves that are emitted via an echographic probe as a wavefront advancing into the eye. The ocular tissues reflect, refract, and scatter these sound waves in a characteristic manner. The reflected components, or echo, are received by the probe's transducer, amplified, filtered, and displayed on a video screen or oscilloscope [134, 135].

Clinical Paradigm

The A- and B-scan ultrasound can be performed on infants and young children. A topical ophthalmic anesthetic is required and a drop of ophthalmic methylcellulose is applied to the probe tip for B-scan ultrasound. If the evaluation is conducted by a skilled examiner, sedation or anesthesia is rarely needed, even in very young patients. Contraindications for A- or B-scan ultrasonography include recent intraocular surgery, perforating injury, or scleral lacerations. Complications of ultrasound include minor corneal abrasions or irritation resulting from the echographic probe, anesthetic, or preservative in the methylcellulose solution [134, 135].

A-Scan Ultrasound

Biometry, or measurement of the eye and its structures, is achieved with the A-scan ultrasound. The echographic probe is placed perpendicular and in light contact with the anesthetized corneal apex. The echoed sound waves transmitted along the optical axis of the eye are plotted as a time-amplitude recording and converted into an electrical distance measure for display on an oscilloscope. Each spike on the graph represents a specific ocular tissue. The measured time intervals between echo spikes can be converted into a measurement (in millimeters) of ocular structures along the optical axis, including axial length. The axial scans in A-scan ultrasound are performed in both the horizontal and vertical directions [134].

A-scan ultrasonography is most commonly used to measure axial length of the eye for the determination of the proper dioptric power for intraocular lens implantation. Other applications include quantifying lesion size, internal structures, and intrinsic vasculature [134]. Figure 7.12 shows the A-scans for the right eye (upper panel) and left eye (lower panel) in a 4-year-old male with the following refractive error: right eye: −18.00 −0.75 x 180; left eye: +1.50 DS. These A-scans were conducted through the child's eyelid due to noncompliance; therefore, the left-most spike normally corresponding to the cornea and front and back lens surfaces are not well differentiated. The right-most spike corresponds to reflections from the retinal and choroidal layers. The interocular difference in axial length is approximately 6 mm. Since 1 mm of axial length corresponds to a 3.00 D change in refractive error, the anisometropia of 18.00 D is well predicted by the A-scan differential.

B-Scan Ultrasound

In B-scan ultrasound, the echogram is displayed as a two-dimensional array in which the horizontal

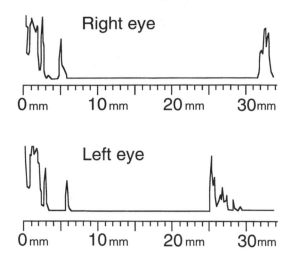

Figure 7.12. A-scan ultrasound indicating a 6-mm difference in axial length between the right and left eye.

axis represents tissue depth and the vertical axis represents the scanned segment of the globe or orbit (Figure 7.13). Several orientations of the echographic probe are used in B-scan ultrasound to allow for transverse, axial, and longitudinal scans. The continuous flow of images as the probe is moved on the eye is evaluated by the examiner during testing and is often videotaped.

B-scan ultrasound is recommended when information is needed about the status of ocular structures posterior to corneal, lens, or vitreous opacities. B-scan localizes lesions and yields information about their configuration and gross reflectivity. A complete B-scan examination is recommended with opaque ocular media, vitreous hemorrhage, retinal detachment, suspected ocular tumors, intraocular foreign bodies, optic disc anomalies, proptosis, and suspected extraocular muscle disease [135].

Clinical Applications of Ultrasound in Pediatric Populations

A-scan ultrasound has been used to study the growth of the eye from birth to puberty [136, 137] and ocular biometry in premature infants [138, 139]. Ultrasound is most commonly used in the pediatric population to make a decision about whether surgical intervention for media opacities is appro-

priate. B-scan ultrasound is used to provide information about the integrity of the vitreous, retina, and posterior pole when a corneal opacity, cataract, or retrolental mass obscures the clinician's view of the fundus. For example, ultrasound is recommended before vitrectomy in ocular trauma to detect retinal detachments or foreign bodies [140]. The differential diagnosis of a retrolental mass includes retinoblastoma, persistent hyperplastic primary vitreous [141] retinopathy of prematurity, dominant exudative vitreoretinopathy, congenital cataracts, posterior uveitis, and retinal dysplasia. Ultrasound and CT are useful in differentiating persistent hyperplastic primary vitreous from retinoblastoma [142], since the characteristic calcification in the retinoblastoma lesion can be detected with both procedures [143]. If the condition is bilateral or there is a positive family history of retinoblastoma, an additional CT scan of the orbit and brain is recommended.

The determination of refractive error in infantile aphakia is aided by measures of axial length with A-scan ultrasound [144]. An A-scan ultrasound is recommended in developmental anterior segment abnormalities if glaucoma is suspected.

Prenatal Diagnosis: Ultrasonic Imaging of the Fetal Brain and Eye

An ultrasound image of structures shielded on all sides by air or by bone more than a few millimeters thick cannot be made. For this reason, ultrasonographic studies of human anatomy are limited to fetuses and infants of up to approximately 9 months of age, when the brain can be assessed through a patent fontanel [145]. The principal clinical concern in fetal cerebral imaging is the identification of major structural abnormalities such as hydrocephalus and holoprosencephaly, the failure of the forebrain to divide into hemispheres. These anomalies are easily identified with ultrasound due to the high contrast of spaces containing cerebrospinal fluid [146]. Additional clinical concerns in neonates are the identification of intracranial hemorrhages, anoxic injury, and infection [145]. Central nervous system lesions associated with toxoplasmosis can be detected with ultrasound pre- and postnatally [147].

Prenatal ultrasound has been used to monitor the development of the fetal eye [148]. The normative data from a study by Achiron et al. that included 450 fetuses from 12 to 37 weeks' gestation may be helpful in the prenatal diagnosis of suspected congenital syndromes that are manifested in ocular growth disturbances such as microphthalmos and anophthalmos. Prenatal ultrasonographic diagnosis of retinal detachment has been demonstrated in Walker-Warburg syndrome, a congenital disorder associated with hydrocephalus and retinal nonattachment [149].

NEUROIMAGING

Computed Tomography

Background

The introduction in 1972 of x-ray CT, also known as computer-assisted tomography, opened up a new era in imaging technology [150]. CT provides a safer, more sensitive way to image soft tissue and bone and is far superior to plain-film x-rays of the orbits and skull. CT can provide images of fine anatomic details of the orbit, oculomotor nerves and muscles, and the central nervous system.

Definition

CT uses multiple x-ray projections and mathematically reconstructs data to create slice images [151]. A layer of any part of the body can be penetrated by narrow x-ray beams that originate from a large number of angles. These multiple transmissions are recorded, and an array of point-by-point relative absorption coefficients is calculated. The absorption coefficient is the representation of the density or substance of the tissue. The resultant image is a gray-scale representation of the array of absorption coefficients. The earliest CT scanners required more than 5 minutes to produce images in an 80×80 matrix containing 29,000 bits of information. Scanning time now has been reduced to less than 1 second per image, with a 512×512 matrix and more than 1,000,000 data points [152].

The cerebral CT scan is a two-dimensional image of a brain slice that can be as thin as 1 mm

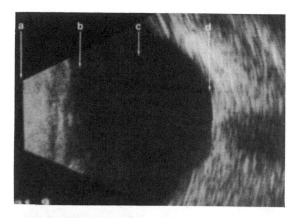

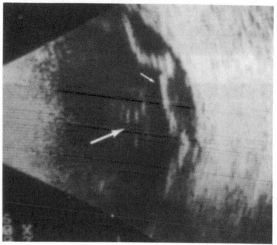

Figure 7.13. B-scan ultrasound in a normal eye (top) and an eye with a vitreous hemorrhage and retinal detachment (bottom). The B-scan image shows tissue-specific reflected echoes. The horizontal axis represents tissue depth and the vertical axis is the scanned segment of the eye. Indicated on the B-scan of the normal eye are echoes from the probe and corneal surface (a), posterior lens surface (b), vitreous (c), and retina (d). The value of the B-scan here lies in the detection of the retinal detachment (small arrow) behind the vitreous hemorrhage (large arrow). (Reprinted with permission from B-Scan Ultrasound: Biometry. In M Fingeret, L Casser, HT Woodcome [eds], Atlas of Primary Eyecare Procedures. East Norwalk, CT: Appleton & Lange, 1990;237.)

[150]. Discrimination of gray from white matter of the brain is achieved due to the high spatial and density resolution of CT scanners. CT can identify structural changes, including cerebral spinal fluid cavities, edema, demyelination, and extravasated

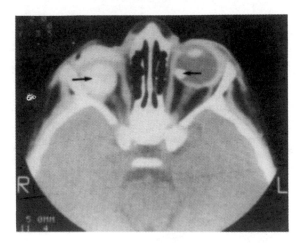

Figure 7.14. Computed tomography scan demonstrating calcification in the left eye due to retinoblastoma (right arrow). The right eye has been enucleated and a prosthesis is present in the right socket. (Reprinted with permission from RA Catalano. Ocular Emergencies. Philadelphia: Saunders, 1992;68.

blood, and can detect the small amounts of calcium that are present in tumoral, granulomatous, and arteriosclerotic calcifications and in Sturge-Weber syndrome.

Application in Pediatric Populations

Because of its excellent imaging of the orbit and bony anatomy, CT is the preferred imaging technique for diagnosis of complex ocular trauma [153] and suspected nonaccidental injury [154]. Calcium deposits within intracranial and intraorbital masses, particularly retinoblastoma, are readily detected with CT (Figure 7.14) [142, 143, 150, 155].

Risks to Pediatric Population

The brief scanning time has significantly reduced the occurrence of CT image degradation secondary to movement in uncooperative patients or children; however, some patients may need to be sedated for the procedure [156]. Intravenous iodine-based contrast enhancement media has been used to enhance the differential diagnostic capability of the CT scan, particularly in evaluation of the optic nerve and its associated sheaths. The side effects of the iodine contrast enhancement media and radiation

exposure should be considered with CT use in infants and children.

Magnetic Resonance Imaging

Background

CT imaging and basic x-rays use propagating rays to interact with biological tissue. Imaging with x-rays is obtained from the scattered or absorbed rays. MRI , however, uses nuclear magnetic resonance to produce tomographic images [157]. MRI has been available for use since the early 1980s and is now accepted as the most sensitive and among the most specific diagnostic imaging tools available for neuro-ophthalmic applications [150].

Definition

MRI encodes image information by using wavelengths of several meters and relying on spatial and time-dependent magnetic fields to excite and modulate the resonance of the hydrogen nuclei in biological tissue [157, 158]. A magnetic resonance instrument uses a strong magnetic field to partially align the hydrogen nuclei, which otherwise would have a naturally random distribution of unpaired nuclear spins. In MRI, specific radiofrequency pulses are used to interact with the hydrogen nucleus in the tissue and transfer energy. The absorbed energy changes the nuclear spin and temporarily distorts the alignment of the hydrogen nuclei. When the radiofrequency pulse is turned off, the nuclei gradually realign with the magnetic field and emit varying radiofrequencies. T1 (longitudinal) and T2 (transverse) relaxation times are the basic parameters used to describe the nuclear realignment and resulting signal pattern. Generally, solids have very short relaxation times, and the relaxation times for tissues increase with increasing fluidity. For example, relaxation times for tumors tend to be longer than those of the host tissue. The differences in relaxation times of tissues enhance the contrast of the magnetic resonance image (Figure 7.15). The T1 or T2 characteristics of various biological tissues can be emphasized by changing the radio frequency pulse repetition time and the signal sampling, or echo, time. T1-weighted images have a short repetition and echo time and therefore result in a high signal-to-noise ratio and relatively short imaging time. T1-weighted image sequences have optimal spatial detail, whereas T2-weighted sequences have optimal tissue contrast.

Fluid is generally dark on T1-weighted images and bright on T2-weighted images. Therefore, T2-weighted images are particularly sensitive to edema. MRI does not image bone well. Fat is seen as a high-intensity (bright) signal on T1-weighted images and may obscure the signal from an adjacent tissue lesion or tumor (e.g., in retrobulbar pathology). Short T1 inversion recovery sequences can be used to decrease the signal from fat. Contrast enhancement can be obtained with the use of intravenous magnetic contrast agents. The primary effect is a T1 shortening that increases the signal on T1-weighted images. The intravenous contrast agent used in MRI is safer and better tolerated than the iodine contrast agents used in CT.

MRI protocols can be varied to optimize diagnostic yield. The most important parameters include imaging plane slice thickness (typically 3–5 mm) and pulse sequence selection. Imaging planes include coronal, transaxial, and sagittal sections. Image contrast and scan protocols can be adjusted to emphasize characteristics of suggested disease states.

Comparison of Magnetic Resonance Imaging and Computed Tomography

There are several advantages of MRI over CT in orbital imaging [157]. MRI has superior imaging performance and the ability to image soft tissue noninvasively. No dose of x-rays is administered; therefore, no orbital tissues are exposed to ionizing radiation. MRI is diagnostic without the use of intravenous iodine-containing contrast agents. When contrast enhancement is needed for diagnostic yield, the gadolinium-containing contrast agent is safe and well tolerated. Also, metallic dental hardware does not degrade the MRI quality. Finally, MRI achieves better imaging than CT of brain stem structures and posterior fossa disease [157]. CT is of limited value in evaluating the posterior fossa due to the beam-hardening artifact of the surrounding bone [150].

There are, however, several disadvantages of MRI compared with CT in orbital imaging. MRI (1) has poor specificity (e.g., tumors, infections, de-

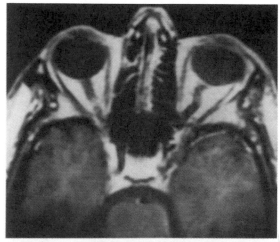

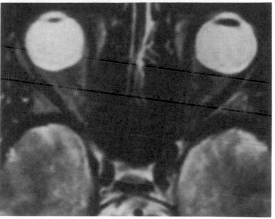

Figure 7.15. The changing signal characteristics of various structures of the normal orbit with T1-weighted axial imaging (top) and T2-weighted axial imaging (bottom). (Reprinted with permission from RG Kamholtz, JJ Abrahams. Magnetic Resonance Imaging of the Orbits and Extraorbital Visual System. In TJ Walsh [ed], Neuro-Ophthalmology: Clinical Signs and Symptoms. Philadelphia: Lea & Febiger, 1992;288.)

myelinating foci, and edematous areas all produce similar signals); (2) has poor detection of calcification within a lesion or tumor, particularly in retinoblastoma; (3) has poor imaging of bony anatomy; (4) has poor detection of bony remodeling or early invasion from an adjacent lesion; (5) provides substandard images resulting from motion artifact; and (6) is time consuming due to the repetition of scan sequences to compensate for motion artifact [157].

Positron Emission Tomography

Background and Definition

PET allows in vivo quantitative measurements of regional physiologic and biochemical processes. In the PET procedure, a tracer is labeled with a positron-emitting radionuclide. The tracer is given intravenously to the subject and the three-dimensional positron activity in the brain is assessed with a positron emission tomograph [159].

PET studies use a variety of tracers to measure local cerebral blood flow, cerebral blood volume, oxygen consumption, glucose consumption, protein synthesis, neurotransmitter receptor properties, tissue proliferation, tissue pH and drug distribution [159]. Research with PET continues on the effects of visual stimulation and cognitive tasks on cerebral glucose metabolism, pathophysiologic events occurring after a stroke, aging and dementia, and grading the malignancy of brain tumors. These studies have significantly increased understanding of the metabolic and physiologic processes of the human brain in normal and pathologic conditions [160].

In pediatric patients, PET has been particularly informative in epilepsy [161, 162]. The PET of local cerebral glucose utilization is highly sensitive in detecting epileptogenic regions [163]. Expanding PET technology provides a new approach that holds great promise in the diagnosis and management of brain disorders in children [163].

Clinical Application of Neuroimaging in the Pediatric Population

Differential Diagnosis for Retinoblastoma

MRI does not detect the calcification in retinoblastoma as well as CT does but may provide information about whether spread along the optic nerve has occurred since the artifact from surrounding bone is reduced [164]. Choroidal melanomas are better detected with MRI than CT because the melanin can cause a paramagnetic effect that enhances the bright signal within the tumor [150]. Magnetic resonance images display certain characteristics in other disorders that aid in the differential diagnosis for retinoblastoma, including (1) Coats' disease, whose clinical signs include retinal telangiectasis with a resultant lipoproteinaceous subretinal exudate; (2) persistent hyperplastic primary vitreous, particularly when accompanied by hemorrhage; and (3) posterior uveitis associated with toxocariasis [158].

Optic Nerve Hypoplasia

CT or MRI should be considered in any case of optic nerve hypoplasia (unilateral or bilateral) associated with a history of neonatal hypoglycemia, seizures, failure to thrive, delayed development, or other neurologic signs. In one study [44] of children with bilateral optic nerve hypoplasia, poor vision, and nystagmus, 39% also had abnormalities shown with neuroimaging. Unilateral optic nerve hypoplasia was associated with intracranial pathologic factors in fewer than 10% of the cases [44]. All infants with optic nerve hypoplasia should also be referred to a pediatric endocrinologist for evaluation. Bilateral optic nerve hypoplasia accompanied by structural abnormalities along the midline of the central nervous system is referred to as *septo-optic dysplasia* or *DeMorsier's syndrome*. Endocrine dysfunction may accompany this disorder, which will result in short stature of the child unless treated [165, 166].

Optic Nerve Atrophy

Optic nerve atrophy is a clinical sign, not a diagnosis. Children presenting at any age with nystagmus and optic atrophy should have a CT or MRI scan to rule out associated conditions. Optic atrophy may be associated with hydrocephalus or anterior visual pathway compression from a suprasellar tumor, including craniopharyngiomas, gliomas, meningiomas, pituitary tumors, metastatic tumors, and arachnoid cysts.

Hydrocephalus is an increased amount of cerebrospinal fluid in the cerebral ventricles resulting from impaired cerebrospinal fluid circulation, reabsorption, or hypersecretion. Hydrocephalus is a common cause of optic atrophy [167], cortical visual impairment, or both in children. Rapid head growth is the most notable clinical finding in hydrocephalus with an onset before 2 years of age. After 2 years of age, various neuro-ophthalmologic abnormalities may present in ocular motility, pupillary responses, optic nerve appearance, vision func-

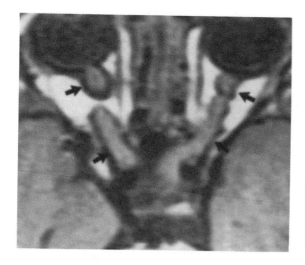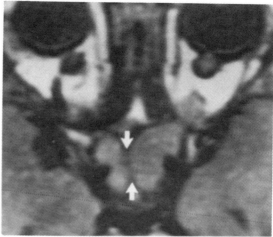

Figure 7.16. Magnetic resonance imaging of the optic nerve glioma. The T1-weighted axial images show fusiform enlargement of both optic nerves (black arrows) extending posteriorly to involve the optic chiasm (white arrows). (Reprinted with permission from RG Kamholtz, JJ Abrahams. Magnetic Resonance Imaging of the Orbits and Extraorbital Visual System. In TJ Walsh [ed], Neuro-Ophthalmology: Clinical Signs and Symptoms. Philadelphia: Lea & Febiger, 1992;299.)

tion, and visual field. CT and MRI are both useful in the diagnosis of hydrocephalus.

Craniopharyngioma is the most common nonglial intracranial tumor of childhood [168]. Children with craniopharyngioma often have only nonspecific symptoms and psychogenic vision loss is often suspected [169]. The vision loss is progressive due to compression of the optic nerves, tracts, or chiasm and resulting optic atrophy. By the time the diagnosis of craniopharyngioma is made, the optic atrophy may be profound. Calcification within the tumor is easily seen on CT scanning or plain skull films.

Optic nerve glioma occurs almost exclusively before 20 years of age and generally occurs in children. The tumor is often associated with neurofibromatosis but may not be detected by ophthalmoscopic examination [170]. MRI is important in all children with neurofibromatosis. With optic gliomas, the most common MRI appearance is fusiform enlargement of the optic nerve (Figure 7.16). Posterior extension through the optic canal with involvement of the chiasm or optic tract can be seen on MRI (see Figure 7.16) [158]. In general, posterior fossa abnormalities, suspected demyelinating processes, and parachiasmal structures are better imaged by MRI [158]. CT is of limited value

in evaluating the posterior fossa due to beam-hardening artifact of the surrounding bone [150].

Brain Tumors

Primary brain tumors are the most common solid neoplasms in children but differ considerably from the adult form in incidence, location, morphology, histology, and natural history [171]. The distribution of brain tumors differs in infants and older children. Vomiting is the most common presenting symptom in all pediatric age groups, but older children are more likely to show localized neurologic signs (e.g., cranial nerve palsy, hemiparesis, clumsiness, ataxia), recurrent headaches, vomiting, and visual complaints, including acute onset of esotropia [171]. The clinician should closely look for papilledema or nystagmus in children with an acute onset of comitant esotropia that does not appear to be an accommodative esotropia [172]. Infants with brain tumors tend to not show focal neurologic deficits due to the immaturity of the brain, but they may have hydrocephalus and papilledema due to increased intracranial pressure [173]. A significant portion of the clinical signs and symptoms in children with brain tumors involves the visual system due to tumor invasion of visual system structures or the mass effects of the tumor (e.g., associated hydrocephalus or secondary compression). MRI and CT and neuro-ophthalmologic evaluation is an important component of follow-up in these children [171].

Cortical Visual Impairment

Neuroimaging is valuable in revealing the structural abnormalities of the central nervous system and is critical to the diagnosis of CVI in infants and children; however, the findings with neuroimaging cannot predict visual function or visual potential. In a study of 30 infants with CVI, all but two infants had abnormalities in the neuroimaging studies. None of the abnormalities demonstrated with neuroimaging correlated with the degree of visual recovery in these infants (except for abnormalities of the optic radiations) [174]. The case of a 20-month-old child who had absent occipital and parietal lobes confirmed by neuroimaging but could use vision to reach for small objects has been reported [175]. Areas that appear nonfunctioning on MRI and CT may have some residual function. Positron emission tomography (PET) and single photon emission computerized tomography (SPECT) studies may be more sensitive and better able to make inferences about visual function, but these are areas of future research [176, 177].

Summary

Neuroimaging studies are indicated in the workup of a possibly blind child when the diagnosis is still uncertain after a careful history, clinical examination, and electrophysiologic testing have been completed [42]. Brodsky et al. [171] recommend neuroimaging studies in (1) infants with congenital nystagmus and optic nerve hypoplasia (to look for CNS anomalies), (2) infants or children with congenital nystagmus and optic atrophy (to rule out hydrocephalus or a congenital suprasellar tumor [craniopharyngioma or chiasmal glioma]), and (3) uncertain diagnoses of congenital nystagmus when the possibility of spasmus nutans exists (to rule out chiasmal gliomas or other suprasellar tumors). Neuroimaging also provides useful information for prognostic and genetic counseling.

Nadel [178] emphasizes that neuroimaging in children is different from that in adults. Important technical considerations include immobilization of the child during imaging, appropriate dosing of radiopharmaceuticals, and appropriate instrumentation. However, new advances in instrumentation, such as multiple detector imaging, the possibility of clinical PET imaging in children, and new radiopharmaceuticals, will further enhance the utility of pediatric imaging.

PHOTOREFRACTION

Background

In the United States, vision disorders are the fourth most common disability and the most prevalent disabling condition in children [179]. For preschool children, these vision disorders include (in decreasing order of prevalence) significant hyperopia, astigmatism, color vision defects, myopia, strabismus, amblyopia, anisometropia, and ocular disease [180, 181]. Although these vision disorders can be readily detected with a vision examination, it has been reported that only 14% of children younger than 6 years of age have received a comprehensive vision examination [179].

Photorefraction is a relatively new technique designed to screen for vision disorders, particularly amblyogenic factors, in infants and young children who are unable to complete the subjective vision tests required in traditional vision screening protocols. Photorefraction uses a camera-based system with a specially placed light source to provide photographic images that can indicate the presence of significant refractive errors, strabismus, media opacities, and ptosis.

Types

There are two principal photorefraction systems: on-axis (co-axial) and off-axis. In the on-axis system, the camera lens and flash are aligned with the subject's visual axis. Three photographs are required to assess refractive error: a focused image for calibration of the pupil and two additional photos with the camera defocused in equal

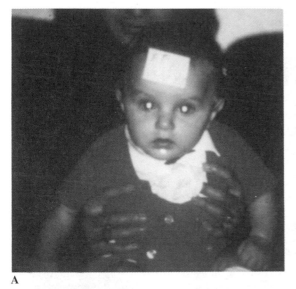

A

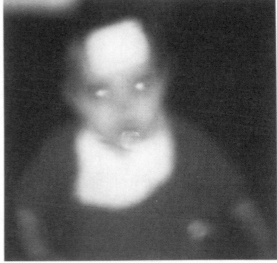

B

Figure 7.17. On-axis photorefraction images with the camera focused at the pupil plane (A) and in front of (B) and behind the pupil plane (C). Comparison of the blur circles in the two defocused images determines the sign and magnitude of the refractive error. (Courtesy of Anthony Norcia, Ph.D.)

C

diopters in front of and behind the pupil plane (Figure 7.17). The sign and magnitude of the spherical and cylindrical errors can be assessed from comparison of the size of the blur circles in the two defocused images. The major axis of the blur ellipse gives the axis of astigmatism for a negative cylinder correction [182].

On-axis photorefraction has several limitations. The apparent size of the blur circle is influenced by fundus pigmentation, pupil size, and the contrast between the subject's face and the blur circle. Scoring the defocused images is difficult and the sub-

ject's direction of gaze, strabismus, and ocular media opacities cannot be detected. Although active fixation on the photographer is encouraged while taking the photos, accommodation to the plane of the camera is not assured; therefore, the presence of significant hyperopia may be masked. The range of refractive errors the camera can detect is from 4.0 D of hyperopia to 4.0 D of myopia [183]. Using an on-axis photorefractor, Hamer et al. [184] reported a sensitivity of 85% and a specificity of 53% in screening for significant refractive error in an infant population.

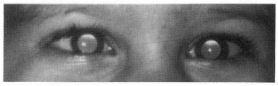
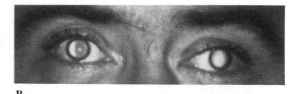

A   **B**

Figure 7.18. Off-axis photorefraction images using a 35-mm camera. Strabismus is determined by interocular comparison of the discrete corneal reflexes shown as (A) right esotropia and (B) left exotropia.

Off-axis photorefraction systems provide more easily interpreted, focused photographs than on-axis systems. In early versions of the off-axis system, a 35-mm camera was equipped with a telephoto lens and the strobe flash was placed directly below the optical axis of the camera lens [185]. These systems only refracted in one orientation and were only sensitive to refractive errors larger than 3 D, depending on the camera aperture and pupil diameter [180]. The next version of off-axis photorefractors substituted a catadioptric (or mirror) telephoto lens and detected refractive errors as small as 0.75 D [186, 187] with a sensitivity range up to 11.0 D for myopia and 7.5 D for hyperopia. Selection of the flash eccentricity determines the range of refractive errors to which the camera is sensitive.

Off-axis photorefraction systems provide a focused image of the pupil and corneal and retinal reflex and therefore overcome many of the limitations of the on-axis systems. A focused image of the corneal reflex (Hirschberg) can be measured to assess fixation and eye alignment. In esotropia the corneal reflex in the deviating eye is displaced temporally and in exotropia the corneal reflex in the deviated eye is displaced nasally (Figure 7.18). The presence of a Bruckner reflex, a unilateral brightening of the red reflex, may indicate either strabismus or significant anisometropia. The clarity of the red fundus reflex can be evaluated to indicate the presence of media opacities. A corneal opacity appears as a bluish haze obscuring the view of the iris and pupil (Plate 7.2A). A cataract or lens opacity appears black or blue within the confines of the pupillary margin (Plate 7.2B). Ametropia is indicated by the presence of a light or yellow crescent within the red reflex. The size of the bright crescent indicates the magnitude of the refractive error and the location of the crescent indicates the direction of the ametropia. The bright crescents of hyperopia are lo-

cated on the opposite side of the camera flash while, myopic crescents are located on the same side as the camera flash. In Plate 7.3, the right eye is myopic along the vertical meridian of the eye and the bright photorefraction crescent is located at the bottom of the pupil margin. The left eye is hyperopic along the vertical meridian and the corresponding bright crescent is located at the upper pupillary margin. Photographs of the child's eyes are taken with the flash oriented both vertically and horizontally to "refract" the 90 degree and 180 degree meridians, respectively. Astigmatism is detected by comparison of the orthogonal crescent with the camera flash oriented vertically and horizontally. In this infant, the hyperopia crescent along the vertical meridian is larger than along the horizontal meridian in each eye, indicating against-the-rule astigmatism (Plates 7.4A and 7.4B).

Current off-axis systems utilize cameras with instant film developing yielding color [188] or black and white images [189, 190]. The advantage of instant camera–based systems is the immediate feedback and compactness and portability of the system.

Clinical Applications

The sensitivity and specificity of off-axis photorefraction as a screening tool has been evaluated by comparison to a clinical vision examination in a few studies [190, 191–195]. These studies included subjects from 3 months to 23 years. The sensitivity and specificity values ranged from 0.41–0.95 to 0.39–0.96, respectively. The lack of standardization of pass versus fail criteria complicates comparison across photorefraction studies. Those studies reporting the highest sensitivity and specificities excluded children for whom analyzable photographs were not obtained [190, 193, 194]. If failure to obtain a readable photograph was counted as an automatic referral, the specificity value in particular would decrease.

Although there is much interest in photorefraction as a screening tool for infants and children, a recent photorefraction study reported that only 58% of the photographs were consistently categorized as pass or fail when scored by a group of health professionals [196]. Further research in photorefraction is needed before routine administration of photoscreening in those groups at greatest risk for vision disorders.

REFERENCES

1. Marmor MF, Arden GB, Nilsson S, Zrenner E. Standard for Clinical Electrophysiology. In JR Heckenlively, GB Arden (eds), Principles and Practice of Clinical Electrophysiology of Vision. St. Louis: Year Book, 1991;283–288.
2. International Society for Clinical Electroretinography (ISCERG). By-laws. Arch Ophthalmol 1989;107:816–819.
3. Burian HM, Allen L. A speculum contact lens electrode for electroretinography. EEG Clin Neurophysiol 1954;6:509–511.
4. Sierpinski-Bart J, Moran A, Hocherman S, et al. Noncorneal electroretinography for pediatric ophthalmology. Metab Ophthalmol 1978;2:387–388.
5. Kriss A. Skin ERGs: their effectiveness in paediatric visual assessment, confounding factors, and comparison with ERGs recorded using various types of corneal electrode. Int J Psychophysiol 1994;16:137–146.
6. Whitacre MM, Ellis PP. Outpatient sedation for ocular examination. Behav Brain Res 1983;10:107–117.
7. Fishman GA, Sokol S. Electrophysiologic Testing in Disorders of the Retina, Optic Nerve, and Visual Pathway. Ophthalmology Monographs 2. San Francisco: American Academy of Ophthalmology, 1990.
8. Zetterstrom B. The Electroretinogram of the Newborn Infant. In A Wirth (ed), Proceedings of the Eighth ISCERG Symposium. Pisa, Italy: Pacini Mariotti, 1972;1–9.
9. Fulton AB. The development of scotopic retinal function in human infants. Doc Ophthalmol 1988;69:101–109.
10. Fulton AB, Hartmann EE, Hansen RM. Electrophysiological testing techniques for children. Doc Ophthalmol 1989;71:341–354.
11. Goethlin GF. Congenital red-green abnormality in color vision and congenital total colour blindness from the point of view of heredity. Acta Ophthalmol 1924;2:15–34.
12. Waardenburg PJ. Achromatopsia Congenita. In PJ Waardenburg, A Franceschetti, DD Klein (eds), Genetics and Ophthalmology (Vol 2). Assen, Netherlands: Royal Van Gorcum, 1963;1695–1725.
13. Haegerstrom-Portnoy G, Schneck ME, Verdon WA, Hewlett SE. Clinical vision characteristics of the congenital achromatopsias. I. Visual acuity, refractive error, and binocular status. Optom Vis Sci 1996;73:446–456.
14. Krill AE. Hereditary Retinal and Choroidal Disease (Vol 2). London: Harper & Row, 1977;335–417.
15. Hansen E. Clinical Aspects of Achromatopsia. In RF Hess, LT Sharpe, K Nordby (eds), Night Vision: Basic, Clinical and Applied Aspects. New York: Cambridge University Press, 1990;316–334.
16. Fonda G, Thomas H. Correction of low visual acuity in achromatopsia: use of corrective lenses as an aid to educational and vocational placement. Arch Ophthalmol 1974;91:20–23.
17. Sloan LL. Ocular Conditions in Which Very High or Very Low Illumination is Required for Maximum Acuity. In LL Sloan (ed), Reading Aids for the Partially Sighted: A Systematic Classification and Procedure for Prescribing. Baltimore: Williams & Wilkins, 1977;109–114.
18. Haegerstrom-Portnoy G, Orel-Bixler D. Light protection and visual acuity development in achromatopsia [abstract]. Optom Vis Sci 1994;71:72.
19. Orel-Bixler D, Haegerstrom-Portnoy G. Acuity Development in Autosomal Recessive Achromatopsia. In Vision Science and its Applications, 1994 Technical Digest Series (Vol 2). Washington DC: Optical Society of America, 1994;348–351.
20. Berson E, Sandberg M, Rosner B, Sullivan PL. Color plates to help identify patients with blue cone monochromatism. Am J Ophthalmol 1983;95:741–747.
21. Haegerstrom-Portnoy G, Schneck ME, Verdon WA, Hewlett SE. Clinical vision characteristics of the congenital achromatopsias. II. Color vision. Optom Vis Sci 1996;73:457–465.
22. Abadi R, Pascal E. The recognition and management of albinism. Ophthalmic Physiol Opt 1989;9:3–15.
23. O'Donnell FE. Congenital Ocular Hypopigmentation. In JD Kilvin (ed), Developmental Abnormalities of the Eye. Boston: Little, Brown, 1984;133–142.
24. Simon JW, Kandel GL, Krohel CB, Nelsen PT. Albinotic characteristics in congenital nystagmus. Am J Ophthalmol 1984;97:320–327.
25. Apkarian P, Reits D, Spekreisje H, van Dorp D. A decisive electrophysiological test for human albinism. Electroencephalogr Clin Neurophysiol 1983;55:513–531.
26. Auerbach E, Godel V, Rowe H. An electrophysiological and psychophysical study of two forms of congenital stationary night blindness. Invest Ophthalmol Vis Sci 1969;8:332.
27. Mikaye Y, Yagasaki K, Horiguchi M, et al. Congenital stationary night-blindness with negative electroretinogram: a new classification. Arch Ophthalmol 1986;104:1013–1020.
28. Carr RE. Electrodiagnostic Tests of the Retina and Higher Centers. In LB Nelson, JH Calhoun, RD Harley (eds), Pediatric Ophthalmology. Philadelphia: Saunders, 1991;78–93.

29. Leber T. Uber retinitis pigmentosa und ungebornene amaurose. Graefes Arch Klin Exp Ophthalmol 1869; 15:1.

30. Foxman SG, Wirtschafter JD, Letson RD. Leber's Congential Amaurosis and High Hyperopia: A Discrete Entity. In Proceedings of the 24th International Congress of Ophthalmology (Vol 1). Philadelphia: Lippincott, 1982;55–58.

31. Lambert SR, Kriss A, Taylor D, et al. Follow-up and diagnostic reappraisal of 75 patients with Leber's congenital amaurosis. Am J Ophthalmol 1989;107: 624–631.

32. Heher KL, Traboulsi EI, Maumenee IH. The natural history of Leber's congenital amaurosis. Ophthalmology 1992;99:241–245.

33. Franceschetti A, Dieterle P. L'importance diagnostique and prognostique de l'électrorétinogramme (ERG) dans les dégénérescence tapetorétiniennes avec retrecissement du champ visual et hemeralopie. Confinia Neurol 1954;14:184.

34. Jan J, Freeman RD, McCormick AQ, et al. Eye pressing by visually impaired children. Dev Med Child Neurol 1993;25:755–762.

35. Joubert M, Eisenring J, Robb JP, et al. Familial agenesis of the cerebellar vermis. Neurology 1969;19:813–825.

36. Heckenlively JR. Retinitis Pigmentosa. Philadelphia: Lippincott, 1988.

37. Usher CH. On a few hereditary eye affections. Trans Ophthalmol Soc U K 1935;55:164–245.

38. Fishman GA, Kumar A, Joseph ME, et al. Usher's syndrome: ophthalmic and neuro-otologic findings suggesting genetic heterogeneity. Arch Ophthalmol 1983;101:1367–1374.

39. Krill AE. The retinal disease of rubella. Arch Ophthalmol 1967;77:445–449.

40. Marks EO. Pigmentary abnormality in children congenitally deaf following maternal German measles. Trans Ophthalmol Soc Aust 1946;6:122–125.

41. Krill AE, Deutman AF. Dominant macular degeneration. The cone dystrophies. Am J Ophthalmol 1972;73:352–359.

42. Fulton AB, Hansen RM, Lambert SR. Workup of the Possibly Blind Child. In SJ Isenberg (ed), The Eye in Infancy. St. Louis: Year Book, 1994;547–560.

43. Francois J, DeRouck A. Electroretinographic study of the hypoplasia of the optic nerve. Ophthalmologica 1976;172:308–330.

44. Skarf B, Hoyt CS. Optic nerve hypoplasia in children. Association with anomalies of the endocrine and CNS. Arch Ophthalmol 1984;102:62–67.

45. Brodsky MC, Baker RS, Hamed LM. Pediatric Neuro-Ophthalmology. New York: Springer, 1996;302–349.

46. Steinberg RH, Griff ER, Linsenmeier RA. The cellular origin of the light peak. Doc Ophthalmol 1983;37:1–11.

47. Arden GB, Barrada A, Kelsey JH. New clinical test of retinal function based upon standing potential of the eye. Br J Ophthalmol 1962;46:449–467.

48. Trimble JL, Ernest JT, Newell FW. Electro-oculography in infants. Invest Ophthalmol Vis Sci 1977; 16:668–670.

49. Kolder HE. Best's Disease. In JR Heckenlively, GB Arden (eds), Principles and Practice of Clinical Electrophysiology of Vision. St. Louis: Year Book, 1991;692–699.

50. Francois L, De Rouck A, Fernandez-Sasso D. Electro-oculography in vitelliform degeneration of the macula. Arch Ophthalmol 1967;77:726–733.

51. Deutman AF. Electro-oculogram in families with vitelliform dystrophy of the fovea: detection of the carrier state. Arch Ophthalmol 1969;81:305–316.

52. Fishman GA. Fundus flavimaculatus: a clinical classification. Arch Ophthalmol 1976;94:2061–2067.

53. Gouras P, Gunkel RD. The EOG in chloroquine and other retinopathies. Arch Ophthalmol 1963;70:629–639.

54. Infante R, Martin DA, Heckenlively JR. Hydroxychloroquine and retinal toxicity. Doc Ophthalmol 1983;37:121–126.

55. Henkes HE, Houtsmuller AJ. Fundus diabeticus: an evaluation of the preretinopathic stage. Am J Ophthalmol 1965;60:662–670.

56. Sokol S. Visually evoked potentials: theory, techniques, and clinical applications. Surv Ophthalmol 1976;21:18.

57. Meredith JT, Celesia GG. Pattern-reversal visual evoked potentials and retinal eccentricity. Electroencephalogr Clin Neurophysiol 1982;53:243.

58. Spekreijse H. Pattern Evoked Potentials: Principles, Methodology and Phenomenology. In C Barber (ed), Evoked Potentials: Proceedings of the International Symposium held in Nottingham U.K. Baltimore: University Park Press, 1980;55–74.

59. Regan D. Human brain electrophysiology: evoked potentials and evoked magnetic fields in science and medicine. New York: Elsevier, 1989.

60. Jeffreys DA, Axford JG. Source locations of pattern-specific components of human visual evoked potentials. II. Component of extrastriate cortical origin. Exp Brain Res 1972;16:22.

61. Apkarian P, Spekreijse H. The Use of the Electroretinogram and Visual Evoked Potentials in Ophthalmogenetics. In JE Desmedt (ed), Visual Evoked Potentials. New York: Elsevier, 1990;169–223.

62. Celesia GG. Steady-state and transient visual evoked potentials in clinical practice. Ann N Y Acad Sci 1982;388:290.

63. Regan D. Speedy assessment of visual acuity in amblyopia by the evoked potential method. Ophthalmologica 1977;175:159–164.

64. Norcia AM, Tyler CW. Spatial frequency sweep VEP: visual acuity during the first year of life. Vision Res 1985;25:1399–1408.

65. Norcia AM, Clarke M, Tyler CW. Digital filtering and robust regression techniques for estimating sensory thresholds from the evoked potential. I.E.E.E. Eng Med Biol 1985;4:26.

66. Campbell FW, Kulikowski JJ. The visual evoked potential as a function of contrast of a grating pattern. J Physiol 1972;222:345.

67. Norcia AM, Tyler CW, Hamer RD, Wesemann W. Measurement of spatial contrast sensitivity with the swept contrast VEP. Vision Res 1989;29:627.

68. Wiener DE, Wellish K, Nelson JI, Kupersmith MJ. Comparisons among Snellen, psychophysical, and evoked potential visual acuity determinations. Am J Optom Physiol Opt 1985;62:669.

69. Orel-Bixler DA. Subjective and visual evoked potential measures of acuity in normal and amblyopic adults and children. Ph.D. diss., University of California at Berkeley, 1989.

70. Norcia AM, Sutter EE, Tyler CW. Electrophysiological evidence for the existence of coarse and fine disparity mechanisms in humans. Vision Res 1985;25:1603.

71. Norcia AM, Manny RE, Wesemann W. Vernier Acuity Measured Using the Sweep VEP. Noninvasive Assessment of the Visual System. In Technical Digest Series (Vol 3). Washington D.C.: Optical Society of America, 1988;151–154.

72. Harter MR, White CT. Effects of contour sharpness and check size on visually evoked potentials. Vision Res 1968;8:701–711.

73. Tyler CW, Apkarian P, Nakayama K, Levi DM. Rapid assessment of visual function: an electronic sweep technique for the pattern VEP. Invest Ophthalmol Vis Sci 1979;18:703–713.

74. de Vries-Khoe LH, Spekreijse H. Maturation of Luminance and Pattern EP's in Man. In G Niemeyer, CH Huber (eds), Docum Ophthal Proc Series 31. The Hague: Junk Publishing, 1982;461–475.

75. Moskowitz A, Sokol S. Developmental changes in the human visual system as reflected by the latency of the pattern reversal VEP. Electroencephalogr Clin Neurophysiol 1983;56:1–15.

76. Teller DV, Movshon JA. Visual development. Vision Res 1987;26:1483.

77. Marg E, Freeman DN, Peltzman P, Goldstein PJ. Visual acuity in human infants: evoked potential measurements. Invest Ophthalmol 1976;15:150–152.

78. Sokol S. Measurement of infant visual acuity from pattern reversal evoked potentials. Vision Res 1978;18:33–39.

79. Orel-Bixler DA, Norcia AM. Differential growth of acuity for steady-state pattern reversal and transient pattern onset-offset VEPs. Clin Vis Sci 1987;2:1–9.

80. Hamer RD, Norcia AM, Tyler CW, Hsu-Winges C. The development of monocular and binocular VEP acuity. Vision Res 1989;29:397–408.

81. Dobson V, Teller DY. Visual acuity in human infants: a review and comparison of behavioral and electrophysiological studies. Vision Res 1978;18:1469.

82. Mayer DL, Fulton AB, Hansen RM. Preferential looking acuity obtained with a staircase procedure in pediatric patients. Invest Ophthalmol Vis Sci 1982;23:538–543.

83. Mayer DL, Dobson V. Assessment of vision in young children: a new operant approach yields estimates of acuity. Invest Ophthalmol Vis Sci 1980;19:566.

84. McDonald M, Sebris SL, Mohn G, et al. Monocular acuity in normal infants: the acuity card procedure. Am J Optom Physiol Opt 1986;63:127.

85. McDonald M, Ankrum C, Preston K, et al. Monocular and binocular acuity estimation in 18- to 36-month-olds: acuity card results. Am J Optom Physiol Opt 1986;63:181.

86. Mayer DL, Beiser AS, Warner AF, et al. Monocular acuity norms for the Teller Acuity Cards between ages one month and four years. Invest Ophthalmol Vis Sci 1995;36:671–685.

87. Birch EE. Infant interocular acuity differences and binocular vision. Vision Res 1985;25:571.

88. Pirchio M, Spinelli D, Fiorentin A, Maffei L. Infant contrast sensitivity evaluated by evoked potentials. Brain Res 1978;141:179–184.

89. Norcia AM, Hamer RD, Tyler CW. Development of contrast sensitivity in the infant. Vision Res 1990;30:1475.

90. Petrig B, Julesz B, Kropfl W, et al. Development of stereopsis and cortical binocularity in human infants: electrophysiological evidence. Science 1981;213:1402–1405.

91. Braddick OJ, Atkinson J, Julesz B, et al. Cortical binocularity in infants. Nature 1980;288:363–365.

92. Allen D, Banks MS, Norcia AM. Does chromatic sensitivity develop more slowly than luminance sensitivity? Vision Res 1993;33:2553–2562.

93. Volbrecht V, Werner J. Isolation of short-wave cone photoreceptors in 4–6 week-old human infants. Vision Res 1987;27:469–478.

94. Adams RJ, Mauer D, Davis M. Newborns' discrimination of chromatic from achromatic stimuli. J Exp Child Psychol 1986;41:267–281.

95. Bieber ML, Volbrecht VJ, Werner JS. Spectral efficiency measured by heterochromatic flicker photometry is similar in human infants and adults. Vision Res 1995;35:1385–1392.

96. Millidot M, Riggs LA. Refraction determined electrophysiologically. Arch Ophthalmol 1970;84:272–278.

97. Levi DM, Harwerth RS. Spatio-temporal interactions in anisometropic and strabismic amblyopia. Invest Ophthalmol Vis Sci 1977;16:90.

98. Levi DM, Harwerth RS. Contrast evoked potentials in strabismic and anisometropic amblyopia. Invest Ophthalmol Vis Sci 1978;17:571.

99. Campos EC, Prampolini ML, Gulli R. Contrast sensitivity differences between strabismic and anisometropic amblyopia: objective correlate by means of visual evoked responses. Doc Ophthalmol 1984;58:45.

100. Sokol S. Visual Evoked Potentials to Checkerboard Pattern Stimuli in Strabismic Amblyopia. In JE Desmedt (ed), Visual Evoked Potentials in Man. Oxford: Clarendon, 1977;410–417.

101. Spekreijse H, Khoe LH, van der Tweel LH. A case of amblyopia: electrophysiological and psychophysics of luminance and contrast. Adv Exp Med Biol 1972; 24:141–156.

102. Arden GB, Barnard WM, Mushin AS. Visually evoked responses in amblyopia. Br J Ophthalmol 1974;58:183.

103. Sokol S, Bloom B. Visually evoked cortical responses of amblyopes to a spatially alternating stimulus. Invest Ophthalmol Vis Sci 1973;12:936–939.

104. Sokol S, Hansen VC, Moskowitz A, et al. Evoked potential and preferential looking estimates of visual acuity in pediatric patients. Ophthalmology 1983; 90:552.

105. Friendly DS, Weiss IP, Barnet AB, et al. Pattern-reversal visual-evoked potentials in the diagnosis of amblyopia in children. Am J Ophthalmol 1986;102:329.

106. Odom JV, Hoyt CS, Marg E. Effect of natural deprivation and unilateral eye patching on visual acuity of infants and children: evoked potential measurements. Arch Ophthalmol 1981;99:1412–1416.

107. Gottlob I, Fendick MG, Guo S, et al. Visual acuity measurements by swept spatial frequency visual-evoked-cortical potentials (VECPs): clinical application in children with various visual disorders. J Pediatr Ophthalmol Strabismus 1990;27:40–47.

108. Gstalder RJ, Green DG. Laser interferometric acuity in amblyopia. J Pediatr Ophthalmol 1971;8:251–265.

109. Selenow A, Cuiffreda KJ, Mozlin R, Rumpf D. Prognostic value of laser interferometric visual acuity in amblyopia therapy. Invest Ophthalmol Vis Sci 1986; 27:273.

110. Mayer DL, Fulton AB, Rodier D. Grating and recognition acuities of pediatric patients. Ophthalmology 1984;91:947–953.

111. Day SH, Orel-Bixler DA, Norcia AM. Abnormal acuity development in infantile esotropia. Invest Ophthalmol Vis Sci 1988;29:327–329.

112. Wilcox LM, Sokol S. Changes in the binocular fixation patterns and the visually evoked potential in the treatment of esotropia with amblyopia. Ophthalmology 1980;87:1273–1281.

113. Beller R, Hoyt CS, Marg E, et al. Good visual function after neo-natal surgery for congenital monocular cataracts. Am J Ophthalmol 1981;91:559–565.

114. Orel-Bixler DA, Haegerstrom-Portnoy G, Hall AP. Visual assessment of the multiply handicapped. Optom Vis Sci 1989;66:530–536.

115. Mackie RT, McCulloch DL, Saunders KJ, et al. Comparison of visual assessment tests in multiply handicapped children. Eye 1995;9:136–141.

116. Bane MC, Birch EE. VEP acuity, FPL acuity, and visual behavior of visually impaired children. J Pediatr Ophthalmol Strabismus 1992;29:202–209.

117. Apkarian P, Spereijse H. The VEP and Misrouted Pathways in Human Albinism. In RQ Craco, I Bodis-Wollner (eds), Evoked Potentials. New York: Allan R Liss, 1986;211–226.

118. Guillery RW, Okoro AN, Witkop CJ Jr. Abnormal visual pathways in the brain of a human albino. Brain Res 1975;96:373–377.

119. Apkarian P. Methodology of Testing for Albinism with Visual Evoked Cortical Potentials. In JR Heckenlively, GB Arden (eds), Principles and Practice of Clinical Electrophysiology of Vision. St. Louis: Year Book, 1991;425–434.

120. Barnett AB, Manson JI, Wilner E. Acute cerebral blindness in children. Neurology 1970;20:1147.

121. Whiting S, Jan JE, Wong PKH, et al. Permanent cortical visual impairment in children. Dev Med Child Neurol 1985;27:730–739.

122. Aduchi-Usami E. Visually Evoked Cortical Potentials in Cortical Blindness. In JR Heckenlively, GB Arden (ed), Principles and Practice of Clinical Electrophysiology of Vision. St. Louis: Year Book, 1991;578–580.

123. Frank Y, Torres F. Visual evoked potentials in the evaluation of "cortical blindness" in children. Ann Neurol 1979;6:126–129.

124. Aldrich MS, Alessi AG, Beck RW, Gilman S. Cortical blindness: etiology, diagnosis and prognosis. Ann Neurol 1987;21:149–158.

125. McCulloch DL, Taylor MJ, Whyte HE. Visual evoked potentials and visual prognosis following perinatal asphyxia. Arch Ophthalmol 1991;109:229.

126. Fiedler AR, Russell-Eggitt IR, Dodd KL, et al. Delayed visual maturation. Trans Ophthalmol Soc U K 1985;104:653–661.

127. Lambert SR, Kriss A, Taylor D. Delayed visual maturation. A longitudinal clinical and electrophysiological assessment. Ophthalmology 1989;96:524–529.

128. Illingworth RS. Delayed visual maturation. Arch Dis Child 1961;36:407–409.

129. Mellor DH, Fielder AR. Dissociated visual development electrodiagnostic studies in infants who are "slow to see." Dev Med Child Neurol 1980;22:327–335.

130. Taylor MJ, McCulloch DL. Visual evoked potentials in infants and children. J Clin Neurophysiol 1992;9: 357–372.

131. Green RL, Byrne SF. Diagnostic Ultrasound. In SJ Ryan, TE Ogden (eds), Retina. St Louis: Mosby, 1989;191–271.

132. Shammus HJ. Atlas of Ophthalmic Ultrasonography and Biometry. St. Louis: Mosby, 1984.

133. Thijssen JM. The History of Ultrasound Techniques in Ophthalmology. In Ultrasound in Medicine and Biology. 1993;19:599–618.

134. A-Scan Ultrasound: Biometry. In Fingeret M, Casser L, Woodcome HT (eds), Atlas of Primary Eyecare Procedures. East Norwalk, CT: Appleton & Lange, 1990; 278–281.

135. B-Scan Ultrasound: Biometry. In Fingeret M, Casser L, Woodcome HT (eds), Atlas of Primary Eyecare Procedures. East Norwalk, CT: Appleton & Lange, 1990; 236–239.

136. Larsen JS. The sagittal growth of the eye. I. Ultrasonic

measurement of the depth of the anterior chamber from birth to puberty. Acta Ophthalmol 1971;49:239–262.

137. Larsen JS. The sagittal growth of the eye. II. Ultrasonic measurement of the axial diameter of the lens and the anterior segment from birth to puberty. Acta Ophthalmol 1971;49:427–452.

138. O'Brien C, Clark D. Ocular biometry in pre-term infants without retinopathy of prematurity. Eye 1994; 8:662–665.

139. Tucker SM, Enzenauer RW, Levin AV, et al. Corneal diameter, axial length, and intraocular pressure in premature infants. Ophthalmology 1992;99:1296–1300.

140. Restori M, McLeod D. Ultrasound in pre-vitrectomy assessment. Trans Ophthalmol Soc U K 1977;97:232–234.

141. Reese AB. Persistence and hyperplasia of the primary vitreous: retrolental fibroplasia—two entities. Arch Ophthalmol 1949;41:527–552.

142. Goldberg MF, Mafee M. Computerized tomography for the diagnosis of persistent hyperplastic primary vitreous. Ophthalmology 1983;90:442–451.

143. Nucci P, Modorati G, Pierro L, et al. Comparative evaluation of echography and C.A.T. in diagnosing retinoblastoma. Minerva Pediatr 1989;41:129–131.

144. Belkin M, Ticho U, Susal A, Levinson A. Ultrasonography in the refraction of aphakic infants. Br J Ophthalmol 1973;57:845–848.

145. Birnholz JC. Ultrasonic Imaging, Human Brain. In G Adelman (ed), Enclopledia of Neuroscience (Vol 2). Boston: Birkhauser, 1987;1249–1250.

146. Birholz JC, Farrell EE. Ultrasound images of human fetal development. Am Sci 1984;72:608–613.

147. Garin JP, Mojon M, Piens MA, Chevalier-Nuttall I. Monitoring and treatment of toxoplasmosis in the pregnant woman, fetus and newborn. Pediatrie 1989;44: 705–712.

148. Achiron R, Gottlieb Z, Yaron Y, et al. The development of the fetal eye: in utero ultrasonographic measurements of the vitreous and lens. Prenat Diagn 1995;15:155–160.

149. Chitayat D, Toi A, Babul R, et al. Prenatal diagnosis of retinal nonattachment in the Walker-Warburg syndrome. Am J Med Genet 1995;56:351–358.

150. McCrary JA. Magnetic resonance imaging applications in ophthalmology. Int Ophthalmol Clin Neuroophthalmol 1991;31:101–115.

151. DiChiro G. Neuroimaging. In G Adelman (ed), Encyclopedia of Neuroscience (Vol 2). Boston: Birkhauser, 1987;795–797.

152. Citrin CM, Alper MG. Computed Tomography in the Evaluation of Retrobulbar Extracranial Causes of Visual Loss. In TJ Walsh (ed), Neuro-Ophthalmology: Clinical Signs and Symptoms. Philadelphia: Lea & Febiger, 1992;217–276.

153. Gilbard SM, Mafee MF, Lagouros PA, et al. Orbital blowout fractures: the prognostic significance of computer tomography. Ophthalmology 1985;92: 1523–1528.

154. Zimmerman RA, Bilaniuk LT. Pediatric head trauma. Neuroimaging Clin N Am 1994;4:349–366.

155. Catalano RA. Ocular Emergencies. Philadelphia: Saunders, 1992.

156. Moseley IF, Sanders MD. Computerized Tomography in Neuro-Ophthalmology. Philadelphia: Saunders, 1982.

157. Redington RW. Magnetic Resonance Imaging (MRI) and Spectroscopy. In G Adelman (ed), Encyclopedia of Neuroscience (Vol 2). Boston: Birkhauser, 1987; 599–600.

158. Kamholtz RG, Abrahams JJ. Magnetic Resonance Imaging of the Orbits and Extraorbital Visual System. In TJ Walsh (ed), Neuro-Ophthalmology: Clinical Signs and Symptoms. Philadelphia: Lea & Febiger, 1992;277–322.

159. Reivich M. Positron Emission Tomography. In G Adelman (ed), Encyclopedia of Neuroscience (Vol 2). Boston: Birkhauser, 1987;958–961.

160. Reivich M, Alavi A. Positron Emission Tomography. New York: Alan R Liss, 1985.

161. Cummings TJ, Chugani DC, Chugani HT. Positron emission tomography in pediatric epilepsy. Neurosurg Clin N Am 1995;6:465–472.

162. Chugani HT. The role of PET in childhood epilepsy. J Child Neurol 1994;9:82–88.

163. Chugani HT. Functional brain imaging in pediatrics. Pediatr Clin N Am 1992;39:777–799.

164. Schulman J, Peyman G, Mafee M, et al. The use of magnetic resonance imaging in the evaluation of retinoblastoma. J Pediatr Ophthalmol Strabismus 1986;23:144–147.

165. Lambert SR, Hoyt CS, Narahara MH. Optic nerve hypoplasia. Surv Ophthalmol 1987;32:1–9.

166. Barkovich AJ, Fram EK, Norman D. Septo-optic dysplasia: MR imaging. Radiology 1989;171:189.

167. Ghose S. Optic nerve changes in hydrocephalus. Trans Ophthalmol Soc U K 1983;103:217–220.

168. Chernikova S, Tzekov H, Karakostov V. Comparative ophthalmologic studies on children and adults with craniopharyngiomas. Ophthalmologica 1990;201:201–205.

169. Miller NR, Solomon S. Retinochoroidal (optociliary) shunt veins, blindness, and optic atrophy: a non-specific sign of chronic optic nerve compression. Aust N Z J Ophthalmol 1991;19:105–109.

170. Lewis RA, Gerson LP, Axelson KA, et al. Von Recklinghausen neurofibromatosis. II. Incidence of optic gliomata. Ophthalmology 1984;91:929–935.

171. Brodsky MC, Baker RS, Hamed LM. Pediatric Neuro-Ophthalmology. New York: Springer, 1996;399–465.

172. Williams AS, Hoyt CS. Acute comitant esotropia in children with brain tumors. Arch Ophthalmol 1989; 107:376–378.

173. Geyer JR. Infant brain tumors. Neurosurg Clin North Am 1992;3:781–791.

174. Lambert SR, Hoyt CS, Jan JE, et al. Visual recovery from hypoxic cortical blindness during childhood.

Computed tomographic and magnetic resonance imaging predictors. Arch Ophthalmol 1987;105:1371–1377.

175. Summers CG, MacDonald JT. After images: vision despite tomographic absence of occipital cortex. Surv Ophthalmol 1990;35:188–190.

176. Uvenbrant P, et al. Single photon emission tomography (SPECT) in neuropediatrics. Neuropediatrics 1991; 22:3.

177. Bosley TM, Rosenquist AC, Koshner M, et al. Ischemic lesions of the occipital cortex and optic radiations: positron emission tomography. Neurology 1985;35:470.

178. Nadel HR. Where are we with nuclear medicine in pediatrics? Eur J Nucl Med 1995;22:1433–1451.

179. Gerali P, Flom MC, Raab EL. Report of Children's Vision Screening Task Force. Report presented at the National Society to Prevent Blindness, Schaumburg, IL, November 1990.

180. Flom MC, Neumaier RW. Prevalence of amblyopia. Public Health Rep 1966;81:329.

181. Erlich MI, Reinecke RD, Simon K. Preschool vision screening for amblyopia and strabismus: programs, methods and guidelines. Surv Ophthalmol 1983;28:145–163.

182. Howland HC. The optics of static photoskiaskopy. Acta Ophthalmol (Copenh) 1980;58:221–227.

183. Atkinson J, Braddick OJ, Durden K, et al. Screening for refractive errors in 6–9 month old infants by photorefraction. Br J Ophthalmol 1984;68:105–112.

184. Hamer RD, Norcia AM, Day SM, et al. Comparison of on- and off-axis photorefraction with cycloplegic retinoscopy in infants. J Pediatr Ophthalmol Strabismus 1992;29:232–239.

185. Kaakinen K. A simple method for screening of children with strabismus, anisometropia or ametropia by simultaneous photography of the corneal and fundus reflexes. Acta Ophthalmol (Copenh) 1979;57:161–171.

186. Hay SH, Kerr JH, Jayroe RR, et al. Retinal reflex photometry as a screening device for amblyopia and pre-

amblyopic states in children. South Med J 1983;76: 309–312.

187. Norcia AM, Zadnik K, Day SH. Photorefraction with a catadioptric lens: improvement on the method of Kaakinen. Acta Ophthalmologica 1986;64:379–385.

188. Hsu-Winges C, Hamer RD, Norcia AM, et al. Polaroid photorefraction of infants: comparison to cycloplegic refraction. J Pediatr Ophthalmol Strabismus 1988; 26:254–260.

189. Freedman HL, Preston KL. Polaroid photoscreening for amblyogenic factors: an improved methodology. Ophthalmology 1992;99:1785–1795.

190. Ottar WL, Scott WE, Holgado SI. Photoscreening for amblyogenic factors. J Pediatr Ophthalmol Strabismus 1995;32:289–295.

191. Duckman RH, Meyer B. Use of photoretinoscopy as a screening technique in the assessment of anisometropia and significant refractive error in infants/toddlers/children and special populations. Am J Optom Physiol Opt 1987;64:604–610.

192. Fern K. A comparison of vision screening techniques in preschool children [abstract]. Invest Ophthalmol Vis Sci 1991;32:2976.

193. Morgan KS, Johnson WD. Clinical evaluation of a commercial photorefractor Arch Ophthalmol 1987; 105:1528–1531.

194. Morris CE, Scott WE, Simon JW, et al. Photorefractive Screening for Amblyogenic Factors: A Three Centre Study. Trans VIIth International Orthoptic Congress, Nurnberg, Germany, 1991;243.

195. Orel-Bixler D, Brodie A. Vision screening of infants and toddlers: photorefraction and stereoacuity [abstract]. Invest Ophthalmol Vis Sci 1995;32:962.

196. Lewis RC, Marsh-Tootle WL. The reliability of interpretation of photoscreening results with the MTI PS-100 in Head Start children. J Am Optom Assoc 1995;66:429–434.

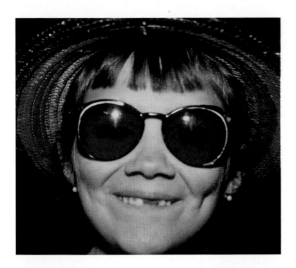

Plate 7.1. The red-tinted spectacle lenses, opaque side shields, and wide-brimmed hat alleviate the significant photophobia in daylight for this child with achromatopsia.

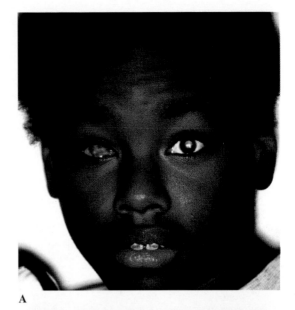

A

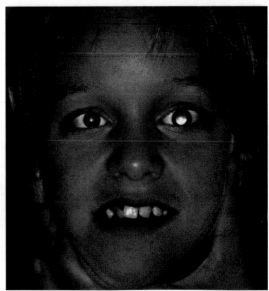

B

Plate 7.2. Media opacities are revealed by the lack of a red fundus reflex, with corneal opacity of the right eye (A) and complete cataract in the right eye (B).

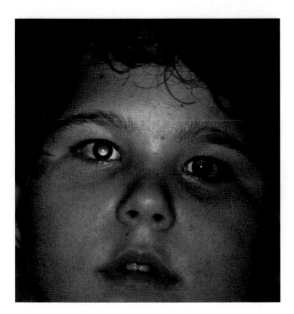

Plate 7.3. Ametropia is indicated by the location of the bright yellow crescent in the pupil margin in each eye. The bright crescent at the bottom of the pupil margin indicates myopia in the right eye. The small bright crescent at the top of the pupil margin indicates hyperopia in the left eye, which is smaller in magnitude than the ametropia in the right eye.

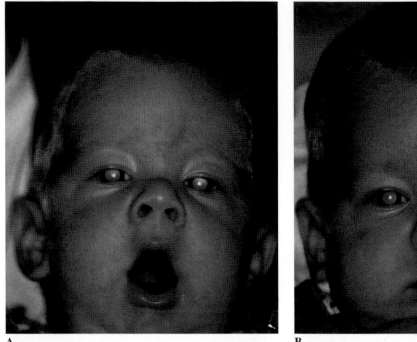

A   B

Plate 7.4. Off-axis photorefraction using a 35-mm camera with the flash oriented vertically (A) and horizontally (B). The location of the bright crescents indicates a hyperopic refractive error. The larger-diameter crescent along the vertical meridian (A) compared with the horizontal meridian (B) indicates with-the-rule astigmatism.

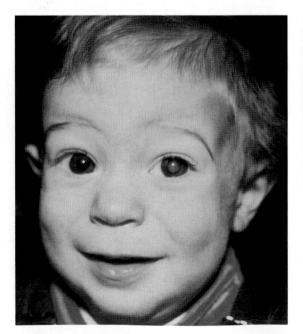

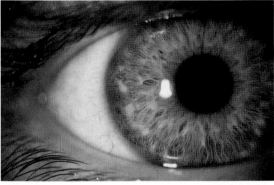

Plate 15.1. Lisch nodule (hypo- or hyperpigmented iris nodules that are found in most patients with neurofibromatosis). They do not affect vision but are useful in arriving at the diagnosis of neurofibromatosis.

Plate 12.1. This patient developed leukocoria suddenly at age 1 year from an idiopathic-acquired unilateral cataract. Surgical removal occurred within days of onset, and the patient developed visual acuity of 20/25 by 5 years of age.

Chapter 8

Strabismus: Detection, Diagnosis, and Classification

Susan A. Cotter and Kelly A. Frantz

Strabismus is the most common eye abnormality in infants and young children, excluding refractive error. When left untreated, strabismus commonly results in poor vision development (amblyopia) and impaired binocularity, or both. Because good binocular vision is required to perform many occupational and avocational tasks accurately and safely, those with strabismus are often prevented from participating in these activities—for example, a child with untreated strabismus (resulting in impaired depth perception) might be unable to become a surgeon, commercial airline pilot, cartographer, or even a police officer or firefighter in many communities. Similarly, patients with strabismus often complain that their sports performance is compromised.

Strabismus may result in delayed developmental milestones within the first 2 years of life [1] and may have a negative impact on the parent-child relationship and the child's psychological development [2–4]. Those with strabismus (particularly those with intermittent deviations) may experience symptoms such as diplopia, headaches, and ocular fatigue, which can result in poor academic or job performance. In addition, a strabismus that is cosmetically displeasing can have a negative effect on a person's self-esteem and personality development. Adverse effects on a person's self-image, interpersonal relationships, schooling, work, and sports activities have been shown to occur throughout life [5].

Despite the significant prevalence of strabismus and potential impact on quality of life, there is an apparent lack of attention to this condition from some eye care practitioners. Until recently, infants and young children were not examined routinely. In fact, many doctors recommended that the child's first eye examination take place at the beginning of school. This philosophy has changed in recent times (and will foreseeably continue to change) for at least two reasons. First, during the past 20–25 years, there has been a wealth of research and new information regarding the dramatic effects of abnormal visual experience on the young visual system during the "sensitive" period (i.e., birth to 7 years). Second, clinical testing methods and procedures have been developed or adapted so that it is now easier to examine young children.

Knowing what we do about the deleterious consequences that strabismus may have on the visual system of young children, as health care providers we would be remiss not to devote time and energy to the early identification and treatment of this condition. By providing prompt diagnosis and treatment, we can offer our young patients the greatest number of occupational and avocational choices as well as improve their quality of life. This chapter addresses the practitioner's initial task—detection and diagnosis of the problem. Before treatment can begin, the proper diagnosis must be made. This chapter begins by reviewing the epidemiology of strabismus. The clinical evaluation of young pa-

Table 8.1. Diagnostic Strategy for Evaluation of Young Children with Strabismus

---

Refractive error and visual acuity (see Chapters 6 and 7)
Ocular health
Evaluation of eye alignment
    Direct observation
    Hirschberg and Kappa tests
    Krimsky test
    Brückner test
    Cover test
    Visuoscopy*
Comitance testing
    Versions and ductions
    Cover test in nine diagnostic fields
Stereopsis testing
    Randot Stereotest
    Random Dot E Stereotest
    Lang Stereotest
Second-degree fusion testing
    Worth four-dot test
    Three-Figure Test

---

*Useful in cases in which microtropia is suspected.

tients having or suspected of having strabismus is described in detail so that the practitioner can arrive at an accurate diagnosis. We then review the most common types of strabismus that occur in infants and young children.

EPIDEMIOLOGIC FEATURES

The prevalence of strabismus in young children is estimated to be 3.7–5.3% [6–10]. In children, esotropia is reported to be approximately three times as frequent as exotropia [7, 8, 10, 11]. Infantile esotropia is the most common form of strabismus [12] and accounts for 28–48% of all esotropia [13, 14].

Although strabismus can develop at any age, it usually develops during early childhood. Two patterns have been described regarding the time of onset of esotropia. Nordlow [8] reported the onset of esotropia to be most frequent (45.3%) during the first year of life, with the incidence diminishing rapidly thereafter, and essentially ceasing by age 7. Others [7, 9, 10, 15], however, have found the incidence of esotropia to be highest in the second or third year of life. Similar to esotropia development, the onset of the majority of exotropias is during in-

fancy or early childhood [8, 15, 16]. The tendency of strabismus to develop in the early years is one reason that it is no longer appropriate for a child's first eye examination to occur when he or she starts school, but rather by 6 months of age (or earlier for "at-risk" children) [17].

EXAMINATION OF THE CHILD WITH STRABISMUS

Although general information about a strabismic deviation can be obtained at the initial examination, we recommend that the first examination focus on obtaining the case history, best visual acuities, refractive status using cycloplegia, and ocular health evaluation, including dilated funduscopy (see Chapters 6 and 7 for discussion of these examination elements). Once the patient has adapted to any significant prescription for approximately 4 weeks, a detailed strabismus evaluation should be performed using this refractive correction. Alternatively, if the examiner is unsure of the effect a proposed refractive correction will have on the strabismus, the patient may be reevaluated after cycloplegia has worn off and measurements can then be made through one or more tentative prescriptions. Measurements of strabismus performed while the patient is cyclopleged should not be considered reliable. Table 8.1 lists the tests commonly used to evaluate children with strabismus.

Evaluating Eye Alignment

Determining the presence, frequency, magnitude, laterality, and direction of any strabismic deviation in a young child is the basis for establishing a prognosis and a treatment plan. Several common tests will reveal these characteristics of strabismus.

Direct Observation

The examination should always begin with direct observation of the child's appearance. Useful information can be obtained when greeting the child, without making him or her apprehensive by approaching too closely with unfamiliar instruments. Noting the child's head posture often provides clues as to the etiology of strabismus. For example, a

Table 8.2. Characteristics Influencing Strabismus Appearance

Factor	Effect on Esotropia	Effect on Exotropia
Epicanthal folds	Exaggerates or produces pseudoesotropia	Masks
Narrow interpupillary distance	Exaggerates	Masks
Wide interpupillary distance	Masks	Exaggerates
Negative angle kappa	Exaggerates	Masks
Positive angle kappa	Masks	Exaggerates
Deep-set eyes	Masks	Masks
Alternating deviation	Exaggerates	Exaggerates
Intermittent deviation	Exaggerates	Exaggerates
Markedly noncomitant deviation	Exaggerates	Exaggerates

Source: Data from MC Flom. Issues in the Clinical Management of Binocular Anomalies. In AA Rosenbloom, MW Morgan (eds), Pediatric Optometry. Philadelphia: Lippincott, 1990;219–244.

head turn to one side may indicate paresis of a horizontally-acting muscle; patients often turn their head into the field of action of the underacting muscle to maintain fusion. Likewise, patients with cyclovertical muscle paresis may manifest a head tilt to one shoulder to compensate for loss of one eye's torsional ability. Tipping the chin up or down can occur in response to an A- or V-pattern strabismus. This head position might permit fusion in the gaze position where the horizontal deviation is smallest in magnitude. One should not, however, be misled by these classic examples; some patients move their head in the direction opposite to that predicted by the involved muscle to move diplopic images farther apart and thus more easily ignore one of them. Other possible reasons for an anomalous head position are uncorrected refractive error, particularly with-the-rule astigmatism, and nystagmus with a null position in a nonprimary gaze. Other characteristics worthy of observation include factors that either mask, exacerbate, or create the false impression of strabismus [18]. These facial features are listed in Table 8.2.

Hirschberg and Kappa Tests

The Hirschberg test is the simplest means to detect strabismus, provided the deviation is sufficiently large. The child simply needs to fixate a penlight or transilluminator briefly. The observer, positioned 33–50 cm from the child, notes the positions of corneal reflexes with respect to the center of the

pupil. An estimate in millimeters is made. In theory, a precise measurement could be made with a millimeter rule, but it is difficult in most cases to bring a millimeter rule close enough to the child's eye (and expect the child to remain adequately still). If the child is not interested in viewing the fixation light, covering it with a finger puppet may hold attention better. For best results, a hole should be made in the puppet's mouth through which the light can shine. Alternatively, reducing the room illumination may attract the child to the light. Making the light "blink" by intermittently placing a finger over it also helps improve attention. Some examiners tell the child to "blow out the light" (like a candle), but it is wise to ascertain that the child has no communicable illnesses before asking him or her to blow toward the examiner's face. When the child has dark irides, it is easier to judge the location of the reflex relative to the pupil border if a direct ophthalmoscope is used. With dim room illumination and a working distance of about 1 m, the Brückner test (discussed in "Brückner Test") can be performed simultaneously.

To interpret the Hirschberg test properly, it is necessary to measure angle lambda (clinically referred to as angle kappa) by observing the corneal reflexes while the child views the light monocularly. The Hirschberg (binocular) part of this sequence should be performed first to avoid disrupting fusion initially. Then each eye is occluded briefly. If the corneal reflexes under monocular conditions appear in the same positions as under binocular conditions, the child is considered not to have strabismus. (Because physiologic asymmetries in angle kappa can occur, this is the most accurate way to interpret the test.) If the reflex position for one eye differs under binocular conditions compared with monocular, that eye is strabismic. For example, if both reflexes are central monocularly, and under binocular conditions the right eye's reflex remains central while the left eye's reflex is now 1 mm temporal, the patient has left esotropia. (The deviating eye's reflex always moves in the opposite direction as the eye.) Research has confirmed that each millimeter of displacement of the corneal reflex is equivalent to approximately 22^Δ of eye misalignment [19–21]. This ratio remains essentially constant from birth [22, 23]. Because of the large ratio, it is unlikely that most examiners will detect strabismus smaller than $10–15^\Delta$ with the Hirschberg test.

One exception to the above interpretation method occurs when one eye has significant eccentric fixation or such poor vision that fixation is impossible. The Hirschberg test can still be performed, but the kappa value from the poorly seeing eye may be unreliable. In this case, the Hirschberg reflexes must both be compared with the kappa value of the better seeing eye; it can be assumed that the poorly seeing eye would have a symmetric angle kappa if normal fixation were possible, unless there is a gross anatomic difference between the eyes.

Krimsky Test

One can quantify the Hirschberg test more precisely by using the Krimsky test after the above sequence has been performed. Once the direction of strabismus is known, an appropriately oriented prism is placed before the fixating eye in an attempt to neutralize the deviation. Meanwhile, the examiner monitors the corneal reflex of the deviating eye as prism power is altered. The end point is reached when the two eyes have symmetric Hirschberg reflexes. The amount of prism used to achieve this endpoint is then recorded as the estimated magnitude of the deviation. Because this modification requires longer fixation by the patient, more cooperation and attention to the target are needed. In addition, research has shown that the value obtained by the Krimsky test is generally smaller than that measured by the cover test [24]. Nevertheless, the Krimsky test is valuable for estimating a stra-

bismic angle at near point in patients having an eye with poor or no vision, because only one eye has to view the target (in contrast to the cover test, discussed in a following section).

Brückner Test

Another simple test of eye alignment is the Brückner test. It can provide information about the presence and laterality of strabismus. This procedure requires the child to fixate a direct ophthalmoscope light in a darkened room. The examiner is positioned approximately 1 m away, so there is less intimidation than with tests requiring the examiner to get close to the child. The examiner merely compares the brightness of the reflected light (i.e., fundus reflex) from the child's two eyes; the whiter and brighter reflex indicates the strabismic eye [25] (Figure 8.1). It is not possible to quantify the strabismic angle unless the Hirschberg reflexes are observed at the same time. The Brückner test is remarkably sensitive in detecting even small angles of strabismus [26]. False-positive interpretations can occur, however, if the patient has media opacities, posterior pole abnormalities, anisocoria, or uncorrected anisometropia. Therefore, the test is best used with the child wearing full refractive correction. Dilated pupils may also invalidate the test. For this reason, the Brückner test should be performed before cycloplegia or dilation [25]. Interestingly, infants less than 2 months of age do not demonstrate the fundus reflex dimming phenomenon that occurs when an eye fixates the ophthalmoscope accurately. In addition, there is an unacceptably high (28%) frequency of asymmetric dimming of fundus reflexes in nonstrabismic infants between 2 and 8 months of age. Thus, it is recommended that the Brückner test not be used to screen for strabismus in infants less than 8 months old [27].

Cover Test

The cover test is the ideal method for detecting as well as quantifying strabismus. Frequency, laterality, and direction of the deviation are also obtained. The cover test, however, requires more cooperation from a child than does the Hirschberg test. It is also necessary for the examiner to ensure that the child can see the selected target with each eye; the smallest possible accommodative target that holds

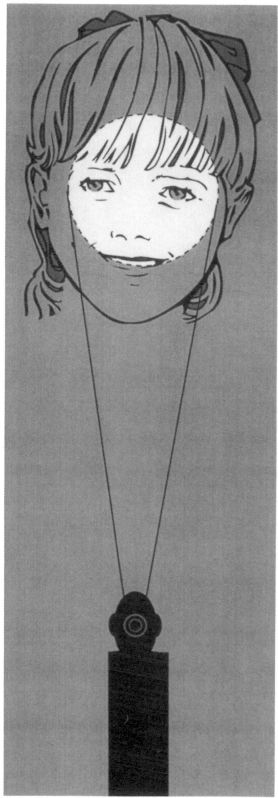

A

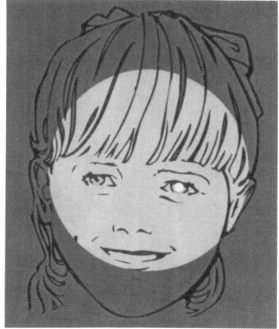

B

Figure 8.1. Brückner test. A. The direct ophthalmoscope is used to illuminate both eyes simultaneously. B. Note the whiter left pupil, indicating left strabismus.

attention should be used. The intent is for accommodation to be postured as close to the plane of the target as possible to allow a more accurate measurement of any phoric or strabismic deviation (Figure 8.2). For infants, illuminated puppets work well. Toddlers respond to large, bright stickers placed on tongue depressors. Older preschoolers with better attention should have their accommodative accuracy controlled by small, detailed stickers or pictures. To keep attention and accommodation on the target, it helps to change targets frequently. If the child will respond, the examiner should ask the child to identify the target's details. Another means of keeping attention is to move the target slowly from side to side, as long as it is stationary at the moment when the cover paddle is repositioned (so that a version movement to follow the target is not mistaken for a refixation by a deviating eye).

It is much easier to maintain interest for a cover test at near point than at a greater distance. Ideally, distance cover testing uses a target at 6 m, but intermediate distances will hold the attention of

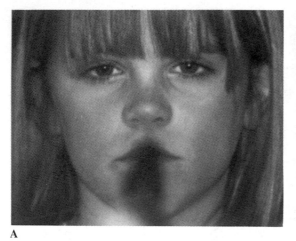
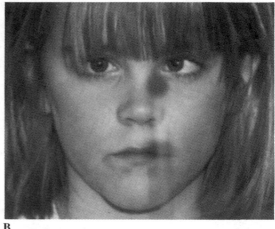

A   B

Figure 8.2. Cover testing. A. Cover testing performed with a nonaccommodative target (transilluminator); no strabismus is present. B. Cover testing with a small accommodative target (single letter "A"); a left esotropia is present.

young children better. It is necessary to have an assistant or parent hold a suitable target and "entertain" the child with it, or to make use of remote-controlled toys that will engage the child's attention. For older preschoolers who can maintain attention better, distance cover testing at 6 m is definitely recommended. Compared with testing at 6 m, testing at 3 m tends to underestimate the magnitude of divergence excess exotropia and to overestimate the magnitude of convergence excess esotropia [28].

During the unilateral cover test (UCT), the direction and laterality (unilateral or alternating) of the strabismus are observed. In addition, the frequency (constant or intermittent) should be determined from the number of times refixation movement occurred on the UCT. It is also useful to estimate the frequency of an intermittent strabismus during casual observation of the child throughout the examination. Frequency of the deviation is critical to the prognosis for successful treatment; intermittent strabismus is more easily and successfully treated [29].

An experienced examiner can estimate the angle of strabismus with the alternating cover test (ACT), but for greatest accuracy, prisms should be used. Personal preference governs the choice of loose prisms or a prism bar. Advantages of loose prisms are that a horizontal and vertical prism can be held together before the eye if needed, and that loose prisms may appear less threatening to a young child, compared to a prism bar. On the other hand, prism bars offer the convenience of not having to interrupt testing to pick up and set down several prisms before the endpoint is reached. Anything that saves time and reduces distractions when testing a child is a definite advantage. In either case, the prism can be presented as a "window" that the child is to look through. Keeping the child attentive to the target during the measurement cannot be overemphasized.

It is also important to hold the prism properly, with its ocular surface perpendicular to the target direction. It must therefore be rotated slightly inward when the child is fixating a near target. The prism should be held as close as possible to the patient's eye. One should avoid stacking two horizontal prisms together over one eye because their total power will be more than their algebraic sum [30].

The movement of the eye *behind* the prism should be neutralized; the fellow eye is designated the fixating eye. If attention permits, strabismus should be neutralized with each eye fixating. A difference of more than 5^Δ between the two measurements suggests noncomitance due to a muscle underaction; the larger of the two angles results when the eye with the underacting muscle is forced to fixate [31, 32]. On the other hand, if the child has uncorrected anisometropia, differing accommodative demands between the two eyes can result in unequal measurements. Thus, if the child has significant refractive error, the cover test ideally should be performed through the refractive correction. However, the examiner should also keep in mind that measurements of strabismus, both horizontal and vertical, will be significantly smaller than the true angle when performed through high plus spectacle lenses, and larger than the true angle through high minus spectacles, due to the prismatic effect of the spectacles [33].

Visuoscopy

Visuoscopy as a test of monocular fixation is important in the diagnosis of microstrabismus. If the patient fixates eccentrically and uses the same retinal site under both monocular and binocular conditions, the examiner would see no movement on the UCT even though strabismus is actually present. In addition, if significant eccentric fixation (EF) is present, any angle of strabismus found with the cover test must be altered by the amount of EF. The amount of EF is simply added algebraically to the measured magnitude of the deviation, with esodeviations and nasal EF designated as (+) and exodeviations and temporal EF as (−). For example, if the ACT measures 20^Δ BO and 3^Δ temporal EF is found on visuoscopy, the true deviation is esotropia of 17^Δ $[(+20) + (−3) = 17^\Delta]$.

To perform visuoscopy, the patient must understand the task adequately. Comprehension can be evaluated by shining the visuoscope grid target on the child's hand and asking him or her to touch the middle of the circle. If the child can accomplish this accurately, the task of looking at the center of the target probably will be performed reliably. It is critical to occlude the eye not being tested and to dim the ophthalmoscope light so that the child can see the target comfortably. For some patients, it is much easier to perform visuoscopy through dilated pupils, so this test is often conducted at the same time as the fundus examination.

Interpretation of visuoscopy results is done by noting what retinal area is seen at the center of the grid, as well as the degree of fixation steadiness. For example, if the center of the target is noted to occupy a location nasal to the fovea but wanders closer to the fovea at times, fixation would be classified as unsteady and nasal. Magnitude is derived from the target's markings; many brands of ophthalmoscopes have marks at 1^Δ intervals with a central circle 2^Δ in diameter.

Evaluating Comitance

Determination of comitance (whether the deviation is equal in all fields of gaze and with either eye fixating) is essential in differentiating functional from pathologic causes of strabismus. Although any recent-onset strabismus should be viewed with suspicion, noncomitance should arouse concern that a cranial nerve or brain lesion might be the cause.

Cover Test in Diagnostic Action Fields

To determine whether an ocular deviation is comitant, the alternate cover test (ACT) provides an objective means of quantifying any changes in magnitude. Ideally the test is performed in nine diagnostic action fields and with each eye fixating. For young children, however, it is more practical to limit testing to primary, up, down, right, and left gazes, all done at one testing distance and with the same eye designated to be fixating (the prism is always before the fellow eye). If these initial measurements suggest that a muscle underaction exists, additional gaze directions can be used to help determine the specific muscle involved. In contrast, evaluation in primary, up, and down gazes is adequate to detect an A- or V-pattern strabismus. After performing the ACT in primary gaze, a near point target is held in each desired gaze position, with the examiner ensuring that it can be seen by each eye. The same prism that neutralized the ACT in primary gaze is used initially for the ACT in the other gazes. It is important to hold plastic prisms with their ocular surface perpendicular to the line of sight for each target position to avoid measurement errors [30, 34]. If 5^Δ or less of movement is seen through the prism that neutralized the movement in primary gaze, the deviation need not be quantified further. Differences of more than 5^Δ usually are considered to be noncomitant [31]. The gaze associated with the greatest deviation narrows the number of possible underacting muscles to two; the direction of the deviation usually enables the examiner to determine which of these two muscles is indeed underacting. For example, if an esodeviation is largest in right gaze (limiting the responsible underacting muscles to the right lateral rectus and the left medial rectus), the underacting muscle would be the right lateral rectus because an underacting medial rectus causes an exodeviation. As another example, consider a child having a right hypertropia of largest magnitude when gaze is directed down and to the left. The muscles responsible for this gaze position are the right superior oblique and the left inferior rectus. However, the underacting muscle must be the right superior oblique because, of these two muscles, only its underaction could lead to a *right* hyperdeviation. One must remember that comitance testing does not determine whether a muscle underaction is due to a lesion in the brain, a cranial nerve paresis, or a muscle restriction. When pathologic etiologies are suspected, neuroimaging techniques (computed tomography or magnetic resonance imaging) should be used as well.

Versions and Ductions

Testing comitance by means of versions (binocular range of motion) and ductions (monocular) is simpler than with the ACT but less sensitive. The examiner is looking for gross muscle underactions in any gaze. Precision can be improved by monitoring the corneal reflexes in each gaze for a change in the strabismic deviation. If ductions show greater movement than do versions, the cause is frequently neurologic. If, however, versions show a muscle underaction and ductions reveal an equal limitation, the cause is most likely restrictive—for example, a tight antagonist muscle or an orbital mass limiting the eye's movement. Confirmatory forced-duction testing is not usually performed on young children without sedation.

At times, an infant or young child may not cooperate for version and duction testing and will appear to have an abduction deficit. Full abduction might be elicited, however, by use of the doll's head maneuver. This can be performed by carefully spinning an infant in a circle or moving him or her quickly to one side. The examiner watches for the vestibular reflex eye movement in the opposite direction of the spin, followed by a saccade in the direction of the spin. In infants with an undeveloped vestibular system, this maneuver will cause a deviation of the eyes in the same direction as the spin. Alternatively, if the child will fixate on the examiner's face or other target, a sudden turning of his head or body by the examiner might reveal full abduction as the child attempts to maintain fixation on the object of interest. Another method that can be used is to patch the apparently unaffected eye and then observe the child in a casual environment outside the examining room. Full abduction of the eye

with a suspected abduction deficit is sometimes noted to occur spontaneously.

Evaluating Stereopsis

Stereopsis testing provides useful information as to the possible presence of strabismus, particularly microstrabismus that might go undetected on a cover test. A positive response to random dot stereopsis (RDS) forms indicates bifoveal fixation and rules out constant strabismus [35]. In addition, positive RDS in a patient with intermittent strabismus implies that the patient has excellent sensory fusion when the eyes are straight.

Randot Stereotest

Children ages 2–3 years and older are usually capable of identifying the shapes of the random dot forms used in the Randot Stereotest (Stereo Optical, Chicago, IL). A demonstration of the required polarized filters on the examiner or a stuffed animal, or placement of the filters in a children's sunglasses frame, often makes the child less hesitant to wear them. To determine whether the test will be usable, the child should first be asked to name the shapes on the front cover of the test, or to point to them as they are called out by the examiner. If identification is possible, the examiner can direct attention to the random dot forms inside. Identification of three or more forms on the Randot test (by naming or matching with the front cover) generally is adequate to consider the child capable of bifoveal fixation.

Because identification of the floating animals on the Randot test reveals only a gross level of stereopsis, it is recommended that the examiner proceed directly to the lateral disparity circles if the child is capable of understanding this part. Having the child "push down the button that is sticking up" may result in a reliable response. It has been suggested that a threshold of less than or equal to 67 seconds of arc indicates that bifoveal fixation is possible [36]. This would translate into responding correctly to at least the first six circles on the Randot test. Because this part of the test demands higher level perceptual and cognitive skills than do the random dot forms, however, a poorer response by a preschooler should not be a concern if the random dot forms have been identified correctly.

Figure 8.3. Random Dot E Stereotest. The patient must differentiate the stereo "E" from the stereo blank.

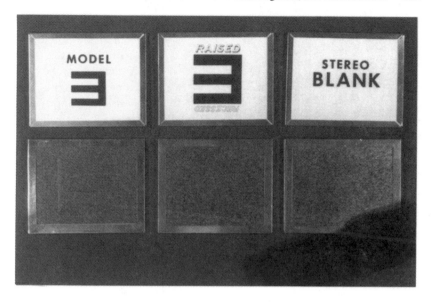

Random Dot E Stereotest

The Random Dot E (Stereo Optical, Chicago, IL) involves differentiating the capital letter "E" from a stereo blank in a forced choice task (Figure 8.3). Bifoveal fixation is needed to perceive the floating E. As with the Randot Stereotest, polarized filters are required. The child can initially be shown the raised model E and told, "This is an E." As long as the child can point reliably to the E when it is shown together with the blank card, the test can be used. It is often performed at a distance of 40 cm, although it has been shown to screen more effectively for amblyopia when performed at 1.5 m [37]. The cards must be shown at least four times, with the E presented randomly on one side or the other of the blank. One must be careful not to allow the child to see the backs of the cards when they are being rearranged, since the labels would reveal where the E is located. Because there is a 50% chance of guessing the location of the E on each presentation, it is necessary for the child to be correct four out of four times, or five of six times, to interpret the results as indicating bifoveal fixation.

Lang Stereotest

The Lang Stereotest (Distributor: Haag-Streit Service, Inc., Waldwick, NJ) has the advantage over the Randot and Random Dot E tests of not requir-

ing polarized filters (Figure 8.4). Again, bifoveal fixation is a prerequisite for identifying the pictures. Although the test does not measure stereopsis threshold, a positive response does provide evidence of normal binocular vision [38]. The test has been used successfully for many children as young as 2 years old, and at that age, it is more usable than the Random Dot E [39]. Because movement of the head or of the test card can allow some perception of the figures, it is critical to hold the test still, in the patient's frontal plane and not to allow the child to move side to side. Good lighting on the front surface of the card is also necessary. The child should merely be asked to identify and point to any pictures seen. If the child is nonverbal or the examiner is unsure whether the child knows these objects, the pictures that accompany the test can be used for matching. It is recommended, however, that these pictures first be cut out and mounted on another piece of paper in a different arrangement from the original drawing because the original is identical to the arrangement on the test card. The clever child might guess that the pictures will be arranged on the test card in the same orientation as the drawing and appear to localize them even if strabismus prevents their being perceived. As an alternative to matching or pointing, the examiner can watch for a child to gaze toward a picture. To interpret the test results as indicating bifoveal fixa-

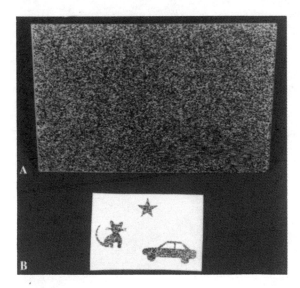

Figure 8.4. Lang Stereotest. A. The Lang Stereotest card. B. The pictures accompanying the test are arranged as they appear in stereo on the test card.

tion, identification or localization of at least two pictures should be achieved [40].

Evaluating Second-Degree Fusion

Because strabismus in a child results in diplopia, suppression, or anomalous correspondence (AC), investigation of second-degree (flat) fusion is useful for inferring the duration of strabismus and for establishing a treatment prognosis. Recent-onset strabismus is likely to produce diplopia, whereas after a period of time (often only 4–6 months [41]) suppression or AC can develop in preschoolers, particularly when the strabismus is constant and unilateral. These adaptations reduce the prognosis for a functional cure [18, 41] and increase the treatment time.

Worth Four-Dot Test

The Worth four-dot test is usable if the child can count to four accurately. The flashlight contains four illuminated dots: one red, two green, and one white, the latter of which can be seen by both eyes and will have a luster appearance when fused (Figure 8.5). It is essential that the child not view the flashlight without anaglyph filters so there is no

prior knowledge of the true number of dots. The child should first put on the filters (conventionally with red on the right eye), and then with one eye covered view the flashlight at near point for the first time. If the child can count two red dots correctly while viewing with the right eye and three green dots while viewing with the left, the examiner can expose both eyes and ask the child to count the dots. If necessary for accuracy, the child can touch each light as he or she counts. This adaptation will only allow testing at near point, however. Ideally, the flashlight is moved away from the child to a distance of 3 m to determine whether the number of dots changes at any distance. The Worth four-dot becomes a more central target as greater testing distances are used.

A number of Worth four-dot test results are possible. A response of four dots can indicate fusion; alternatively, it suggests AC if strabismus is present at the time of the response. To differentiate normal fusion from AC in a strabismic patient, it is necessary either to observe the eyes for obvious strabismus during the test, or to perform the UCT while the patient observes the white dot (this dot being chosen so that the fixated dot does not disappear when an eye is covered). This dot should be described by its location rather than by color, however, because it will not appear white through anaglyph filters. During the UCT, any refixation movement of either eye on covering the fellow eye would indicate the presence of strabismus and AC; no movement of either eye would indicate normal fusion.

A response of two or three dots reveals suppression of the eye that cannot see the dots corresponding to the color of its filter. Five dots would indicate diplopia. An attempt should be made to neutralize diplopia with prism; the child can raise his or her right or left hand to show which side the red dots are on. If the orientation of the diplopia corresponds to the direction of strabismus found by the cover test or Hirschberg test, the initial prism power to attempt neutralization can be based on the previously measured strabismus magnitude. It can be difficult to find the correct neutralizing prism for a child's diplopia, but if true second-degree fusion can be achieved, this boosts the prognosis significantly [18, 41]. This test is helpful in determining whether a prism correction would be appropriate for a child with constant strabismus. Caution should be used if the subjective prism value to produce four dots dif-

Figure 8.5. Worth four-dot test (left) and Three-Figure Test (right). These flashlights project red, green, and white dots or pictures, and are used with anaglyph filters for evaluation of second-degree fusion. The Three-Figure Test is useful for patients who cannot count reliably.

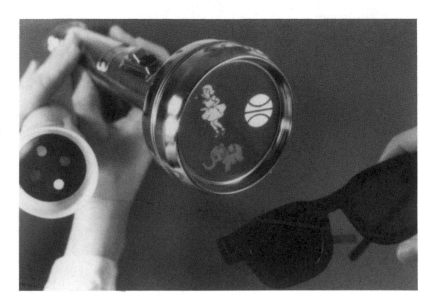

fers from the objective magnitude of the deviation. The patient may be using fusional vergence to achieve fusion with less than full neutralization of the angle, or AC may be present. Again, to differentiate the two conditions, the UCT should be performed as discussed in the previous paragraph.

Three-Figure Test

For children too young to count dots accurately, the Three-Figure Test (Bernell Corp., South Bend, IN) can be substituted (see Figure 8.5). The flashlight contains a red girl, a green elephant, and a white ball. A testing procedure similar to that for the Worth four-dot test should be used, except that the child merely tells the examiner what pictures are seen. Interpretation is similar to the Worth four-dot; a "fusion" response must be differentiated from AC in a child with strabismus. A diplopic response would consist of a red girl, a green elephant, and one ball of each color. Absence of one picture would indicate suppression. Because of the relatively large size of the pictures, however, only peripheral suppression can be revealed.

Additional Tests of Sensory Fusion

The polarized Child's Vectographic Slide (Reichert Ophthalmic Instruments, Buffalo, NY) has

been found to be a sensitive test of suppression for children age 3 years and older [42]. This distance projector slide contains two sets of identical polarized pictures positioned side by side. One set of pictures is polarized for each eye. The patient must wear polarized filters and indicate whether two of each picture are seen. Failure to see two of each picture can be interpreted as absent bifixation [42].

The major amblyoscope is extremely valuable for evaluating correspondence and sensory fusion in many patients. In addition to using stereopsis tests and the Worth four-dot test, in-instrument evaluation is advisable (when possible) for a complete analysis of strabismus. Although some preschoolers cannot sit still nor give sufficiently reliable responses in this instrument, it yields useful information in many, especially for children 4 years of age and older.

Lastly, the four prism diopter base-out test has been recommended for diagnosis of suppression or lack of binocular fixation [43]. However, we have recently found the test not to be repeatable and to yield numerous atypical responses in both normal subjects and those without binocular vision [44]. For these reasons, diagnosis of suppression is better made with the Worth four-dot test or polarized vectographic slide [36] and suspected microstrabismus should be evaluated with the cover test, visuoscopy [43], and RDS testing [35].

Table 8.3. Classification of Common Forms of Strabismus in Young Children

Esotropias in young children
    Pseudoesotropia
    Congenital esotropia
    Accommodative esotropia
    Partially accommodative esotropia
    Acute-onset comitant esotropia
    Nystagmus blockage syndrome
    Cyclic esotropia
    Sensory esotropia
Exotropias in young children
    Congenital
    Intermittent exotropia
Special forms of noncomitant strabismus
    Paralytic
        Oculomotor paresis
        Trochlear paresis
        Abducens paresis
    Nonparalytic
        Duane's retraction syndrome
        Brown's syndrome

CLASSIFICATION OF STRABISMUS

Strabismus, in general, is caused by a mechanical, optical, or innervational factor (or combination thereof) [41]. Mechanical origins include abnormalities of the extraocular muscles, ligaments, tendons, orbital contents, or fractures of the orbital bones. Optical causes include high refractive error, anisometropia, and media opacities. Innervational factors may involve muscle tonus changes resulting from trauma or disease and innervational anomalies (which may include high or low accommodative convergence–accommodation [AC/A] ratios).

Table 8.3 includes the most common forms of strabismus that occur in infants and young children. Categories of classification include esotropia, exotropia, and special forms of noncomitant strabismus. Although this system is useful for clinical purposes, one should note that not all existing types of strabismus are included. In addition, some uncommon types are included because of the importance of differentiating them from the more prevalent forms of strabismus.

Pseudoesotropia

Pseudostrabismus is the condition in which an individual appears to have a strabismus but in fact does not. Of the possible types of pseudostrabismus, pseudoesotropia is the most prevalent. It is most commonly seen in infants and young children who have wide, flat nasal bridges, prominent or asymmetrical epicanthal folds, and small interpupillary distances. In addition, children with temporally-displaced angles kappa (i.e., angles lambda) may also appear to have an esotropia.

The reduced amount of visible sclera nasally, secondary to prominent or asymmetrical epicanthal folds, often is the culprit. It creates the impression that the eye is turned inward, especially when the child looks to the side. Parents often report that the child's eye almost disappears completely from view when this occurs. As the child becomes older, the esotropic appearance generally disappears because the bridge of the nose becomes more prominent and displaces the epicanthal folds so that the medial aspect of the sclera appears proportional to that visible laterally. Some individuals, such as those of Asian descent, may maintain the appearance of pseudoesotropia because of the tendency of their bridges to remain flat and their epicanthal folds to persist.

Pseudoesotropia is commonly seen in infants and toddlers. Costenbader [14] reported that in a consecutive group of 753 children with the presenting complaint of the apparent esotropia, nearly half were pseudoesotropic. This percentage, however, does not reflect our clinical experience. In fact, most of our young patients that present with a suspicion of esotropia are indeed strabismic. Costenbader admitted that the large number of pseudostrabismic patients who presented for examination might have been encouraged because the data was collected in a "squint-conscious community and an ophthalmic office treating a large percentage of strabismus." Interestingly, others [45] have reported that parents are often remarkably good at identifying strabismus in their young children.

When evaluating the child, the cover test, Hirschberg test, and Brückner test should be used to assess whether the child's eyes are aligned or indeed esotropic. If the child is old enough, one of the aforementioned random dot stereotests may also be used.

It is wise to perform a cycloplegic refraction to rule out latent hyperopia that might be causing accommodative esotropia that is occurring intermittently. Even when one is rather certain that the young child has a pseudoesotropia, it is prudent to follow the child closely until one is absolutely certain there is no strabismus. The child should be evaluated at least one or two additional times within the year. A 3- to 4-month follow-up is recommended. Provided that the doctor does not find an esotropia at this visit, another follow-up in 6 months is reasonable. Asking the parents to bring photographs of the child, especially pictures with the child looking straight ahead, is often helpful for evaluation and documentation.

Table 8.4. Characteristics of Congenital Esotropia

Consistent
  Onset before 6 months of age
  Large, relatively stable angle, usually 30–70$^\Delta$
  Normal central nervous system
Variable
  Dissociated vertical deviation
  Overacting inferior oblique muscles
  A- or V-patterns
  Latent or manifest-latent nystagmus [12, 46]
  Amblyopia
  Apparently defective abduction
  Crossed fixation

Congenital Esotropia

A large-angle, constant esotropia with an onset during the first 6 months of life in an otherwise neurologically normal infant has historically been referred to as congenital esotropia. However, there has been considerable discussion and controversy in recent years regarding the appropriate terminology to describe this clinical entity. Some have proposed that *infantile* or *essential infantile* may be more appropriate terms because the esotropia is not actually present at birth, as the term *congenital* would imply [12, 46]. Others object to the term *infantile* because (1) many different forms of strabismus can be included in this heterogeneous classification [47] and (2) infancy describes the first 2 years of life, and congenital esotropia has its onset in the first 6 months of life [48].

Nixon and colleagues [49] examined 1,219 newborn infants in an attempt to determine whether esotropia is present at birth or develops later. Interestingly, they were unable to find a single infant who had typical findings of congenital esotropia at birth. In another study, Archer and coworkers [50] found only 0.7% of 3,316 neonates had esodeviations at birth. Furthermore, most of these deviations were intermittent and follow-up showed that the esotropias subsequently resolved. Of the three infants who were eventually diagnosed with congenital esotropia, all originally had an exodeviation or orthotropia at birth and did not develop the esotropia until several months after birth. These studies have established that esotropia is infrequently present at

birth but probably develops in the first few months of life, likely between 2–4 months of age [49–51].

Despite the fact that congenital esotropia is not connatal (although many parents report observing the esotropia since birth) and the term may not be semantically accurate, it remains in common usage. We (as well as others) [47, 48] prefer to use this terminology because it remains a widely accepted designation, describing a specific strabismic entity that is easily distinguished from other forms of acquired infantile esotropia. As a separate entity with its own etiology and clinical characteristics, congenital esotropia is just one form of a heterogeneous group of esodeviations with an onset before 1 year of age (i.e., infantile esotropia).

Congenital esotropia is a common form of strabismus, accounting for approximately 28–48% of all esotropia [13, 14]. The etiology of congenital esotropia is unknown, although there are probably multiple causes. A positive family history for strabismus is commonly found, suggesting an element of heritability. The mode of transmission, however, is by no means clear although some believe it is multifactorial (i.e., polygenic and environmental interaction) [52].

Clinical Features

Essential characteristics of congenital esotropia are an esotropia in a neurologically normal child, with a documented onset by 6 months of age, that remains despite correction of any hyperopia (Table 8.4) [53].

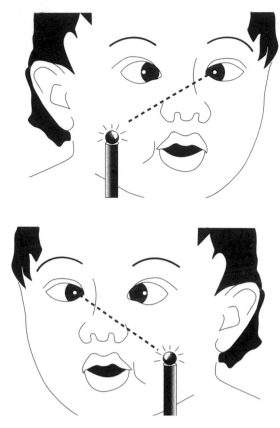

Figure 8.6. Crossed fixation. The left eye fixates in the right field of gaze (top), and the right eye fixates in the left field of gaze (bottom).

The significance and prevalence of other clinical characteristics vary among different studies; however, there is general agreement that consistent clinical findings include a constant, large-angle esotropia that is usually greater than 30^Δ [54], with averages reported in the range of $40–60^\Delta$ [14, 55, 56]. Typically, the magnitude of the angle with near and far fixation is approximately the same, indicating a normal AC/A ratio. The angle is often described as stable (i.e., not changing in size during the examination or at subsequent visits [12]). Ing [57] recently reported, however, that the majority (25 of 41) of his patients with congenital esotropia demonstrated a progressive increase of 10^Δ or more in esotropia magnitude when followed for a period of several months.

Variable associated clinical findings can be found in Table 8.4. Dissociated vertical deviations

(DVDs) are found in approximately 50–75% of patients with congenital esotropia [54, 58], but rarely before 2–3 years of age. A DVD presents as a spontaneous drifting upward of either eye when an individual is daydreaming or fatigued or, more commonly, when one eye of a patient is covered. Clinically, the practitioner will usually first see this phenomenon when attempting to neutralize the ACT. When the cover is removed, the elevated eye will move slowly downward to settle in the primary position. (If the eso component is already neutralized with base-out prism, the eye will move straight down. If the eso is not neutralized, one will see each eye move down as well as outward). This phenomenon will happen with both eyes—thus, the term *double hyper* or DVD. The amount of elevation when the eye is under cover is usually variable and asymmetric between the eyes. A DVD is notoriously difficult to neutralize with prism.

The incidence of unilateral or bilateral overacting inferior oblique muscles has been reported to be as high as 72% in congenital esotropia [56, 59], but this feature is rarely detected before age 1. This upshoot in adduction is best noted during version testing. The bilateral form is characterized by a right hyperdeviation in left gaze and a left hyperdeviation in right gaze. There is no vertical deviation in primary gaze.

An apparent deficiency of abduction is not uncommon. The practitioner, however, must differentiate whether the child is truly *unable* to abduct or is *unwilling* to abduct. Using the aforementioned doll's head maneuver or patching the fixating eye for several days will help to determine if there is a true abduction paresis present. Typically, one finds that the child has full abduction abilities.

Although many infants with congenital esotropia initially cross-fixate (i.e., view targets in the left field of gaze with the right eye and view targets in the right field of gaze with the left eye, as illustrated in Figure 8.6) a significant number of these will later exhibit a fixation preference for one eye with subsequent amblyopia development. Amblyopia is reported to develop in approximately 35% [54] to 72% [60] of patients with congenital esotropia and may even occur among those who cross-fixate [61]. Latent or manifest-latent nystagmus as well as A or V patterns may also be present.

In contrast to accommodative esotropia, which is often accompanied by significant hyperopia, the refractive error distribution in congenital esotropia is skewed toward low hyperopia (i.e., <2.00 D); however, approximately 40–50% have hyperopia in excess of 2.00 D [14]. The notion that congenital esotropia is nonaccommodative is disputed by Réthy and Gal [62] and Réthy [63], who assert that many of the infants who are diagnosed as having congenital esotropia in fact have accommodative esotropia. They suggest one should routinely cycloplege these patients and prescribe the full hyperopic correction with an additional 0.50–1.00 D of plus. Whenever additional, latent hyperopia becomes manifest, they recommend the prescription be increased. Their belief is that unless this type of prescribing regimen is instituted at an early age, the increased accommodative tonus and the associated convergence will become stable and then resistant to therapeutic intervention.

Differential Diagnosis

In addition to congenital esotropia, there are several other forms of esotropia that can have an onset at birth or during infancy (Table 8.5). Sixth nerve paresis, early-onset accommodative esotropia, nystagmus blockage syndrome (NBS), pseudoesotropia, sensory esotropia, Möbius' syndrome, Duane's retraction syndrome (DRS) type I, and esotropia with neurologic impairment are presented as separate classifications of esotropia that are discussed independently in following sections. Additional differentials include the esotropias seen in children with Möbius' syndrome and with other neurologic impairments, and are discussed below. Because the prognosis and treatment are different for each of these entities, it is imperative that the practitioner be able to accurately differentiate them.

Möbius' Syndrome.   Möbius' syndrome is a rare congenital condition characterized by a nonprogressive facial diplegia and bilateral abducens paralysis (i.e., abduction deficit) presenting with multisystem involvement. In addition to VI and VII cranial nerve involvement, other physical abnormalities, such as partial atrophy of the tongue, deafness, webbed fingers or toes, orofacial anomalies and congenital limb amputation, are commonly present. The child's eyelids may be fixed open or have the inability to close completely. It is estimated that approximately 40% of these children have an es-

Table 8.5. Differential Diagnosis of Congenital Esotropia

Pseudoesotropia
Duane's retraction syndrome type I
Möbius' syndrome
Nystagmus blockage syndrome
Sixth nerve paresis
Sensory esotropia
Early-onset accommodative esotropia
Esotropia associated with neurologic impairment

otropia [64] that is usually 50^Δ or greater [65]. Typically, there is a positive history of sucking and feeding problems. With their characteristically abnormal facial appearance and associated systemic abnormalities, children with Möbius' syndrome are not difficult to differentiate from those with other forms of infantile esotropia.

Esotropia Associated with Neurologic Impairment.   Neurologically impaired children with conditions such as Down syndrome, cerebral palsy, meningomyelocele (spina bifida), hydrocephalus, and intraventricular hemorrhage are at increased risk for esotropia, as well as for other forms of strabismus [66–68]. Manifest nystagmus is often associated with the strabismus. These esotropias, many of which are clinically similar in presentation to congenital esotropia, are considered separately because different etiologies are probably involved. The management of these children is usually more complicated and the results of treatment less predictable [69].

Prognosis

Regardless of the form of treatment prescribed, treatment should be initiated as soon as possible. However, because of the propensity among pediatricians to "wait and see if the child outgrows the esotropia" as well as the established referral patterns between pediatricians and pediatric ophthalmologists, optometrists often do not see these patients at an early age. It makes one wonder if this delay may account for some of the poor treatment results obtained. Nevertheless, one should attempt to educate all pediatricians and parents that any esotropia persisting beyond 2–3 months of age is probably abnormal and therefore the patient should be referred for a comprehensive eye examination immediately [12, 51]. The prognosis for achieving completely normal binocularity (with RDS) in patients with congenital esotropia is considered to be poor [46, 70, 71], although there are a few isolated reports of bifixation with stereoacuity being achieved [72–74]. Generally, a post-treatment result of subnormal binocular vision, microtropia [12], or monofixation syndrome [36] is considered to be a success.

Accommodative Esotropia

Definition and Clinical Features

An acquired convergent strabismus that is associated with the activation of accommodation is called an *accommodative esotropia*. The child has either uncorrected hyperopia, an abnormally high AC/A ratio, or a combination of the two. The average age of onset is 2.5–3.0 years of age with a range generally of 6 months to 7 years [75, 76]; however, accommodative esotropia has been documented in infants before 6 months of age [76, 77].

Characteristically, the deviation has an intermittent onset and gradually increases in frequency. If treatment is delayed or not given, the esotropia generally becomes constant. The deviation usually occurs first at near point and is frequently seen when a child is tired. Typically, the esodeviation is variable and depends on the physical state of the patient and the amount of accommodation exerted; the magnitude is of moderate size (approximately $20–40^\Delta$). Dependent on the AC/A ratio, the esotropia at near point may be the same size or larger than the magnitude at far point.

Signs and symptoms include intermittent diplopia, asthenopia, and closing one eye when performing close work. We have had the experience of examining a 2-year-old child who screamed and cried whenever her eye turned in; however, the majority of young children with accommodative esotropia do not verbalize any symptoms or complaints to their parents. In our experience, the most common presenting complaint is that the parent notices the child's eye turning in. Frequently, there is a positive family history of hyperopia and esotropia.

Provided the accommodative esotropia is in the intermittent stage, sensory adaptations such as am-

blyopia, deep suppression, and AC do not develop. Once the deviation becomes constant, however, one can expect the development of suppression or AC, as well as amblyopia if the esotropia is unilateral.

Accommodative esotropia can be subdivided into refractive and nonrefractive entities. Refractive accommodative esotropia results from partially or totally uncorrected hyperopia that is generally in the range of 2.00–6.00 D, with an average of approximately 4.75 D [75]. The esotropia is eliminated and bifixation is attained when an optical correction to compensate for the underlying uncorrected hyperopia is prescribed. Many children with higher amounts of uncorrected hyperopia do not demonstrate accommodative esotropia, presumably because the effort to accommodate the amount necessary to achieve clear vision is too great.

Nonrefractive accommodative esotropia is an esodeviation that is greater at near than far and is unrelated to uncorrected hyperopia, instead resulting from a high AC/A ratio. It can occur in children with emmetropia, hyperopia, or myopia. The average amount of hyperopia is approximately +2.25 D [75]. The diagnosis is made when one finds esotropia at near while performing the cover test on a patient who is fixating an accommodative target and whose refractive error is fully corrected. Obviously, an accommodative esotropia can result from a combination of uncorrected hyperopia and a high AC/A ratio (Figure 8.7).

The importance of performing a cover test with an accommodative target cannot be overemphasized. A practitioner who uses only a penlight or other nonaccommodative stimulus is likely to miss a good number of accommodative esotropias. This is illustrated in Figure 8.2. Once a diagnosis is made, cover testing should be repeated through the full hyperopic correction and through a plus addition for near, if needed, to determine if lenses will reduce or eliminate the esotropia.

From a practice management standpoint, it is wise to forewarn the child's parents that when the child removes his or her glasses, the esotropia may appear to be worse than it was before receiving the prescription. Parents frequently report that their child only had a small eye turn and they saw it only occasionally before the child received glasses, whereas the esotropia appears to be larger in magnitude or occur more frequently (when the child's

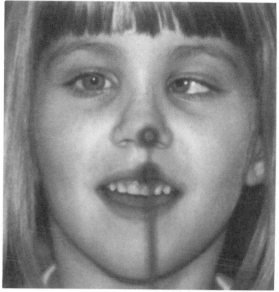

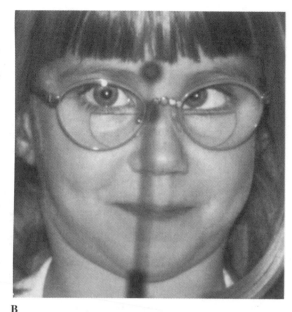

A

B

Figure 8.7. Accommodative esotropia: Uncorrected hyper-opia and high AC/A ratio. A. Constant left esotropia is present at distance and near without correction. B. Full distance refractive correction of +4.50 –100 x 090 (OU) eliminates the esotropia at distance and decreases the angle at near (note Hirschberg reflexes), but a residual esotropia remains at near despite the distance correction. C. When patient views through a +3.00 OU bifocal add at near, the esotropia is fully eliminated.

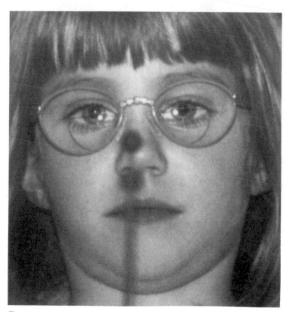

C

glasses are removed) now that the child has been wearing glasses. Parents sometimes think that the increased deviation is because of the glasses and that the child is becoming "dependent" on the glasses. One can easily explain this phenomenon on the basis that the child no longer has to use excessive accommodation ("focusing") in order to see clearly because the glasses relieve the accommodative demand. The child has become accustomed to seeing clearly through the glasses and desires to keep things clear when the glasses are removed. Therefore, he or she accommodates in order to properly bring things into clear focus, and suddenly the parents see an esotropia. Understandably, it is better to counsel the parents on this beforehand rather than after the fact.

Prognosis

The prognosis for accommodative esotropia is good provided the child is given the appropriate refractive correction to straighten the eyes before the esotropia becomes constant. In these cases, bifixation should be maintained and the development of amblyopia, suppression, or AC is unlikely [78]. Clinically, we see a number of children with constant esotropias and significant amounts of uncorrected hyperopia whose parents report an initial presentation of an intermittent esotropia at 2–3 years of age that gradually became more frequent, and finally constant. Many of the parents waited (sometimes on the advice of their pediatrician) several months or even years before bringing the child to an eye care practitioner. We find it is not unusual for a residual small angle of esotropia to remain after providing the full refractive correction. This could be indicative that the esotropia is "partially accommodative" (i.e., the convergent strabismus is reduced with the optical correction but a residual esotropia remains). We have the impression, however, that many of these esotropias were initially intermittent and fully accommodative, but there was too long a time between the onset of the strabismus and treatment. According to Parks [79], single binocular vision with bifixation can be permanently lost after 2–3 months of nonuse. In the patients just described, sometimes it appears that this may be the case. Therefore, it is extremely important that evaluation not be delayed after the onset of a strabismus, even if the deviation initially presents as an intermittent one. Development of sensory adaptations makes it much more difficult or even impossible to reestablish normal sensory-motor fusion.

Partially Accommodative Esotropia

When accommodative factors contribute to but do not account entirely for an esotropia, the strabismus is referred to as a *partially accommodative esotropia*. The esotropic angle becomes smaller, with full correction of hyperopia or additional plus at near, yet a residual esotropic angle remains. Many children with esotropia have this type of deviation. In some cases, it appears that the child initially has a congenital esotropia and then an accommodative element develops later, becoming superimposed on the original esotropia as the child grows older [12]. Repeated cycloplegic refractions should be performed because they sometimes reveal additional hyperopia, particularly if the child has worn his or her hyperopic correction for a month or two. Correction of this additional hyperopia may help to control the esotropia.

Acute-Onset Comitant Esotropia

Acquired during early childhood, a comitant esotropia of acute onset always deserves special attention because it can be the first indication of serious central nervous system pathology. The onset of the strabismus is often sudden but the deviation can be variable and intermittent over several weeks. Typically, the angle is relatively large, refractive error is insignificant, and AC/A ratio is normal. Diplopia is likely, although most young children do not report double vision to their parents, presumably because of their lack of realization that diplopia is an unnatural occurrence. Parents sometimes will notice that their child is closing or winking one eye, presumably to avoid diplopia.

If there has been disruption of fusion (e.g., occlusion for therapeutic reasons), one may suspect this as the cause of an acute-onset comitant esotropia. If there has been no fusion disruption, however, the doctor is obligated to investigate further. A careful and thorough ocular motility examination is necessary to determine whether the deviation is comitant or noncomitant. A noncomitant esotropia would suggest a sixth cranial nerve paresis (discussed in a following section).

Until recently, most authorities thought that an acute-onset comitant esotropia was benign and had no risk of being associated with any serious underlying neurologic pathology. It has become apparent, however, that this is not true—comitance in an acute-onset esotropia does not rule out underlying neurologic disease; it can be indicative of intracranial pathology, particularly tumors of the brain stem or cerebellum [80–82]. Therefore, these patients prove to be a diagnostic dilemma as well as a management quandary. One must decide if the patient should be referred for a neurologic or neuroradiologic evaluation, or both. Obviously, any associated findings, such as headaches, papilledema, an afferent pupillary defect, unusual clumsiness, and so forth, would warrant a neurologic evaluation. Other definite causes for referral are the presence of nystagmus or the inability to demonstrate sensory fusion with prism or in the major amblyoscope [80, 81].

The pathogenesis of these esotropias is unknown. Accommodation is not a factor. Physical or emotional stress is sometimes a precursor. The prognosis for restoration of normal binocular vision (provided there is no underlying central nervous system pathology) is very good because the patient has presumably enjoyed normal binocular vision before the esotropia's appearance. Assuming a fairly recent onset, sensory adaptations will not have had an opportunity to develop.

Nystagmus Blockage (Compensation) Syndrome

NBS, or nystagmus compensation syndrome, is an entity that should be distinguished from other forms of infantile esotropia with and without nystagmus. It is characterized by an esotropia of early onset that is preceded by nystagmus, a pseudoabducens paresis, head turn elicited by covering either eye, and manifest nystagmus as the fixating eye moves from adduction toward abduction. The etiologic theory is that an infant with primary congenital nystagmus discovers that he or she can "block" the nystagmus by adduction or stimulation of convergence (presumably to increase visual acuity) [83]. The esotropia may initially be intermittent but eventually becomes constant because of sustained convergence efforts and resulting hypertonicity of the medial recti [84].

The nystagmus is horizontal and generally reduced or absent in adduction. As the adducted viewing eye follows a target moving laterally toward primary position, nystagmus generally occurs before the eye reaches midline and steadily increases as the eye abducts. Therefore, the amplitude of the nystagmus increases as the esotropia magnitude decreases [83].

Several clinical scenarios are possible. Both eyes may be adducted, resulting in a head turned toward the side of the fixating adducted eye. When only one eye is adducted and it is the fixating eye, the infant develops a head turn in the direction of the dominant fixating eye (which then remains adducted). This allows the patient to view an object straight ahead with the dominant eye in adduction.

The head turn will persist even if the other eye is occluded because this allows the patient to continue fixating in adduction. Strabismic amblyopia often develops. If the adducted eye is the nonfixating eye, there is usually no abnormal head position; however, one may be elicited by occluding the fixating eye. The infant will ordinarily turn his or her face toward the uncovered eye in order to keep it in adduction. If the patient does not demonstrate a strong ocular dominance, fixation may alternate between the eyes. Consequently, the head turn will vary according to which eye is used for fixation and amblyopia development is less likely.

Two findings can be used to differentiate patients with NBS from those with congenital esotropia. First, whereas congenital nystagmus may be present in patients with congenital esotropia, it occurs in all positions of gaze. NBS patients will not demonstrate nystagmus in adduction and will show an increasing nystagmus as the eye abducts (which should also be distinguished from an end-position nystagmus that appears *only* in abduction). Second, patching of either eye will cause the head to be turned toward the uncovered eye so that the eye can remain in the adducted position. This will not happen when a child with congenital esotropia is patched even if the child is a cross-fixator.

There has been considerable controversy regarding the prevalence and diagnostic criteria for NBS because most diagnoses are based solely on clinical observation rather than oculographic recordings. Dell'Osso and colleagues [85] provided some insight by using quantitative oculography. They propose that the esotropia is truly a "blockage" of an ongoing congenital nystagmus present when both eyes are parallel. Furthermore, they believe that there may be different mechanisms that underlie NBS in different patients. Accommodative convergence, however, is not thought to be one of them. There are those who maintain that there should be no evidence of pupillary constriction during the esotropia phase [84, 85] and others who report that it occurs at times [86].

Cyclic Esotropia

Cyclic, or circadian, strabismus, a very rare form of strabismus with unknown etiology, is characterized by alternating periods of straight eyes and a large-angle strabismic deviation, usually esotropia. The most common cycle is a 48-hour cycle. The child's eyes are straight, with normal binocularity for 24 hours, followed by a 24-hour period during which there is a manifest esotropia. The angle is often as large as 40–50$^\Delta$. Cyclic strabismus is usually acquired in early childhood, most commonly occurring during the mid-preschool years [87]. After several months (or even years) the cycle breaks, and the esotropia becomes constant. This form of strabismus appears to be idiopathic, and there is no known relationship to refractive error or visual acuity [88].

Cyclic esotropia must be differentiated from intermittent esotropia, the latter being much more irregular in its time pattern, as well as manifesting an esodeviation on the ACT whether or not strabismus occurs during a UCT. In addition, the cyclic type is unrelated to visual activity or illness. If parents ever report that their child has an intermittent esotropia that is present only some days, one should request that the parents mark the days that the child exhibits the deviation on a calendar. Alternatively, one can evaluate the child for several consecutive days to determine if there is a cyclic pattern.

Sensory Strabismus

Sensory strabismus is a deviation of one eye secondary to a severe reduction or loss of vision caused by an abnormality in that eye. The significantly reduced monocular visual acuity is considered to be the primary deficit that acts as a sensory obstacle to fusion. Because the potential for sensory fusion is limited, the visually impaired eye changes its position relative to the fixating eye and drifts either inward or outward. The resulting strabismus, the sensory esotropia or exotropia, is a direct consequence of the vision loss caused by the ocular abnormality.

Various vision-depriving factors may lead to a sensory strabismus. Common causative conditions in children that limit visual acuity in one eye and thereby can lead to a sensory strabismus include uncorrected anisometropia, congenital and traumatic cataracts, corneal opacities, optic nerve lesions, retinal lesions, and macular disease [89, 90]. The degree of monocular visual impairment is usually severe but can range from 20/60 to light perception

[89]. In addition, functional amblyopia may be superimposed on the organically caused loss of vision, resulting in a further decrease in vision [91, 92].

Esotropia and exotropia are encountered with almost equal frequency when the monocular visual impairment occurs at birth or between birth and 5 years of age, whereas exotropia tends to predominate in older children and adults [89]. The magnitude of the deviation can vary from relatively small to very large. The factors that determine the resultant direction and magnitude of sensory strabismus are unclear.

An accompanying vertical deviation is present in approximately one-third of the cases [89]. Overaction of the inferior oblique muscle of the involved eye is most frequently found, followed by bilateral inferior oblique overaction; superior oblique overaction in one or both eyes is less commonly found. The etiology of the overacting oblique muscles is unknown. DVDs have been reported to be present in approximately 12.5% of patients having sensory strabismus [90].

When first evaluating infants and young children with a constant, unilateral strabismus, one should consider the possibility that the deviation is a sensory manifestation of an underlying pathologic process. Any constant, unilateral strabismus could be the first clinical sign of poor visual acuity or blindness of that eye. For example, esotropia has been reported to be the second most common presenting sign of retinoblastoma [93]. Therefore, any young child with constant, unilateral strabismus should be evaluated immediately to determine if there is an organic cause for the strabismus. There is great urgency in infants with congenital cataracts; cataracts need to be removed within the first weeks or months of life for optimal development of visual acuity and binocular vision development [94, 95]. Therefore, it is imperative that a complete eye health examination, including a dilated fundus evaluation, be a component of the initial vision examination of every strabismic child. Fortunately, sensory strabismus in infants and young children is not common.

Congenital (Infantile) Exotropia

Congenital exotropia is often associated with neurologic syndromes or with craniofacial anomalies. The presence of an idiopathic or primary, isolated constant exotropia in an otherwise normal and healthy child younger than 1 year of age is uncommon [96, 97]. It is estimated that this condition occurs in only 1 of 30,000 individuals in the general population [98]. It is von Noorden's [12] impression (as well as ours) that this condition is more common in black individuals than in white individuals.

Congenital idiopathic exotropia is characterized by a large, constant (usually alternating) exotropic deviation at distance and near that presents during the first year of life. It must be differentiated from the transient intermittent exotropias commonly seen in the first few months of life [49, 51] as well as from sensory exotropia secondary to poor vision in one eye caused by ocular disease. Its onset is probably at about the same time as that of congenital esotropia, which is 2–4 months of age [50].

Clinical characteristics include a magnitude that generally ranges from 25^Δ to 80^Δ, with a mean of $35–50^\Delta$ [96, 99]; the angle may increase in size over time. A DVD is often associated with the exodeviation [96, 99]. Refractive error does not differ from that expected for nonstrabismic children of the same age.

Because congenital exotropia is more often associated with significant ocular disease or neurologic syndromes, the doctor should always consider the possibility of a coexistent neurologic disorder, such as cerebral palsy, before making the diagnosis of idiopathic congenital exotropia. Because most of these children alternate fixation, amblyopia is not common; however, the early-onset constant strabismus severely interferes with development of normal binocular vision.

Intermittent Exotropia

Intermittent exotropia is characterized by an exodeviation that is controlled so that the eyes are aligned and bifixation is present part of the time, whereas at other times it spontaneously breaks down into a manifest exotropia. A small, intermittent exotropia is normal in many newborns [49, 51]. In fact, in a study of 1,219 newborns, Nixon and coworkers [49] found that 22% of the infants had an intermittent exotropia. This particular type of intermittent exotropia is usually transient, however, and typically resolves by 2–6 months of age [51]. Therefore, one could consider these intermittent exotropias developmentally normal up to 6 months of age. However, these are not the intermittent exotropias that the optometrist routinely sees in practice. Nevertheless, and contrary to common belief, the majority of intermittent exotropic deviations seen later in life usually have their onset during infancy or early childhood [8, 15, 16].

The manifest phase of intermittent exotropia is aggravated by daydreaming, visual disinterest, fatigue, illness, and distance viewing. A tendency to close one eye in bright light (particularly sunlight) is commonly associated with intermittent exotropia; however, the reason for this phenomenon remains unclear [100]. Young children rarely complain of symptoms (e.g., blurred vision, tired eyes, and diplopia) often seen in older children and adults with intermittent exotropia.

Because of its intermittent occurrence and relationship to the patient's general health, alertness, and attention span, there may be a wide variation in the degree of control of the deviation from one examination to the next. Therefore, repeated examinations under varying conditions of attentiveness and fatigue may be necessary for the proper diagnosis. If a parent gives the history of an eye wandering out and the examiner does not detect an exotropia on examination, it is prudent to schedule an appointment with the child on another day, preferably at a time of day when he or she might be tired. In addition, one should discreetly monitor the child's eye alignment while speaking to the parent during the history or consultation. Sometimes this is the only time that the examiner may see the deviation. Because the angle is often variable and dependent on attention and fatigue, a prolonged ACT should be performed, making sure always to have one eye covered and to measure to reversal. In this way, one is more likely to measure the angle at its largest. In addition, when possible, the child should fixate at a distance of 6 m or greater in order to disclose the full distance exodeviation, especially when the angle is larger with distance fixation than with near fixation [28].

The natural history of intermittent exotropia is unknown. Valid longitudinal studies of untreated patients observed over a period of years are not available. The results of the most frequently cited study by Hiles and colleagues [101] were questioned when Friendly [102] reported that "about

81% of these patients received orthoptic therapy." At best, we know that in the majority of untreated cases, intermittent exotropia does not improve, and only in rare cases does it spontaneously resolve. Clinical experience suggests that once the intermittent exotropia is manifest, it either remains the same or it gradually deteriorates to a more frequently occurring exotropia and in some cases to a constant exotropia. Therefore, it is important to monitor and evaluate these children over a period of time to ascertain whether the condition is progressing.

The presence of an intermittent exotropia is rarely considered to be an urgent matter provided the deviation remains intermittent. In most cases, these children are monitored carefully until they are old enough to participate in a vision therapy program. Simple gross convergence exercises, passive anti-suppression procedures (e.g., TV trainer), or a temporary over-minus prescription may be prescribed in the interim to encourage more frequent fusion [41].

Oculomotor (Third Cranial Nerve) Paresis

Third cranial nerve paresis in children is uncommon and usually is congenital [103, 104]. Congenital oculomotor nerve paresis has been reported to exist in isolation without associated neurologic abnormalities [104], but has also been found to be associated with other disturbances of the central nervous system [105, 106]. Perinatal injury to the peripheral nerve during delivery is considered to be a possible mechanism in the development of congenital oculomotor paresis, especially if it is not accompanied by any other abnormalities [104]. It appears that central brain stem lesions may also account for some cases of congenital third nerve paresis, particularly in children who show signs of associated neurologic damage [106].

Causes of acquired oculomotor paresis in children are different than those found commonly in adults (e.g., diabetes, aneurysms, trauma, and metastatic tumors). In children, acquired third nerve paresis is most likely caused by trauma, tumors, infectious processes, and ophthalmic migraines [103, 107, 108]. Trauma is the most frequent acquired cause; significant head injury sustained in a motor vehicle accident is often the culprit.

Third cranial nerve paresis may be unilateral, bilateral, complete, or incomplete. The child with a total third nerve paresis classically presents with a large exotropia, small hypotropia, and nonreactive pupil, all hidden behind a ptotic lid. Deficient adduction, elevation, and depression of the involved eye are present on version testing. An incomplete third nerve paresis may involve only the nerve's superior division (innervating the levator and superior rectus muscle) or inferior division (innervating the inferior rectus, inferior oblique, medial rectus, pupil, and ciliary body). Acquired isolated paresis of a single extraocular muscle is very infrequent. Amblyopia and the absence of binocular vision are commonly found in congenital third nerve pareses [104]. In addition, aberrant regeneration and abnormal pupil reactions or sizes are often present [106, 107].

Although a congenital third cranial nerve paresis is often benign and isolated, Balkan and Hoyt [106] recommend that all infants with this condition be evaluated by a pediatric neurologist for other signs of focal neurologic damage. The degree of associated central nervous system involvement can range from very mild to severe. Mild neurologic damage may be difficult to detect in early infancy; therefore, caution should be used in advising parents of their child's general prognosis. Generalized developmental delay has been reported [105, 106].

Trochlear (Fourth Cranial Nerve) Paresis

The most common isolated cyclovertical muscle paresis [109], as well as the most common form of paralytic strabismus found in children in a primary care setting [110], is a fourth cranial (trochlear) nerve paresis. Because the trochlear nerve innervates the superior oblique muscle, the child will present with a hyperdeviation of the involved eye. This deviation can be a phoria or strabismus. Regardless, the magnitude should increase with the affected eye in adduction and be maximal when the eye is placed in the field of action (i.e., adduction and depression) of the involved superior oblique. Abnormal head positions are commonly present. In the case of a unilateral paresis, the head is usually tilted toward the shoulder opposite the eye with the paresis, and the chin is depressed.

If the vertical deviation is a phoria, the head tilt may be the only sign that a superior oblique paresis is present. Therefore, it is always wise for the practitioner to be alert for anomalous head positions and to consider a muscle paresis as a possible etiology. Likewise, when a head tilt is present, it is prudent to first determine if it is an *ocular* or congenital *nonocular* torticollis. A torticollis that is congenital usually results from a musculoskeletal anomaly secondary to a congenital shortening of the sternocleidomastoid muscle. On palpation this muscle would feel tight and firm, and one could not passively tilt the child's head to the opposite shoulder. In contrast, the head can be tilted passively to the opposite (from the habitual) shoulder in children with ocular torticollis. In addition, the vertical deviation is larger when the head is tilted to the shoulder on the same side as the paretic superior oblique muscle; this is referred to as a positive Bielschowsky head-tilt test. The "patch test" can also help differentiate ocular from congenital torticollis. Typically, the anomalous head tilt disappears when the paretic eye is patched (except in long-standing cases in which muscular changes have occurred). Some children are misdiagnosed as having orthopedic problems and undergo extensive physical therapy when, in fact, the causative factor is visual.

The child usually adopts the head tilt to position his or her eyes away from the field of action of the involved superior oblique. The tilt allows the eye to extort and use the muscles that are still functional. This often allows normal sensory fusion to occur. Many of these patients bifixate when using their abnormal head position. Because the tilt usually facilitates fusion, it is rare for amblyopia to develop.

Version testing typically reveals an underaction of the affected superior oblique and overaction of the ipsilateral antagonist inferior oblique. Although the spread of comitance may occur with time and mask the diagnosis in some cases, the three-step test usually remains diagnostic for an isolated superior oblique paresis. The ACT reveals a hyperdeviation that is greater when the affected eye is adducted (versus in the abducted position) and when the head is tilted toward the shoulder on the same side as the involved eye (versus tilted toward the shoulder opposite the affected eye). Although double Maddox rod testing is usually unreliable in young children, a cyclodeviation can be noted objectively using binocular indirect ophthalmoscopy or fundus photography (comparing the relative positions of disk and macula) [111].

Superior oblique paresis may be congenital or acquired. Congenital causes are more commonly encountered in a general practitioner's office [110, 112] and include birth trauma, developmental anomalies of the trochlear nerve, and perinatal infections. The ensuing paresis may remain well compensated for during childhood, either by enlarged vertical vergence ranges or a head tilt. Congenital pareses usually remain stable. Nonetheless, congenital latent paretic deviations can decompensate during childhood as well as in adulthood. Early childhood photographs that demonstrate a consistent head tilt are usually indicative of a long-standing or congenital paresis.

The most common known cause of acquired trochlear nerve paresis is closed head trauma [108]; however, many times no definitive cause can be established [108, 112]. Acquired paresis may resolve or become more comitant with time. Kodsi and Younge [108] found a complete recovery rate of 31.6% with a mean recovery time of 2.3 months in their pediatric sample. Recovery may take as long as 6–8 months.

Trochlear nerve paresis may be unilateral or bilateral. Bilateral cases are rarely congenital, and most often result from head trauma [110]. Involvement is usually asymmetrical. Diagnostic features distinguishing a bilateral paresis from a unilateral one are the presence of a right hypertropia in levoversion and a left hypertropia in dextroversion, and a positive Bielschowsky head-tilt test on tilting the head toward either shoulder [110]. The absence of these two features, however, does not rule out bilateral involvement.

Abducens (Sixth Cranial Nerve) Paresis

Clinical characteristics of an abducens or sixth cranial nerve paresis include a noncomitant deviation with an esotropia in primary gaze and limited abduction of the affected eye. The esotropia is largest when the patient attempts to abduct the paretic eye. The paresis can be unilateral or bilateral. In unilateral cases, the child usually adopts a compensatory horizontal face turn toward the involved eye if binocularity can be attained.

An abducens paresis can be congenital or acquired. Congenital sixth nerve paresis in children is rare (when DRS and Möbius' syndrome are not included [109]); however, transient neonatal paresis is estimated to occur in one of every 182 births (i.e.,

0.5 %) [113]. These transient palsies usually resolve in approximately 6 weeks [113].

In contrast, acquired sixth nerve impairment in a young child can be an ominous sign. Etiologies include trauma, tumor, inflammation, infection, hydrocephalus or shunt malfunction, as well as other miscellaneous and idiopathic causes. Trauma (28–42%) followed by tumors (19–27%) have been found to be the major causes in children younger than 16–18 years of age [108, 112, 114]. There may be age-related differences between children 7 years of age and younger and those older than 7 years, however, because Aroichane and Repka [115] found that tumor was most common, followed by hydrocephalus and then trauma in children 7 years of age and younger.

Because of the high association between lateral rectus paresis and intracranial tumors, one should always be concerned that an isolated sixth nerve paresis may be the first sign of an intracranial neoplasm. From a differential diagnostic standpoint, most of these children invariably have other neurologic signs, such as papilledema, optic neuropathy, hemiparesis, ataxia, dysarthria, or a previous history of metastatic cancer [108, 115]. Therefore, if there are any symptoms of neurologic dysfunction other than diplopia, the child should be referred immediately so that elevated intracranial pressure and intracranial neoplasms can be ruled out. If one suspects that head trauma is the cause of the sixth nerve impairment, the child's head, neck, and face should be carefully examined for signs of child abuse.

Another type of sixth nerve paresis develops in children 2–3 weeks after a nonspecific febrile or upper respiratory illness [116, 117] or immunization [118]. These are benign and usually resolve spontaneously within 10 weeks [116]; however, they can recur. Sixth nerve paresis has been reported to recur 2 to 11 times in the same child [119, 120].

Spontaneous recovery in young children is more common with idiopathic and infectious etiologies [115], as well as trauma [115, 121]. Recovery is less common with tumors [115, 121] and hydrocephalus [115]. Due to residual strabismus in many of these patients, prophylactic treatment for amblyopia should be instituted.

Children with sixth nerve paresis must be differentiated from those with DRS type I, congenital esotropia with crossed fixation, and Möbius' syndrome. All of these present with esotropia and an apparent abduction deficit; however, there are other clinical characteristics that distinguish one from the other. Children with DRS have a narrowing of the palpebral fissure and retraction of the globe on attempted adduction, which is absent with abducens paresis. The additional associated ocular and systemic abnormalities associated with Möbius' syndrome are absent in those with isolated lateral rectus paresis. Apparent abduction deficits in congenital esotropic patients who cross-fixate can be differentiated from the true abduction deficits caused by sixth nerve palsies either by using the aforementioned doll's head maneuver or by patching an eye for an hour or sometimes even a day or two. With either of these methods, one should be able to elicit abduction in the patient with congenital esotropia who cross-fixates.

Duane's Retraction Syndrome

DRS is a congenital disorder of ocular motility that is characterized most commonly by (1) limitation of abduction, (2) narrowing of the palpebral fissure and retraction of the globe on adduction, (3) slight or no limitation of adduction, and (4) upshoot or downshoot on adduction. A classic example is shown in Figure 8.8. DRS can be unilateral or bilateral. There is a female preponderance and a predilection for the left eye. Approximately 1–4% of the general strabismic population has DRS [122].

Three types of DRS have been identified. In type I, the most common form, there is limited or absent abduction with normal or a slight deficiency of adduction. Type II DRS patients have limited or absent adduction with relatively normal abduction; many have an exotropia in primary gaze. Type III is characterized by limited or absent adduction and abduction. Common to all three types is narrowing of the palpebral fissure and retraction of the globe with attempted adduction. These characteristics are summarized in Table 8.6.

Type I DRS is the form that can be confused with congenital esotropia or a sixth-nerve paresis. Although a heterophoria may be present in primary position, an esotropia is often present. Similar to those with sixth-nerve palsies, these patients often adopt a compensatory head turn toward the in-

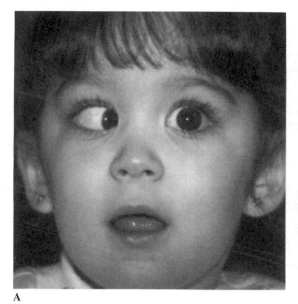

A

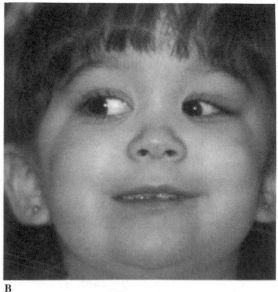

B

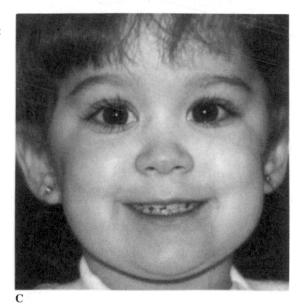

C

Figure 8.8. Duane's retraction syndrome type I of the left eye. A. Significant abduction deficit of the left eye and right eye esotropia noted in left gaze. B. Narrowing of the left eye's palpebral fissure and retraction of the globe are seen with left eye in adduction. C. No strabismus in primary gaze.

volved eye to maintain single binocular vision. Because of the abduction deficiency, there is usually a prominent esotropia when the child attempts to abduct the affected eye (see Figure 8.8). For example, in the case of an affected left eye, if the child turns his or her eyes to the left (rather than the head), one typically sees an obvious esotropia. This is what often prompts the parents to bring the child in for an evaluation.

There are numerous theories concerning the etiology and pathogenesis of DRS. Mechanical, innervational, and central nervous system anomalies have all been implicated [122]. At present, there is no general consensus among researchers. It is possible that a spectrum of various mechanical, innervational, and central nervous system defects present with a similar clinical picture that has been classified as a distinct entity—that is, DRS [122].

Table 8.6. Duane's Retraction Syndrome Classification

Clinical Finding	Type I	Type II	Type III
Abduction	Marked limitation	Normal or slight limitation	Limitation
Adduction	Minimally defective or normal	Marked limitation	Limitation
Palpebral fissure	Narrowing on adduction	Narrowing on adduction	Narrowing on adduction
Globe retraction	With adduction	With adduction	With adduction

There is a frequent association of DRS with other congenital anomalies and malformations. Pfaffenbach and colleagues [123] found that those with DRS had a 10–20 times greater incidence of congenital facial anomalies, ear and hearing anomalies, roentgenographic abnormalities, and skeletal deformities than the general population. DRS has also been associated with syndromes such as Klippel-Feil, Wildervanck's, Okihiro, Holt-Oram, and Goldenhar's [122]. Therefore, besides differentiating DRS from the other forms of infantile esotropia, the examiner should also look for additional malformations. Nevertheless, in the vast majority of DRS patients that we have seen, DRS has been an isolated finding.

Brown's Syndrome

Brown's syndrome is a classic disorder of ocular motility that is characterized by the inability of the affected eye to elevate in adduction, either actively (i.e., on version testing) or passively (i.e., with forced-duction testing). Typically, there is less elevation deficiency when the eye is in midline and no deficiency in abduction. Figure 8.9 shows a child with a typical Brown's syndrome. Often, there is divergence in up-gaze resulting in a V-pattern exodeviation. A widening of the palpebral fissure may be present in adduction.

Most patients with Brown's syndrome have normal eye alignment in primary gaze. Rarely does the patient present with a conspicuously abnormal head posture or a manifest hypotropia in primary gaze. In addition, there is usually no overaction of the ipsilateral superior oblique muscle. The most common clinical characteristics are listed in Table 8.7. However, a positive forced-duction test (i.e.,

restriction to passive movement) is essential for the diagnosis to be made unequivocally.

Brown's syndrome can be congenital or acquired. It can be further classified as constant or intermittent depending on its course. The original designation given to the condition by Harold Whaley Brown [124, 125], the "superior oblique tendon sheath syndrome," is no longer used because it has been determined that there is no abnormality of the tendon sheath itself. Although multiple causes (e.g., trauma, inflammation, or anomalous development of the tendon) may be responsible for this condition, the common denominator is some defect in the trochlea/tendon complex that hinders normal movement of the tendon through the trochlea. The prevalence of Brown's syndrome has been estimated to be approximately 0.23% of strabismic cases [126]. Although a hereditary influence has been suspected, most cases appear to be sporadic and no mode of inheritance has been identified [127].

Differential diagnosis includes inferior oblique paresis, blow-out fracture, congenital fibrosis syndrome, monocular elevation deficiency, and adherence syndromes. Brown's syndrome can be easily distinguished from the less common inferior oblique paresis, with or without superior oblique overaction, by the forced-duction test. In Brown's syndrome, the test will unequivocally demonstrate restricted passive elevation in adduction, whereas passive elevation will be possible when the individual has a paretic inferior oblique muscle.

Because congenital fibrosis syndromes usually affect multiple extraocular muscles, including the levator, the presence of a ptosis or elevation deficiency in abduction as well as adduction easily differentiates this from Brown's syndrome. In the case of a blow-out fracture, there should be a history of

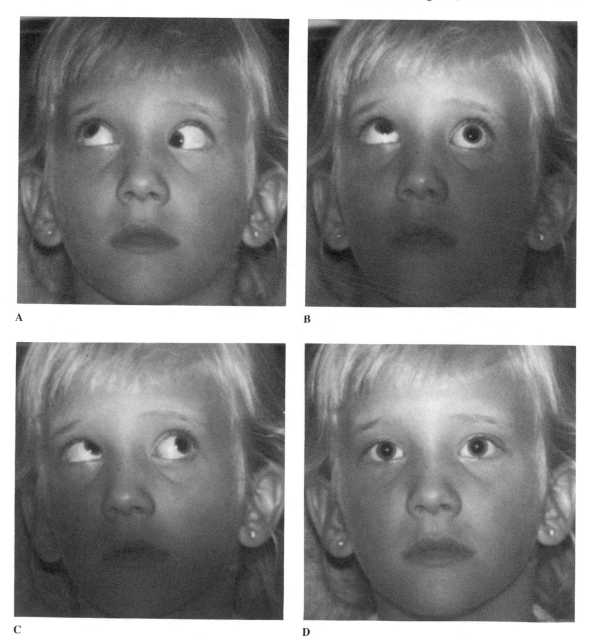

A
B
C
D

Figure 8.9. Brown's syndrome. A. Left eye demonstrates deficient elevation in adduction. A widening of the left eye palpebral fissure is also apparent. B. Less elevation deficiency in midline. C. Minimal elevation deficit in abduction. D. Absence of vertical strabismus in primary gaze; patient bifixates.

orbital trauma as well as restriction of elevation in both abduction and adduction. In the instance of an adherence syndrome, there should be a history of muscle surgery on the inferior oblique muscle and a hypotropia in primary position.

Because a vertical strabismus is rarely found in primary gaze and most patients are asymptomatic, the most common form of management is nothing more than observation and parental reassurance. Some believe that spontaneous resolution of the

Table 8.7. Brown's Syndrome:
Characteristic Features

Restriction of elevation in adduction
Less elevation restriction in midline
Minimal or no elevation restriction in abduction
Minimal or no overaction of the ipsilateral superior oblique
V-pattern resulting from divergence in up-gaze
Positive forced-duction test

condition occurs more often than is recognized [127]. This may account for the clinical observation that Brown's syndrome is seen more often in children than in teenagers and adults. Surgery is usually reserved for patients having a primary hypotropia or a bothersome anomalous head position, or both.

MANAGEMENT OF STRABISMUS

Once an appropriate evaluation has been performed and a diagnosis made, various management options must be considered. Obviously, if neurologic disease is the etiology of the strabismus, medical or surgical management, or both, of the underlying cause is usually indicated. In the great majority of cases, however, no disease process is involved, and management centers around the judicious use of lenses, prisms, occlusion, simple vision therapy techniques, pharmaceuticals (e.g., miotics for accommodative esotropia), and extraocular muscle surgery. It is important to keep the treatment as simple as possible for infants and preschoolers. Thus, the first consideration should be the use of a lens prescription to reduce the size of the strabismic angle, possibly including a bifocal addition for patients with a high AC/A ratio who have a strabismus in which the magnitude differs with near and far fixation. If suppression is not severe and normal correspondence is present, a prismatic prescription may enable the patient to achieve stable binocular vision. Occlusion can be used as a passive means to prevent suppression and AC, in addition to its use in amblyopia treatment. Unilateral occlusion must be used with caution in infants and young children, however, due to the possibility of causing occlusion amblyopia [128]. There also exist excellent passive vision therapy techniques to

develop sensory and motor fusion ability in young children. Our approach is to use these noninvasive treatment methods to promote fusion whenever possible. If the patient has a cosmetically unacceptable strabismic angle and a poor prognosis for achieving a functional cure, or if the strabismus magnitude is too great to allow stable fusion without long-term wear of a large amount of prism, we refer the patient to a pediatric ophthalmologist for extraocular muscle surgery. After surgery, it is important to reevaluate the patient and continue with any appropriate management, with the goal of achieving the best possible functional as well as cosmetic result. There are a number of excellent resources that discuss the use of these management options in greater detail [31, 41, 129–134].

CONCLUSION

Strabismus is a prevalent childhood visual anomaly that often has deleterious effects on the visual system of infants and young children. As primary health care providers, optometrists will be called on to clinically evaluate these young patients to detect strabismus and provide an early diagnosis. Prompt diagnosis may prevent secondary visual conditions, such as amblyopia, AC, and suppression, from developing. Restoration of normal binocular vision should be more easily obtained. As part of the clinical evaluation and differential diagnosis, the eye care practitioner will rule out sight-threatening (e.g., retinal detachment) or life-threatening conditions (e.g., tumors) that cause some types of strabismus. Optometry's commitment to the early diagnosis and treatment of infants and young children with strabismus will benefit these children from cosmetic, functional, and psychological standpoints.

REFERENCES

1. Prosser PC. Infantile development: strabismic and normal children compared. Ophthalmic Optician 1979; 19:681–683.
2. Tolchin JG, Lederman ME. Congenital (infantile) esotropia: psychiatric aspects. J Pediatr Ophthalmol Strabismus 1978;15:160–163.
3. Tonge BJ, Lipton GL, Crawford G. Psychological and educational correlates of strabismus in school children. Aust N Z J Psychiatry 1984;18:71–77.

4. Lipton EL. A study of psychological effects of strabismus. Psychosocial Study Child 1970;25:146–174.

5. Satterfield D, Keltner JL, Morrison TL. Psychological aspects of strabismus study. Arch Ophthalmol 1993;111:1100–1105.

6. Roberts J, Rowland M. Refractive Status and Motility Defects of Persons 4–74 Years, United States 1971–1972. In Vital and Health Statistics (Series No. 11). DHEW publication (PHS) 78-1654. Hyattsville, MD: National Center for Health Statistics, 1978.

7. Frandsen AD. Occurrence of squint: a clinical-statistical study on the prevalence of squint and associated signs in different groups and ages of the Danish population. Acta Ophthalmol Scand [Suppl] (Copenh) 1960;62:1–158.

8. Nordlow W. Squint—the frequency of onset at different ages, and the incidence of some associated defects in a Swedish population. Acta Ophthalmol 1964;42:1015–1037.

9. Adelstein AM, Scully J. Epidemiological aspects of squint. BMJ 1967;58:334–338.

10. Graham PA. Epidemiology of strabismus. Br J Ophthalmol 1974;58:224–231.

11. Friedman Z, Neumann E, Hyams SW, Peleg B. Ophthalmic screening of 38,000 children, age 1 to 2 1/2 years, in child welfare clinics. J Pediatr Ophthalmol Strabismus 1980;17:261–267.

12. von Noorden GK. Binocular Vision and Ocular Motility—Theory and Management of Strabismus (5th ed). St. Louis: Mosby, 1996;299–337, 344.

13. Scobee RG. Esotropia—incidence, etiology, and results of therapy. Am J Ophthalmol 1951;34:817–833.

14. Costenbader FD. Infantile esotropia. Trans Am Ophthalmol Soc 1961;59:397–429.

15. Hall IB. Primary divergent strabismus: analysis of aetiological factors. Br Orthopt J 1961;18:106–109.

16. Costenbader FD. The Physiology and Management of Divergent Strabismus. In JH Allen (ed), Strabismic Ophthalmic Symposium I. St. Louis: Mosby, 1950; 349–366.

17. Scheiman MM, Amos CS, Ciner EB, et al. Pediatric Eye and Vision Examination: Optometric Clinical Practice Guideline. St. Louis: American Optometric Association, 1994.

18. Flom MC. Issues in the Clinical Management of Binocular Anomalies. In AA Rosenbloom, MW Morgan (eds), Pediatric Optometry. Philadelphia: Lippincott, 1990;219–244.

19. Jones R, Eskridge JB. The Hirschberg test—a re-evaluation. Am J Optom Arch Am Acad Optom 1970; 47:105–114.

20. Brodie SE. Photographic calibration of the Hirschberg test. Invest Ophthalmol Vis Sci 1987;28:736–742.

21. Eskridge JB, Wick B, Perrigin D. The Hirschberg test: a double-masked clinical evaluation. Am J Optom Physiol Opt 1988;65:745–750.

22. Wick B, London R. The Hirschberg test: analysis from birth to age 5. J Am Optom Assoc 1980;51:1009–1010.

23. Riddell PM, Hainline L, Abramov I. Calibration of the Hirschberg test in human infants. Invest Ophthalmol Vis Sci 1994;35:538–543.

24. Aouchiche K, Dankner SR. What's the difference? Krimsky vs alternate cover testing. Am Orthopt J 1988;38:148–150.

25. Tongue AC, Cibis GW. Brückner test. Ophthalmology 1981;88:1041–1044.

26. Griffin JR, Cotter SA. The Brückner test: evaluation of clinical usefulness. Am J Optom Physiol Opt 1986; 63:957–961.

27. Archer SM. Developmental aspects of the Brückner test. Ophthalmology 1988;95:1098–1101.

28. Kushner BJ, Morton G. Measurement of strabismus in shortened exam lanes versus the 20-foot lane. Ann Ophthalmol 1982;14:86–89.

29. Ziegler D, Huff D, Rouse MW. Success in strabismus therapy: a literature review. J Am Optom Assoc 1982; 53:979–983.

30. Thompson JT, Guyton DL. Ophthalmic prisms: deviant behavior at near. Ophthalmology 1985;92:684–690.

31. Griffin JR, Grisham JD. Binocular Anomalies: Diagnosis and Vision Therapy (3rd ed). Boston: Butterworth–Heinemann, 1995;108–111.

32. Repka MX, Kelman S, Guyton DL. Prism measurement of incomitant strabismus. Binoc Vis 1985;1:45–49.

33. Hansen VC. Common pitfalls in measuring strabismic patients. Am Orthopt J 1989;39:3–11.

34. Repka MX, Arnoldi KA. Lateral incomitance in exotropia: fact or artifact? J Pediatr Ophthalmol Strabismus 1991;28:125–128.

35. Cooper J, Feldman J. Random-dot-stereogram performance by strabismic, amblyopic, and ocular-pathology patients in an operant-discrimination task. Am J Optom Physiol Opt 1978;55:599–609.

36. Parks MM. The monofixation syndrome. Trans Am Ophthalmol Soc 1969;67:609–657.

37. Rosner J. The effectiveness of the random dot E stereotest as a preschool vision screening instrument. J Am Optom Assoc 1978;49:1121–1124.

38. Manny RE, Martinez AT, Fern KD. Testing stereopsis in the preschool child: is it clinically useful? J Pediatr Ophthalmol Strabismus 1991;28:223–231.

39. Cotter SA, Pass AF. A comparison of the Random Dot-E and Lang stereotests in screening young children. Am J Optom Physiol Opt 1987;64:68P.

40. Cotter SA, Scharre JE. The Lang stereotest: performance by strabismic, amblyopic, and visually normal patients. Am J Optom Physiol Opt 1987;64:68P.

41. Caloroso EE, Rouse MW. Clinical Management of Strabismus. Boston: Butterworth–Heinemann, 1993;27, 59–61, 233–234, 295–352.

42. Eustis HS, MacPhee A. Screening for "absent bifixation" (monofixation syndrome): the superiority of the distance Polaroid®™ Vectograph test for suppression over near stereotests, in 246 children. Binoc Vis Eye Muscle Surg Q 1993;8:83–89.

43. von Noorden GK. Atlas of Strabismus (4th ed). St. Louis: Mosby, 1983;72–89.

44. Frantz KA, Cotter SA, Wick B. Re-evaluation of the four prism diopter base-out test. Optom Vis Sci 1992;69:777–786.

45. Rosner J, Rosner J. Parents as screeners for strabismus in their children. J Visual Impair 1988:5:193–94.

46. von Noorden GK. Current concepts of infantile esotropia (Bowman lecture). Eye 1988;2:343–357.

47. Parks MM. Congenital esotropia vs. infantile esotropia. Graefe's Arch Clin Exp Ophthalmol 1988;226:106–107.

48. Lang J. Congenital or infantile, that is the question. Binoc Vis 1988;3:116–117.

49. Nixon RB, Helveston EM, Miller K, et al. Incidence of strabismus in neonates. Am J Ophthalmol 1985; 100:798–801.

50. Archer SM, Sondhi N, Helveston EM. Strabismus in infancy. Ophthalmology 1989;96:133–137.

51. Sondhi N, Archer SM, Helveston EM. Development of normal ocular alignment. J Pediatr Ophthalmol Strabismus 1988;25:210–211.

52. Paul TO, Hardage LK. The heritability of strabismus. Ophthalmic Genet 1994;15:1–18.

53. Helveston EM. 19th annual Frank Costenbader lecture—the origins of congenital esotropia. J Pediatr Ophthalmol Strabismus 1993;30:215–232.

54. von Noorden GK. A reassessment of infantile esotropia (XLIV Edward Jackson Memorial lecture). Am J Ophthalmol 1988;105:1–10.

55. Helveston EM, Ellis FD, Schott J, Mitchelson J, et al. Surgical treatment of congenital esotropia. Am J Ophthalmol 1983;96:218–228.

56. Hiles DA, Watson BA, Biglan AW. Characteristics of infantile esotropia following early bimedial rectus recession. Arch Ophthalmol 1980;98:697–703.

57. Ing MR. Progressive increase in the angle of deviation in congenital esotropia. Trans Am Ophthalmol Soc 1994;92:117–131.

58. Helveston EM. Dissociated vertical deviation: a clinical and laboratory study. Trans Am Ophthalmol Soc 1980;78:734–779.

59. Wilson ME, Parks MM. Primary inferior oblique overaction in congenital esotropia, accommodative esotropia, and intermittent exotropia. Ophthalmology 1989;96:950–957.

60. Robb RM, Rodier DW. The variable clinical characteristics and course of early infantile esotropia. J Pediatr Ophthalmol Strabismus 1987;24:276–281.

61. Dickey CF, Scott WE. Amblyopia—The Prevalence in Congenital Esotropia Versus Partially Accommodative Esotropia—Diagnosis and Results of Treatment. In M Lenk-Schäfer (ed), Orthoptic Horizons: Transactions of the Sixth International Orthoptic Congress. Harrogate, Great Britain: 1987;106–112.

62. Réthy I, Gal Z. Results and principles of a new method of optical correction of hypermetropia in cases of esotropia. Acta Ophthalmol 1968;46:757–766.

63. Réthy S. Mistake of strabismology. Audiotape #2 of papers presented at the 25th meeting of the College of Optometrists in Vision Development, Palm Springs, CA, October 1995. Coeur D'Alene, CO: Insta-Tapes.

64. Henderson JL. The congenital facial diplegia syndrome: clinical features, pathology and aetiology. Brain 1939;62:381–403.

65. Nelson LB, Wagner RS, Simon JW, Harley RD. Congenital esotropia. Surv Ophthalmol 1987;31:363–383.

66. Wesson MD, Maino DM. Oculovisual Findings in Children with Down Syndrome, Cerebral Palsy, and Mental Retardation without Specific Etiology. In DM Maino (ed), Diagnosis and Management of Special Populations. St Louis: Mosby, 1995;17–54.

67. Clements DB, Kaushal K. A study of the ocular complications of hydrocephalus and meningomyelocele. Trans Ophthalmol Soc U K 1970;90:383–390.

68. Bankes JLK, Thornhill DM, Corr PE, et al. The Management and Binocular Achievement of Mentally Handicapped Children with Squint. In S Moore, J Mein, L Stockbridge (eds), Orthoptics: Past, Present, Future. New York: Grune & Stratton, 1976;293–298.

69. Holman RE, Merritt JC. Infantile esotropia: results in the neurologic impaired and "normal" child at NCMH (six years). J Pediatr Ophthalmol Strabismus 1986; 23:41–45.

70. Scheiman M, Ciner E, Gallaway M. Surgical success rates in infantile esotropia. J Am Optom Assoc 1989;60:22–31.

71. Taylor DM. Is congenital esotropia functionally curable? Trans Am Ophthalmol Soc 1972;70:529–576.

72. Parks MM. Congenital esotropia with a bifixation result: report of a case. Doc Ophthalmol 1984;58:109–114.

73. van Selm JL. Primary infantile-onset esotropia—20 years later. Graefe's Arch Clin Exp Ophthalmol 1988;226:122–125.

74. Wright KW, Edelman PM, McVey JH, et al. High-grade stereo acuity after early surgery for congenital esotropia. Arch Ophthalmol 1994;112:913–919.

75. Parks MM. Abnormal accommodative convergence in squint. Arch Ophthalmol 1958;59:364–380.

76. Baker JD, Parks MM. Early-onset accommodative esotropia. Am J Ophthalmol 1980;90:11–18.

77. Pollard ZF. Accommodative esotropia during the first year of life. Arch Ophthalmol 1976;94:1912–1913.

78. Wilson ME, Bluestein EC, Parks MM. Binocularity in accommodative esotropia. J Pediatr Ophthalmol Strabismus 1993;30:233–236.

79. Parks MM. After the eyes are straightened what is the ophthalmologist's responsibility? Ophthalmology 1986;93:1020–1022.

80. Hoyt CS, Good WV. Acute onset concomitant esotropia: when is it a sign of serious neurological disease? Br J Ophthalmol 1995;79:498–501.

81. Williams AS, Hoyt CS. Acute comitant esotropia in children with brain tumors. Arch Ophthalmol 1989; 107:376–378.

82. Timms C, Taylor D. Intracranial Pathology in Children Presenting as Concomitant Strabismus. In G Lennerstrand (ed), Update on Strabismus and Pediatric Ophthalmology. Proceedings of the Joint Congess June 19–23, 1994. Boca Raton, FL: CRC Press, 1995; 593–596.

83. von Noorden GK, Avilla CW. Nystagmus Blockage Syndrome: Revisited. In RD Reinecke (ed), Strabismus II. Proceedings of the Fourth Meeting of the International Strabismological Association, October 25–29, 1982. New York: Grune & Stratton, 1984;75–82.

84. Adelstein F. Cüppers C. Zum Problem der echten und scheinbaren Abducenslähmung (das sogenannte "Blockierungssyndrom"). In EF Stuttgart (ed), Augenmuskellähmungen, Büchd Augenarzt Heft 46 1966;271–278, as cited in von Noorden GK. The nystagmus compensation (blockage) syndrome. Am J Ophthalmol 1976;82:283–290.

85. Dell'Osso LF, Ellenberger C, Abel LA, Flynn JT. The nystagmus blockage syndrome: congenital nystagmus, manifest latent nystagmus, or both? Invest Ophthalmol Vis Sci 1983;24:1580–1587.

86. von Noorden GK, Munoz M, Wong SY. Compensatory mechanisms in congenital nystagmus. Am J Ophthalmol 1987;104:387–397.

87. Helveston EM. Cyclic strabismus. Am Orthopt J 1973;23:48–51.

88. Parlato CJ, Nelson LB, Harley RD. Cyclic strabismus. Ann Ophthalmol 1983;15:1126–1129.

89. Sidikaro Y, von Noorden GK. Observations in sensory heterotropia. J Pediatr Ophthalmol Strabismus 1982;19:12–19.

90. Kutluk S, Avilla CW, von Noorden GK. The prevalence of dissociated vertical deviation in patients with sensory heterotropia. Am J Ophthalmol 1995;119: 744–747.

91. Kushner BJ. Functional amblyopia associated with organic ocular disease. Am J Ophthalmol 1981;91:39–45.

92. Bradford GM, Kutschke PJ, Scott WE. Results of amblyopia therapy in eyes with unilateral structural abnormalities. Ophthalmology 1992;99:1616–1621.

93. Ellsworth RM. The practical management of retinoblastoma. Trans Am Ophthalmol Soc 1969;67:462–534.

94. Moore BD. Pediatric cataracts—diagnosis and treatment. Optom Vis Sci 1994;71:168–173.

95. Drummond GT, Scott WE, Keech RV. Management of monocular congenital cataracts. Arch Ophthalmol 1989;107:45–51.

96. Moore S, Cohen RL. Congenital exotropia. Am Orthopt J 1985;35:68–70.

97. Tychsen L. Pediatric ocular motility disorders of neuroophthalmic significance. Ophthalmol Clin North Am 1991;4:615–643.

98. Biedner B, Marcus M, David R, Yassur Y. Congenital constant exotropia: surgical results in six patients. Binoc Vis Eye Muscle Surg Q 1993;8:137–140.

99. Rubin SE, Nelson LB, Wagner RS, et al. Infantile exotropia in healthy children. Ophthal Surg 1988; 19:792–794.

100. Wiggins RE, von Noorden GK. Monocular eye closure in sunlight. J Pediatr Ophthalmol Strabismus 1990; 27:16–20.

101. Hiles DA, Davies GT, Costenbader FD. Long term observations on unoperated intermittent exotropia. Arch Ophthalmol 1968;80:436–442.

102. Friendly DS. Surgical and nonsurgical management of intermittent exotropia. Ophthalmol Clin North Am 1992;5:23–30.

103. Miller NR. Solitary oculomotor nerve palsy in childhood. Am J Ophthalmol 1977;83:106–111.

104. Victor DI. The diagnosis of congenital unilateral thirdnerve palsy. Brain 1976;99:711–718.

105. Keith CG. Oculomotor nerve palsy in childhood. Aust N Z J Ophthalmol 1987;15:181–184.

106. Balkan R, Hoyt CS. Associated neurologic abnormalities in congenital third nerve palsies. Am J Ophthalmol 1984;97:315–319.

107. Ing EB, Sullivan TJ, Clarke MP, Buncic JR. Oculomotor nerve palsies in children. J Pediatr Ophthalmol Strabismus 1992;29:331–336.

108. Kodsi SR, Younge BR. Acquired oculomotor, trochlear and abducent cranial nerve palsies in pediatric patients. Am J Ophthalmol 1992;114:568–574.

109. Parks MM, Mitchell PR. Cranial Nerve Palsies. In TD Duane, EA Jaeger (eds), Clinical Ophthalmology (Vol 1, Chapter 19). Philadelphia: Lippincott, 1986.

110. von Noorden GK, Murray E, Wong SY. Superior oblique paralysis: a review of 270 cases. Arch Ophthalmol 1986;104:1771–1776.

111. Morton GV, Lucchese N, Kushner BJ. The role of funduscopy and fundus photography in strabismus diagnosis. Ophthalmology 1983;90:1186–1191.

112. Harley RD. Paralytic strabismus in children. Etiologic incidence and management of the third, fourth, and sixth nerve palsies. Ophthalmology 1980;87:24–43.

113. Reisner SH, Perlman M, Ben-Tovim N, Dubrawski C. Transient lateral rectus muscle paresis in the newborn infant. J Pediatr 1971;78:461–465.

114. Afifi AK, Bell WE, Menezes AH. Etiology of lateral rectus palsy in infancy and childhood. J Child Neurol 1992;7:295–299.

115. Aroichane M, Repka MX. Outcome of sixth nerve palsy or paresis in young children. J Pediatr Ophthalmol Strabismus 1995;32:152–156.

116. Knox DL, Clark DB, Schuster FF. Benign VI nerve palsies in children. Pediatrics 1967;40:560–564.

117. Bixenman WW, von Noorden GK. Benign recurrent VI nerve palsy in childhood. J Pediatr Ophthalmol Strabismus 1981;18:29–34.

118. Werner DB, Savino PJ, Schatz NJ. Benign recurrent sixth nerve palsies in childhood secondary to immunization or viral illness. Arch Ophthalmol 1983;101: 607–608.

119. Boger WP, Puliafito CA, Magoon EH, et al. Recurrent

isolated sixth nerve palsy in children. Ann Ophthalmol 1984;16:237–244.

120. Sullivan SC. Benign recurrent isolated VI nerve palsy of childhood. Clin Pediatr 1985;24:160–161.

121. Robertson DM, Hines JD, Rucker CW. Acquired sixth-nerve paresis in children. Arch Ophthalmol 1970; 83:574–579.

122. DeRespinis PA, Caputo AR, Wagner RS, Guo S. Duane's retraction syndrome. Surv Ophthalmol 1993; 38:257–288.

123. Pfaffenbach DD, Cross HE, Kearns TP. Congenital anomalies in Duane's retraction syndrome. Arch Ophthalmol 1972;88:635–639.

124. Brown HW. Congenital Structural Muscle Anomalies. In JH Allen (ed), Strabismus Ophthalmic Symposium I. St. Louis: Mosby, 1950;205–236.

125. Brown HW. Congenital Structural Anomalies of the Muscles. In JH Allen (ed), Strabismus Ophthalmic Symposium II. St. Louis: Mosby, 1950;391–427.

126. Crosswell HH, Haldi BA. The superior oblique tendon sheath syndrome, a report of two bilateral cases. J Pediatr Ophthalmol 1967;4:8–12.

127. Wilson ME, Eustis HS, Parks MM. Brown's syndrome. Surv Ophthalmol 1989;34:153–172.

128. Levi DM. Occlusion amblyopia. Am J Optom Physiol Opt 1976;53:16–19.

129. Cotter SA (ed). Clinical Uses of Prism: A Spectrum of Applications. St. Louis: Mosby, 1995.

130. Wick B. Vision Therapy for Very Young Children. In MM Scheiman (ed), Problems in Optometry: Pediatric Optometry. Philadelphia: Lippincott, 1990;354–364.

131. Garzia RP. Management of Amblyopia in Infants, Toddlers, and Preschool Children. In MM Scheiman (ed), Problems in Optometry: Pediatric Optometry. Philadelphia: Lippincott, 1990;438–458.

132. London R. Passive Treatments for Early Onset Strabismus. In MM Scheiman (ed), Problems in Optometry: Pediatric Optometry. Philadelphia: Lippincott, 1990; 480–495.

133. Scheiman MM, Wick B. Optometric Management of Infantile Esotropia. In MM Scheiman (ed), Problems in Optometry: Pediatric Optometry. Philadelphia: Lippincott, 1990;459–479.

134. Rutstein RP. Evaluation and Treatment of Incomitant Deviations in Children. In MM Scheiman (ed), Problems in Optometry: Pediatric Optometry. Philadelphia: Lippincott, 1990;528–561.

Chapter 9
Vision Therapy for Amblyopia

Leonard J. Press and Paul Kohl

Amblyopia may be defined as reduced visual acuity not improvable solely by optical correction and not caused by structural ocular abnormalities. There are three main types of amblyopia: form deprivation, refractive, and strabismic. The adverse effects resulting from amblyopia include not only decreased visual acuity, but also abnormalities of contour interaction, the accommodative and ocular systems, and pupillary responses. Moderate and high hyperopia, oblique astigmatism, strabismus, premature birth and low birth weight, birth defects, mental retardation, and a myriad of hereditary factors and ophthalmic diseases are all significant risk factors for the development of amblyopia.

Deprivation amblyopia is the most severe form of amblyopia, but fortunately the rarest. It is primarily due to media opacities present at birth. Strabismic amblyopia results from constant or near-constant strabismus, usually esotropia. It often results in poorer visual acuity than refractive amblyopia and is more refractory to treatment. Refractive amblyopia is usually the result of anisometropia, but isoametropic amblyopia is occasionally noted in previously uncorrected high bilateral hyperopes and astigmats. It is generally considered to be the type of amblyopia most easily treated.

This chapter is primarily directed at the optometric treatment of amblyopia. For a detailed discussion of the physiology and diagnosis of amblyopia, the reader is directed to *Amblyopia: Basic and Clinical Aspects*, edited by KJ Ciuffreda, DM Levi, and A Selenow and published by Butterworth–Heinemann, and *Problems in Optometry: Amblyopia*, edited by R Rutstein and published by Lippincott.

Amblyopia occurs in approximately 2.5% of the population and is responsible for loss of vision in more children than any other form of ocular disease [1]. The image degradation associated with amblyopia results in profound changes in the entire visual system. These changes are exhibited morphologically, neurophysiologically, and psychophysically, and therefore cause concern about the development and function of the visual pathways. Amblyopia involves a decrement in virtually all areas of visual function, including accommodative accuracy and facility, fixational stability, pursuit and saccadic accuracy, localization in space, and contrast sensitivity.

The subtypes of amblyopia are reviewed in Table 9.1. Amblyopia therapy should not begin without the possibility of occult ocular disease being addressed. Successful amblyopia therapy depends on optimally timed intervention to enhance visual information processing and efficiency as well as binocular vision. This therapy should take into account the periods of visual development: the critical, sensitive, and susceptible periods and a period of residual plasticity (Table 9.2). For pediatric patients, the critical and sensitive periods are most relevant in the consideration of developmental timelines for amblyopia and its remediation. Following a rationale for therapeutic intervention in amblyopia, this chapter focuses on the types of activities used in amblyopia vision therapy.

Table 9.1. Clinical Classification of Amblyopia

Organic
Strabismic
Refractive
    Isometropic (bilateral blur)
    Anisometropic (unilateral blur)
Form deprivation
Iatrogenic (occlusion-induced)

Table 9.2. Developmental Periods in Amblyopia

Critical period
    Birth to 6 months
    Aggressive treatment required
    Lack of treatment results in legal blindness and
        nystagmus
Sensitive period
    6 months to 8 years
    Upper age limit for onset of amblyopia
    Aggressive treatment required
    Lack of treatment results in visual impairment
Susceptible period
    8 years to 18 years
    Aggressive treatment indicated if patient is compliant
    If amblyogenic risk factor is still present, amblyopia
        can recur
Residual plasticity period
    18 years to adulthood
    Treatment can be successful if patient is compliant and
        prognosis optimal
    Amblyopia not likely to recur even if amblyogenic risk
        factor still present

Sensitive and critical periods in the development of sensory-motor function are common to all neurobiological systems in many species. The ultimate goal of guidance and intervention is to establish normal vision during the early, malleable period of life [2]. Because the way the brain is used will play a part in determining its biochemical and neurophysiologic status, the modifiability of visual circuitry is a function of usage and learning as well as age [3]. As cited by Scott, Elliott Forrest explains that "maturity of vision develops from exposure to movement at the proper time and place [4]. In the absence of proper developmental exposure, substitute exposure at a different time and place can also enhance the movement patterns of the organism, although certainly not to the same extent as it would have been if done at its proper biological time. Nevertheless, it would be far more efficient than if the learning were not done at all" [4].

The degree to which amblyopia is a developmental, or adaptive, process is subject to debate [5]. It is clear, however, that the emphasis on the ocular component of amblyopia masks the globality of developmental and adaptive processes. Kavner and Suchoff [6] noted that inhibition of the amblyopic eye is expressed in a reorganization of the spatial values of the nonfixating eye. They observed that the end result of the adaptive process involved a different directional orientation and localization that was not confined to the retina. Spatial localization is ocularly determined only to a limited degree in humans. Treatment of amblyopia should therefore incorporate the concept of body image and proper cues from the different senses, including the inner ear and gravitation. Gross motor activities involving balance, coordination, and laterality are therefore indicated to help infants, toddlers, and preschoolers learn to overcome poor visual spatial localization caused by amblyopic viewing [7].

Treatment regimens for amblyopia vary in their intensity because the models on which they are based vary. If amblyopia is seen as merely a difference between the two eyes in visual acuity, occlusion is the treatment of choice. Occlusion alone, however, is problematic. Children rarely comply with occlusion therapy and are likely to "cheat" by creating a peephole or removing the patch entirely when critical visual information processing tasks must be executed. It is easy to understand why children do not understand the purpose of occlusion treatment, especially when they are able to see perfectly with both eyes open. The explanation that "the better eye is being patched to make the weaker eye stronger" is difficult for a child to understand and accept.

During the sensitive period of visual development in early childhood, gains made during amblyopic therapy are rapid. This has led to the observation that intervention is most effective at an age when the child is least able to appreciate it. However, children do show progressively less resistance to occlusion and monocular therapy activities as the visual function of the amblyopic eye rapidly improves.

Patients with refractive amblyopia exhibit a greater degree of binocular integration than patients with strabismic amblyopia. They generally require a shorter period of occlusion therapy. Gains made during the early phases of monocular therapy are readily assimilated into the binocular state. Refractive amblyopes must be encouraged to wear their prescriptive lenses full time. Younger patients especially need encouragement since they feel they can see just as well with lenses as without.

THERAPEUTIC SEQUENCE

Vision therapy for amblyopia is implemented in a specific sequence (Figure 9.1).

1. Prescribe an appropriate prescription. Ciner's guidelines for prescribing lenses are widely accepted (Table 9.3). Sherman [8] has advocated a prescription system that keeps lens power at an absolute minimum. Regardless of the prescription guidelines used, frequent retinoscopy and subjective refinement should be mandatory because of the lability of the young child's refractive status.

2. Implement occlusion therapy for strabismic amblyopia. Occlusion remains the cornerstone of conventional amblyopia therapy [9]. It is less important in cases of refractive amblyopia, in alternating strabismus, or when fusion is present under some viewing conditions. Patching is mandatory in all cases of unilateral strabismic amblyopia.

3. Prescribe an active vision therapy program to augment occlusion therapy. In most cases, occlusion is an adjunct to lenses and active vision therapy rather than a passive cure-all.

4. Assess prescription power and visual acuity with appropriate frequency. Because of the lability of the young child's refractive status, young children in active vision therapy should be reevaluated at least once monthly. Visual acuity must be monitored regularly. Table 9.4 outlines a suggested reexamination schedule.

Very different results may be obtained from different acuity tests. As children grow older, different tests will be used to assess their visual acuity. An infant who is initially tested with preferential looking (PL) cards will later be tested with Cardiff cards, picture cards (Allen or Lighthouse), the Broken Wheel test, tumbling E, and finally, the Snellen test. Studies have shown poor correlation between PL, Cardiff, and Snellen acuities when these tests

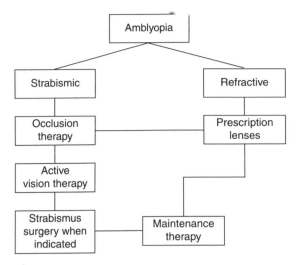

Figure 9.1. Sequencing amblyopia therapy.

were administered to adults [10]. A gross overestimation of visual acuity was found for both PL and Cardiff tests. Parents should therefore be advised that as the demand of the acuity test changes, the child's visual acuity may appear to be decreasing when in fact the amblyopic status has remained unchanged with time or improved with intervention.

5. Consider strabismus surgery when appropriate. The best way to maintain improvement in visual function of the strabismic amblyopic eye is to develop binocular integration. When significant regression is noted after vision therapy is terminated, strabismus surgery should be considered. The ideal time for strabismus surgery is when the visual function of the amblyopic eye has attained maximum improvement through nonsurgical means.

6. Monitor compliance with prescription and maintenance activities. Treatment of the pediatric patient not only requires the development of a positive, trusting relationship with the patient, but also necessitates the full cooperation of the parents. The parents must be educated on amblyopia, its impact on their child, therapy methods, and their role in the child's treatment. Success is dependent on both the child's and parents' compliance.

The clinician should try to ascertain the level of compliance before judging the success of a prescriptive approach or of a particular set of home activities. Children vary widely in their compliance with a prescription and parents also vary in their dili-

Table 9.3. Guidelines for Prescribing to Minimize Amblyopia

Refractive Status	Refractive Error at Which Amblyopia Concern Is Indicated	Prescription Guidelines
Isometropia		
Myopia	>5.00 D OU	Consider bifocal or under minus if there is evidence of a functional component.
Hyperopia	>2.00 D OU	Full prescription adjusted for age, amount of hyperopia, AC/A ratio, and phoria.
Astigmatism	>1.25 D OU	Oblique cylinders are more ambylogenic and warrant full prescription. If the patient is older than 8 years and this is a first prescription, use trial frames to monitor adaptation.
Anisometropia		
Myopia	>4.00 D	Full prescription with contact lenses OU or one lens for more myopic eye. Patient may adapt using monovision if anisometropia is <4.0 D using more myopic eye for near. If so, undercorrect and keep higher myopic eye for near.
Hyperopia	>1.00 D	Full prescription with spectacle lenses. Consider contact lenses if anisometropia is >4.0 D.
Astigmatism	>1.00 D	Full prescription indicated. If cylinder is cut, try to preserve the spherical equivalent.

OU = both eyes; AC/A = accommodative convergence to accommodation.
Source: Adapted from EB Ciner. Refractive error in young children: evaluation and prescription. Pract Optom 1992;3:182–190.

Table 9.4. Patching Schedule

Age (Years)	Quality-Time Schedule	Full-Time Schedule	Minimum Examination Frequency
1	Four 60-min periods	1 day on, 1 day off	Weekly
2	Three 30-min periods	2 days on, 1 day off	Every 2 wks
3	Three 30-min periods	3 days on, 1 day off	Every 3 wks
4	Two 60-min periods	4 days on, 1 day off	Every 4 wks
5	Two 60-min periods	5 days on, 1 day off	Every 5 wks
6	Two 60-min periods	6 days on, 1 day off	Every 6 wks

gence at ensuring that a prescription is used and that home activities prescribed for the child are completed. It is often easier to elicit the truth about compliance with glasses and home activities by checking with the child and the parent independently. Overall, the authors have found that parents and children are generally truthful about compliance with home activities. Children are less straightforward about whether or not they have been wearing their glasses in school. Although some parents can attest to whether their child is wearing glasses at home, rarely can they confirm whether the glasses are being used in school.

OCCLUSION THERAPY

Constant occlusion, although the fastest way to improve vision of the amblyopic eye with central fixation, carries with it the concern of occlusion amblyopia during the sensitive period. A form of deprivation amblyopia, occlusion amblyopia occurs when the vision of the nonamblyopic eye drops as a result of patching. The younger the child, the more likely this is to occur. The risk is greatest when the patient does not return to the office for regular monitoring of visual acuity or fixation preference patterns.

This problem can be addressed by limiting the number of days of consecutive occlusion to the number of years in age of the child being treated (see Table 9.4). For example, if a child with amblyopia of the right eye is 3 years of age, the left eye should be patched for 3 consecutive days and the patch left off on the fourth day. Then, patching should be resumed using the same regimen. If the child has strabismic amblyopia, particularly with eccentric fixation, indirect patching is done on the "off" day. In this instance, the child would have the right eye patched on the fourth day and eighth days. Occlusion amblyopia is a clinical concern until 7 years of age.

Occlusion amblyopia is not necessarily an untoward occurrence. It occurs only if the caretaker and child are compliant with full-time occlusion, and in most cases it can be readily reversed. The authors suspect that the rare cases of occlusion amblyopia resulting in profound visual loss are instances in which the child's vision was not monitored regularly by the prescribing clinician. When amblyopia occurs without constant strabismus, "quality-time patching" suffices. During quality-time occlusion, the child is engaged in visual activities that challenge the threshold level of resolution and stimulate accommodation, as well as the other information processing skills of the amblyopic eye, rather than leaving stimulation to chance. In cases of intermittent strabismus, refractive amblyopia, or both, part-time occlusion is usually successful. Table 9.4 can be used as a guide for the scheduling of part-time occlusion.

The most effective patch is one applied directly to the skin. The Coverlet (Beiersdorf) patches are much more adhesive than the Opticlude (3M) patches but potentially more irritating. The more adhesive patch should be used if the patch is to be left in place for several days. If the patch will be taken on and off frequently, the Opticlude patch suffices. The best time to apply the patch over the eye of an infant or toddler is during a nap. For preschoolers, the operant conditioning approach of associating the patch with a reward may be helpful. Parents who threaten or scream are rarely successful in ensuring long-term compliance. Children who are self-conscious about their appearance with the patch or who are teased by other children can begin by wearing the patch at home.

Patches applied to the glasses are less effective than adhesive eye patches, but must be used in some instances. Felt patches that also block visual input from the side of the frame may be slipped around the temple. These are available from Patch Works in colorful designs that young children readily accept. For the address of Patch Works and other companies whose products are recommended, see Chapter Appendix 9A. Standard clip-on patches that clip to the front of the lens are available, but often dislodge accidentally or with assistance. Elastic band patches may also be used. When the child does not wear prescriptive lenses, an elastic band patch that has a soft sponge inside for comfort (available from the Bernell Corporation) should be used.

Refractive amblyopes who already exhibit bilateral integration (as demonstrated in binocular performance tests such as random dot stereopsis) should wear prescriptive lenses for 2 months before occlusion therapy is begun. Occlusion need not be considered if visual acuity is improving. If improvement does not occur or there are diminishing returns, occlusion therapy should begin. Generally full-time occlusion should not be necessary unless amblyopia is coupled with constant strabismus [11]. When the binocular system is fragile, overzealous occlusion can convert a latent strabismus into a constant strabismus, or a small-angle strabismus to a larger-angle strabismus.

Partial Occlusion Therapy

The three forms of partial occlusion therapy are form deprivation through occlusion foil, image degradation through optical blurring, and pharmacologic penalization.

Occlusion Foils

Bangerter occlusion foils (available from the Fresnel Prism and Lens Company) are a series of translucent membranes that are applied in a manner similar to Fresnel prisms. They are applied directly to the lens surface with moisture and reduce acuity of the nonamblyopic eye. They are available in eight levels of image degradation, from 0.8 (approximately 20/40) to less than 0.1 (less than 20/200). The 0.0 foil is dense and provides an effect equivalent to that obtained when translucent tape is applied to the surface of a lens. These foils have been used for many years by orthoptists in European countries to create partial occlusion, referred to as *einshleich occlusion* or *occlusion partielle*. The minimum amount of image degradation that decreases acuity of the nonamblyopic eye to a level below that of the amblyopic eye is used initially. The density of the foil in front of the nonamblyopic eye is gradually reduced as the performance of the amblyopic eye improves. Although the application of graded occlusion requires more professional time, cost, and decision making than conventional occlusion, it is now more commonly used by vision therapy practitioners in the United States [12].

Optical Blurring

Optical blurring can also be used to degrade the image of the nonamblyopic eye. A contact or spectacle lens can be prescribed to decrease the visual function of the nonamblyopic eye to a level below that of the amblyopic eye. Theoretically, the child will then prefer to use the amblyopic eye for tasks involving visual resolution beyond the level of the blurred nonamblyopic eye. Compliance with wearing the lens that fogs the nonamblyopic eye is the essential element of success with this approach.

The initial fogging lens power induces the child to prefer use of the amblyopic eye. The behavior of the child should be vigilantly observed. A high-plus fog lens in front of the nonamblyopic eye will ensure distance blur, but a close near point viewing distance may afford enough conjugacy to favor use of the nonamblyopic eye at near. Conversely, a young child may have enough accommodative ability to override the potential blurring effect of a high-minus lens at distance. The authors favor use of a high-plus fog lens for optical blurring, and application of a Fresnel lens so that the intensity of the fog can be easily reduced.

For children younger than 1 year of age, vision is centered at near. Optical blur should therefore be prescribed. Multiple prescriptions designed for near, intermediate, and far distance conditions may be considered. If a fogging lens does not appear to encourage fixation with the amblyopic eye at the dis-

tance desired, occlusion foils of sufficient density should be used.

Penalization

Penalization is an effective form of partial, or graded, occlusion [13]. Atropine (1%) is administered to the nonamblyopic eye, inducing blur at near. This procedure works best when the child is significantly hyperopic in the amblyopic eye. In such cases, a plano lens is prescribed for the nonamblyopic eye, which ensures blur at distance as well. When the child has refractive amblyopia, improvement in visual function is signaled by rapid improvement in visual acuity. When strabismus coexists with amblyopia, the patient may begin to exhibit fixation preference with the formerly nondominant eye. As with standard occlusion, the refractive amblyopia improves quickly as long as the patient is compliant with wearing prescriptive lenses. The strabismic amblyope may need to have pharmacologic penalization tapered from 1% atropine to 1% cyclopentolate. The schedule for "weaning the patient" from penalization varies with the degree of binocular integration that can be attained. If the patient is too young or unable to cooperate with active therapy, a "holding pattern" of alternation is maintained.

Penalization has proven to be an excellent alternative to occlusion when the child is noncompliant [14]. Penalization is more than a substitution for total occlusion—it actually serves as a form of central monocular stimulation of the amblyopic eye within the peripheral context of the fellow eye. In this sense, it reverses the visual relationship that previously existed between the two eyes. It is more cosmetically acceptable than a patch and does not rely on the child's compliance (other than for cycloplegic instillation). It has the added bonus of being operative during all waking hours and ensuring that the child cannot cheat. The image of the fellow eye is degraded; therefore, the amblyopic eye is activated for visual judgments normally made by the nonamblyopic eye.

Modifying Occlusion in Bilateral Amblyopia

In all forms of occlusion, complete or partial, the assumption is made that visual function of one eye is considerably better than that of the fellow eye. In some instances, bilateral amblyopia is present, but to a greater extent in one eye than the fellow eye. In such cases, binocular stimulation is initiated as soon as visual performance has equalized in the two eyes. This will occur at a level of visual processing that is not yet normal in either eye. For example, taking acuity as the sine qua non function, let us assume that the initial acuities are 20/40 with the right eye and 20/100 with the left eye. The goal is not for the acuity of the left eye to be 20/40 or better before occlusion is switched to the left eye. Rather, binocular therapy should be implemented as soon as the acuity of the left eye approaches 20/40 or, in the case of strabismus, when fixation preference has switched from the right eye to the left eye.

VISION THERAPY ACTIVITIES

The need to combine occlusion therapy with prescribed vision activities to gain and maintain optimal visual outcomes has been well documented in the literature [15, 16]. Gillie and Lindsay note that occlusion alone is incomplete [17]. Pratt-Johnson and Tillson concur that occlusion is more effective when combined with guided visual activities that challenge visual resolution, such as coloring, tracing, playing video games, or watching television programs [18]. Studies have established that structured, guided visual stimulation not only accelerates the rate of improvement in vision [19, 20] but can also be used successfully in cases of occlusion therapy failure [21, 22]. The limitations of occlusion therapy can be traced to three main sources:

1. Most children are noncompliant with occlusion to at least some degree and therefore do not experience maximum improvement. Full-time occlusion alone often creates behavioral problems and becomes a serious point of contention between parent and child.

2. Full-time occlusion is difficult for children with initial amblyopic acuity below 20/70 who are in a preschool or kindergarten program in which adequate performance requires good visual acuity.

3. Full-time occlusion as the only treatment of strabismic amblyopia will result in frequent backsliding in acuity as soon as patching is terminated. Acuity must be closely monitored after patching is

stopped. Parents as well as practitioners can be lulled into a false sense of security that the improved acuity will maintain itself. Acuity apparently decreases again because the improved amblyopic function is not integrated with the fellow eye and suppression ensues as soon as the patch is removed.

Because young children often resist occlusion therapy, it is important for the caretaker to engage the infant, toddler, or preschool child in appropriate activities when the patch is worn. The challenge for the clinician is to select activities appropriate for the child's developmental level. Garzia [23] developed a comprehensive listing of activities for children from 4 months through 5 years of age, which we have expanded (Tables 9.5–9.8). We consider these activities to be a developmental menu from which procedures are selected à la carte to suit the desired vision demand, the capabilities of the child, and the child's willingness to engage in various activities on demand. Our mentor, Dr. Arnold Sherman, once remarked: "If a child can't do the activity, you've selected the wrong activity."

The activities listed in these tables for infants are useful for general vision development, even if amblyopia is not a concern. In general, activities that are most effective for amblyopic children visually engage the child by involving both motility and fine fixations, requiring overt motor responses (such as reaching, grabbing, pointing, kicking), and stimulating the accuracy of accommodative responses. The difference in performance when the amblyopic eye is used instead of the nonamblyopic eye should be carefully observed. Chapter Appendix 9B includes further information on developmental vision activities that can be used monocularly to improve visual information processing through the child's amblyopic eye.

High-contrast, low–spatial frequency targets, such as those used in vision stimulation with low-vision infants, are helpful when amblyopia is dense. Precision Vision Company (of Wimmer-Ferguson, Inc.) distributes a wide variety of testing and training materials for the child with low vision, including a multimedia vision enhancement kit with high-contrast dolls, puzzles, books, videos, and computerized training software. These materials serve as excellent visual stimulation targets for children with amblyopia. Johnson & Johnson makes a number of toys for infants that capture visual attention. Because of

Table 9.5. Direct Occlusion Activities
for the Infant

---

4 months
    Lifting head when prone
    Propping body on forearms
    Supported sitting
    Using walker
    Carriage riding
    Pursuing a moving object
    Paying attention to parents' faces or soft, noise-making
      toys
    Head rotations produce doll's eye movement
    Swiping at small toys
    Playing with cradle gym
    Searching visually for sounds
6 months
    Creeping
    Peek-a-boo
    Imitating facial expressions
    Tracking face-like targets
    Paying attention to noise-making crib toys and mobiles
    Playing in mirror
    Reaching for toys
    Tracking small objects of different sizes, shapes
    Picking up dropped objects
8 months
    Crawling on stomach using shoulders and elbows
    Sitting with hands free to reach and play
    Reaching for toys
    Crawling toward a toy placed out of reach
    Stacking or banging blocks of different sizes
    Peek-a-boo
    Playing with jack-in-the-box toys, mirrors, and stuffed
      toys
    Looking at things upside down
    Placing larger, colored wooden blocks into a large jar
10 months
    Creeping on hands and knees with abdomen raised
    Standing with support
    Walking holding two hands
    Playing with stuffed animals
    Feeding and dressing self
    Crumbling paper
    Rolling ball
    Stacking rings
    Matching blocks
    Pat-a-cake

---

habituation, the therapist must be prepared with a large variety of stimuli to choose from to maintain the child's interest and participation.

The subtitle of *Highlights* magazine is "Fun with a Purpose," and that is the order of the day when en-

gaging toddlers or preschoolers in therapy activities with occlusion. Many of the materials listed in Table 9.5 are commercially available. *Highlights* magazine and various jumbo activity books can be found in toy stores and educational stores. In all activities listed in Table 9.5 and Chapter Appendix 9B, the patient must use repeated visual scanning and demonstrate figure-ground discriminability. The following guidelines should be used when engaging the child in vision development activities:

1. Whenever possible, present the activity to the child without use of occlusion to make sure that it is within his or her cognitive level of understanding and developmental level of performance.

2. Whenever possible, first attempt the activity with the amblyopic eye occluded to determine what effect monocularity has on performance.

3. These guidelines are suggestions. Behavioral pragmatism should predominate over clinical theory. If it is difficult just to get the child to wear a patch and fun activity is reserved for times when the patch is worn, the patch should not be taken off just because it is recommended that activities be first done binocularly.

Activities that involve identifying similarities and differences are always fun and challenging. For example, *Highlights* magazine presents a feature called "Check...and Double Check," which asks the child to identify at least 12 differences between two corresponding pictures. Sedan's excellent book reproduces a number of these activities [24]. A contemporary version of this activity, developed by Vogel, is included in Bernell Corporation's Visual Skills software for IBM-compatible systems.

A wonderful advantage of homemade or commercially available targets is that they can be enlarged or reduced with a photocopier to suit the acuity level of the child. Younger children will require larger spacing and, perhaps, enlargement if the amblyopia is dense. As visual skills and acuity improve, smaller materials may be used, or the original materials may be reduced.

Therapy Activities Under Monocular Conditions

Many activities can be modified for use with young patients with amblyopia. We credit Patricia Pollack,

Table 9.6. Direct Occlusion Activities for the Early Toddler

12–14 months	**18 months** (*continued*)
Walking	Spontaneous scribbling
Crawling over low barriers	Working simple inset puzzles
Playing chase and catch games	Ball throwing and catching
Pouring water with bath toys	Playing with pull toys
Playing with inflatable beach ball	Stringing large, colored beads
Looking at book with stiff pages	Working with hammer-peg workbench
Rolling a ball	Putting shapes into a shape-sorting toy
Playing with pots, pans, nesting cups, or mixing bowls	**20 months**
Finding toys under box, cup, or pillow	Jumping forward
Building towers after demonstration	Running
Tearing pages from a book or magazine	Ball kicking
16 months	Pushing a sit-in–wheeled toy
Standing on one foot with help	Sand and water play (pouring from one cup to another)
Playing with pull and push toys	Stringing beads
Playing with stacking toys	Pounding bench
Playing in a sandbox	Throwing a small ball
Tossing a ball while standing	Playing with take-apart toys
Imitating scribbling	Playing the "what's that?" game
Putting round block in form board	Working with circle, square, and triangle form board
Bouncing Ping-Pong ball on hardwood floor	**22 months**
Turning pages of books	Riding small tricycle
Bringing a specific toy on request	Ball kicking
18 months	Tossing a ball at target
Fast walking	Balloon bop and toss
Jumping with two feet	Blowing, catching, and popping bubbles
Imitating ball kicking motion	Playing with pop-it beads
Identifying objects	Playing with blocks or train of cubes
Naming pictures in books	Playing with toy animals
Putting round and square blocks in form board	Inserting pencil into hollow tube

a vision therapy assistant who works with one of the authors for the following innovative modifications.

Pencil-in-Tube

The stick-in-straw activity is too precise for many young children to perform, particularly when amblyopia is dense. One way to lessen the demand of the procedure is to substitute objects with larger visual subtense, which facilitates visual localization. We substitute a tube from an empty roll of toilet tissue for the straw. For the pointer, we substitute an unsharpened pencil.

The procedure is performed with the examiner holding the tube. The Z axis is usually easiest, so we have the child try to insert the pencil in the tube from the "outside-in" direction first. When this is mastered we progress to the Y axis, with the child

approaching the hole from above. Lastly we attempt the X axis, with the child inserting the pencil into the tube from the side.

As with older children, some of the preschool children will be more accurate when they hold the tube in one hand and the pencil in the other. For preschoolers this will probably be too unwieldy, but should be attempted if localization is grossly inaccurate when the therapist holds the tube.

Modified Michigan Tracking (Happy Faces)

The goal in standard letter-tracking activities is to execute a visual search for a specific letter and point to or circle the letter. Although saccadic fixation is used during the tracking activity, figure-ground discriminability is also involved in the visual search. Toddlers and many preschoolers do not have ade-

Table 9.7. Direct Occlusion Activities for the Older Toddler

24 months
- Obstacle course when walking
- Walking a path (e.g., a line on floor with masking tape)
- Walk on short walls or curbs with assistance
- Balancing on one foot
- Rocking chair, swing
- Dancing
- Television viewing (e.g., Sesame Street)
- Playing with toy cars and trucks
- Playing in a sandbox (filling and emptying containers)
- Playing a "show me" game
- Scribbling
- Solitary book reading

2–2½ years
- Tricycle riding
- Climbing
- Tunnel crawl
- Playing with wagons or push trucks
- Building with blocks
- Cutting with small scissors
- Inserting pegs into pegboard
- Putting together jigsaw puzzles (2–5 pieces)
- Cutting objects
- Helping with household chores
- Modeling clay
- Using paints, crayons
- Playing with giant dominoes

2½–3 years
- Standing on one foot
- Walking on 2-in. line
- Hopping on one foot
- High jump
- Tower building with cubes
- Looking at picture books
- Finger painting
- Easel painting
- Crayons and paper drawing
- Paper folding
- 1-in. bead or macaroni stringing
- Playing with sewing cards
- Jigsaw puzzles (12–15 pieces)
- Playing with plastic building sets
- Picking up and matching colored M&Ms, Fruit Loops, or buttons
- Placing stick into holes punched in paper

Table 9.8. Direct Occlusion Activities for the Preschooler

3–5 years
- Modified Hart chart saccadics (pictures or easy letters)
- Modified Michigan tracking (smiley faces)
- Marble in cup
- Pie pan rotations
- Flashlight tag
- Beanbag toss
- Ball throwing, catching, bouncing
- Bowling (plastic ball and pins)
- Obstacle course
- Coloring books
- Dot-to-dot games
- Pounding nails
- Tic-tac-toe
- Filling in O's
- Lite-Brite
- Pegboard rotator (static, then dynamic)
- Stringing small objects or cereal with holes
- Shooting candle flame with water pistol
- Playing jacks
- Playing Bingo
- Mazes progressing from large to small
- Groffman tracings
- Picking up small objects with tweezers
- Marsden ball tracking
- Balancing on balance board
- Walking on walking rail
- Cutting and pasting as fine motor tasks
- Line tracing
- Letter or picture symbol searching
- Finding hidden pictures
- Where's Waldo?
- Typing or keyboarding
- Matching memory cards
- Card matching (e.g., Sherman card games)
- Chalkboard activities
- Stick and straw
- Pick-up sticks
- Stacking dominoes
- Playing video games progressing from simple to complex
- Wayne saccadic fixator
- Tachistoscopic projection
- Educational computer software

Figure 9.2. Happy face (modified Michigan) tracking sheet.

j☺lk whin fleg v☺s pexy liat br☺mp duz

yip culn m☺g dist huk zerp s☺y wuth n☺st

fig☺r quap z☺t bivy whax kl☺m tiput w☺lk

capy raj stek d☺zer lub duc fraz mup

sart nad☺w thef byst zabid yeb chiw epat

duk gleq frud mish yeld thib jum ceval

w☺nk fing jilk beh ax☺p marf ebel y☺la

gif hald perd grup bac mits tarf zuber☺

quate alphanumeric knowledge to use commercially available series such as the Michigan (Ann Arbor) Tracking workbooks. We have modified the activity so that each letter *O* contains a smiling face. (Figure 9.2). The smiling face becomes the key feature in the visual search.

This activity can be varied so that some of the faces are smiling and some frowning. If the child has good fine eye-hand coordination skills, the therapist can allow the child to begin with unaltered *O's* and draw his or her own happy or sad faces. As the child becomes more proficient in the activity, the therapist should reduce the sheets so that the resolution demand of the target increases commensurate with the improving level of acuity and visual skills.

Hart Chart Fixations: Modification 1

A standard Hart Chart is a grid of 10 rows of 10 letters each. Because number knowledge usually precedes letter knowledge, a chart modified to consist solely of numbers is useful. Because young children with normal vision exhibit crowding-like behavior when reading eye charts [25], charts should be constructed with fewer numbers and increased spacing between characters. As with other procedures, the nonamblyopic eye serves as a control for what the child is expected to be capable of with the amblyopic eye when this activity is successfully completed. When the child begins to learn the alphabet, remember that certain letters are identified earlier than others, and take this into consideration in design of the near-far charts [26].

Hart Chart Fixations: Modification 2

An easy way to modify the Hart Chart for older toddlers is to use the Lighthouse acuity chart symbols of apple, house, and umbrella. We begin with a large chart in a 3 × 4 grid format (Figure 9.3) with a matching reduced-size near point chart (Figure 9.4). Remember that toddlers and preschoolers will not usually maintain attention on visual stimuli at a distance of more than 10 feet [27].

Monocular Activities in a Binocular Field

For strabismic amblyopes, bridging the gap between monocular and binocular activities is crucial [28]. Strabismic therapy incorporating monocular activities in a binocular field (MFBF) theory is useful in bridging this gap. Some of the more common MFBF procedures are reviewed in this section. Because of the expense involved, the vectogram, Macular Integrity Trainer (MIT), saccadic fixator, and computer activities are usually reserved for office use. The remainder are suitable for home use as well.

Figure 9.3. Modified Lighthouse Distance Accommodative Rock Chart.

Anaglyphic Television Trainer

In this activity, available from the Bernell Corporation, a red filter is placed in the center of a television screen, with the amblyopic eye viewing through the red side of the anaglyphic glasses. A computer screen may also be used instead of a television, with well-spaced numbers typed onto the screen at the beginning of the activity. A red filter can be used on the screen with any educational software suitable for young children or optometric software adapted for this purpose.

Sherman Vision Therapy Playing Cards

Use only the cards (available from the Bernell Corporation) that can be seen by the amblyopic eye when the anaglyphic glasses are in place. Play card games suitable for the child's level of comprehension. Play a simple game first without the red-green filters to be certain that the child understands what to do. Let the child win often.

Lens Rock with Single Vectogram or Tranaglyph

The Clown vectogram is an excellent target because the block letters have a subtense of 20/200 at 16 in. (approximately 40 cm). If, for example, the right eye is amblyopic, use only the slide marked "right eye" at the bottom. The left eye will see the surrounding field, and the right eye sees all of the detail. Tranaglyphs, the red and green analog of polarized vectograms, can be used in a similar manner to counteract suppression of the amblyopic eye. The Clown tranaglyph (Bernell) and the Circus tranaglyphs (Optomatters) are both available through the Bernell Corporation. Some preschoolers will also be responsive to plus and minus lens accommodative rock therapy used in conjunction with a single vectogram or tranaglyph.

Anaglyphic Wayne Saccadic Fixator or Lite-Brite

Place the red filter in front of the amblyopic eye so that only that eye will be able to see the red light-emitting diode (LED) lights. The saccadic fixator (available from Wayne Engineering) is a favorite activity for most preschoolers, so we usually save it as a reward for when the child has behaved well for most of the session.

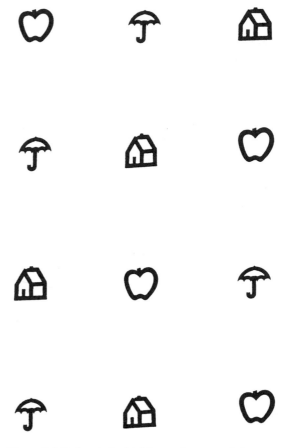

Figure 9.4. Reduced-size Lighthouse Accommodative Rock Chart.

Lite-Brite is a commercially available toy that can be used in a similar manner. Use the red pegs only, with the amblyopic eye viewing through the red filter. Arrange the pegs on the board in various patterns and have the child remove the pegs as quickly as possible. Even young children like to play this version of "beat the clock."

Anaglyphic Tracing

Place the red filter in front of the nonamblyopic eye. The amblyopic eye views red printed ink in workbooks or coloring books available through Bernell Corporation or Midwest Vision Therapy. The eye viewing through the red filter sees red light, but cannot see red printed ink. The therapist should always check the cancellation, particularly when self-made targets are used. Doctors and therapists have been known to scour the aisles at toy stores with anaglyph glasses in hand, looking for items that cancel through red or green filters.

Haidinger Brush and Macular Integrity Trainer Mazes

Initially use the blue filter in front of the amblyopic eye and the black filter in front of the nonamblyopic eye to make certain that the child can see the Haidinger Brush with the amblyopic eye. Then convert to the blue-clear filter combination, thereby creating monocular stimulation through the Haidinger Brush in the binocular field of the MIT. Many preschoolers can perform the standard MIT activities of pointing and accommodative rock with Plexiglas plate letters. MIT mazes are available with letters ranging in subtense from 20/400 to 20/20, thereby allowing the patient to combine pursuits, fixations, and eye-hand coordination with accommodative feedback. Preschoolers and some older toddlers can work with amblyo-maze targets that feature sports figures, airplanes, insects, or animals. Haidinger Brush and MIT Mazes are available from Bernell.

Perforated Form Board Kit

The perforated form board kit, available through Midwest Vision Therapy, contains a series of targets suitable for young children. Holes are placed around an 8-in. × 10-in. laminated page. The activity can first be done as a straw-piercing task with the nonamblyopic eye occluded. Red/clear filters are then used so that the hole is seen by the nonamblyopic eye, but the detail of the picture is seen only by the amblyopic eye. The patient is then directed to insert the pointer into the hole at various locations on the picture.

The Pierce Light

1. Remove the cap of a large lantern or flashlight and cut a piece of black construction paper to fit underneath it. Then cut out a square shape from the edge of the paper and tape green acetate to the back side of the remaining construction paper. When the light is turned on, a green square will glow. The green side of the anaglyphic glasses should be in front of the nondominant strabismic eye [29, 30].

2. After the patient reports no difficulty seeing the square, unscrew the cap and modify the target. Cut a round circle in the center of the paper and add red acetate so that a red light shines through the center. Simultaneous perception is easier to attain initially when the amblyopic eye views the periphery. If this proves difficult, have the patient move closer or further to see if he or she can see both the red and green portions of the flashlight simultaneously, and try to move the light to different positions of gaze. When simultaneous perception is stable, switch the filters so that the nondominant eye now views the central red circle. Repeat the procedure of moving the flashlight in and out, rotating both clockwise and counterclockwise. Toddlers and preschoolers may respond better if animal shapes are used in the center of the light instead of the red circle.

Black Felt Blanket Games

It is very challenging to work with children 6–18 months old. It can be especially difficult to get them to play while wearing red-green glasses for monocular activities in a binocular field. If the child wears a prescription, the filters can be taped onto his or her glasses. If the child does not wear a prescription, the flexible anaglyphic glasses with elastic bands work well.

Red stimuli must be selected so that they cancel with the green filter and the child is able to view only the object through the amblyopic eye. Rolling a red ball, chasing a red flashlight beam, finding red beads, and searching for red Fruit Loops or gelatin pieces is both fun and therapeutic (in encouraging the use of the amblyopic eye) for this age group. When selecting any object for the first time, first look through the green filter to ascertain that the object is difficult if not impossible to see through the filter. Then, have the child wear the red and green glasses with the green filter in front of the nonamblyopic eye.

CONCLUSION

Amblyopia therapy for infants, toddlers, and preschool children is challenging. In many instances, frequent monitoring of the appropriate lens prescription and compliance with occlusion activities is all that is needed to ensure normal visual development. In other instances, structured activities must be prescribed with appropriate guidance for home use. Young children vary widely in their ability to perform in-office therapy that is instrument bound. We have therefore limited the developmental menu of activities to those procedures that most children can do most of the time at the ages indicated.

The material presented in this chapter should be used to spur further thought on appropriate treatment methods. Most of the concepts discussed should serve as useful guidelines for that thought process. The optometrist or optometric vision therapy technician should be prepared with a list of many possibilities before each appointment. Each child must be treated as an individual. No two doctors, optometric vision therapy technicians, caretakers, or children are exactly alike; therefore, no two cases are exactly alike. When using amblyopia therapy with young children, ingenuity is the order of the day.

REFERENCES

1. Boothe RG, Dobson V, Teller DY. Postnatal development of vision in human and nonhuman primates. Ann Rev Neurosci 1985;8:495–545.
2. Spitzer NC. Development, Regeneration, and Plasticity. In MJ Cohen, F Strumwasser (eds), Comparative Neurobiology: Modes of Communication in the Nervous System. New York: Wiley, 1985.
3. Cynader MS. Mechanisms of brain development and their role in health and well-being. Proc Am Acad Art Sci 1994;123(4):155–165.
4. Scott CL. The Vision Development Process. In A Barber (ed), Vision Therapist: Infant and Toddler Vision. Santa Ana, CA: Optometric Extension Program, 1993;1–9.
5. Flom MC, Bedell HE, Barbeito R. Spatial Mechanisms for Visual Acuity Deficits in Strabismic and Anisometropic Amblyopia—Developmental Failure or Adaptation? In EL Keller, DS Zee (eds), Adaptive Processes in Visual and Oculomotor Systems. New York: Pergamon, 1986.
6. Kavner RS, Suchoff IB. Pleoptics Handbook. New York: Optometric Center of New York, 1969.
7. Griffin JR. Binocular Anomalies: Procedures for Vision Therapy. Chicago: Professional Press, 1982;184.
8. Sherman A. Treatment of amblyopia without full refractive correction or occlusion. J Behav Optom 1995;6:15.
9. Cotter SA. Conventional therapy for amblyopia. Probl Optom 1991;3:312–330.
10. Kohl P, Bass JL, Ramsey CS, Robertson BD. A Clinical Comparison of Visual Acuity Between the Cardiff Acuity Test and the Teller Acuity and Snellen Acuity Tests in an Adult Population. Forest Grove, OR: Pacific University; 1995.Thesis.
11. Ciuffreda KJ, Levi DM, Selenow A. Amblyopia: Basic and Clinical Aspects. Boston: Butterworth–Heinemann, 1991.
12. Bosse JC, Lederer PJ. Contemporary diagnostics: Thoughts on the use of graded occlusion. J Optom Vis Dev 1991;22(4):13–16.
13. Rutstein RP. Alternative treatment for amblyopia. Probl Optom 1991;3:331–354
14. Lam GC, Repka MX, Guyton DL. The efficacy of optical and pharmacological penalization. Ophthalmology 1993;100:1751–1756.
15. Garzia RP. Efficacy of vision therapy in amblyopia: A literature review. Am J Optom Physiol Opt 1987;64:393–404.
16. Press LJ. Amblyopia. J Optom Vis Dev 1988;19:2–15.
17. Gillie JC, Lindsay J. Orthoptics: A Discussion of Binocular Anomalies. London: Hatton Press, 1969.
18. Pratt-Johnson JA, Tillson G. Management of Strabismus and Amblyopia: A Practical Guide. New York: Thieme, 1994;86–90.
19. Francois J, James M. Comparative study of amblyopic treatment. Am Orthoptic J 1955;5:61–64.
20. Callahan WP, Berry D. The value of visual stimulation during constant and direct occlusion. Am Orthoptic J 1968;18:73–74.
21. Shipman S. Video games and amblyopia treatment. Am Orthoptic J 1985;35:2–5.
22. von Noorden GK, Romano P, Parks M, Springer F. Home therapy for amblyopia. Am Orthoptic J 1970;20:46–50.
23. Garzia RP. Management of amblyopia in infants, toddlers, and preschool children. Probl Optom 1990;2:438–458.
24. Sedan J. Reeducative Treatment of Suppression Amblyopia [translated by TK Lyle, C Douthwaite, J Wilkinson]. Edinburgh: E&S Livingston, 1960.
25. Marsh-Tootle WL. Clinical methods of testing visual acuity in amblyopia. Probl Optom 1991;3:208–236.
26. Press LJ. Examination of the Preschool Child. In LJ Press, BD Moore (eds), Clinical Pediatric Optometry. Boston: Butterworth–Heinemann, 1993;52.
27. Richman JE. Assessment of visual acuity in preschool children. Probl Optom 1990;2:319–332.
28. Cohen AH. Monocular fixation in a binocular field. J Am Optom Assoc 1981;52:801–806.
29. Getz DJ. Strabismus and Amblyopia. Santa Ana, CA: Optometric Extension Program, 1990.
30. McGraw LG. Guiding Strabismus Therapy. Santa Ana, CA: Optometric Extension Program, 1991.

Appendix 9A

Companies That Produce Products Useful in Amblyopia Therapy

Patch Works
7655 Scribner Drive
Citrus Heights, CA 95610
(916) 726-9649

The Bernell Corporation
750 Lincolnway East
P.O. Box 4637
South Bend, IN 46634

The Fresnel Prism and Lens Company
24996 State Road 35
Siren, WI 54872
(800) 544-4760

Wimmer-Ferguson, Inc.
P.O. Box 100427
Denver, CO 80250

Wayne Engineering
1825 Willow Road
Northfield, IL 60093

Midwest Vision Therapy Equipment Co., Inc.
P.O. Box 949
Cicero, IN 46034-0949
(800) 757-6620

Dimensions
34 State Street
Ossining, NY 10562

Appendix 9B

Developmental Vision Program for Infants

(From Claude Valenti, O.D.)

The material in this appendix was originally written for parents who engage their infants in general programs of vision enhancement and development. We found these guidelines so useful that we have included them as principles to incorporate when applying vision activities specific to amblyopia therapy.

GENERAL RULES

Scheduling Vision Activities

Feeding, sleeping, and elimination occur in cycles, and parents learn that their schedule conforms to the infant's. The same is true in vision therapy. By 3 months of age, infants have begun to incorporate a time for exploring and playing in their schedule. Vision therapy is best accomplished during these times. Vision therapy attempted when the infant is hungry, sleepy, or cranky will not be productive. The ideal time for vision therapy is just after the bath, which is usually the infant's most enjoyable experience.

Duration of Vision Activities

A parent must use intuition to determine when to begin and end an activity. Activities for infants should generally last 5–15 minutes. The parent should tell the infant when the activity is over, rather than the infant telling the parent by fussing or activity avoidance. These activities are most effective when they are done on a daily basis as opposed to doing them for long stretches sporadically. It is not always necessary to do each activity every day if several are prescribed. Use judgment and work on the activity that the infant seems to enjoy at that moment. More than one activity session can be done per day, but the infant should be closely monitored for signs of fatigue. These guidelines should apply unless the clinician outlines a specific activity schedule.

Record Keeping

To properly monitor changes, a record of the activities must be kept. Be sure to record the activity performed, the time of day, the duration of the activity, general observations, and specific visual observations. Look for alignment, brightness, and movements of the eyes; pupil changes; head movement; shifting of visual attention; and blinking. The clinician should instruct the parent on specific observations to be made for specific procedures.

Making Sounds and Having Fun

Infants have an intrinsic alerting and orienting response to sounds. If the activity calls for the infant's eyes to be directed toward a certain place (e.g., eye contact with the parent), the addition of clucking and cooing sounds will help to bring the eyes to gaze in the proper direction. Make the sounds continuously and then introduce a sudden discontinuous sound. With older infants, keeping up a banter will work as well. Parents know the routine that their infants respond to best. Generally, when the parent is having fun, the infant will have fun.

ACTIVITIES

Marble-in-Cup

Purpose

The infant initially learns to calibrate space through the interaction of the visual system with hand manipulation. By observing an object fall through space, the infant learns that two areas can be visually related without being in direct physical contact. In addition, hand activities provide opportunities for effective, sustained development of visual fixation under binocular control.

Procedure

Seat the infant comfortably in your lap. Give the infant a large marble to hold in one hand. Hold a large, clear plastic cup directly underneath the hand holding the marble, and encourage the infant to drop the marble into the clear plastic cup. The sound from the marble dropping into the cup and appropriately timed reinforcement (e.g., "Ooh! What was that? The marble [show] went into the cup?" [shake]) will help the infant understand visual relations in space.

As the infant becomes more involved, hold the cup off to the left side of the infant and then off to the right. Keep alternating from side to side. In addition, lower the cup further down from the infant's hand so the marble can fall a greater distance through space. At all times, encourage the infant to look toward the marble as it drops.

Bed Trampoline

Purpose

Good coordination using both eyes depends on good balance between the two sides of the body.

Activities that require a simultaneous activation of muscles by each half of the body will help the infant develop bilateral body coordination.

Procedure

Have the infant stand on the edge of the bed while you extend your two forefingers for the infant to firmly grasp. Raise your hands so the infant's arms extend fully overhead. Depending on the height of the bed, it may be desirable for you to stand on a stool so the infant can be more easily supported. Next, slowly lift the infant from the bed while being careful to ensure that both of the infant's arms are pulling equally on your fingers. After lifting the infant 6–12 inches off the bed, slowly lower the infant back down to the bed. Repeat this cycle slowly several times.

As the infant begins to feel more comfortable supporting him- or herself, encourage him or her to push off with both legs equally by speeding up the rhythm and gently bouncing off the bed. If the infant tends to pull more with one hand or push more with one leg, provide a differing amount of arm support to make the infant use the weaker side more.

Near Point of Convergence Push-Up

Purpose

As objects move closer to the infant, the two eyes should coordinate to move inward. This is known as convergence. This activity has the infant make a convergence movement with the eyes and develop visual response to moving objects coming toward the infant.

Procedure

Hold the infant above your head with your arms extended. Make eye contact and slowly lower the infant closer and closer to your face until you actually touch noses. Maintain eye contact during the entire movement and observe the convergence movement with the eyes as the infant approaches. Do the procedure in reverse, starting up close with noses touching and slowly pushing the infant up and away until your arms are extended.

Repeat the procedure with the infant slightly torqued to one side or the other to promote an asymmetric convergence, unless directed otherwise by the doctor or therapist. This activity can also be carried out with the infant reclining and the parent slowly approaching inward while maintaining eye contact.

Visual Sit-Up

Purpose

There are many direct nerve connections between the visual system and the muscles in the upper neck. The infant needs to relate certain feelings in the neck to proper visual alignment. The posture of the neck muscles will influence the alignment of the eyes.

Procedure

Carry out the procedure in a well-lit room that is filled with objects, but not too cluttered. Place the infant on his or her back while you are on your knees by the infant's feet, directly facing the infant. Grasp the infant by the hands firmly, and encourage the infant to grasp your fingers. Slowly raise the infant to a sitting posture while taking care not to cause a jerking of the neck. Maintain eye contact with the infant while he or she is being raised. Watch for proper alignment of the eyes and a brightness to the eyes, which indicates that proper focusing is occurring.

Once the infant is in a sitting position, repeat the process in reverse by slowly lowering the infant to the reclining position. Encourage the infant to maintain his or her head in the erect position.

Face Target

Purpose

Infants should exhibit steady fixation and smooth pursuit development by the third month of life. Symmetric eye tracking ability is necessary for normal binocular development and the use of both eyes simultaneously, accurately, and efficiently. Infants are captivated by targets that exhibit the properties of facial contours.

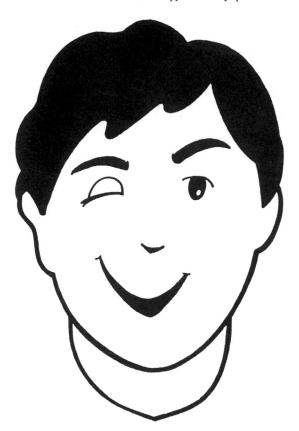

Figure 9B.1. Face target to develop fixation and following ability.

Procedure

Have the infant comfortably seated in someone's lap or secured in a high chair. Remove any other distracting sights or sounds from the area. Present the face target (Figure 9B.1) at a distance of 25 cm (10 in.). Move the target slowly so that you can observe that the infant is following the target. The normal extent of tracking will occur to 30 degrees off the midline. The infant will use head rotation to assist eye movements. Watch the eyes closely to make sure that both eyes are tracking as a team. If you are emphasizing the movements of one eye that has worse vision than the other, drop your thumb down inconspicuously to cover the better eye. After side-to-side movements are developed, work on up-and-down and diagonal movements.

Chapter 10

Screening for the Vision Problems
of Young Children

Paulette P. Schmidt

The ideal way to identify vision problems in children is to clinically examine the vision of each child. Vision examinations are not available to all children in the United States, however. Vision screening, a procedure that, at best, is a rudimentary observation to detect the presence or absence of general categories of vision problems, is often advocated as a cost-effective way to identify those unexamined children in need of further vision care and is required for preschool children by Head Start and by 28 states [1].

Vision screening should not be confused with a vision examination. Each procedure produces distinctly different results. A clinical examination is conducted under conditions in which control can be exercised (e.g., control of lighting during visual acuity testing or cover test through the patient's precise refractive correction), is conducted by a professional, and is a diagnostic procedure, whereas screening is conducted on an as-is basis (e.g., visual acuity testing through scratched lenses), may be conducted in part or in total by lay personnel, and is nondiagnostic. The fact that screening procedures are nondiagnostic is an illusory concept, at best, for the public. People may infer (incorrectly) that anyone who "passes" a screening program has no vision problem. The vision of those screened may be compromised, especially if the screening mechanism is of questionable or unknown effectiveness. The limitations of vision screening programs must

be recognized, and the effectiveness of a screening method merits close scrutiny.

Public service–oriented people and organizations frequently recruit clinicians to help develop guidelines for screening the vision of children and to advise what specific screening methods should be used. These well-motivated citizens and professionals can fall into the false belief that a combination of tests, usually completed by or under the supervision of trained professionals, can be adapted for the screening environment and effectively used to detect vision problems. Well-intentioned people can erroneously conclude that "something is better than nothing" for those unexamined children who do not have access to clinical vision examinations. Thus, across the country, public service organizations, governmental agencies, and professional organizations have adopted or are adopting vision screening guidelines for use in preschool populations. But is the premise "something is better than nothing"— that is, a test or combinations of tests adopted for the purpose of screening vision rather than no screening—valid? This chapter discusses the rationale for the early detection of and the public health significance of vision disorders in infants and toddlers; defines appropriate goals for screening the vision of infants and young children; and discusses currently prescribed or promoted vision screening procedures as well as their effectiveness, or lack thereof.

RATIONALE FOR EARLY DETECTION OF VISION PROBLEMS

The visual system is immature at birth and develops rapidly during infancy and early childhood [2, 3]. Health care professionals, recognizing the need to identify ocular conditions, such as cataract and infantile strabismus that might prevent the development of normal vision, do advocate eye examination of newborns and young infants to detect specific conditions [4–9]. The identification by examination of these early vision problems occurs most frequently in the hospital setting. Because the prevalence of ocular disease other than amblyopia and strabismus is collectively less than 1% and the magnitude of infantile strabismus deviations cause them to be overtly obvious, these particular conditions do not constitute public health issues necessitating mass screening. Amblyo- and strabismogenic refractive errors have been targeted by some groups for identification in infancy. Yet screening for refractive error is of uncertain value because serious questions remain as to whether correcting refractive error in infancy may interfere with the emmetropization process, as to what magnitude of the refractive error should be corrected, and as to the effectiveness of noncycloplegic evaluations of refractive error in infancy.

Although eye examinations in early infancy are important and useful, they cannot predict the occurrence of conditions, such as accommodative esotropia, that often appear after infancy. Moreover, infants cannot perform many of the examination procedures, such as recognition visual acuity, that are classically used to measure functional vision loss. After infancy, vision examinations are next recommended at approximately age 3 years [10]. By then, additional vision problems may have occurred, and 3-year-olds will possess the cognitive and communication skills necessary to respond to vision assessment procedures similar to those used in adult examinations. Also, and most important, detection of vision problems in this age group allows intervention at a time when the problems are highly amenable to treatment [11].

In summary, early vision problems, such as cataract and infantile strabismus, are targeted for detection in the hospital at birth, and there is general agreement among national professional and service organizations that 3-year-olds should be targeted for vision screening to detect vision problems of public health significance so that they can be treated in time for vision to development normally.

PUBLIC HEALTH SIGNIFICANCE OF CHILDREN'S VISION PROBLEMS

In the United States, vision disorders are the fourth most common disability of children and the leading cause of handicapping conditions in childhood [12]. In children in their preschool years, these vision disorders include amblyopia, strabismus, significant refractive error, ocular disease, and color vision deficits [13, 14]. The public health significance of each of these conditions is reviewed in the following sections. The prevalence, negative associations, and intervention strategies for each condition is summarized in Table 10.1.

Amblyopia

Amblyopia is responsible for loss of vision in more people younger than 45 years than all other ocular diseases and trauma combined [15]. The most frequent causes of amblyopia are the presence in early childhood of significant uncorrected refractive error, strabismus, and media opacities [16–23]. One review of leading research results concluded that if the risk factors for amblyopia development are detected in infancy or early childhood, amblyopia, "in principle at least, is completely preventable" [24]. It has also been shown that if amblyopia does develop, treatment is highly effective in early childhood [11, 14, 25]. Notwithstanding this potential for minimization of the incidence of amblyopia, six million Americans have vision loss due to amblyopia; and an additional 75,000 3-year-olds develop amblyopia each year [15].

Strabismus

The most common forms of strabismus in children are infantile esotropia, with a prevalence of 1–2%, and accommodative esotropia, with a prevalence of 2.0–2.5% [17, 26–34]. Onset of infantile esotropia

Table 10.1. Prevalent Childhood Vision Disorders

General Vision Disorder	Prevalence %	Negative Associations	Intervention Strategies
Amblyopia	2–3% [99, 121, 242–249]	Visual impairment Loss of stereopsis Occupational limitations	Patching Spectacles Vision therapy
Strabismus	3–4% [26–32]	Amblyopia Cosmesis Binocular dysfunction Loss of stereopsis Occupational limitations	Prism Spectacles Surgery Vision therapy
Refractive errors	15–30% [45–98]	Amblyopia Binocular dysfunction Loss of stereopsis Delayed perceptual skills Decreased reading abilities	Contact lenses Spectacles
Ocular disease	<1% [100–109]	Visual impairment Illness or loss of life Vision rehabilitation	Low-vision devices Medical or surgical
Color vision defects	8–10% (of males) [111–113]	Loss of learning potential Occupational restrictions	Education

occurs before 6 months of age and is characterized by an obvious deviation. The typical age of onset for accommodative esotropia is between 2 and 3 years of age [15]; it is often correctable with spectacles [17, 33–66]. The longer strabismus, in any form, is present without treatment, the more severe the sensory anomalies, such as amblyopia and suppression, become [35, 36]. Furthermore, the longer strabismus is present, the less likely it is that either a functional or cosmetic cure can be achieved [37, 38]. Overall, success in achieving cure rates for treatment of strabismus in young children ranges from 60% to 90% depending on whether the goal is a functional or merely cosmetic cure and on the type of strabismus and associated conditions found [39–41].

Refractive Errors

Refractive errors include myopia, hyperopia, astigmatism, and anisometropia and are the most prevalent, correctable vision problems found in the preschool population [44–98]. The prevalence of significant refractive errors in the preschool population ranges from 4% for myopia to 20% for hyperopia [45–73, 97, 98]. Approximately 10% of 3- to 4-year-olds have clinically significant astigmatism, and less than 1% of 5-year-olds have significant anisometropia [74–96]. The refractive errors that are most amblyo- and strabismogenic are anisometropia, astigmatism, and hyperopia. Treatment of refractive error in infants and children younger than 3 years may prevent amblyopia and strabismus [11, 42–44, 96]. However, there remain unanswered questions as to (1) whether prescribing refractive correction in these early years may interfere with the emmetropization process, and (2) what the magnitude of the appropriate refractive correction should be.

Ocular Disease

Ocular disease (other than amblyopia and strabismus) encompasses a wide range of disorders in isolation or associated with other systemic conditions. These include developmental anomalies of the eye (e.g., microphthalmia, aniridia, and coloboma), retinal anomalies (e.g., retinopathy of prematurity and retinoblastoma), media opacities (e.g., cataracts), and optic nerve anomalies. Ocular and congenital anomalies occur in less than 1% of children younger than 4 years of age, but the prevalence is considerably higher in certain subgroups (e.g., premature, multihandicapped, or drug-exposed) [99–110]. Failure to detect and treat these conditions may result in permanent visual impairment or, in the case of retinoblastoma, loss of life. However, the low prevalence of these conditions does not meet the currently prescribed public health criteria for the mass screening of general populations of young children.

Abnormal Color Vision

Abnormal color vision includes X-linked recessive protan and deutan (red-green) deficits, which occur in 8–10% of males and less than 0.5% of females; and other rare deficits, which affect up to 0.007% of both males and females [111]. Identification of color vision deficiency before school age is extremely important, since a large part of the early educational process involves the use of color identification and discrimination [112, 113]. Furthermore, changes in color vision capabilities may be an early indicator of retinal or optic nerve disorder.

Summary

In summary, the vision screening process should identify children with vision conditions or potential conditions that represent significant public health problems and that are not obvious, including amblyopia, strabismus, significant refractive error, and abnormal color vision.

GOALS OF PUBLIC HEALTH VISION SCREENING

Screening is an established public health strategy for the detection of people *with* or *at risk of developing* significant health problems and is used when the signs and symptoms of those problems are not obvious. The vision screening procedure is nondiagnostic and is used to divide the screened population into two groups—those with or at risk for vision problems and those who are not. Amblyopia, strabismus, significant refractive error, ocular dis-

ease, and color vision anomalies are frequent causes of visual impairment in childhood.

Table 10.1 lists the prevalence, negative associations, and intervention strategies for each of these vision disorders. The low prevalence rates of ocular disease in preschool children do not meet the public health criteria for the mass screening of general populations; however, the prevalence of amblyopia, color vision deficits, refractive error, and strabismus and their asymptomatic nature warrants the use of mass screening strategies to identify them in preschool children. Although there are accepted treatments and interventions for each of these conditions when they appear during early childhood, questions remain about the effects of some forms of intervention during infancy.

VISION SCREENING POLICY AND GUIDELINES RECOMMENDED FOR USE WITH PRESCHOOL CHILDREN

The vision problems of the preschool child, described in the previous sections, are detectable with a comprehensive vision examination. It is estimated, however, that only 14% of children younger than 6 years of age receive a comprehensive vision examination [114]. Vision screening has been recommended to identify young children who would benefit most from a complete eye examination and who probably would not otherwise receive one [12, 115].

In Public Law 99-457, the federal government requires a statement about health status, including vision, for each child who enters an early intervention program, such as Head Start [116]. Twenty-eight states also recommend or require vision screening of preschool children, although in the majority of these states neither the tests to be used nor the referral criteria are specified [117].

Guidelines for vision screening programs, including specific tests to be used, have been issued by a number of organizations [4–9]. Table 10.2 lists the ages, vision anomalies, and associated methods recommended for detecting those vision problems by four nationally recognized organizations or programs. The American Academy of Pediatrics, American Academy of Ophthalmology, American Association of Pediatric Ophthalmology and Strabismus, American Optometric Association, Prevent

Table 10.2. Recommended Guidelines for Preschool Vision Screening Programs

Organization	Age	Vision Anomalies	Method
American Academy of Pediatrics American Academy of Ophthalmology American Association of Pediatric Ophthalmology and Strabismus	3–5 yrs	Reduced visual acuity	*(any of the following)* Snellen letters Snellen numbers Tumbling E HOTV test Picture tests Allen figures Lighthouse test (all at 3 m)
		Ocular misalignment	Unilateral cover test (at 3 m) *or* Random Dot E Stereotest (at 40 cm)
American Optometric Association	2–6 yrs	Amblyopia High refractive error	Monocular visual acuity Patient history Brückner test Monocular visual acuity Plus lens test
		Ocular misalignment or strabismus	Patient history Observation Brückner test Hirschberg test Cover test
Prevent Blindness America	3–4 yrs	Color vision deficiencies Eye health Reduced visual acuity	Ishihara plates or equivalent Observation and questions LEA chart (at 3 m) Linear symbols
		Other (unspecified)	Optional tests include cover test, corneas reflection test, stereopsis tests, and plus lens tests, although they are not recommended. State recommendations may vary.
Head Start Program	3 yrs	Reduced visual acuity Strabismus	Tumbling E (at 3 m) Cover test Hirschberg test

Blindness America, and the Head Start Program each currently provide guidelines for use in preschool vision screening programs. No comparable guidelines exist for infants and toddlers.

SCREENING PRACTICES IN THE UNITED STATES

Although both laws and guidelines exist for the screening of preschool children, only 21% of preschool children currently are screened for vision problems [11, 117]. This is despite implementation of programs that fund vision screening, such as the Early and Periodic Screening Diagnosis and Treatment Program (EPSDT) and the Crippled Children's Program of the Institute of Maternal and Child Health [118, 119]. In a sample of 102 private pediatric practices, vision screening was attempted on only 38% of 3-year-old children [120]. Thus, although there is general agreement that 3-year-old children are the appropriate age group to screen, 3-year-old children are not being widely tested.

PUBLIC CONFUSION ABOUT THE DIFFERENCES BETWEEN VISION SCREENING AND CLINICAL EXAMINATION

The vision screening process is consistently confused with an examination despite clear statements that screenings are nondiagnostic procedures that do not substitute for a vision examination and are meant only to divide children into two groups—those who need a complete vision examination because of some vision disorder potentially disclosed by the screening and those who do not. Vision screenings are not intended to diagnose or identify specific vision disorders.

Furthermore, young children frequently cannot tell us how they see, do not know how they should see, and do not experience alarm-giving pain from the vision problems. Also, parents may incorrectly assume, to the child's ultimate detriment, that the screening procedure is broadly effective because it has been adopted for use by a reputable state or local agency, profession group, or service organization.

Therefore, public agencies and groups must give the vision welfare of the citizenry, especially very young children, the top priority and select only vision screening procedures with known effectiveness. Any state or local agency and professional or service organization conducting vision screenings for children implies that children who pass the screening do not have, or are not at risk for, developing a visually handicapping condition and that those who fail the screening have a vision problem or are at risk for developing one. The visual welfare of the children during these critical years of visual development depends on the accuracy (effectiveness) of the screening procedure adopted. Therefore, adoption of a screening method must be based solely on its known or proven effectiveness.

EFFECTIVENESS OF VISION SCREENING

Sensitivity is a particularly critical measure of screening effectiveness because it documents the percentage of children who will be missed by the screening method (100% − sensitivity [%] = % under-referred). Specificity is the percentage who will be over-referred (100% − specificity [%] = % over-referred). The percentage of under-referrals is vastly more important than over-referrals. Both over- and under-referrals need to be kept to small percentages but under-referrals are those children with, or at risk for, significant vision problems who are missed and are not referred for vision examination. Therefore, under-referral rates must be known before an organization or agency can properly evaluate and adopt screening methodologies. For further discussion of the measures of effectivity, sensitivity, specificity, etc., of screening methods, see Schmidt 1990 [121].

Studies that reported quantitative results (e.g., effectiveness of the vision screening tests used) include studies of photorefraction, the Modified Clinical Technique (MCT—a combination of procedures, including visual acuity assessment, cover test, retinoscopy, and ophthalmoscopy), stereoacuity, or visual acuity measurement. Those studies also indicated the level of training of the personnel conducting the screening procedure.

RESEARCH ON VISION SCREENING METHODS

A review of the vision screening literature from 1952 to 1995 disclosed more than 450 vision screening studies; however, only a few of them reported the results in a form other than rates of referral [14, 122–212]. A battery of tests known as the MCT is often referred to as the "gold standard" for vision screening in school-age children. The MCT identifies reduced visual acuity, significant refractive errors, ocular disease, and eye misalignment. When the MCT and other screening procedures (visual acuity; combinations procedures incorporated into a single instrument, such as the Telebinocular, etc.) were compared with the results obtained in comprehensive vision examinations conducted by optometrists and ophthalmologists, the sensitivity of the MCT was 0.96 and the specificity was 0.98, with the result that 97.2% of the 1,163 school-age children screened were correctly identified; other procedures correctly identified 42.3–77.8% of the children but missed up to 21.2% [145, 149, 150].

Recently, several studies have evaluated modified versions of the MCT in preschool populations with differing results. Fern compared the results of the MCT with the results of a comprehensive eye examination in 102 18- to 71-month-old preschool children [124]. The MCT was modified to use the HOTV chart rather than the tumbling E test for acuity screening. Results indicated a sensitivity of 0.87 and a specificity of 0.66. Marsh-Tootle et al. compared the results of the MCT, with the addition of the Random Dot E stereo test, with the results of a comprehensive eye examination of 61 3- to 5-year-old children who had failed the MCT and of an age-matched sample of 45 children who passed the MCT [126]. Sensitivity was 0.49 and specificity was 0.79, with 70% of those diagnosed by examination being correctly identified using the MCT. Although these studies suggest that the MCT is less effective for screening preschoolers than for school-age children, the comparison is tainted by the fact that the MCT in the preschool studies was administered by students, whereas in the Orinda study the MCT was administered by licensed eye care practitioners [145]. Furthermore, these low sensitivity and specificity values may have resulted from difficulties that preschool children had with the tumbling E acuity test. Schmidt demonstrated improved effectiveness of the MCT procedure among 119 preschool children (mean age = 3.51 years) when age-appropriate tests were used to decrease screening failures that resulted from an inability to complete one of the screening tasks [196].

The MCT may be useful in screening preschool children if age-appropriate, valid tests are selected for the battery; however, the MCT may not be cost-effective or feasible in many preschool settings because it must be administered in part by a health care professional. Therefore, screening methods appropriate for lay personnel have been suggested. Such methods include visual acuity, photorefraction, and stereoacuity.

Stereoacuity screening has been evaluated; five of the studies include quantitative results [124, 129–133, 157, 185, 188–193, 213–219]. Reports of the value of a Random Dot E stereo test in screening preschool children have varied from unusable to high sensitivity, specificity, and testability when pretraining is used [124, 126, 133]. Some studies have demonstrated the usefulness of stereoacuity alone or in combination with visual acuity or retinoscopy in screening preschool children; others have shown poor sensitivity or reduced testability [124, 131–133, 185, 193]. In a small group ($n = 30$) of 3-year-old (± 1 month) children at high risk for amblyopia, strabismus, and refractive error (10 very low birth weight), Schmidt compared the results of screening with the Random Dot E stereo test after a pretraining session with results of complete vision examination [133]. When screening by a professional and by an untrained screener was compared with comprehensive vision examination of all children, results showed a single test of stereoacuity to have a sensitivity of 0.77 and specificity of 0.88, with 83.3% correctly identified. Testability was 86.7%; but the four children who were untestable failed the vision examination due to vision problems. Marsh-Tootle et al. also reported an increased usefulness in stereo testing with 3-year-old children when a brief pretraining session was conducted [126]. Orel-Bixler and Brodie have reported similar sensitivities and specificities for Mr. Stereo Smile stereoacuity (0.52 and 0.82) and noncycloplegic photorefraction (0.57 and 0.84) in a small study of young children up to 3 years of age [129]. Furthermore, related investigations have demonstrated the greater sensitivity of stereoacuity over visual acuity to binocularly or monocularly blurred vision resulting from optical blur or anisometropic amblyopia [213, 214]. Random dot stereoacuity testing demonstrates the potential for being a sensitive and inexpensive test for vision screening, especially when combined with screening for refractive error [133].

Assessment of visual acuity remains the most widely used vision screening test [25, 97, 120–123, 131, 145, 154, 202, 203, 212–215, 220–222]. However, under-referrals have been a consistent problem with visual acuity screening procedures [119–123]. For example, in older children able to be tested with monocular measures of Snellen recognition acuity, use of the standard 20/40 referral cutoff has resulted in under-referral rates of 21.2% [145]. In the preschool population, results of a large-scale screening program reported a prevalence of 0.43% for amblyopia and 0.61% for strabismus, far below the prevalence rates of 2% and 4%, respectively, that have been reported for the general population by Ehrlich et al. [122]. They argue that the low prevalence rates found in screening reflect inadequacies in methods used to screen—that is, isolated symbol acuity is not effective in detecting amblyopia, and observation and cover tests, when administered by lay screeners, are not effective in detecting strabismus [131, 203]. Other studies also support that visual acuity testing in children is unreliable [120, 179]. To avoid difficulties experienced by preschoolers in performing complex letter acuity tasks, some researchers have used picture-naming acuity tasks or assessment of grating acuity using the Teller acuity card procedure [154, 196]. Both picture acuity and grating acuity tasks can greatly overestimate visual acuity, however, and lead to high under-referral rates [220, 221]. Photorefraction is being promoted for lay screening of preschool children because it is quick and requires little cooperation. It is being recommended for the detection of media opacities, strabismus, and refractive error [44, 69, 75, 79, 82, 87, 89, 98, 123, 125, 127–130, 138–140, 164–169, 173, 223–240]. Results from 13 photorefraction screening studies show the following limitations with the procedure [69, 98, 123–125, 127–130, 231, 239, 240, 241].

1. All 13 studies reporting quantitative results (sensitivity, specificity, etc.) were conducted by highly trained professionals or technicians, not by lay personnel.

2. Of the 13 studies, only six used commercially available photorefractors or videophotorefractors (or the prototypes of the commercially available instruments).

3. Studies that report the results of photorefraction when cycloplegia is used demonstrate fewer under-referrals than those without the use of cycloplegia.

4. Several reports that assess commercially available instruments reported that sensitivity is high; however, the estimates of sensitivity are not based on all children; only children for whom analyzable photos were obtained were included in the results [127, 128, 130].

5. Although the under-referrals for all refractive errors (anisometropia, astigmatism, hyperopia, and myopia) were reported collectively as 0–38%, in the three studies (all with commercially available instruments or prototypes) that reported referral rates by individual refractive error type and without benefit of cycloplegia, the under-referrals var-

ied greatly by type: hyperopia, 53–88%; astigmatism, 47–71%; anisometropia, 17–46%; and myopia, 7–38% [69, 125, 223].

6. Little information is available about the ability of the instrumentation to detect strabismic conditions that are not cosmetically obvious (less than 10 prism diopters).

7. When photos were scored by a group of health professionals, only 58% of the photos were consistently categorized as pass or fail [173].

Therefore, the studies fail to document the effectiveness of photorefraction screening for the detection of nonobvious amblyo- and strabismogenic conditions.

SCREENING PERSONNEL

Studies that demonstrate the use of stereoacuity screening report the results of screening by professionals and untrained screening personnel [115, 131–133, 173, 185, 188, 189, 192, 193, 198, 200–204, 213, 216]. All other studies report the results only when professionals conduct the screening tests. The effectiveness of screening procedures in the hands of lay personnel has not been established. Yet, to implement a nationwide program of preschool vision screening, many groups will expect to depend on lay volunteers.

CONCLUSION

In summary, there is no validated, highly effective method for vision screening of preschool children that is comparable with the MCT that is used with the school-age population.

Recently, several tests have been developed that (1) can be completed by a large proportion of preschool-age children and (2) meet standards that have been set for measures of vision used for adults.

To conduct valid public health screenings of vision in an ethically responsible way and in a manner that can validly and correctly be relied on by parents and other interested parties, there is a need to develop and test a preschool vision screening battery of tests that is easy to administer to the target population (3-year-olds) in a preschool setting and that has a high sensitivity and specificity when compared to the "gold standard" of vision examination. Additionally, in the interest of minimizing health care costs, the ideal battery of tests would be one that can be administered by lay persons.

Although new testing procedures make the widespread screening of 3-year-olds potentially viable, until such a battery of tests is validated, one cannot conduct a public health vision screening of preschool children. The critical elements of under- and over-referral rates are not known; therefore, the purported screening procedure is not a valid, scientifically reliable screening. If a "screening procedure" is adopted before validation, the agency or group implicitly warrants that the procedure is effective in identifying the vision problems for which preschoolers are at greatest risk. In this case, "something may be worse than nothing" because the number of children having a possibly remediable disorder missed by the procedure will be unknown and perhaps significant; and, at the same time, the child, parent, or guardian may be given a false sense of security that vision is developing normally and may fail to seek care that would detect and allow for intervention to occur during the critical periods of visual development. Adopting unvalidated procedures for screening of vision of preschool children would help to ensure that vision disorders remain the leading cause of handicapping conditions in childhood.

Acknowledgments

The author wishes to express her sincere appreciation to the Preschool Children's Vision Screening Study Group for sharing information and references critical to the substance of this chapter. Members of the group include Dale Allen, O.D., Ph.D.; Elise Ciner, O.D.; Lynn Cyert, Ph.D., O.D.; Velma Dobson, Ph.D.; Maureen Maguire, Ph.D.; Bruce Moore, O.D.; Deborah Orel-Bixler, Ph.D., O.D.; Paulette P. Schmidt, O.D., M.S.; and Janet Schultz, C.P.N.P.

REFERENCES

1. Ciner E, Schmidt P. Orel-Bixler D, et al. Vision screening of preschool children: evaluating the past, looking toward the future. Optom Vis Sci 1998; 75:571–84.
2. Isenberg SJ (ed). The Eye in Infancy. St. Louis: Mosby, 1994.
3. Daw NW. Visual Development. New York: Plenum, 1995.
4. Anonymous. Proposed vision screening guidelines. Am Acad Pediatr News 1995;11(1):25.
5. American Foundation for Vision Awareness. Children's vision and literacy campaign position paper. St. Louis: American Foundation for Vision Awareness, 1993.
6. American Optometric Association Clinical Care Guide: Guidelines for Preventive Eye Care. St. Louis:American Optometric Association, 1994.
7. American Optometric Association. National Survey of Vision Screening of the Preschool and School Age Child: The Results of the American Optometric Association 1989–1990 Survey. St. Louis: American Optometric Association, 1992;49(23), 49(46).
8. American Optometric Association Vision and School Health Committee. The American Optometric Association Guidelines on Vision Screening, St. Louis: Optometric Development Enterprises, 1979.
9. Healthcare Standards 1996. Plymouth Meeting, PA. ECRI. 1974.
10. Foster B. Board recommends eye exam schedule. American Optometric Association News 1993;32(2):1,6.
11. Sjostrand J, Abrahamsson M. Screening for Amblyopia. In C Bisantis, EC Campos, MR Angi (eds), Crescita Dell'Occhio E Sviluppo Della Visione Nel Bambino. Padova, 1991.
12. Gerali P, Flom MC, Raab EL. Report of Children's Vision Screening Task Force. Schaumburg, IL: National Society to Prevent Blindness, 1990.
13. Von Noorden GK. Stimulus deprivation amblyopia. Am J Ophthalmol 1981;92:416.
14. Ciuffreda K, Levi J, Selenow DM. Amblyopia: Basic and Clinical Aspects. Boston: Butterworth–Heinemann, 1991.
15. Dell W. The epidemiology of amblyopia. Probl Optom 1991;3(2):195.
16. Sjostrand J, Abrahamsson M. Risk factors in amblyopia. Eye 1990;4:787–93.
17. Ingram RM, Walker C. Refraction as a means of predicting squint or amblyopia in preschool siblings of children known to have these defects. Br J Ophthalmol 1979;63:238.
18. Glover LP, Brewer WR. An ophthalmologic review of more than 20,000 men at the Altoona Induction Center. Am J Ophthalmol 1944;27:346.
19. Downing AH. Ocular defects in 60,000 selectees. Arch Ophthalmol 1945;33:137–143.
20. Jampolsky A, Flom BC, Weymouth FW, et al. Unequal corrected visual acuity as related to anisometropia. Arch Ophthalmol 1955;54:893.
21. Phillips CI. Strabismus,anisometropia, and amblyopia. Br J Ophthalmol 1959;43:449.

22. Horwith H. Anisometropic amblyopia. Am Orthoptic J 1964;14:99.
23. Gwiazda J, Bauer J, Thorn F, et al. Meridional amblyopia does result from astigmatism in early childhood. Clin Vis Sci 1986;1:145.
24. National Advisory Eye Council. Vision Research. A National Plan: 1994–1998. A Report of the National Advisory Eye Council. Washington, DC: U.S Department of Health and Human Services (PHS), National Eye Institute (NIH Publication No. 93-3186), 1993.
25. Flynn J, Cassady J. Current trends in amblyopia treatment. Trans Am Acad Ophthalmol Otolaryngol 1978; 85:428.
26. Chew E, Remaley NA, Tamboli A, et al. Risk factors for esotropia and exotropia. Arch Ophthalmol 1994; 112:1349.
27. Friedman L, Biedner B, David R, et al. Screening for refractive errors, strabismus, and other anomalies from age 6 months to 3 years. J Ped Ophthalmol Strabismus 1977;17:315.
28. Graham PA. Epidemiology of strabismus. Br J Ophthalmol 1974;58:224.
29. Woodruff ME. Vision and refractive status among grade 1 children of the province of New Brunswick. Am J Optom Physiol Opt 1986;63:545.
30. Flom MC, Bedell HE. Identifying amblyopia using associated conditions, acuity, and nonacuity features. Am J Optom Physiol Opt 1985;62:153.
31. Nixon RB, Helveston EM, Miller K, et al. Incidence of strabismus in neonates. Am J Ophthalmol 1985; 100:798.
32. Von Noorden GK. Infantile esotropia: a continuing riddle. Am Orthoptic J 1984;34:52.
33. Burian HM. Thoughts on the nature of amblyopia ex anopsia. Am Orthoptic J 1956;6:5.
34. Ciner E. Management of Refractive Error in Infants, Toddlers and Preschool Children. Probl Optom 1990;2(3):294.
35. Flom M. Issues in Clinical Management of Binocular Anomalies. In AA Rosenbloom, MW Morgan (eds), Principles and Practice of Pediatric Optometry. Philadelphia: Lippincott, 1990.
36. Flom M, Wick B. A Model for Treating Binocular Anomalies. In AA Rosenbloom, MW Morgan (eds), Principles and Practice of Pediatric Optometry. Philadelphia: Lippincott, 1990.
37. Caloroso EE, Rouse MW. Clinical Management of Strabismus. Boston: Butterworth–Heinemann, 1993;60.
38. Oliver M, Neumann R, Chaimovitch Y, et al. Compliance and results of treatment for amblyopia in children more than 8 years old. Am J Ophthalmol 1986;102:340.
39. Scheiman M, Ciner E, Gallaway M. Surgical success rates in infantile esotropia. J Am Optom Assoc 1989; 60(1):22.
40. Flax N, Selenow A. Results of surgical treatment of intermittent divergent strabismus. Am J Optom Physiol Opt 1985;62(2):100.
41. Flax N, Duckman RH. Orthoptic treatment of strabismus. J Am Optom Assoc 1978;49(12):53
42. Ingram R, Walker C. Prediction of amblyopia and squint by means of refraction at age 1 year. Br J Ophthalmol 1985;69:851.
43. Ingram R, Arnold P, Dally S, Lucas J. The results of a randomised trial of treating abnormal hypermetropia from the age of 6 months. Br J Ophthalmol 1990; 74:158.
44. Atkinson J, Braddick O, Wattam-Bell J, et al. Photorefractive screening of infants and effects of refractive correction. Invest Ophthalmol Vis Sci 1987:28(4) Suppl:339.
45. Abrahamsson M, Sjostrom A, Sjostrand J. A longitudinal study of changes in infantile anisometropia [abstract 83]. Invest Ophthalmol Vis Sci 1989;30(Suppl):141.
46. Banks MS. Infant refraction and accommodation. Int Ophthalmol Clin 1979;20:205.
47. Banks MS, Aslin RN. Sensitive period for the development of human binocular vision. Science 1975; 190:675.
48. Fledelius H. Prematurity and the eye: opththalmic 10-year follow-up of children of low and normal birth weight. Acta Ophthalmol Suppl 1976;128:47–97, 127–157.
49. Shapero M, Yanko L, Nawratzki I, et al. Refractive power of premature children at infancy and early childhood. Am J Ophthalmol 1980;90:234.
50. Goldschmidt E. Refraction in the newborn. Acta Ophthalmol (Copenh) 1969;47:570.
51. Garner L, Grosvenor T, McKellor M, et al. Refraction and its components in Melanesian school children in Vanuatu. Am J Optom Physiol Opt 1988;65:182–189.
52. Althaus K, Bischoff P. Videorefraktionsmessung im ersten lebensjahr. Klin Monatsbl Augenheilkd 1994; 205:133.
53. Cook RG, Glasscock RE. Refractive and ocular findings in the newborn. Am J Ophthalmol 1951;34:1407
54. Wibaut F. Uber die emmetropisation und den ursprung der spharischen refracktionsanomalien. Graefes Arch Clin Exp Ophthalmol 1926;116:596.
55. Ingram RM, Barr A. Changes in refraction between the ages of 1 and 3 years. Br J Ophthalmol 1979;63:339.
56. Kalogiera T. Refractive error in Yugoslav urban children aged between 3 and 7 years. Child Care Health Dev 1979;5:439.
57. Fletcher MC, Brandom S. Myopia of prematurity. Am J Ophthalmol 1955;40:474.
58. Graham MV, Gray OP. Refraction of premature babies' eyes. Br Med J 1963;1:1452.
59. Gwiazda J, Thorn F, Bauer J, et al. Prediction of school age myopia from infant refractive errors. Invest Ophthalmol Vis Sci 1990;31:233.
60. Scharf J, Zonis S, Zeltzer M. Refraction in Israeli premature babies. J Pediatr Ophthalmol 1975;12:193.
61. Mohindra I, Held R. Refraction in humans from birth to five years. Doc Ophthalmol 1981;28:19.
62. Fulton AB, Hanson R, Peterson R. The relation of my-

opia and astigmatism in developing eyes. J Ophthalmol 1982;89:298.

63. Ingram R, Barr A. Refraction of 1 year old children after cycloplegia with 1% cyclopentolate: comparison with finding after atropinization. Br J Ophthalmol 1979;63:348.

64. Fulton A, Dobson V, Salem D, et al. Cycloplegic refractions in infants and young children. Am J Ophthalmol 1980;90:239.

65. Santanastaso A. La refraziene oculare nei primi anni de vita. Annu Ottal Clin Ocul (Italy) 1930;58:852.

66. Angle J, Wissmann DA. The epidemiology of myopia. Am J Epidemiol 1980;3:220.

67. Woodruff ME. Cross-sectional studies of corneal and astigmatic characteristics of children between the twenty-fourth and seventy-second months of life. Am J Optom Physiol Opt 1971;48:650.

68. Kitchen WH, Rickards A, Ryan MM, et al. A longitudinal study of very low-birthweight infants. II. Results of controlled trial of intensive care and incidence of handicaps. Develop Med Child Neurol 1979;21:582.

69. Hodi S. Screening of infants for significant refractive error using video refraction. Ophthal Physiol Opt 1994;14(7):310.

70. Gwiazda J, Mohindra I, Brill S, et al. Infant astigmatism and meridional amblyopia. Vision Res 1985; 25:1269.

71. Saunders KJ, Westall CA. Comparisons between near retinoscopy and cycloplegic retinoscopy of infants and children. Optom Vis Sci 1992;69(8):615.

72. Schallig-Delfos NE. The development of myopia in premature infants with and without retinopathy of prematurity. Invest Ophthalmol Vis Sci 1992; 33(4)Suppl:2981.

73. Brown EVL, Kronfeld P. Net average yearly changes in refraction of atropinized eyes from birth to beyond middle life. Arch Ophthalmol 1938;19:719.

74. Abrahamsson M, Fabian G, Sjostrand J. Changes in astigmatism between the ages of 1 and 4 years: a longitudinal study. Br J Ophthalmol 1988;72:145.

75. Howland HC, Atkinson J, Braddick O, et al. Infant astigmatism measured by photorefraction. Science 1978;202:331.

76. Gwiazda JE, Scheiman M, Mohindra I, et al. Astigmatism in children: changes in axis and amount from birth to six years. Invest Ophthalmol Vis Sci 1984;25:88.

77. Dobson V, Howland HC, Moss C, et al. Photorefraction of normal and astigmatic infants during viewing of patterned stimuli. Vision Res 1983;10:1043.

78. Gwiazda JE, Scheiman M, Held R: Meridional amblyopia in former astigmats. Invest Ophthalmol Vis Sci 1984;22(4)Suppl:88.

79. Atkinson J, Braddick O, French J. Infant astigmatism: its disappearance with age. Vision Res 1980;20:891.

80. Mohindra I, Held R, Gwiazda J, et al. Astigmatism in infants. Science 1978;202:329.

81. Dobson V, Fulton AB, Manning K, et al. Cycloplegic refractions of premature infants. Am J Ophthalmol 1981;91:490.

82. Howland HC, Sayles N. Photorefractive measurement of astigmatism in infants and young children. Invest Ophthalmol Vis Sci 1984;25:93.

83. Lyle WM. Changes in corneal astigmatism with age. Am J Optom Arch Am Acad Optom 1971;48:467.

84. Hirsch MJ. Changes in astigmatism during the first eight years of school—an interim report from the Ojai longitudinal study. Am J Optom Arch Am Acad Optom 1963;40:127.

85. Gwiazda J, Thorn F, Bauer J, et al. Prediction of school age myopia from infant refractive errors. Invest Ophthalmol Vis Sci 1984;31:233.

86. Fulton AB, Hansen RM, Petersen RA. The relation of myopia and astigmatism in developing eyes. Ophthalmology 1982;89:298.

87. Howland HC, Sayles N. Photokeratometric and photorefractive measurements of astigmatism in infants and young children. Vision Res 1985;25:73.

88. Shapiro M. Amblyopia. Philadelphia: Chilton Book Co., 1971;267.

89. Howland HC. Infant eye: optics and accommodation. Current Eye Res 1982;2:217.

90. Dobson V, Fulton, Sebris SL. Cycloplegic refractions of infants and young children: the axis of astigmatism. Invest Ophthalmol Vis Sci 1984;25:83.

91. Fulton AB. Screening preschool children to detect visual and ocular disorders [editorial]. Arch Ophthalmol 1992;110:1553.

92. Anstice J. Astigmatism—its components and their changes with age. Am J Optom Physiol Opt 1971;48:1001.

93. Dobson V, Fulton, Sebris SL. Cycloplegic refractions of infants and young children: the axis of astigmatism. Invest Ophthalmol Vis Sci 1984;25:83.

94. Jampolsky A, Flom BC, Weymouth FW, et al. Unequal corrected visual acuity as related to anisometropia. Arch Ophthalmol 1955;54:893.

95. Ingram R, Traynar M, Walker C, Wilson J. Screening for refractive errors at age 1 year. A pilot study. Br J Ophthalmol 1979;63:243.

96. Abrahamsson M, Fabian G, Sjostrand J. A longitudinal study of a population based sample of astigmatic children. II. The changeability of anisometropia. Acta Ophthalmol (Copenh) 1990;68:435.

97. Friedman Z, Neumann E, Hyams SW, et al. Ophthalmic screening of 38,000 children, age 1 to 2 years, in child welfare clinics. J Pediatr Ophthalmol Strabismus 1976;17:261.

98. Atkinson J, Braddick OJ, Durden K et al. Screening for refractive errors in 6–9 month old infants by photorefraction. Br J Ophthalmol 1984;68:105.

99. Edmonds LD, James LM. Temporal trends in the prevalence of congenital malformation at birth based on the Birth Defects Monitoring Program, United States, 1979–1987. MMWR CDC Surveill Summ 1990; 39(SS4):19.

100. Stagno S, Pass RF, Alford CA. Perinatal Infections and Maldevelopment. In AD Bloom, LS James (eds), The Fetus and the Newborn. New York: Alan R Liss, 1981;31.

101. Snowe RJ, Wilfert CM. Epidemic reappearance of gonococcal ophthalmia neonatorum. Pediatrics 1973; 51:110.

102. Magni R, Pierro L, Brancato R. Microphthalmus with colobomatous orbital cyst in Trisomy 13. Ophthalmic Pediatr Genet 1990;12:39.

103. DeLuise VP, Anderson DR. Primary infantile glaucoma. Surv Ophthalmol 1983;28:1.

104. Abel EL, Sokol RJ. A revised conservative estimate of the incidence of FAS and its economic impact. Alcohol Clin Exp Res 1991;15:514.

105. Frank DA, Zuckerman BS, Amaro H, et al. Cocaine use during pregnancy: prevalence and correlates. Pediatrics 1988;82:888.

106. Pe'er J, Braun JJ. Ocular pathology in trisomy 18 (Edward's syndrome). Ophthalmologica 1986;192:176.

107. Devessa SS. The incidence of retinoblastoma. Am J Ophthalmol 1975;80:263.

108. Palmer EA, Flynn JT, Hardy RJ, et al. Incidence and early course of retinopathy of prematurity. Ophthalmology 1991;98:1628.

109. Billmire ME, Myers PA. Serious head injury in infants: accident or abuse? Pediatrics 1985;75:340.

110. Cassady JV. Dacryocystitis of infancy. Am J Ophthalmol 1948;31:773.

111. Krill AE. Congenital Color Vision Defects. In AE Krill, DB Archer (eds), Krill's Hereditary Retinal and Choroidal Diseases (Vol II). Clinical Characteristics. Hagerstown, MD: Harper & Row, 1977.

112. Heath GG. The handicap of color blindness. J Am Optom Assoc 1974;45(1):62.

113. Mandola J. The handicap of color anomalies in elementary school achievement. J Sch Health 1969;39:633.

114. Poe GS. Eye Care Visits and Use of Eyeglasses or Contact Lenses. United States 1979 and 1980. Vital and Health Statistics (Series 10, No. 145). DHHS Publication (PHS) 841573, Hyattsville, MD: DHHS, August 1984.

115. Navon SE, McKeown CS. Amblyopia. Int Ophthalmol Clin 1992;22(1):35.

116. U.S. Department of Health and Human Services. Public Law 99-457.

117. U.S. Department of Health and Human Services. Head Start—A Child Development Program. Washington, DC: U.S. Department of Health and Human Services Publication No. 8131092 (OHDS), 1981.

118. Austin C. Mass preschool vision screening. Children 1959;6:58.

119. Frankenburg W, North A. A Guide to Screening for the Early and Periodic Screening, Diagnosis and Treatment Program. U.S. Department of Health, Education and Welfare Publication No. (SRS) 74-24516. Washington, DC: U.S. Department of Health, Education and Welfare

in cooperation with the American Academy of Pediatrics, 1974.

120. Wasserman RC, Croft CA, Brotherton SE. Preschool vision screening in pediatric practice: a study from the pediatric research in office setting (PROS) network. Pediatrics 1992;89:834.

121. Schmidt PP. Vision Screening. In Rosenbloom AA, Morgan M (eds), Principles and Practice of Pediatric Optometry. Philadelphia: Lippincott, 1990;467–485.

122. Ehrlich MI, Reinecke RD, Simons K. Preschool vision screening for amblyopia and strabismus: programs, methods, and guidelines, 1983. Surv Ophthalmol 1983;28:145.

123. Duckman RH, Meyer B. Use of photoretinoscopy as a screening technique in the assessment of anisometropia and significant refractive error in infants/toddlers/children and special populations. Am J Optom Physiol Opt 1985;62(9):621.

124. Fern K. A comparison of vision screening techniques in preschool children. Invest Ophthalmol Vis Sci 1991;32(4)Suppl:3976.

125. Freedman HL, Preston KL. Polaroid photoscreening for amblyogenic factors. Ophthalmol 1993;99:1785.

126. Marsh-Tootle W, Corliss DA, Alvarez S, et al. A statistical analysis of Modified Clinical Technique vision screening of preschoolers by optometry students. Optom Vis Sci 1994;71(10):593.

127. Morgan KS, Johnson WD. Clinical evaluation of a commercial photorefractor. Arch Ophthalmol 1987;105 (11):1528.

128. Morris CEA, Scott WE, Simon JW, et al. Photorefractive Screening for Amblyogenic Factors: A Three Centre Study. In G Tillson (ed), Trans VIIth Int Orthoptic Congress. Nürnberg, Germany: Fahner Verlag 1991; 243–247.

129. Orel-Bixler D, Brodie A. Vision screening of infants and toddlers: photorefraction and stereoacuity. Invest Ophthalmol Vis Sci 32(4)Suppl:962.

130. Ottar WL, Scott WE, Hogado SI. Photoscreening for amblyogenic factors. J Pediatr Ophthalmol Strabismus 1995;32:289.

131. Rosner J. The effectiveness of the random dot E stereotest as a preschool vision screening instrument. J Am Optom Assoc 1978;49:1121.

132. Ruttum MS, Nelson DB. Stereopsis testing to reduce overreferral in preschool vision screening. J. Pediatr Ophthalmol Strabismus 1991;28(3):131.

133. Schmidt P. Vision screening with the RDE stereotest in pediatric populations. Optom Vis Sci 1994;71(4):273.

134. Allen HF. A new picture series for preschool vision testing. Am J Ophthalmol 1957;44:38.

135. Almeder LM, Peck LB, Howland HC. Prevalence of anisometropia in volunteer laboratory and school screening populations. Invest Ophthalmol Vis Sci 1990;31:2448.

136. Atkinson J, Anker S, Evans C, McIntyre A. The Cam-

bridge Crowding Cards for Preschool Visual Acuity Testing. In M Lenk-Schäfer (ed), Trans Sixth International Orthoptic Congress. Harrogate, Great Britain, 1987;482–486.

137. Atkinson J, Braddick O. Assessment of vision in infants. Trans Ophthalmol Soc U K 1979;99:338.

138. Atkinson J, Braddick O. The use of isotropic photorefraction for screening in infants. Acta Ophthalmol Suppl 1983;157:36–45.

139. Atkinson J, Braddick O, Pimm-Smith E, Durden K. Refractive screening of infants. Am J Ophthalmol 1982;93:372.

140. Atkinson J, Braddick O. Vision screening and photorefraction—the relation of refractive errors to strabismus and amblyopia. Behav Brain Res 1983;10:71.

141. Austin C. Mass preschool vision screening. Children 1959;6:58.

142. Avilla CW, von Noorden GK. Limitation of the TNO random dot stereo test for visual screening. Am Orthoptic J 1981;31:87.

143. Barker J, Barmatz H. Eye Function. In WK Frankenburg, BW Camp (eds), Pediatric Screening Tests. Springfield, IL: Thomas, 1975.

144. Blackhurst RT, Radke E. Vision screening procedures used with mentally retarded children. A second report. Sight Sav Rev 1967;38:84.

145. Blum H, Peters HB, Bettman JW. Vision Screening for Elementary Schools: The Orinda Study. Berkeley, CA: University of California Press, 1959.

146. Burman ML. Vision screening of preschool children in Prince George's County, Maryland, nursery schools. J Natl Med Assoc 1969;61:352.

147. Cohen AH, Lieberman S, Stolzberg M, Ritty JM. The NYSOA vision screening battery—a total approach. J Am Optom Assoc 1983;54:979.

148. Colasuonno TM. Preschool vision screening study in Douglas County, Oregon. Sight Sav Rev 1958;28:156.

149. Crane MM, Scobee RG, Foote FM, Green EL. Study of procedures for screening elementary school children for visual defects. Referrals by screening procedures - vs- ophthalmological findings. Sight Sav Rev 1952;22:141.

150. Crane MM, Foote FM, Scobee RG, et al. Screening school children for visual defects. Children's Bureau Publication No. 345. Washington, DC: Government Printing Office, 1954.

151. Cunningham F. Preschool vision screening. Sight Sav Rev 1957;27:90.

152. Davens E. The nationwide alert to preschool screening. Sight Sav Rev 1966;36:13.

153. Diskan SM. A new visual screening test for children. Am J Ophthalmol 1955;39:369.

154. Fern KD, Manny RE. Visual acuity of the preschool child: a review. Am J Optom Physiol Opt 1986;63(5):319.

155. Fink WH. Testing visual acuity of the preschool child. Minn Med 1950;42:23.

156. Gruber J, Dickey P, Rosner J. Comparison of a modified (two-item) Frisby with the standard Frisby and random dot E stereotests when used with preschool children. Am J Optom Physiol Opt 1985;62(5):349.

157. Hammond RS, Schmidt PP. A random dot E stereogram for the vision screening of children. Arch Ophthalmol 1986;104:54.

158. Hatfield EM. A year's record. Sight Sav Rev 1966;36(1):18.

159. Hatfield EM. Methods and standards for screening preschool children. Sight Sav Rev 1979;49:71.

160. Hilton AF, Stark DJ, Biggs AB, O'Hara V. Preschool vision screening—a pilot study. Aust J Ophthalmol 1982;10:199.

161. Hyams SW, Neumann E. Picture cube for vision screening of preschool children. Br J Ophthalmol 1972;56:572.

162. Ingram RM. The problem of screening children for visual defects. Br J Ophthalmol 1977;61:4.

163. Ingram RM. Refraction as a basis for screening children for squint and amblyopia. Br J Ophthalmol 1977;61:8.

164. Kaakinen K. A simple method for screening children with strabismus, anisometropia or ametropia by simultaneous photography of corneal and fundus reflexes. Acta Ophthalmol 1979;57:161.

165. Kaakinen K. Photographic screening for strabismus and high refractive errors of children aged 1 to 4 years. Acta Ophthalmol 1981;59:38.

166. Kaakinen K. Simultaneous two flash static photoskiascope. Acta Ophthalmol 1981;59:378.

167. Kaakinen K, Tommila V. A clinical study on the detection of strabismus, anisometropia or ametropia of children by simultaneous photography of corneal and fundus reflexes. Acta Ophthalmol 1979;57:600.

168. Kaivonen M, Koskenoja M. Visual screening for children aged four years and preliminary experience from its application in practice (a preliminary report). Acta Ophthalmol 1963;41:785.

169. Kelley CR. Visual Screening and Child Development: The North Carolina Study. Raleigh, NC: North Carolina State College, 1957.

170. Kohler L, Stigmar G. Vision screening of four-year-old children. Acta Paediatr Scand 1973;62:17.

171. Kozaki M, Iwai H, Mikami C. Vision screening of three year old children. Jpn J Ophthalmol 1973;17:60.

172. Leverett HM. A school vision health study in Danbury, Connecticut. Am J. Ophthalmol 1955;39:527.

173. Lewis RC, Marsh-Tootle WL. The reliability of interpretation of photoscreening results with the MTI PS-100 in Head Start preschool children. J Am Optom Assoc 1995;66(7):429.

174. Lieberman S, Cohen AH, Stolzberg M, Ritty JM. Validation study of the New York Optometric Association (NYSOA) screening battery. Am J Optom Physiol Opt 1985;62(3):165.

175. Lin-Fu JS. Vision Screening of Children. Washington, DC: U.S. Maternal and Child Health Service, 1971.

176. Lippmann O. Vision screening of young children. Am J Public Health 1971;61:1586.

177. LoCascio GP. Preschool-age vision screening. Am J Optom Arch Am Acad Optom 1971;48:1044.

178. Marcinak JF, Werntz Yount SC. Evaluation of vision screening practices of Illinois pediatricians. Clin Pediatr 1995;34(7):353–357.

179. Macpherson H, Braunstein J, La Roche GR. Utilizing basic screening principles in the design and evaluation of vision screening programs. Am Orthoptic J 1991;41:110–121.

180. Moran CT. Preschool vision screening in Louisville. Sight Sav Rev 1958;28:92.

181. Morgan AL, Crawford JS, Pashby TJ, Gaby JR. A survey of methods used to reveal eye defects in school children. Can Med Assoc J 1952;67(1):29.

182. Nordlow W, Joachimsson S. A screening test for visual acuity in four-year-old children. Acta Ophthalmol 1962;40:453.

183. O'Shea JB. Optometric visual survey in schools of four Massachusetts towns. J Am Optom Assoc 1946;17:253.

184. Patz A, Hoover RE. Protection of Vision in Children. Springfield, IL: Thomas, 1969;3.

185. Peduti-Cuhna TA, Caldeira JAF. Stereopsis testing in preschool vision screening programs. Binoc Vis Q 1990; 5(2):65.

186. Peters HB. Vision Screening. In MJ Hirsch, RE Wick (eds), Vision of Children. Philadelphia: Chilton, 1969.

187. Pugmire GE, Sheridan MD. Revised vision screening chart for very young or retarded children. Med Officer 1957;98:53.

188. Reinecke RD. Screening 3 year olds for visual problems. Arch Ophthalmol 1986;104:33.

189. Reinecke R, Simons K. A new stereoscopic test for amblyopia screening. Am J Ophthalmol 1974;78:714.

190. Reinecke R. Current concepts in ophthalmology—strabismus N Engl J Med 1979;300:1139.

191. Russell EL, Kada JM, Hufhines DM. Orange County vision screening project. II. Ophthalmological evaluation. Sight Sav Rec 1961;31:215.

192. Ruttum MS. Visual screening with random dot stereograms. Semin Ophthalmol 1988;3(3):175.

193. Ruttum MS, Bence SM, Alcorn D. Stereopsis testing in preschool vision screening programs. J Pediatr Ophthalmol Strabismus 1986;23(6):298.

194. Savitz RA, Reed RB, Valadian I. Testability of preschool children for vision screening. J Pediatr Ophthalmol 1964;1:15.

195. Savitz RA, Reed RB, Valadian I. Vision Screening of the Preschool Child: Report of a Study. Washington, DC: U.S. Department of Health, Education and Welfare, Welfare Administration, Children's Bureau, 1964.

196. Schmidt P. Effectiveness of vision screening in preschool populations with preferential-looking cards used for assessment of visual acuity. Optom Vis Sci 1991;68(3):210.

197. Schmidt PP. Effectiveness of vision-screening with the modified clinical technique when preferential-looking cards are used to measure visual acuity. Am J Optom Physiol Opt 1986;63(10):108.

198. Schmidt PP, Hammond RD. School vision-screening using a random dot stereogram. Invest Ophthalmol Vis Sci 1985;26(3):309.

199. Shaffer TE. Study of vision testing procedure. Am J Public Health 1948;38:1141.

200. Simons K. A glasses-free random element stereogram test for preschool and infant vision screening. Invest Ophthalmol Vis Sci 1988;29:10.

201. Simons K. Stereoacuity norms in young children. Arch Ophthalmol 1981;99:439–45.

202. Simons K, Reinecke RD. A new stereoscopic test for amblyopia screening. Am J Ophthalmol 1974;78(4):707.

203. Simons K, Reinecke R. Amblyopia Screening and Stereopsis. In E Helveston (ed), Symposium on Strabismus: Transactions of the New Orleans Academy of Ophthalmology. St. Louis: Mosby, 1978;15.

204. Simons K, Reinecke R. A reconsideration of amblyopia screening and stereopsis. Am J Ophthalmol 1974; 78:707.

205. Sloane AE, Gallagher JR. A comparison of vision screening tests with clinical examination results. Am J Ophthalmol 1952;35(6):819.

206. Sloane AE, Gallagher RJ. A vision test for pediatrician's use. J Pediatr 1946;28:140.

207. Sloane AE, Rosenthal P. School vision testing. Arch Ophthalmol 1960;64:763.

208. Stump NF. Report on Webster study—the modified Ortho-Rater compared with the Massachusetts vision tests [unpublished report]. Rochester, NY: Bausch and Lomb Optical Co., 1955.

209. Sulzman JH, Davis CJ. The New York school vision tester. N Y State J Med 1958;58:833.

210. Trotter RR, Phillips RM, Shaffer K. Measurement of visual acuity of preschool children by their parents. Sight Sav Rev 1966;36:80.

211. Vellayappan K. Visual acuity in pre-school children. J Singapore Paediatr Soc 1979;21:70.

212. Yasuna ER, Green LR. An evaluation of the Massachusetts vision test for visual screening of school children. Am J Ophthalmol 1952;35(2):235.

213. Schmidt PP. Sensitivity of RDE stereoacuity and Snellen acuity to optical blur. Optom Vis Sci 1994; 71(7):466.

214. Schmidt PP, White RF. Comparisons of stereoacuity in children with and without refractive amblyopia. Invest Ophthalmol Vis Sci 1995;36(4)Suppl:45.

215. National Research Council Committee on Vision. Recommended standard procedures for the clinical measurement and specification of visual acuity 1979. Adv Ophthalmol 1980;41:103.

216. Ciner EB, Schanel-Klitsch E, Herzberg C. Stereoacuity development: 6 months to 5 years. A new tool for testing and screening. Optom Vis Sci 1996;73(1):43–48.

217. Ciner EB, Scheiman MM, Schanel-Klitsch E. Stereopsis testing in 18- to 35-month-old children using operant preferential looking. Optom Vis Sci 1989;66: 782–787.

218. Ciner EB, Schanel-Klitsch E, Schuman M. Stereoacuity development in young children. Optom Vis Sci 1991;68:533.

219. Schanel-Klitsch E, Ciner EB, Schuman M. Stereopsis assessment in young children: a comparison of three tests. Binoc Vis Q 1996;11(2):125.

220. Friendly DS, Jaafar MS, Morillo DL. A comparative study of grating and recognition visual acuity testing in children with anisometropia amblyopia without strabismus. Am J Ophthalmol 1990;110(3):293.

221. Schmidt P. Allen figure and broken wheel acuity measurement in preschool children. J Am Optom Assoc 1992;63(2):124.

222. Schmidt PP. Comparisons of testability of preliterate visual acuity tests in preschool children. Binoc Vis Q 1991;6(1):37.

223. Wood ICJ, Hodi S. Comparison of the techniques of video refraction and static retinoscopy in the measurement of refractive error in infants. Ophthal Physiol Opt 1994; 14(1):20.

224. Olver JM. Simple retinoscopic screening. Eye 1988;2:309.

225. Atkinson J. Infant Vision Screening: Prediction and Prevention of Strabismus and Amblyopia from Refractive Screening in the Cambridge Photorefraction Programme. In K Simons, DL Guyton (eds), Handbook of Infant Vision: Laboratory and Clinical Research. Oxford: Oxford University Press, 1993;335–348.

226. Preslan MW, Simmerman E. Photorefraction screening in premature infants. Ophthalmology 1993;100:762–68.

227. Duckman R. Using Photorefraction to Evaluate Refractive Error, Ocular Alignment, and Accommodation in Infants, Toddlers, and Multiply Handicapped Children. In M Mitchell, M Scheiman (eds), Problems in Optometry: Pediatric Optometry. Philadelphia: Lippincott, 1990;333–53.

228. Abramov I, Hainline L, Duckman RH. Screening infant vision with paraxial photorefraction. Optom Vis Sci 1990;67:538–45.

229. Wanger P, Waern G. Instant photographic refractometry in children. Acta Ophthalmol 1988;66:165–69.

230. Hoyt CS. Photorefraction [editorial]. Arch Ophthalmol 1987;105:1497–8.

231. Day SH, Norcia AM. Photographic detection of amblyogenic factors. Ophthalmology 1986;93:25–28.

232. Kirn T. Medical news and perspectives. JAMA 1987;257(8):1026.

233. Bobier WR, Braddick OJ. Eccentric photorefraction: optical analysis and empirical measures. Am J Optom Physiol Opt 1985;62(9):614–20.

234. Howland HC. Optics of photoretinscopy: results from ray tracing. Am J Optom Physiol Opt 1985;62(9):621–25.

235. Howland HC, Braddick O, Atkinson J, Howland B. Optics of photorefraction: orthogonal and isotropic methods. J Opt Soc Am 1983;73:1701–8.

236. Howland HC, Sayles N. Photorefractive studies of normal and handicapped infants and children. Behav Brain Res 1983;10:81–85.

237. Braddick O, Atkinson J, French J, Howland HC. A photorefractive study of infant accommodation. Vision Res 1979;19:1319–30.

238. Howland HC, Howland B. Optics of photorefraction. J Opt Soc Am 1974;64:240–49.

238. Kennedy RA, Sheps S. A comparison of photoscreening techniques for amblyogenic factors in children. Can J Ophthalmol 1989;24(6):259–64.

240. Smellie TJ, Tovey J, Deutsch J. Photorefraction—A Comparative Study. In G Tillson (ed), Trans VIIth Int Orthoptic Congress. Nürnberg, Germany: Fahner Verlag, 1991;232–36.

241. Angi MR, Bergamo L, Bisantis C. The binocular videorefractoscope for visual screening in infancy. J Ophthalmol [Germany] 1993;2:182–188.

242. Nawratzki I, Oliver M, Neumann E. Screening for amblyopia in children under three years of age in Israel. Isr J Med Sci 1972;8:1469.

243. Theodore FH, Johnson RM, Miles NE, et al. Causes of impaired vision in recently inducted soldiers. Arch Ophthalmol 1946;31:399.

244. Helveston EM. The incidence of amblyopia ex anopsia in young adult males in Minnesota in 1962–1963. Am J Ophthalmol 1965;60:75.

245. Cole RBW. The problems of unilateral amblyopia: a preliminary study of 10,000 national health patients. Br Med J 1959;1:202.

246. Cholst MR, Cohen LJ, Losty MA. Evaluation of amblyopia problems in the child. N Y J Med 1962; 62:3927.

247. Thompson JR, Woodruff G, Hiscox FA, et al. The incidence and prevalence of amblyopia detected in childhood. Br J Ophthalmol 1991;105:455.

248. Vinding T, Gregersen E, Jensen A, et al. Prevalence of amblyopia in old people without previous screening and treatment. An evaluation of the present prophylactic procedures among children in Denmark. Acta Ophthalmol (Copenh) 1991;69:796.

249. Flom MC, Neumaier RW. Prevalence of amblyopia. Public Health Rep 1966;81:329.

Chapter 11
Pediatric Ocular Pharmacology

Bruce D. Moore

This chapter discusses some of the significant differences in the use of diagnostic and therapeutic pharmacologic agents between children and adults. It is clinically oriented to the young child. A much more thorough treatise on general ocular pharmacology may be found in Bartlett and Jaanus' *Clinical Ocular Pharmacology*, third edition, to which the reader is directed.

Particular care must be exercised in the use of pharmacologic agents in young children because of the increased risk of potentially catastrophic adverse reactions due to their small size and their immature mechanisms for drug excretion and biotransformation.

DRUG EXCRETION AND BIOTRANSFORMATION

Drug excretion and biotransformation differ in young children from adults, particularly for neonates. It is essential to consider these differences when using and prescribing drugs in the pediatric population to reduce the risk of adverse drug effects.

The kidneys are the major site of drug excretion from the body. The renal glomerular filtration rate does not reach full function until approximately 1 year of age, although there is considerable variability. Renal tubular secretion is reduced during the neonatal period but is usually well developed by 6 months of age. Young children with medical problems may exhibit impairment of drug excretion through the kidneys. This is especially true in children that are dehydrated. The decreased rate of excretion increases the period of bioavailability of the drug, potentially exaggerating the effects of the drug and increasing the risk of toxicity. Drugs that are excreted primarily through the kidneys must be given in lower dosages and less frequently in neonates than adults to reduce these toxicity risks.

The primary organ responsible for drug metabolism (especially of lipid-soluble drugs) is the liver, through its microsomal enzyme system. The activity of the microsomal enzyme system is reduced in normal neonates and further reduced in premature infants and those with medical problems affecting the liver. The microsomal enzyme system reaches adult levels of function by about 1 year of age. The nonmicrosomal enzyme system, although involved in the biotransformation of fewer drugs than the microsomal enzyme system, is important for certain drugs (particularly aspirin and sulfa drugs). This system is also immature in young children.

Plasma protein binding of drugs within the serum is important both in the distribution of the drugs throughout the body and in their bioavailability. Infants have significantly reduced plasma protein binding compared with adults, which affects the distribution and activity of certain drugs, in particular aspirin, phenytoin (Dilantin), and phenobarbital. The fluid composition relative to total body mass of young children is greater than in adults, necessitating somewhat higher dosages for certain drugs than would be estimated from a simple ratio of adult body weight. An additional factor that is important in arriving at the proper dosage of certain drugs is the decreased effectiveness of the blood-brain barrier in young children. This may lead to increased drug effect on the central nervous system.

DETERMINING PEDIATRIC DRUG DOSAGE

Several formulas have been developed to derive the proper pediatric dosage of pharmaceutical agents from those used for adults. All have inherent inaccuracies and should be used cautiously. Young's rule is based on the child's age. Since there are such wide differences in a child's size at any given age, this rule is clinically useless. Clark's rule is based on the child's weight but may be inaccurate because it does not take into account a child's proportionally higher fluid weight than that in adults, which is of great importance in determining the actual clinical effectiveness of a drug. Augsberger's rule is similar but has been modified to be more accurate for infants. Somewhat more accurate is a determination of pediatric dosage that is based on a child's surface area. This is arrived at by looking up in a table the approximate relationship between the child's weight and the child's surface area as a percentage of adult values. This may be the most clinically useful method arrived at by formula for determining the correct pediatric dosage but still may have clinical limitations that could be problematic for certain patients.

By far the safest approach to pediatric drug dosage is to follow the recommendations that the manufacturers have arrived at as part of the U.S. Food and Drug Administration (FDA) clinical evaluations for each individual drug. These recommended dosages are generally conservative and minimize the potential for adverse drug effects. Many drugs, however, have not been evaluated specifically for pediatric use and consequently there will not be any recommendations for pediatric dosages. Optometrists should generally not use or prescribe any pharmaceutical agent that has not been FDA-approved for pediatric use unless there are very specific reasons to do so. One example of this would be the pediatric use of beta-blockers for the treatment of glaucoma. None of this class of agents is currently approved for pediatric usage, although they are routinely used in this population.

ADMINISTRATION

The two main routes of drug administration by optometrists are topical and oral. Topical vehicles are divided into ointments and liquids (which include drops, suspensions, and solutions). There are advantages and disadvantages of each vehicle. Drops (including the other liquid vehicles) are often easier to instill than ointments (at least in cooperative children), are less messy, and have only a minimal and transitory effect on vision after instillation. Drops have a somewhat greater potential of systemic absorption via the nasolacrimal duct if the punctum is not blocked, and therefore possess an increased risk of systemic toxicity. Drops also have a minimal contact time with the cornea before the drug is effectively diluted and then removed by tearing. This is obviously hastened by the child's crying. The effect of this minimal contact time is to reduce the absorption into and through the cornea, reducing the drug's efficacy. In addition, there may be uncertainty whether the drop actually gets into the eye of a struggling, hysterical child.

A case has been made to use an atomized spray of cycloplegic or mydriatic agents applied to the area around closed eyelids, in lieu of eyedrops, on young children to prevent upsetting the child. This may prove useful in some children, but it is difficult to be certain that an adequate dosage of the drug reaches the eye and accomplishes the intended purpose. There may also be some potential for increased absorption of the drug directly into the respiratory tract through inhalation of the atomized mist. Personal experience strongly suggests that standard instillation of ocular pharmaceutical agents via drops applied directly through the open eyelids is effective and possible in all but the rarest child and does not cause significant behavioral problems that make completion of the examination difficult or impossible.

Ointments may have reduced potential of systemic toxicity because they pass through the nasolacrimal duct more slowly than do drops. It is important to note that they have a longer contact time on the cornea, thus ensuring that more of the drug arrives at the desired location. Ointments therefore may have improved pharmacologic effect than drops, particularly in the case of antibiotics and steroids required to penetrate the cornea and reach the anterior chamber. It is also more apparent that an ointment has gotten onto the eye than a drop. Potential disadvantages of ointments are transiently blurred vision, increased potential of contact dermatitis, and a question (largely put to rest today) of retardation of corneal epithelial healing. In general, ointments are preferred for therapeutic purposes in young children, when that option is available.

There are two categories of oral pharmacologic agents: liquid, in the form of suspensions and solutions, and solid, in pill, capsule, or tablet form. Solids are usually more difficult for children to swallow than liquids and hence not the first choice when liquids are available. Commonly used oral agents that are prescribed by optometrists include antihistamines, decongestants, and antibiotics.

DIAGNOSTIC AGENTS

By far the most commonly used ocular pharmacologic agents by optometrists are diagnostic drugs for the purpose of dilation, cycloplegia, and tonometry. Although optometrists are generally familiar with the use of pharmaceutical agents in the adult population, many are less experienced with their use in the pediatric population. An overview of their clinical use is therefore presented here.

Anesthetics

There are several indications for the use of anesthetic agents in children. Although routine applanation tonometry measurements are not as necessary for children as for adults, they are advisable when possible. The technique of applanation tonometry in older children is identical to that of adults. The technique is different in younger or less cooperative children and is not generally necessary unless there is a suspicion of glaucoma or the child requires topical steroids for an extended period of time. In these younger patients, a hand-held applanation or air-puff tonometer is used instead of the slit-lamp mounted applanation tonometer. A drop of a combination anesthetic and fluorescein agent is instilled in the eye before applanation. The anesthetic is usually 0.4% benoxinate or 0.5% proparacaine. There is an increased risk of a corneal abrasion in these younger patients because it is less likely that the child will maintain steady gaze and will sit still during the procedure. It is wise to check for abrasions with a cobalt blue filter on the slit-lamp or with a hand-held ultraviolet light after completing the technique. If there is a deep abrasion, patching and prophylactic antibiotics may be indicated.

An additional indication for the use of an anesthetic is to reduce ocular irritation before instillation of ocular diagnostic agents, such as mydriatics and cycloplegics. The discomfort from the second and later drops is reduced after anesthetic instillation, but the initial discomfort from the anesthetic itself remains a problem for many children. This discomfort from the initial anesthetic drop may cause behavioral difficulty with instillation of the mydriatic or cycloplegic agents themselves. An important effect of anesthetic use is to disrupt the corneal surface, increasing absorption of any subsequent drops and potentiating their effects. In addition, if the child rubs an anesthetized eye, there is a risk of abrading the already "softened-up" cornea.

The routine use of an anesthetic agent before instillation of other diagnostic agents varies from practitioner to practitioner. Some do not think that its use significantly lessens the physical or emotional trauma of eyedrop instillation and that there is increased potential for adverse effects. Children who become upset at the use of eyedrops will become upset with or without an anesthetic. If the child does become upset from use of the drop, he or she will invariably become calm within minutes. Other practitioners prefer to use anesthetics in the belief that it lessens the trauma of cycloplegia by reducing the level and duration of stinging from the other drops. It would seem that the use of anesthetics for this purpose is a decision best left to the experience of the practitioner.

Dilating Agents

Dilating agents aid in the examination of the anterior and posterior segments of the eye. Dilation is particularly important in young children because they will not tolerate the length of the typical ophthalmoscopic or slit-lamp examination performed on adults. The examiner must be able to obtain a satisfactory view as quickly as possible. Dilation is essential in order to rule out serious pathologic entities in patients with strabismus and amblyopia.

There are several clinically useful dilating agents. Phenylephrine hydrochloride is the only useful, direct-acting adrenergic agonist (also sometimes categorized as a sympathomimetic agent). Hydroxyamphetamine is an indirect-acting adrenergic agonist that was unavailable until recently, and has become a very useful dilating agent when used in conjunction with tropicamide.

Phenylephrine is a widely used drug, particularly in adults. Phenylephrine provides rapid dilation without any cycloplegic effect. It has a relatively short period of action, except in patients with light irides. Its use in children, especially young children, must proceed with caution because of the potential for cardiovascular side effects. There have been documented cases of rapid and dangerous increases in heart rate and blood pressure in premature infants, and even in adults with higher dosages. Pediatric use should be restricted to no more than 2 drops of the 2½% concentration spaced 5 minutes apart. Never use the 10% concentration. Use in children younger than 3 years of age and in children with a history of cardiovascular problems should be restricted. Phenylephrine may be used with appropriate cycloplegic agents when both cycloplegia and maximum dilation is required. There is a somewhat greater risk of potentially adverse reaction with phenylephrine than with the cycloplegic agents.

Although tropicamide is technically a cycloplegic agent (a cholinergic antagonist), its cycloplegic effect is weak and unpredictable, and best thought of as a useful dilating agent. It is the safest dilating agent available. The dosage is 1 drop of 0.5% or 1% tropicamide repeated 5 minutes later. It performs well as a short-acting and short-duration mydriatic agent in patients with light irides, and is a very effective dilating agent for binocular indirect ophthalmoscopy in patients with darker irides when used in conjunction with hydroxyamphetamine hydrobromide (Paredrine) in the combination hydroxyamphetamine hydrobromide/tropicamide ophthalmic solution (Paremyd).

Paremyd is a combination of 0.25% tropicamide and 1% hydroxyamphetamine hydrobromide. The reduced dosage of tropicamide causes minimal cycloplegia, except on those with the lightest irides.

Hydroxyamphetamine causes the release of norepinephrine from receptor sites of the adrenergic system. The onset is rapid, with good mydriasis reached within 30 minutes, and the duration is relatively short, generally less than 2–4 hours. Surprisingly, it usually provides excellent mydriasis even on patients with dark irides. It has become a dilating agent of choice for many practitioners. If it proves ineffective for maximum dilation, 2½% phenylephrine hydrochloride (Neo-Synephrine) and a stronger cholinergic antagonist, such as cyclopentolate hydrochloride (Cyclogyl) or even atropine, may be considered on subsequent examination.

Dapiprazole hydrochloride (Rev-Eyes), an alpha adrenergic blocking agent, is used to reverse mydriasis produced by phenylephrine on adult patients. There have been reports of its efficacy in reversing mydriasis from both tropicamide and hydroxyamphetamine. Dapiprazole is not currently approved for use in children. Furthermore, there is little plausible rationale for reversing mydriasis in children, even if the drug was approved for use in this population.

Cycloplegic Agents

The mode of action of cycloplegic agents (cholinergic antagonists) is to block the neurotransmitter acetylcholine at receptor sites of the ciliary body and iris. Cholinergic antagonists are used primarily for the purpose of cycloplegic refraction. This is a fundamental procedure in the diagnostic workup of a child with strabismus, amblyopia, or significant refractive error. Although noncycloplegic refraction techniques are useful and acceptable in older patients, cycloplegic refraction and binocular indirect ophthalmoscopy is essential in ruling out the presence of potentially serious ocular abnormalities in younger patients.

Two agents (cholinergic antagonists) are largely of historical interest for the purpose of cycloplegic refraction [1]. Scopolamine has properties that are similar to atropine but is somewhat less predictable and less effective in action. It is still used in the treatment of uveitis but is not generally used for cycloplegic refraction, since it has no advantage over atropine when a strong agent is required. Similarly, homatropine resembles cyclopentolate but is less predictable and possibly has greater risk of adverse effects. Both scopolamine and homatropine have little to recommend their use in lieu of atropine and cyclopentolate, respectively.

Although tropicamide is less predictable than atropine or cyclopentalate, it rarely causes adverse effects, making its use acceptable under certain circumstances. It should not be used in the presence of amblyopia, strabismus, or hyperopia, because of its relative weakness as a cycloplegic agent. In addition, when it is used, the limited window of effectiveness, maximum at 30 minutes, must be considered.

Atropine is the strongest cycloplegic agent with the longest and most predictable action. It is not the best agent to use routinely because its duration of action is longer than clinically required, lasting up to 2 weeks in some patients. It is best to restrict its use to those patients that are inadequately cycloplegic with cyclopentolate due to darkly pigmented irides, those patients with high hyperopia or accommodative esotropia, and those few patients in whom the use of an in-office drop will preclude by their behavior an adequate examination after instillation. When used, the ointment form is preferred to minimize systemic absorption through the nasolacrimal duct and reduce the risk of adverse reactions. The 0.5% or 1% atropine ointment is used once or twice a day for the 3 days before the examination, to be instilled by the parents at home. No medication is used on the day of the examination to prevent the ointment from affecting the clarity of the retinoscopic reflex. Parents must be both clearly warned and given a written instruction sheet describing the potential adverse reactions from atropine. Clinically, this is usually restricted to mild fever and irritability, but potentially could be more dramatic. If reactions occur, parents are instructed to call immediately. These more serious problems are certainly of concern but actually happen only rarely.

The cycloplegic drug of choice for in-office use is cyclopentolate. This is a rapidly acting agent with a duration of action that is usually on the order of 6–12 hours, but longer in patients with light irides or increased sensitivity to the drug. Although somewhat less complete in action than atropine, it is effective enough for most patients. There may be slightly more residual accommodation remaining than with atropine. Clinically, 1 drop of the 1% solution is repeated after about 5 minutes by a second drop. A third drop may be administered at least 45 minutes

later in older patients that are not adequately cycloplegic but should not be added in younger children. The 2% drop has a much higher incidence of adverse effects and should not be used. It is important to note that the degree of mydriasis does not necessarily correlate with the degree of cycloplegia (this is true for all cycloplegics). The eyes may therefore be well dilated but poorly cycloplegic, or vice versa. The degree of cycloplegia is best checked by assessing the consistency of appearance of the retinoscopic reflex, and not the degree of pupillary dilation.

The most common adverse effect of cycloplegic agents is what is described as a "transient psychotic episode," where the child exhibits bizarre behavior and hyperactivity for a short time. This is self-limited and not a cause for inordinate concern, as it leaves no significant long-term effects, but is certainly quite dramatic for the parents and the optometrist. Antidotes are not required. More commonly, patients may exhibit fever and irritability, particularly in younger and smaller children. The best way to minimize any of these adverse effects is to carefully block the punctum when instilling the drops to minimize systemic absorption through the nasolacrimal duct, and to never use more than 2 drops of 1% solution. Certain categories of patients may exhibit increased sensitivity to anticholinergic agents. Included are children with a variety of neurologic disorders, those with Down syndrome (trisomy 21), and those that are lightly pigmented. For a thorough review of ocular drug toxicity in children, please see the chapter by Apt and Gaffney in *Duane's Foundation of Clinical Ophthalmology* [2].

Cyclopentolate used alone provides both effective cycloplegia and mydriasis for most patients. It can be used concurrently with phenylephrine or Paremyd when maximum dilation in patients with very dark irides is required for binocular indirect ophthalmoscopy of slit-lamp examination. The effect of cycloplegia that is so disturbing to adult patients is generally not much of an issue with children. It is worth mentioning to the parents that the child will be somewhat blurred for the rest of the day at near, and that reading and homework may be impossible.

THERAPEUTIC AGENTS

This section on therapeutic ocular pharmaceutical agents discusses only those areas in which there are significant differences in ophthalmic drug use between adults and children. For the most part, there is close similarity in the use of antimicrobials and anti-inflammatory agents in children and adults. Dosages must be carefully considered, as the potential for adverse effects in children is greater than with adults. Ointments are preferable to solutions because they allow for a longer contact time on the cornea, thus guaranteeing a greater concentration of the drug actually getting to the intended ocular structure. Since many anti-inflammatory agents are not available in ointment form, the specific choice of agents may be restricted. Dexamethasone is available as an ointment and is therefore a good choice as a steroid agent for young children. There are wider choices with antibiotics. Both bacitracin and erythromycin are available only in ointment form, although other excellent agents are available only in drop form. Trimethoprim sulfate and polymyxin B sulfate (Polytrim) is widely considered to be an excellent first-line, antibacterial agent for use in children due to its broad spectrum and rare adverse effects. If culture and sensitivity reports indicate the choice of an agent that is not available in ointment form, the use of that drop is clearly warranted.

The pharmacologic treatment of glaucoma is quite different in children than adults. With few exceptions, the treatment of congenital and early-onset glaucoma requires surgical intervention, usually at an early stage [3]. Open-angle glaucoma in adults is almost always initially treated medically. The reason for these different treatment modalities lies in the difference in etiologic factors of the glaucomas. Early childhood glaucoma is generally caused by anatomic abnormalities in the structure of the angle that are not treatable by medication. Various filtering procedures or cryotherapy are often used along with the use of oral acetazolamide (Diamox) to decrease aqueous production. Acetazolamide is a useful and widely prescribed antiglaucoma agent in young children, and often used for an extended period of time. An important side effect of acetazolamide involves gastrointestinal upset, which in young children may lead to failure to thrive. This possibility must be monitored carefully. A topical form has recently become available that reduces some of these adverse effects.

Miotic agents, such as pilocarpine, and adrenergic agonists, such as epinephrine and dipivefrin, although useful in adults, are not used much in young children. The beta-blockers, in spite of the fact that they are not currently FDA-approved for use in children, are widely used [4]. Although there has been concern about the beta 2 effect in children with asthma, both timolol (both beta 1 and 2) and betaxolol (beta 1 only) are used in children with glaucoma, particularly in older children, where the concerns are not as great. It must be stated again that the more definitive treatment for many pediatric patients with glaucoma is surgical, and not medical.

PHARMACOLOGIC TREATMENT OF STRABISMUS

Anticholinergics or Cholinergic Antagonists

Ocular anticholinergic agents are occasionally used in the treatment of accommodative esotropia by nature of its cycloplegic effects. Their actions mimic the use of maximum plus-power spectacle lenses by paralyzing accommodation and convergence. Theoretically, atropine could be used by itself without refractive correction to reduce or eliminate accommodative esotropia in affected patients, but because of the significant optical blur caused by the cycloplegia, atropine is almost always used in conjunction with refractive correction [5].

A common usage of atropine in the treatment of strabismus or amblyopia is to "encourage" the hyperopic child to accept the wearing of high plus-power spectacle lenses. When high-plus spectacles are first dispensed, the child initially may have difficulty in relaxing his or her level of habitual accommodation, and the child's vision will be blurred. The child may then reject the use of the correction. To facilitate acceptance of the spectacles, atropine may be used for a period of several weeks in both eyes to provide cycloplegia. The only way to obtain clear vision under cycloplegia in the moderate to high hyperopic patient will be through the use of spectacles. This technique can prove very effective in getting the child to accept the spectacles. After acceptance has been gained, the atropine is discontinued. The child will usually continue to wear the spectacles, even after the effects of the atropine have completely worn off.

It is important to keep in mind that in patients with significant degrees of hyperopia found under cycloplegia, more residual hyperopia is to be expected weeks or months later, after the child adapts to the spectacle correction and is re-refracted under cycloplegia. The refractive prescription may then need to be increased, especially if there is still some residual accommodative esotropia.

Another potential use of cycloplegic agents in the treatment of amblyopia is in the technique of penalization [6]. Atropine (or a shorter acting agent such as cyclopentolate) is instilled in the nonamblyopic eye to blur the acuity of that eye to a level below that of the amblyopic eye. Since the cycloplegia will prevent any accommodation, the eye will be blurred at one or more distances, depending on the underlying refractive error. If the patient is hyperopic in the nonamblyopic eye, the drug will blur near vision more than far and no correction may be required in the nonamblyopic eye. If the eye is myopic, there will be little if any effect beyond that present without the drug. Atropine penalization is useful only when the level of amblyopia is relatively mild. If the amblyopia is severe, there is usually little if any benefit, since the degree of blur brought about by the drug is invariably less than that present in the amblyopic eye. Spectacles are usually used in conjunction with the cycloplegic agent.

Cholinergic Agonists or Anticholinesterase Agents

There are two long-acting anticholinergic agents that are used in the treatment of accommodative esotropia, diisopropyl fluorophosphate (DFP) and echothiophate iodide (Phospholine Iodide [PI]). Their pharmacologic action increases the effectiveness of acetylcholine by inactivation of acetylcholinesterase, thereby stimulating accommodation and miosis, as well as increasing aqueous output.

The important effect of this class of drugs on patients with accommodative esotropia is to reduce the accommodative convergence/accommodation (AC/A) ratio. The reduction in accommodative effort results in a decrease in accommodative convergence, thereby reducing the esotropic deviation at near. There may also be a slight further effect caused by induced miosis increasing the depth of focus of the eye, thereby reducing the stimulus to accommodation, but this has not been confirmed [7].

Clinically, miotic agents may convert an accommodative esotropia into a phoria, allowing for restoration of binocularity. Most authorities stipulate that miotics should not be continued in the absence of some degree of binocularity. Miotics may be indicated in patients who will not tolerate wearing bifocal spectacles. Some authorities believe that miotics are preferable to spectacles, because the patients may become overly reliant on the glasses. This argument seems to ignore the possibility of adverse side effects from the drug itself, especially when used over a long period of time.

Patients that may potentially benefit from the use of miotics generally have high AC/A ratios and are usually hyperopic. The patient should be placed on a trial of the medication for about 2 weeks. If there is a significant decrease in the angle of deviation at near or especially if there is a restoration of binocularity, a continuation of the medical treatment is warranted if there are no adverse effects from the drug itself. If there is not a significant reduction in the angle of deviation, it is likely that the underlying cause of the esotropia is not accommodative, and miotics are contraindicated.

Because more severe miosis occurs with DFP, PI is usually the drug of choice. The starting dosage is generally 1 drop of 0.125% or 0.06% solution each evening before bedtime. If there is a good response to this dosage, the concentration and the frequency of use can be decreased to the lowest dosage that maintains adequate effect.

Miotics may cause the development of iris cysts. Phenylephrine hydrochloride drops are often used concurrently with the miotic as a preventive measure for these cysts. The usual dosage is 1 or 2 drops of 2.5% phenylephrine per day, although some authorities recommend that the pharmacist formulate a single solution combining both the PI and phenylephrine. Any patient that is on miotic therapy must be monitored frequently for the development of these iris cysts or other adverse side effects, as well as for the state of the strabismus and visual acuity.

Side Effects of Anticholinergic Agents

Anticholinergic agents are potent drugs with a host of potential side effects. As mentioned in the previous section, the formation of iris cysts has been associated with the prolonged use of both drugs, but perhaps somewhat more readily with DFP. These epithelial cysts are located at the inner margin of the pupil and can extend into the pupillary aperture, occasionally progressing to the point of occluding the pupil if miotic therapy is inadvertently continued long-term. Phenylephrine hydrochloride has been found to prevent, or at least minimize, this hypertrophy of the iris.

More worrisome is the effect that anticholinesterase drugs have on cholinesterase levels in red blood cells and in plasma. These agents decrease the rate of hydrolysis of succinylcholine, a drug used to facilitate general anesthesia. If a child who is on miotic therapy undergoes emergency surgery and the use of succinylcholine in the anesthesia, respiratory paralysis may ensue. Parents must be clearly made aware of this potential risk.

Systemic side effects in the form of excessive salivation, lacrimation, urination, defecation or diarrhea, and sweating (the acronym SLUDS) may be encountered, but they usually are not clinically significant in the absence of overdosage. Ocular effects include iris cysts and the theoretical possibility of retinal detachment and cataracts, which have not been reported in children. Photophobia, headache, and browache have been noted. A "miotic upper respiratory syndrome" consisting of rhinorrhea, a sensation of chest constriction, cough, and conjunctival injection has also been reported [8].

Botulinum Toxin

In the late 1970s, Dr. Alan Scott began investigating the pharmacologic treatment of strabismus [9, 10]. He experimented with the direct injection of various neurotoxins into the extraocular muscles. The theory being, that by causing a temporary paralysis of an extraocular muscle, a change in the alignment of the eye could be produced. This would be analogous to the acute esotropia that occurs in a sixth cranial nerve palsy. Botulinum toxin type A has proven to be useful as a substitute for, or as an adjunct to, strabismus surgery in many cases [9]. After a 10-year investigational period under FDA regulation, during which time more than 8,000 injections were given, the drug is now available for clinical use under the trade name Oculinum.

Botulinum toxin is a large protein molecule that, after intramuscular injection, is bound at the receptor sites on motor nerve terminals within 24 hours. The toxin remains at the nerve terminal for several days to weeks. Here it interferes with the release of the neurotransmitter acetylcholine. When injected in therapeutic doses, the effect remains localized to the injection region, which results in a denervation muscle paralysis with the onset 3–5 days after injection. The duration of total extraocular muscle paralysis can last from 2 to 8 weeks, with eventual recovery. The purpose of botulinum therapy in strabismus is to achieve lasting improvement through secondary effects of the toxin-induced paralysis. Toxin-induced paralysis lasting for several weeks can result in permanently changed ocular alignment as the injected muscle lengthens and its antagonist contracts.

For this to work, the antagonist must be a functioning muscle and not restricted due to scar formation. If the patient has the potential for binocular vision, the change in alignment produced by the toxin is more likely to be permanent.

Indications for treatment of strabismus with botulinum toxin include horizontal strabismus of less than 40 prism diopters. Botulinum toxin is also used for the treatment of postoperative residual strabismus. Injection can be combined with strabismus surgery when there is reluctance to operate on more than two extraocular muscles in the same eye to avoid anterior segment ischemia. One of the best indications for the use of botulinum toxin is for the treatment of esotropia resulting from sixth nerve palsy [11]. In these cases, the antagonist medial rectus muscle is injected in the eye with the palsy. This can balance the paralysis and straighten the eye to correct primary gaze diplopia and prevent secondary contracture of the medial rectus muscle. Future surgery may be obviated in such cases.

Relative contraindications to the use of botulinum toxin include large deviations of more than 40 diopters and restrictive strabismus as occurs in Duane's syndrome or in some postoperative cases.

Complications that have been reported with the use of botulinum toxin include scleral perforation, retrobulbar hemorrhage, and local conjunctival inflammation. The toxin can diffuse into adjacent muscles and produce an unwanted, vertical deviation. Transient ptosis lasting for a few weeks has been reported in as many as 16% of patients injected. No systemic illness has been produced after injection of the toxin [10]. Many patients report having diplopia during the first few weeks after the injection. This is usually short-lived as there is frequently a temporary overcorrection. This is desirable for fusion in many cases.

Although not considered a complication, patients must be warned that the effect of the toxin may not be permanent and that the strabismus may not be totally corrected. Some patients may then require additional injections or strabismus surgery.

Results in the injection of children have shown that 63% of those injected achieved a deviation of 10 prism diopters or less. Exotropia in children was the most common undercorrected strabismus category. A study of 72 children injected between the ages of 4 months and 13 years reported that 85% had 10 prism diopters or less of deviation at the time of the last examination [12]. In this study, complications included transient ptosis and hyperdeviations, which always resolved in 6 months and usually resolved several weeks following injection.

There is a great deal of interest in the treatment of congenital esotropia by injecting the medial rectus muscle in the first year of life [13]. These children often adopt a horizontal face turn following paralysis of the muscle with botulinum. This is evidence that some patients may have fusional potential. Such treatment has been associated with long-term stability of alignment in some patients.

REFERENCES

1. Moore BD. Cycloplegic refraction of young children. N E J Optometry 1988;41:10–15.
2. Apt L, Gaffney WL. Toxic Effects of Topical Eye Medication in Infants and Children. In W Tasman, EA Jaeger (eds), Duane's Foundation of Clinical Ophthalmology (Vol 1). Philadelphia: Lippincott, 1990;1–21.
3. DeLuise VP, Anderson DR. Primary infantile glaucoma (congenital glaucoma). Surv Ophthalmol 1983;28:1–19.
4. Boger WP, Walton DS. Timolol in uncontrolled childhood glaucoma surgery. Ophthalmology 1981;88:253–258.
5. Rethy I. Stabilized Accommodative Factors in Esotropia. In OM Ferrer (ed), Ocular Motility. Int Ophthalmol Clin 1971;11;27.
6. Rutstein R. Alternative treatment for amblyopia. Probl Optometry 1991;3:331–354.
7. Ripps H, Chin NB, Siegel IM, Breinin GM. The effect of pupil size on accommodative convergence, and the AC/A ratio. Invest Ophthalmol 1962;1:127–135.
8. Fraunfelder FT. Ocular Toxicology. In CA Weisbecker, FT Fraunfelder, AA Gold (eds), Physicians Desk Reference for Ophthalmology. Oradell, NJ: Medical Economics Co., 1997;17–20.
9. Scott AB. Botulinum toxin injection of eye muscles to correct strabismus. Trans Am Ophthalmol Soc 1981;79:734–770.
10. Scott AB. Botulinum toxin treatment of strabismus. Clin Modules Ophthalmologists 1989;7:1–11.
11. Wagner RS, Frohman LP. Long-term results: botulinum for sixth nerve palsy. J Pediatr Ophthalmol Strabismus 1989;26:106–108.
12. Magoon EH. Chemodenervation of strabismic children. Ophthalmology 1989;96:931–934.
13. Magoon EH. Botulinum toxin chemo-denervation for strabismus in infants and children. J Pediatr Ophthalmol Strabismus 1984;21:110–113.

Chapter 12

Diseases of the Orbit and Anterior Segment

Bruce D. Moore

Many abnormalities affecting the orbit and globe are readily apparent to the parent and clinician. Detecting the presence of these conditions is often easier than correctly diagnosing them. Because the early stages of orbital inflammation and proptosis are often occult, careful history and physical examination of the child are essential. Diagnostic imaging by x-ray, computed tomography (CT), or magnetic resonance imaging (MRI) are invaluable in discerning the problem. Several of the underlying causes of proptosis and orbital inflammation are potentially life threatening and require prompt diagnosis and treatment.

CONGENITAL ORBITAL ABNORMALITIES

Size Abnormalities

Both the orbits and globes are normally about equal in size and configuration. Many ocular and systemic conditions are associated with asymmetry in the size of the eyes, the orbits, or both (Table 12.1).

Clinical anophthalmia, the apparent absence of the eye, is a rare condition. The specific cause is variable, and patients are likely to have additional birth defects. Anophthalmia is an extreme manifestation of the more common condition of microphthalmia.

Microphthalmia occurs in about 1 in 2,000 births [1]. It may be unilateral or bilateral and varies widely in severity. Microphthalmia may be isolated or associated with other ocular and systemic conditions, including persistent hyperplastic primary vitreous, congenital cataracts, maternal rubella and toxoplasmosis, trisomy 13, colobomata, and high hyperopia. Developmental glaucoma is a late complication. The orbits and the optic foramina are usually reduced in size. The growth of the orbit is affected by the bulk of the orbital contents. Patients with severe microphthalmia or anophthalmia and blindness may benefit from fitting with an inert orbital expander after enucleation to stimulate orbital growth during subsequent development and improve cosmesis.

An enlarged globe (megalophthalmia) in a patient must be assumed to be due to congenital glaucoma until proven otherwise. The more likely causes of megalophthalmia are high myopia, Marfan's syndrome, or a hereditary familial pattern. Patients with megalocornea, which must be differentiated from megalophthalmia, may appear to have an enlarged globe, but it is only the cornea and not the globe that is enlarged. The appearance of an enlarged globe may actually be due to proptosis.

Craniofacial Abnormalities

Normal children obviously have a wide range of facial appearances. Dysmorphology is often difficult to determine. Facial abnormalities are even more difficult to distinguish in infancy, becoming less so

Table 12.1. Causes of Congenital
Orbital Abnormalities

Size abnormalities
   Anophthalmia
   Microphthalmia
   Megalophthalmia
Craniofacial abnormalities
   Crouzon's syndrome
   Apert's syndrome
   Plagiocephaly
   Hypertelorism
   Treacher Collins syndrome
   Goldenhar's syndrome
   Fetal alcohol syndrome
   Orbital dermoids

as the child matures and the physical appearance changes. Observing the general appearance of parents and siblings is helpful in arriving at the correct diagnosis.

In general, dysmorphic appearances that are of limited functional or cosmetic significance need little if any intervention. Malformations that are of functional or cosmetic concern require attention. A myriad of abnormalities of the facies may be seen by the clinician (see Table 12.1). The description of these conditions and the determination of the proper treatment required (if any) is complex and requires the help of clinicians from other specialties.

The craniosynostosis syndromes are among the more commonly encountered groups of craniofacial abnormalities. They are due to a premature closure of one or more cranial sutures, causing reduced skull growth perpendicular to the fused suture and increased growth parallel to the fused suture. As a result, the skull grows in an abnormal configuration. The sutures normally do not completely fuse until around late puberty, allowing for continued growth in the volume of the cranium and the brain. Restricted growth of the bony structures may cause neurologic problems and mental retardation, along with a host of ocular complications. The calvarium is the area of the brain that is most frequently affected.

Crouzon's syndrome is a craniosynostosis with marked midface hypoplasia and oxycephaly ("tower skull" or increased height of the skull in relation to its width or length) and brachycephaly (increased width of the head in comparison to its length). Affected individuals also exhibit a beaked-shaped nose, hypertelorism, shallow orbits, maxillary hypoplasia, and an abnormal inferiorly displaced position of the lateral palpebral ligaments, which results in an anti-mongoloid slant to the eyelids.

Patients with Apert's syndrome have a somewhat similar appearance to those with Crouzon's, with the addition of greater oxycephaly, greater incidence of cleft palate, and, of diagnostic importance, syndactyly of the hands and feet and fusion of the digits. Patients with Apert's and Crouzon's syndromes may present with a V-pattern exotropia due to harlequin-shaped, shallow orbits. Proptosis from the abnormal shape of the orbits is common, occasionally resulting in corneal exposure and corneal scarring. High refractive errors requiring optical correction and attention to amblyopia are common [2]. Fitting glasses to these patients may occasionally prove difficult or impossible, necessitating the use of contact lenses. The optic nerves may be involved, especially after surgical treatment of the facial abnormalities. Both Crouzon's and Apert's syndrome are autosomal dominantly inherited, with variable expressivity and what appears to be a relatively high rate of new mutations.

Plagiocephaly is a craniofacial abnormality caused by a unilateral fusion of a coronal suture [3]. Many of these patients have a form of strabismus that simulates a fourth cranial nerve paresis, but is actually due to an underaction of the superior oblique muscle caused by the abnormal configuration of the orbit [4]. These oculomotor abnormalities persist even after craniofacial surgery, and patients may require additional ophthalmic intervention for amblyopia and strabismus.

Hypertelorism, a greater than normal horizontal separation of the orbits, occurs in a number of conditions. An increase in the width of the ethmoid results in an increased interpupillary distance, sometimes as great as 80 mm. An exotropia is usually present due to the increased pupillary distance or to abnormalities in the shape of the orbits. This is similar to the exotropia seen in Apert's and Crouzon's syndromes, but occasionally an esotropia may be present.

Treacher Collins syndrome (mandibulofacial dysostosis) is a condition with a number of skeletal and facial abnormalities, including depressed cheek bones, small jaw, beaked nose, abnormally shaped ears, hearing loss, dental abnormalities, and cleft palate. The palpebral fissures slant downward (antimongoloid slant), producing a characteristic facial appearance. Also, medial eyelashes may be absent, and ectropion and a coloboma of the lower lid may occur. The condition is transmitted in an autosomal dominant pattern, with variable penetrance and expressivity.

Goldenhar's syndrome is also called hemifacial microsomia or first and second branchial arch syndrome. It is usually unilateral, but a small number of patients may show bilateral deformity. Goldenhar's syndrome results in a hypoplastic facial abnormality that affects the area of the cheek and jaw, along with prominent epibulbar dermoids and lipodermoids, small, low-set ears, inferior anomalous auricular tags, and vertebral skeletal abnormalities. An associated coloboma of the upper lid and, less commonly, strabismus and microphthalmia are also seen. The limbal dermoids may cause anisometropic astigmatism and amblyopia in a few patients.

The surgical treatment of choice in patients with craniofacial abnormalities is a series of complex and extensive midface procedures named after Paul Tessier [5], a French surgeon who first attempted treatment of these conditions. Ocular complications may result from the extensive surgical shifting of the facial bones [6], including residual strabismus (especially exotropia), optic nerve damage, ptosis, corneal exposure, and enophthalmos. The cosmetic improvement for the patient can range from minimal to dramatic, depending on individual factors.

Fetal Alcohol Syndrome and Substance Abuse

Fetal alcohol syndrome is a multisystem congenital disorder typically arising from heavy maternal consumption of alcohol [7]. Binge drinkers place their fetuses at highest risk. Some evidence has been found that alcohol in any amount may present a risk to the developing fetus [8]. The risk appears to decrease if drinking is stopped during the pregnancy. Fetal alcohol syndrome affects the infants of approximately 4.3% of mothers who drink heavily during pregnancy and occurs in 1 per 1,000 live births in the United States [9]. This is a rate four times higher than in Europe and appears to be related, at least in part, to socioeconomic sta-

tus. Alcohol is the specific teratogenic factor behind these abnormalities, but the actual mechanism by which they are produced is not yet known. Professional intervention in maternal behavior during pregnancy is the only way of reducing the risk to the infant.

The systemic manifestations include growth retardation; central nervous system disorders; developmental delay; mental retardation; and urogenital, cardiopulmonary, and skeletal abnormalities. The typical facial dysmorphology includes microcephaly, a flat maxilla, thin upper lip, and small palpebral apertures. Affected individuals exhibit marked variability in the extent of their abnormalities.

The ocular manifestations are also quite variable. They include ptosis, anterior chamber cleavage syndrome, reduced palpebral aperture, epicanthal folds, telecanthus, strabismus, optic nerve hypoplasia, cataracts, and high myopic and astigmatic refractive errors [10].

The recent, dramatic increase in the number of infants born to women who are addicted to crack cocaine has become a major medical and social problem. Many of these pregnant women receive little or no prenatal care, are poorly nourished, and face a myriad of medical and social problems. Affected infants have a high rate of prematurity and all of its attendant medical problems. The children have a high incidence of neurologic, developmental, and learning problems. Oculomotor and optic nerve abnormalities may be due to the fetal exposure to crack cocaine [11]. The incidence of retinopathy of prematurity is high among these children. Other abnormalities include high refractive error, strabismus, and amblyopia. The association of all forms of substance abuse to increased risk of neonatal human immunodeficiency virus infection has become all too obvious. It is impossible to pinpoint the specific cause of these birth and developmental abnormalities, since the pregnant women whose children are affected are frequently multisubstance abusers whose lifestyles increase the risk of many types of abnormalities in their offspring. Regardless of the etiologies, these children require careful neonatal evaluation, early and intensive social service support, and close monitoring during early childhood.

Nicotine has also been implicated as a significant risk factor in fetal abnormalities. The most sig-

Table 12.2. Congenital Eyelid Abnormalities

Abnormality	Description
Size or shape abnormalities	
Coloboma	Absence of a portion of the lid
Epiblepharon	Extra skin fold causing entropion
Entropion	Inward turning of the lid
Ectropion	Outward turning of the lid
Blepharophimosis	Small palpebral aperture
Telecanthus	Increased intercanthal distance
Epicanthus	Extra skin fold at inner canthus
Ptosis	Upper lid drooping
Vascular tumors	
Hemangioma	Endothelial proliferation
Port-wine stain	Finding associated with Sturge-Weber syndrome
Nevus flammeus	More benign condition not associated with Sturge-Weber syndrome

nificant effects appear to be reduced birth weight, an increased risk of prematurity, and fetal hypoxia, which increases the incidence of cerebral palsy. In the future, much more will be learned about the effects of maternal smoking.

Orbital Dermoids

Orbital dermoid cysts are the most common pediatric orbital tumor. Many orbital dermoids are not noted at birth, but become more apparent over the next 20–30 years as they grow in size or become inflamed due to various causes. Most orbital dermoids are located superiorly. They may cause proptosis, ptosis, and restriction of ocular motility that requires surgical excision.

EYELIDS

Many of the conditions affecting the eyelids will be immediately apparent to the parents or clinician. Congenital abnormalities are likely noted in the newborn nursery. Conditions affecting the maintenance of the tear film frequently cause red eyes and recurrent episodes of inflammation. Many of the less severe eyelid disorders need to be followed closely for signs of ocular inflammation, but most will require little if any treatment. Patients with

marked ptosis must be monitored for the possibility of deprivation amblyopia.

Vascular eyelid abnormalities that develop in the first few months of infancy, such as eyelid hemangiomas, will be alarming to parents and will generate a quick referral. These cases need to be managed by someone experienced with this disorder. Patients with nevus flammeus need referral to their pediatrician for evaluation for Sturge-Weber syndrome. Simple observation is most important in making the correct diagnosis for patients with eyelid abnormalities.

Congenital Abnormalities of Size and Shape

Many congenital abnormalities affect the size or shape of the eyelids (Table 12.2). Some are only of cosmetic importance, but others affect the function and health of the eye. Many of these abnormalities are associated with other congenital malformations. The appearance of any single abnormality should arouse suspicion of additional ocular and systemic problems, requiring a thorough internal and external ocular examination. An important consideration in any patient with eyelid problems is the effect on the maintenance of the tear film and corneal clarity.

Colobomas of the eyelids occur most frequently on the nasal aspect of the upper eyelids, and somewhat less commonly on the temporal side of the lower lid. The degree of involvement is quite variable, from a slight indentation of a small portion of one lid to complete absence of one or both lids. Only rarely are there multiple colobomas on the same eyelid. Patients may also have additional colobomas or structural abnormalities of the eyes or face. Surgery is preferred treatment of eyelid colobomas if either the cosmetic appearance of the patient or the proper maintenance of the tear film is compromised.

Epiblepharon appears as an extra horizontal fold of tissue across the lower eyelid. It may lead to an entropion or turning inward of the lashes in infants. Johnson [12] has noted that differentiation between epiblepharon and entropion is important because the treatment is different. The appearance of epiblepharon generally changes over the first years of life as the face and eyelids grow. The condition frequently resolves completely during childhood. It is found most often in

Asians and may be familial. Surgical treatment is required only if the epiblepharon causes problems in the corneal integrity.

Congenital entropion and ectropion rarely occur as isolated findings. When there is true entropion, the condition tends to worsen with age, whereas the opposite tends to be true in patients with epiblepharon. Associated problems of the lids or facies are common in patients with entropion. Ectropion may also be associated with trisomy 21 and blepharophimosis.

Patients with blepharophimosis have a horizontal and vertical narrowing of the palpebral aperture and an absence of the transverse fold of the upper lid. The medial canthus is shifted, and the nasal bridge is flattened. Ptosis, epicanthus, telecanthus, and hypertelorism may occur. Cosmetic surgery may be performed, especially if deprivation amblyopia is a threat or an anomalous head position is required for vision in severely affected patients. Telecanthus appears as an exaggerated intercanthal distance with an essentially normal interpupillary distance. It may be isolated or occur along with epicanthus and blepharophimosis.

Epicanthus appears as an extra fold of the eyelid at the medial aspect of the inner canthus at the semilunaris. One fairly common type of epicanthus may be associated with blepharophimosis, but most patients have a simple isolated form. Epicanthus is of considerable clinical importance because it is frequently the cause of pseudoesotropia, one of the more common conditions for which parents bring infants to the optometrist's office. In pseudoesotropia, the child appears to have esotropia, especially with the eyes in slight lateral gaze. Examination shows only epicanthal folds paralleling the bridge of the nose. This facial appearance almost always changes by 6–8 years of age as the face, and especially the bridge of the nose, grow. Treatment is not required, but actual strabismus must be carefully ruled out by repeat examination.

Congenital Ptosis

Congenital ptosis is a common abnormality that affects the position and function of the upper eyelid. It may be unilateral or bilateral, and can be isolated or associated with paresis of the superior rectus muscle, Marcus Gunn jaw-winking syndrome, epi-

canthus, or blepharophimosis. The heredity pattern may be autosomal dominant.

Visual acuity may be impaired in a few patients with severe ptosis if the pupillary axis is effectively blocked by the lid, leading to deprivation amblyopia in the affected eye(s). Individuals with marked ptosis may assume a position with the head thrust back in order to maintain binocularity. Many of these patients become adept at using the orbicularis muscle to elevate the lids. More commonly, the ptosis is less marked and only of cosmetic concern.

The typical form of congenital ptosis is due to dysplasia of the levator palpebrae muscle. The skin of the upper eyelid is smooth because it lacks the tarsal fold caused by the presence of the levator. Treatment, when required, is surgery. A commonly used procedure to treat ptosis uses autogenous fascia lata slings of one or both eyes.

Marcus Gunn jaw-winking syndrome is a type of congenital ptosis that is due to a miswiring of the nerves responsible for the muscle actions of the jaw and the eyelids. Either a retraction or relaxation of the eyelid via the levator muscle occurs when the jaw moves. This action is most readily observed when the child is sucking a bottle and tends to become less noticeable over time. Marcus Gunn jaw-winking syndrome is generally a unilateral condition with considerable variation in appearance among patients. It may produce a significant social problem requiring surgical intervention in some patients.

Eyelid Abnormalities Due to Vascular Tumors

Capillary Hemangioma

Capillary hemangiomas are vascular tumors that develop rapidly and dramatically soon after birth. They often cause cosmetic, structural, and functional problems for affected infants (see Chapter 14 for a more detailed discussion of hemangiomas).

Port-Wine Stains and Nevus Flammeus

The terms *port-wine stains* and *nevus flammeus* have been used interchangeably but are properly considered to be two different types of vascular malformations (see Table 12.2). The port-wine stain is a vascular lesion of the upper eyelid and adjacent facial regions that is often associated with Sturge-Weber syndrome [13]. The lesion is composed of masses of dilated capillaries within the skin and differs from hemangiomas in that it does not have any abnormal endothelial proliferation. It is a flat, purplish lesion (in contrast to eyelid hemangiomas, which are elevated) over the distribution of the trigeminal nerve, up to but not usually extending beyond the midline. Port-wine stains darken when the child cries. These lesions are of ocular importance because of their association with choroidal hemangiomas and glaucoma and the systemic effects of Sturge-Weber syndrome. Treatment includes the use of the argon laser to improve cosmesis. Surgery is not indicated for the skin lesions. All patients with port-wine stains must be monitored closely for the development of glaucoma and choroidal hemangiomas, which can cause hyperopic anisometropia and amblyopia.

Nevus flammeus is a term that should probably be restricted to a much more benign type of skin lesion that is very common in infants. These occur most often on the face and neck and do not necessarily follow the distribution of the trigeminal nerve. They often fade in the first few years of life, but may remain into the adult years. Treatment is generally not indicated.

LACRIMAL APPARATUS

Dry eyes of the type commonly seen in adults are rare in young children. Obviously, wet eyes and epiphora may indicate the presence of a nasolacrimal duct obstruction. Conservative treatment is generally preferred for most patients.

Alacrima

Alacrima is the rare absence or severe reduction of aqueous tear production. Neonates may not tear for several weeks after birth [14], but should exhibit at least some tear production by 1 month of age and normal tearing by 3 months of age. Alacrima may be due to a true absence or hypoplasia of the lacrimal gland, to neurologic abnormalities, or to a blockage of tear flow into the eye. It is usually bilateral, but may be unilateral.

The eyes of these patients look dry and have a reduced corneal light reflex. Photophobia, corneal staining and scarring, and bulbar and palpebral conjunctival injection are associated problems. Schirmer's or Jones' tests (instillation of fluorescein into the conjunctival sac and a cotton swab in the nose to catch the dye after it has traversed the nasolacrimal duct) will confirm a lack of tear production or drainage. Rose bengal staining may be evident.

Treatment is difficult and is directed at conserving whatever limited tear output is available. Any occlusion of the tear production and delivery systems (although very rare) requires surgical intervention to facilitate output. Various brands of artificial tears should be tried until the most effective is found. Ointments should be used at night and at other times if they are tolerated. Punctal occlusion, therapeutic and collagen contact lenses, swim goggles and other moisture barriers, and tarsorrhaphy may be considered when lubricants fail to prevent further corneal scarring and photophobia.

Alacrima is an important manifestation of the Riley-Day syndrome, a multisystem autosomal recessive disease. Patients have a reduced, but still present, tear production along with greatly diminished corneal sensitivity. This results in corneal scarring, ulceration, or perforation [15]. Patients may have a tonic pupil. Systemic manifestations include lability of blood pressure, skin blotching during emotional distress, and greatly reduced pain threshold. Affected children may exhibit hyperactivity and unusual behavior. The basic defect is unknown, but the decreased tearing seems to be due to abnormal parasympathetic innervation of the lacrimal gland. Ocular treatment can be very difficult due to the child's behavior and is directed at keeping the corneas moist and preventing corneal injury.

Other Causes of Dry Eyes

The form of keratitis sicca commonly found in adults is rare in otherwise healthy children. Tear production, particularly of the aqueous layer, tends to be high in most children. A few systemic and ocular conditions can adversely affect this, occasionally leading to corneal problems. Blepharitis and other external ocular inflammations can result in toxicity to the corneal surface. Patients with cystic fibrosis may have an abnormal mucoid secretion in their tears. This can cause heavy coating of contact lenses.

Patients who have been treated with radiation for leukemia and other neoplastic diseases frequently exhibit signs and symptoms of ocular surface drying. This is due to direct damage to the structures that produce the components of the tear film and to effects on the corneal epithelium. These patients often develop cataracts as a result of the radiation treatment, requiring use of aphakic contact lenses. The ability to successfully wear the contact lenses may be adversely affected by the decreased tear production and compromised corneal epithelium. Supplemental ocular lubrication may be required.

Nasolacrimal Duct Obstruction

This obstruction is a common, unilateral or bilateral blockage of the lacrimal drainage system, usually at the nasal end of the duct. Patients present with epiphora over one or both cheeks, a "wet" appearance to the eye, and a recurrent conjunctivitis. The blockage may be complete or partial and somewhat intermittent. The Jones' test will indicate an absence or significant decrease in tear outflow to the nose. Many full-term neonates do not have a patent duct, but patency develops in most infants within the first few weeks or months of life, thus spontaneously resolving the problem of epiphora and infection. Parents tend to be acutely sensitive to the presence of nasolacrimal duct obstruction and want immediate treatment. The best treatment, however, is to delay use of a probing procedure until at least 6–8 months of age [16]. Spontaneous resolution may be aided by daily massage of the duct between the lower punctum and the nose. Episodic use of antibiotic ointments to control purulent conjunctivitis may be necessary. Others have advocated early treatment [17]. Probing is usually performed under anesthesia to prevent the child from struggling and to minimize trauma to the area, but some surgeons feel comfortable performing the procedure in a sedated child in the office setting. Probing is successful in 90% of cases [18] and, if not successful initially, may be repeated as needed.

Dacryocystitis may be a complication of chronic nasolacrimal duct obstruction. The swelling and

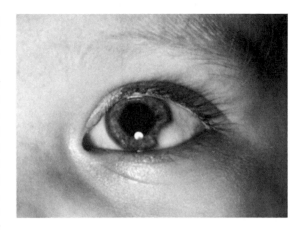

Figure 12.1. Typical limbal dermoid extending onto the cornea. A significant degree of irregular astigmatism is often associated with this type of dermoid. (Reprinted with permission from LJ Press, BD Moore. Clinical Pediatric Optometry. Boston: Butterworth–Heinemann, 1993;106.)

tenderness that develop inferonasally to the lower punctum may be extensive, requiring antibiotics and possibly drainage.

CORNEA AND CONJUNCTIVA

Infections of the cornea and conjunctiva are discussed in Chapter 14. Limbal dermoids are usually easy to diagnose because of their characteristic appearance and size (Figure 12.1). Unilateral abnormalities of corneal diameter are also easily seen, but mild bilateral size inequalities may be less obvious. These patients must have a full ocular evaluation to rule out other potentially serious problems, such as glaucoma and cataracts.

Corneal opacities, both congenital and acquired, are among the most difficult of all pediatric eye disorders to accurately diagnose. Careful biomicroscopy is essential in categorization of corneal opacities. Since most causes of corneal opacities are rare, referral to a corneal specialist is necessary.

Dermoid Cysts

Dermoid cysts are histologically classified as choristomas, normal tissue that is abnormally located.

Dermoids are relatively common tumors that are composed primarily of connective tissue with a keratinized epithelial surface. Lipids, bony material, hair follicles, and sebaceous glands are also sometimes present. Dermoids may be found in various locations in and around the eyes or eyelids, especially the orbit and limbus. The size is variable, but can be quite large. The color is usually whitish or yellowish.

Conjunctival dermoid cysts are most often located at the temporal aspect of the limbus and may extend several millimeters onto the cornea. Dermoids may be very deep and arise from the bones of the orbit in some cases. They may be congenital or become clinically apparent later in life. The mass of the dermoid can cause a deformation of the globe, inducing irregular astigmatism and amblyopia. Therefore, early treatment of the refractive error and occlusion therapy are required.

Limbal dermoids may be associated with either microphthalmia or Goldenhar's syndrome, which is characterized by auricular abnormalities, epibulbar dermoids, and vertebral malformations [19]. Most dermoids are sporadic in nature, but there is evidence of infrequent autosomal recessive inheritance. Dermoids that are not of functional or cosmetic concern are generally left untreated, but they may be surgically removed if desired. Care must be taken to prevent rupture of the cyst, which can cause a serious inflammatory response. Because dermoids sometimes extend very deeply into the surrounding ocular tissue, surgical complications during excision may occur.

Corneal Size Abnormalities

The normal horizontal corneal diameter in a neonate is 9–10 mm. The normal adult diameter of 11.5–12.0 mm is normally reached by 3–4 years of age. The increase in corneal diameter is accompanied by an increase in the corneal vault (also sometimes called the corneal sagitta). The central corneal curvature is steep at birth, but due to the minimal corneal vault, the corneal plane is very similar to that of the sclera. By 6 months of age, however, the cornea rises out of the plane of the sclera, assuming a more adult-like configuration by 3–4 years of age. The central corneal curvature flattens during early childhood [20]. Simultaneous growth changes in the structure of the entire anterior segment occur as well.

Megalocornea is defined as a corneal diameter greater than 11.5–12.0 mm in an infant or greater than 13 mm in a fully grown eye. Other ocular parameters are often normal. The most important etiology to consider is congenital glaucoma. Congenital glaucoma may be unilateral or bilateral. The initial presentation is a steamy cornea, prominent photophobia and tearing, and increased corneal diameter, which should not be confused with true megalocornea. Affected infants may have abnormal visual behavior. Megalocornea is almost always a bilateral condition. The most common heredity is X-linked recessive, but other patterns of heredity exist. The megalocornea form known as anterior megalophthalmus is characterized by the presence of a number of associated ocular abnormalities, including high refractive errors, iridodonesis, iris atrophy, cataracts, and ectopia lentis. Megalocornea is usually nonprogressive and in itself is not visually threatening. Patients with typical megalocornea possess a normal corneal endothelial cell density, whereas patients with congenital glaucoma have a reduced endothelial cell density [21]. Enlarged corneal diameter is commonly seen in patients with Marfan's syndrome. Ectopia lentis, extreme degrees of myopia, and retinal detachments are also possible complications of Marfan's syndrome. All patients with large corneas should have a thorough eye examination to check for corneal clouding, increased intraocular pressure, myopia, lens changes, and retinal problems.

Microcornea is defined as a corneal diameter of less than 9 mm at birth or asymmetric corneal diameters at a later age with one or both corneal diameters smaller than normal. Microcornea may occur as an isolated finding in otherwise normal eyes. Inheritance pattern may be autosomal dominant or recessive. It is most frequently seen, however, in patients with persistent hyperplastic primary vitreous, congenital cataracts, or both. These patients possess abnormalities of the eyes in addition to microcornea. Microcorneas may also occur in the anterior chamber cleavage syndromes, often along with a central corneal leukoma in the variant known as Peter's anomaly.

Corneal Opacities

The conditions that cause corneal opacification in children are both numerous and individually quite rare. Only the more commonly encountered conditions that cause corneal opacities in young children are discussed (Table 12.3).

Sclerocornea is a nonspecific type of congenital corneal opacification with vascularization that is essentially continuous with the sclera. Most patients with sclerocornea have bilateral, nonprogressive opacifications. The limbus is usually poorly defined, but the central cornea may be somewhat clearer than the periphery. The major defect is in the stroma, with a disruption of the typical lamellar structure and an appearance quite similar to that of the sclera. There may also be disorganization of other corneal layers, especially of the endothelium and Descemet's membrane. Individuals may have one of the many variations of sclerocornea, including otherwise relatively normal eyes with at least a modest level of vision; eyes with small, very flat corneas and anterior segments; microphthalmic eyes; anterior chamber cleavage syndrome; and eyes with completely white, opaque corneas and no vision. Visual prognosis depends on the degree of opacification. Penetrating keratoplasties can be attempted on patients with potential for visual rehabilitation, especially if the condition is bilateral and asymmetric. In this case, the eye with worse vision may be operated on to give the infant at least a chance at achieving functional vision. These cases are very difficult to treat because of deprivation amblyopia and the irregular corneal surfaces resulting from the surgery. Early intervention is critical. The use of rigid contact lenses for subsequent optical correction provides the most regular corneal surface possible.

Tears or opacification of Descemet's membrane and the endothelium may be caused by birth trauma and congenital glaucoma. Injuries from birth trauma may be caused by the use of forceps to aid in the delivery of the infant [22]. These injuries are unilateral, appearing as vertical striae in Descemet's membrane. Decreased visual acuity results directly from both the opacities and astigmatism and the induced amblyopia.

Only a few corneal dystrophies are seen at birth. Congenital hereditary endothelial dystrophy (CHED)

Table 12.3. Causes of Neonatal Corneal Opacities

Sclerocornea
Birth trauma
Glaucoma
Congenital hereditary endothelial dystrophy
Congenital hereditary stromal dystrophy
Infection
Mucopolysaccharidosis
Mucolipidosis
Fabry's disease

is thought to be an autosomal recessive inherited condition presenting as variable, bilateral corneal clouding and sensory nystagmus, if the opacities are dense enough to severely impair vision. In contrast to congenital glaucoma, there is minimal photophobia, blepharospasm, or tearing, and corneal diameters are normal. The dominantly inherited form is more progressive and more symptomatic than the recessive form [23]. Penetrating keratoplasty should be considered if vision is severely compromised.

Congenital hereditary stromal dystrophy is less common than CHED. It is an autosomal dominantly inherited condition appearing as a dense, central stromal opacification and somewhat clearer periphery. Vision may be affected less than with CHED because of the possibility of some degree of vision through the relatively clearer peripheral cornea.

A number of other conditions rarely cause corneal opacities in the neonate, but do occur more often somewhat later in life. Corneal infection by the herpes simplex virus is a major cause of corneal opacity, but is seen only rarely in neonates, mainly as a sequelae of disseminated congenital herpes. Several common and usually mild systemic diseases of later life, such as cytomegalovirus and rubella, can have devastating effects if the infection is congenital. Certain types of mucopolysaccharidosis, mucolipidosis, and tyrosinemia, all of them very rare, may manifest corneal opacities at birth. Fabry's disease may initially present in patients with an unusual, whorl-like corneal opacity [24]. There may be a similar whorl-like or propeller-like opacification of the lens as well. The differentiation of these conditions is very complex. Peter's anomaly, the central corneal manifestation of the anterior chamber cleavage syndrome, is clinically the most

Table 12.4. Congenital Uveal Abnormalities

Anterior chamber cleavage syndrome
Aniridia
Coloboma
Pupillary anomalies
Albinism

common cause of dense, central corneal opacities in neonates.

IRIS AND CILIARY BODY

Congenital uveal abnormalities such as aniridia, iris coloboma, and oculocutaneous albinism may sometimes be detected and diagnosed by observation alone (Table 12.4). Those conditions associated with foveal hypoplasia result in early-onset nystagmus and reduced vision.

Anterior Chamber Cleavage Syndrome

The anterior chamber cleavage syndrome includes a diverse group of congenital mesodermal abnormalities of the anterior segment of the eye. Various systemic abnormalities are sometimes present also.

Waring et al. [25] devised a stepladder classification scheme for the anterior chamber cleavage syndrome that is useful in its categorization.

The abnormalities associated with anterior chamber cleavage syndrome are classified as either central or peripheral defects. A third group consists of a combination of the two. Peripheral abnormalities are the easiest to identify. Central abnormalities may be difficult to see because of obscuration by central corneal opacities. The ocular abnormalities may be unilateral, but more frequently are bilateral and asymmetric. The cause of these defects is unclear, but is probably related to intrauterine inflammation or a developmental abnormality. Several of the variants have an autosomal dominant inheritance pattern.

The least significant of the peripheral defects is a prominent Schwalbe's line (posterior embryotoxon) (Figure 12.2). It appears as a whitish ring within the cornea just inside the limbus and may be separated from the limbus by a lucid interval. The ring may be incomplete, with the most visible ones located temporally. Posterior embryotoxon is usually a common and harmless finding and is not often associated with the true anterior chamber cleavage syndrome and its many serious ocular complications.

A prominent Schwalbe's line coupled with fine attachments inserting onto the iris is known as Axenfeld's anomaly (see Figure 12.2). The appearance

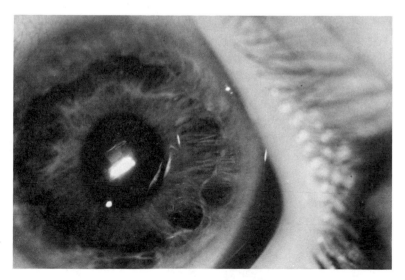

Figure 12.2. This patient has a prominent anteriorly displaced Schwalbe's line with fibers extending to the iris and hypoplasia of the anterior iris stroma. The risk of later-onset glaucoma is greatly increased in these patients. (Reprinted with permission from LJ Press, BD Moore. Clinical Pediatric Optometry. Boston: Butterworth–Heinemann, 1993;114.)

of these iris strands is quite variable, ranging from small numbers of intermittent, fine fibers, to thick, almost continuous membranes extending around the entire angle. Patients [26] with Axenfeld's anomaly have an increased risk of glaucoma, resulting in the entity known as Axenfeld's syndrome. The glaucoma may develop at a young age, making early diagnosis and treatment difficult and resulting in significant visual loss that may occur early or as late as the second decade of life.

Like Axenfeld's anomaly, Reiger's anomaly is characterized by hypoplasia of the anterior iris stroma. The iris appears stringy without the normal architecture of the collarette and iris stroma. The pupil is often irregular. Glaucoma is common, appearing anytime from early childhood to middle age. Reiger's anomaly is usually inherited in an autosomal dominant pattern, with high penetrance and variable expressivity. When facial and dental abnormalities are associated, the condition is called Reiger's syndrome [27]. Neurologic, cardiologic, and skeletal abnormalities may also be present. A variant of Reiger's syndrome is iridogoniodysgenesis, which has a similar presentation except for an absence of the prominent Schwalbe's line and a greater associated tendency for megalocornea.

The central defect of the anterior chamber cleavage syndrome is a corneal opacity caused by an absence or hypoplasia of the central corneal endothelium and Descemet's membrane. The peripheral cornea often appears normal. The appearance of this corneal opacity may change considerably after birth, either clearing somewhat or becoming denser and vascularized. There is a wide spectrum of central abnormalities that may be encountered, with the effect on visual acuity also quite variable. Peter's anomaly is a central corneal leukoma, with iris strands arising from the iris collarette and attaching to the posterior surface of the leukoma. The density and configuration of the iris strands are variable, as is the size and density of the leukoma. Microphthalmia or microcornea may also be present.

Posterior keratoconus appears as a central posterior corneal depression accompanied by an area of hazy corneal stroma located anteriorly to the posterior defect. This condition is very different from the typical anterior corneal keratoconus, which is a degeneration of the anterior cornea. It may be unilateral and vision is often only mildly affected.

The major ocular complications resulting from the anterior chamber cleavage syndrome are visual loss secondary to the central corneal leukoma and an associated high risk for the development of glaucoma. All patients, even those with only the minor characteristics of the condition, must be closely monitored for glaucoma, particularly during the early years. Examination under anesthesia should be performed early if adequate office-based examination is not possible. Attention should be paid to measurement of the intraocular pressure, the clarity of the media, and the configuration of the anterior angle. Patients with bilateral dense corneal leukomas must be evaluated early for consideration of corneal transplantation in order to preserve some level of vision. Management (particularly surgical) of this condition is difficult, but prompt intervention may be the only way to forestall the development of bilateral deprivation amblyopia and severe visual impairment.

Aniridia

The term *aniridia* is a misnomer because it implies the absence of an iris. Actually, patients with aniridia retain at least a small residual iris root that may not be difficult to visualize behind the corneal-scleral junction (Figure 12.3). There are a host of other ocular abnormalities that may be associated with aniridia, including foveal and macular hypoplasia, keratopathy, optic nerve hypoplasia, anterior polar cataracts, ectopia lentis, persistent pupillary membrane, sensory nystagmus, and photophobia. Patients are invariably legally blind.

Abnormalities of aqueous drainage and the anterior angle result in a high incidence of developmental glaucoma, sometimes with late onset. This may be due to trabeculodysgenesis or occlusion of the trabeculum from hyperplasia of the iris stroma. It is very difficult to treat. A corneal dystrophy develops in the anterior layers of the peripheral cornea, along with slowly advancing pannus. The central cornea is usually relatively clear, even late in the course of the disorder.

Familial aniridia is inherited in an autosomal dominant pattern, with high penetrance and variable expressivity. The sporadic form, present in approximately 20–35% of infants with aniridia, is

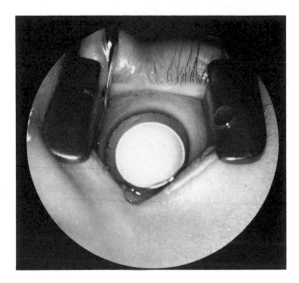

Figure 12.3. A thin rim of iris tissue is easily visible in this aniridia patient. Although aniridia is often thought of as the absence of the iris, there is always at least some evidence of hypoplastic iris tissue in these patients. (Reprinted with permission from LJ Press, BD Moore. Clinical Pediatric Optometry. Boston: Butterworth–Heinemann, 1993;115.)

Affected individuals often have high hyperopic astigmatism, which is probably associated with the foveal hypoplasia and aberrant emmetropization. Contact lenses may prove beneficial for optical purposes in those patients with high refractive error and nystagmus.

Iris Coloboma

Colobomas of the iris are relatively common and may be associated with other ocular colobomas of the choroid, ciliary body, lens, retina, and optic nerve. The heredity pattern may be autosomal dominant. The typical position of an iris coloboma is inferonasal, which corresponds to the last area of closure of the fetal fissure. Visual acuity is usually relatively unaffected, unless there is an associated coloboma of the posterior segment of the eye that includes the macula or the optic nerve head. Colobomas may be of cosmetic concern in some patients, and if large enough, can be a source of photophobia. Cosmetic-tinted contact lenses may be helpful for these patients.

associated with Wilm's tumor of the kidneys. Most of these patients are found to have a deletion of the short arm of chromosome 11 [28]. Since this tumor can develop at any time in childhood, especially in the first 3–4 years of life, all infants and children with aniridia must be closely followed by a pediatrician to watch for any signs of development of this tumor. Infants with aniridia should have a chromosome analysis to help in the diagnosis. Infants with the sporadic form of aniridia may also be at risk for a host of systemic abnormalities, including mental retardation, craniofacial abnormalities, microcephaly, and genitourinary disorders.

Attempts have been made to fit darkly tinted contact lenses to patients with aniridia as early as possible in order to help in the development of visual acuity. This technique is based on the hypothesis that excessive light to the retina is a prime cause of the decreased acuity, but there is no confirming evidence that this does improve the potential for vision. It is likely that much of the reduced visual acuity is due to foveal and macular hypoplasia and not to photophobia.

Pupillary Abnormalities

A great variety of abnormalities in the shape, position, and size of the pupil may occur. These pupillary abnormalities may be congenital or acquired and due to trauma or infection. The congenital iris abnormalities are often sporadic in nature, but may in some cases be hereditary. Partial forms of aniridia can cause multiple aberrant pupils (polycoria) due to iris aplasia. There is also a wide spectrum of persistent pupillary fibers, ranging from a few fine iris fibers across the pupil to thick fibers that cause an anomalous pupil shape (corectopia) and under rare circumstances can effectively block the visual axis, resulting in varying degrees of deprivation amblyopia. Anterior or posterior synechiae may be associated. Treatment of pupillary abnormalities is generally not indicated.

Albinism

Albinism is an abnormality of pigmentation that is due to an inborn error of metabolism. The uvea is the most obviously affected ocular structure. Other structures, including the nervous system connecting the retina to the visual cortex, are also grossly abnormal. Albinism is classified as either generalized (oculocutaneous) albinism or ocular albinism.

Oculocutaneous albinism is fairly common, occurring in 1 of 20,000 people, but is much more common in certain isolated populations and ethnic groups. It is thought to be an autosomally inherited condition, usually as a recessive trait. Many subtypes of oculocutaneous albinism are determined by certain genotypic and phenotypic characteristics, but a classification system based on the presence or absence of tyrosinase in the hair bulbs is the one most commonly used today. The tyrosinase-negative group of patients lack the enzyme tyrosinase. When their hair bulbs are incubated in tyrosinase, they are unable to produce melanin. The tyrosinase-positive group is able to produce melanin in the presence of tyrosinase. Other subtypes have been identified that have variations of these tyrosinase findings, including the yellow mutant variant found in the Amish. In general, the tyrosinase-negative patients have a greater deficit of pigmentation and greater severity of ocular abnormalities. The tyrosinase-positive patients usually retain some degree of pigmentation and have less severe visual loss.

Ocular albinism is thought to be primarily an X-linked condition, but some subtypes exhibit an autosomal recessive pattern of inheritance. Skin pigmentation is usually normal or near normal, but a disturbance of melanosome production has been noted in the skin, indicating that this is actually a more systemic disorder than previously assumed [29]. Certain patients may possess enough ocular pigmentation that they do not exhibit obvious iris transillumination and may even have brown iris coloration (Figure 12.4).

A number of abnormalities occur in the eye as a result of albinism. Transillumination of the iris is always present. A bright light shined through the sclera is visible through the iris and the sclera in a completely darkened room. The eye shows a bright red reflex through the iris and pupil, whereas a normally pigmented eye will not. The color of the iris is usually blue to minimally pigmented. It is less pigmented in tyrosinase-negative individuals than in those with some residual pigmentation. There may be a pupillary hippus. Foveal hypoplasia, which is the major cause of decreased visual acuity and nys-

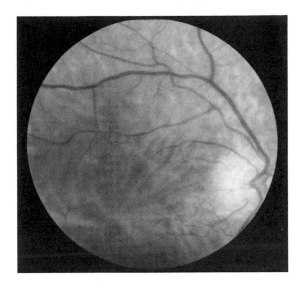

Figure 12.4. The fundus in this patient with albinism retains a considerable degree of fundus pigmentation. Foveal hypoplasia, which is a hallmark of albinism, is present. Patients with partial albinism may maintain a surprisingly good level of visual acuity. (Reprinted with permission from LJ Press, BD Moore. Clinical Pediatric Optometry. Boston: Butterworth–Heinemann, 1993;118.)

tagmus, is almost always present. Foveal hypoplasia ophthalmoscopically appears as a decrease in macular pigmentation and foveal light reflex (see Figure 12.4). The cones in the foveal region resemble those normally present in parafoveal areas [30]. The foveal pit is reduced or invisible due to a continuation of the ganglion cell layer through the macular region, where it should not normally be present.

Many patients have moderately high hyperopic and astigmatic refractive errors [31]. The absence of the fovea may play some role in this breakdown of emmetropization. Strabismus is common and is due in large measure to the nondecussation of nerve fibers at the chiasm [32]. Corrective strabismus surgery is relatively unsuccessful because of this anatomic defect; albinos do not have a simple misalignment of the eyes that can be mechanically corrected. Photophobia is present because of the lack of normal pigmentation, but is often less significant than expected. Photophobia was previously thought to be the main cause of decreased visual acuity, but it is now understood that foveal hypoplasia is more at fault. Color vision is often relatively normal, as is the electroretinogram response. Some patients

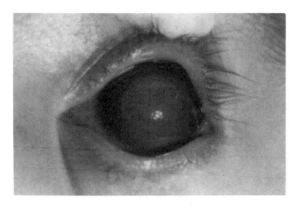

Figure 12.5. The cloudy, enlarged cornea in this patient is typical of infants with congenital glaucoma. (Reprinted with permission from LJ Press, BD Moore. Clinical Pediatric Optometry. Boston: Butterworth–Heinemann, 1993;124.)

may have surprisingly good visual acuity (the authors have seen patients with ocular albinism with visual acuity of 20/25 or better) and an absence of nystagmus and strabismus and a partial foveal light reflex. These patients are sometimes classified as albinoid as opposed to albinotic.

It is important to carefully correct the high refractive error. Since most albinos have nystagmus, glasses do not provide the optimal mode of correction. Contact lenses move with the eye during the nystagmoid eye movements, allowing the pupillary axis of the eye to coincide with the optic center of the lens and minimize the prismatic effects caused by off-axis viewing through glasses. Contact lenses can be tinted to decrease the intensity of ambient light, sometimes reducing photophobia and its adverse effects on visual acuity. Strabismus surgery is of less value, except for cosmesis. Oculocutaneous albinos should use effective skin protection against ultraviolet light exposure in order to prevent severe sunburn and the increased risk of skin cancers. Accommodation is often abnormal, requiring the use of high near adds.

GLAUCOMA

Congenital Glaucoma

The detection of congenital and early-onset glaucoma is usually easy, but the treatment is difficult.

Once the diagnosis of congenital glaucoma is made, these patients are best managed by a specialist in pediatric glaucoma.

Signs and Symptoms

Open-angle glaucoma in adults, the most prevalent type of glaucoma in that age group, often requires extensive examination to detect and diagnose. This is not the case with glaucoma in infants. Most infants with congenital glaucoma have an obvious ocular problem; there is little question that something is seriously wrong.

Infantile glaucoma is marked by several cardinal signs and symptoms. The cornea exhibits a number of abnormalities as a result of congenital glaucoma. Most apparent is increased corneal diameter. Megalocornea in young children can be caused by other factors, including primary hereditary megalocornea and Marfan's syndrome, but enlarged corneal diameter in the infant should immediately arouse suspicion of glaucoma. Furthermore, increased corneal diameter may indicate enlargement of the eye itself. Many patients with congenital glaucoma and megalocornea will be myopic as well [33]. In unilateral or asymmetric bilateral cases, this may lead to anisometropia and amblyopia, even in those patients whose glaucoma is controlled early and effectively.

Corneal clouding is a common sign of congenital glaucoma (Figure 12.5). Many other conditions cause corneal clouding, but the combination of enlarged and cloudy corneas is highly suggestive of congenital glaucoma. Both of these signs can be rapidly progressive and quite dramatic in appearance if only one eye is affected. Horizontal breaks in Descemet's membrane, called Haab's striae, may be seen. This is accompanied by a flow of aqueous into the cornea through the corneal endothelium. These breaks in Descemet's membrane occur only with onset of glaucoma in the first year or two of life and are a valuable diagnostic indicator in later years of the presence of congenital glaucoma. The ruptures in Descemet's membrane tend to greatly exacerbate the severity of symptoms in these patients.

Patients with congenital glaucoma frequently exhibit distinct behavioral patterns that aid in the diagnosis. Photophobia tends to be extreme. It is typical on initial examination to have the parent and child present with the child's head buried in the parent's shoulder, trying to block any light from getting to the eyes. This is accompanied by intense blepharospasm and epiphora, making attempts at examination very difficult. Eye rubbing may also be seen. This behavior tends to worsen before treatment is instituted and the pressure brought under control. It is often this reclusive behavior, more than any physical signs, that brings the parent and child in for evaluation.

Other, less apparent signs of congenital glaucoma visible only on examination under anesthesia include a deep anterior chamber and surprisingly extensive glaucomatous optic disc cupping. The optic nerve head of infants is much less able to resist the effects of increased intraocular pressure than adults and cupping develops rapidly. This cupping can regress if the pressure is brought under control before optic atrophy ensues [34]. This change may occur in only a matter of days. Increased intraocular pressure is another important finding in congenital glaucoma, but the degree of elevated pressure may be much less than generally found in open-angle glaucoma in adults.

Etiology

The basic etiology of congenital glaucoma lies in abnormalities of the filtering angle of the eye. In general, it is the outflow of aqueous that is abnormal, not the inflow. Several theories have been advanced as to the specific defect. One concept is that there is some sort of film or membrane (Barkan's membrane) that covers the trabecular meshwork, impairing the drainage of aqueous. Another implicates an absence or maldevelopment of Schlemm's canal. Other patients with primary congenital glaucoma have been found to have a type of trabeculodysgenesis. This may take several forms, with either an anomalous, anteriorly displaced insertion of the iris into the trabecular meshwork at the scleral spur as opposed to its normal insertion posterior to the scleral spur, or an anomalous configuration of the iris itself at the point of insertion into the trabeculum [35]. The iris may show additional abnormalities of the anterior stroma and iris vessels. It is likely that each of these mechanisms, along with additional ones, are responsible for cases of congenital glaucoma.

Examination of Infants with Congenital Glaucoma

A comprehensive examination of every infant with presumed congenital glaucoma is the first step in diagnosis. A complete history, including family history, perinatal history, and general medical history must be obtained. While eliciting this information, the infant's behavior should be closely observed. Visual acuity testing using an objective technique, such as preferential looking (PL) or visual evoked potential (VEP), should be done. Any asymmetry in acuities between eyes should be looked for carefully. If this is not possible, assessing fixation behavior will suffice at this time. An external ocular examination of the pupils, lids, cornea, anterior chamber, and tearing should be performed. If possible, a hand-held slit-lamp should be used. Depending on the intensity of photophobia, this may be difficult or impossible. Retinoscopy and direct ophthalmoscopy, in part to evaluate the presence and appearance of a red reflex, should be done. A measurement of intraocular pressure should be obtained with a hand-held applanation tonometer. With the help of the parent or an assistant, reasonably accurate pressures can usually be obtained. Schiötz tonometry is less useful than applanation tonometry. The likelihood of abrading the cornea with the metal footplate and differences in the scleral rigidity factor between infants and adults (the sclera is much softer and more pliable in infants, giving a different rigidity function) lead to potentially inaccurate results. Koeppe gonioscopy should be attempted to evaluate the anterior angle if the cornea is relatively clear and the child can be adequately restrained for the procedure.

An examination while the child is under anesthesia should be scheduled. This will allow a more thorough and less traumatic examination to be performed than may be possible in an office setting. A good view of the anterior segment of the eye with the aid of a slit-lamp or operating microscope is invaluable. Measurement of intraocular pressure while under anesthesia may differ from that obtained in the office because of the effects of the anesthesia medication itself [36]. The pressure can be much lower while under anesthesia, with readings that would be considered normal in the office indicating high pressures under anesthesia. Differences in intraocular pressure are especially important under these circumstances. Thorough examination of the anterior angle and the fundus with gonioscopy and the indirect ophthalmoscope should follow.

The last step in the examination of infants with congenital glaucoma is to send the patient back to his or her pediatrician for a thorough physical examination to check for the presence of systemic disease that may be associated with the glaucoma. After all this has been done, a proper diagnosis can be made and a treatment plan developed. While awaiting completion of the evaluation, initial medical treatment can be instituted.

Conditions Causing Congenital Glaucoma

Primary Congenital Open-Angle Glaucoma. The most frequent cause of congenital glaucoma is primary congenital open-angle glaucoma. This is usually a sporadic, primary ocular condition without systemic manifestations, although a small percentage of cases appear to be hereditary in nature. Approximately 10% of patients have an autosomal recessive hereditary pattern. In 75% of cases, the condition is bilateral. Congenital glaucoma is somewhat more prevalent in males (about 65% of cases). The estimated incidence of the disease is approximately 1 in 10,000 births [37]. The primary presenting signs and symptoms are enlarged and cloudy corneas, photophobia, epiphora, and optic disc cupping, which is usually present in the first year of life. The etiology of primary congenital glaucoma is related to structural and functional abnormalities of the drainage angle.

Treatment of congenital glaucoma is eventually surgical in nature because the antiglaucoma drugs typically used in adults are only of limited utility. However, carbonic anhydrase inhibitors (both topical and systemic) may be somewhat effective on an interim basis in selected patients. Many patients with congenital glaucoma will require multiple surgical procedures before the intraocular pressure is brought under reasonable control. It is important to understand that congenital glaucoma is a very difficult disease to treat. Many patients will never achieve adequate control of the increased intraocular pressure and will eventually develop significant visual loss. For these reasons, glaucoma is best treated by an experienced pediatric glaucoma specialist, not a general practitioner.

Other Causes of Congenital Glaucoma. Congenital glaucoma is a manifestation of many ocular and systemic conditions. In addition to iris hypoplasia, patients with aniridia have a 50% incidence of congenital or early-onset glaucoma. This is due to either a physical blockage of the trabecula by the remnant of the iris or trabeculodysgenesis, which is typically seen in primary congenital open-angle glaucoma. Glaucoma secondary to aniridia is a particularly difficult type of congenital glaucoma to treat [38]. Goniotomy surgery and medical therapy are the best treatments currently available. Aniridia patients without early-onset glaucoma must still be closely followed throughout life because of the high risk of developing glaucoma later.

Patients with variants of the anterior chamber cleavage syndrome are also susceptible to congenital or early-onset glaucoma. A number of abnormalities of the anterior angle occur, including anteriorly displaced Schwalbe's line, adhesions between the iris and Schwalbe's line, and iris hypoplasia. Glaucoma may be present in approximately 50% of these patients [25]. All patients with the anterior chamber cleavage syndrome must be followed throughout life for possible late development of glaucoma. Treatment is initially by medication, with surgery indicated later if the medical therapy is ineffective.

Two of the phakomatoses, Sturge-Weber syndrome and neurofibromatosis (von Recklinghausen's disease), have a significant incidence of congenital and early-onset glaucoma. Sturge-Weber syndrome causes glaucoma in 30–50% of patients, most often in those having the typical port-wine stain on one side of the face with its distribution following the course of the fifth (trigeminal) cranial nerve. Sturge-Weber syndrome is associated with a hemangioma of the leptomeninges of the affected side [39]. Sturge-Weber syndrome is the most prevalent systemic disorder causing congenital glaucoma. The angle is affected by what is thought to be a membranous film over the trabecula. Additional abnormalities of the uveal vasculature that may limit the ability of the trabecula to pass aqueous are usually present, but the mechanism of the glaucoma is not yet known for certain. This type of glaucoma is also difficult to treat.

Glaucoma secondary to neurofibromatosis is often associated with plexiform neuromas of the eyelids on the affected side. The cornea may become greatly enlarged in congenital cases. The etiology of the glaucoma is variable but may include trabeculodysgenesis, synechiae, or a membranous covering over the trabecula.

A number of less common causes of congenital glaucoma occur. Patients with Marfan's syndrome and homocystinuria may develop early glaucoma from pupillary block of a dislocated lens or as a result of abnormalities of the drainage angle. Patients with Lowe's syndrome, Hurler's syndrome, Weill-Marchesani syndrome, and Pierre Robin syndrome also have a significant risk of the development of congenital glaucoma.

Acquired Glaucoma

The conditions discussed above that cause congenital glaucoma may not become manifest until some time after birth, thus technically falling into the category of acquired glaucoma. This is true especially of the phakomatoses. The detection and diagnosis of these secondary glaucomas is not very different than that of the congenital types. It is easier to examine these older patients than neonates and it is likely that examination under anesthesia will not be required as often as in younger patients.

Trauma is the leading cause of all glaucomas in children, with hyphema being the single most important predisposing event. Several specific factors increase the risk of development of secondary glaucoma: the size of the hyphema, the occurrence of rebleeds, and the presence and degree of angle recession. Treatment includes paracentesis of the anterior chamber and trabeculectomy along with medical treatment. Angle recession without hyphema may cause glaucoma soon after the injury or many years later. The greater circumference of angle that is recessed, the greater the risk of glaucoma. If three-fourths of the angle is involved, glaucoma at some point in the future is almost assured.

Glaucoma secondary to chronic or acute uveitis is also a significant cause of acquired glaucoma in children. It can occur as a result of blockage of the trabeculum by inflammatory cells and debris or by neovascularization of the angle. Iris bombe and angle closure due to inflammation may also cause secondary glaucoma. Juvenile rheumatoid arthritis is a frequent cause of this type of glaucoma [40]. The primary treatment for most forms of uveitis is administration of topical or systemic steroids,

Table 12.5. Causes of Lens Abnormalities

Ectopia lentis
  Marfan's syndrome
  Homocystinuria
  Ehlers-Danlos syndrome
  Weill-Marchesani syndrome
  Hyperlysinemia
  Sulfite-oxidase deficiency
  Trauma
Cataracts
  Unknown etiology
  Autosomal dominant inherited condition
  Congenital infection
  Prematurity
  Galactosemia
  Fabry's disease
  Refsum's disease
  Hypoglycemia
  Hypocalcemia
  Hallerman-Streiff syndrome
  Conradi's syndrome
  Stickler's syndrome
  Zellweger's syndrome
  Lowe's syndrome
  Persistent hyperplastic primary vitreous
  Uveitis, especially juvenile rheumatoid arthritis
  Steroids and other drugs
  Atopic disease
  Radiation
  Trauma

which itself can cause glaucoma. This can make it somewhat unclear if it is the uveitis, the treatment, or, more likely, a combination of both that precipitates the glaucoma. Regardless of the cause, the treatment consists initially of medical therapy followed by surgical intervention if necessary.

Additional causes of secondary glaucoma in children include that resulting from cataract extraction, even many years after surgery, retinopathy of prematurity, congenital systemic infections with ocular sequelae, and ocular neoplasms.

LENS

Ectopia lentis, or dislocated lens, is a not uncommon finding in children. It is important to correctly diagnose these patients because of the potentially serious systemic manifestations of many of its causes (Table 12.5). For example, early diagnosis of aortic aneurysms in patients with Marfan's syndrome may prevent premature death.

Congenital and early-onset cataracts in young children often are impossible to categorize. Many of the uncommon systemic disorders that cause cataracts can be diagnosed by careful evaluation (see Table 12.5). Early detection and treatment of these cataracts greatly enhance a favorable outcome, whereas late treatment virtually guarantees failure. These patients should be referred to an appropriate facility for treatment as expeditiously as possible.

Ectopia Lentis

Ectopia lentis, or dislocation of the anatomic lens, occurs as a result of trauma, as part of a systemic disease syndrome, or as an isolated ocular event [41]. The lens is normally held in position by the zonules, which are fine, elastic fibers that connect the ciliary body muscle to the vicinity of the equator of the lens. Several types of zonular fibers originate in different geographic areas of the ciliary body and terminate either exactly at the equator or just anterior or posterior to the equator of the lens. Weakness, trauma, or absence of any or all groups of these zonules determines the direction and the magnitude of the lens dislocation.

Irregular refractive error resulting from the malpositioned crystalline lens is a major consequence of this condition. The lens may be tilted or displaced out of its normal position. Light rays traverse the lens in either a nonparaxial orientation or through a peripheral region of the lens. This induces an irregular form of astigmatism and myopia that cannot be adequately corrected with glasses or contact lenses. Patients with ectopia lentis are difficult to refract because of the aberrant retinoscopic reflexes caused by the malpositioned lens and poor endpoint of subjective refraction, especially in young children. Visual acuity is adversely affected. In addition, patients with early onset of ectopia lentis are subject to refractive amblyopia. The refractive error may fluctuate as the crystalline lens continues to dislocate. Occasionally, the dislocation is so extreme that the eye becomes effectively aphakic. These patients can then be corrected with a standard aphakic refractive correction, often obtaining a higher level of visual acuity than that previously reached when the eye was functionally phakic.

Several other important sequelae are associated with ectopia lentis. Uveitis due to direct contact of the lens with the iris or ciliary body occurs [42]. Rarely, a ruptured lens may cause a phacolytic uveitis. Glaucoma can result from pupillary block secondary to chronic uveitis or displacement into the anterior chamber. Anterior chamber displacement may damage the corneal endothelium and lead to corneal opacification. Retinal detachment is the most frequent serious complication and is difficult to treat. Iridodonesis is also found in patients with ectopia lentis, regardless of the etiology.

Management

The goal of management is to provide the best refractive correction possible and identify early the more serious ocular complications. Determining the refractive error by objective means (i.e., retinoscopy) is difficult and requires skill and patience. Extreme myopia and irregular astigmatism are typical. Unilateral or asymmetric bilateral ectopia lentis produces anisometropia and amblyopia. Repeat refractions are required since the refractive error may be quite unstable.

Patients with ectopia lentis need careful and repeat retinal examination because of the risk of retinal detachment. Instillation of miotic drops after dilation reduces the risk of anterior lens displacement. The risk of inducing glaucoma should be considered.

Clear lens extraction is a controversial treatment modality for patients with ectopia lentis. Currently, most experts believe that lensectomy should be performed only when there is a specific indication, such as recurrent anterior chamber displacement, cataract, and phacolytic uveitis. Lensectomy performed on these patients carries a greater than normal risk of retinal detachment, glaucoma, and cystoid macular edema.

Anteriorly Displaced Ectopia Lentis

Although uncommon, the crystalline lens can dislocate into the anterior chamber. Patients may present without symptoms or may complain of blurred vision or ocular or periocular pain. The cornea may be mildly to severely hazy, depending on the duration and extent of contact between the lens and corneal endothelium. This may on initial examination appear remarkably like an anterior chamber intraocular lens. The pupil will probably be mid-dilated and fixed.

Repositioning of the lens into the posterior chamber should be attempted to minimize damage to the corneal endothelium and reduce the risk of glaucoma. If the pupil is not already dilated, a short-acting mydriatic agent such as tropicamide (Mydriacyl) should be instilled while the patient lies quietly on his or her back. The lens may spontaneously reposition itself into the posterior chamber. If this occurs, the pupil should be constricted with pilocarpine to maintain the lens position. The intraocular pressure should be checked and the angle evaluated by gonioscopy. Then the clinician must decide whether to keep the patient on a miotic agent to prevent recurrence of the anterior lens displacement or remove the lens surgically. If there is any indication that the anterior lens displacement is recurrent, as evidenced by history or the appearance of corneal endothelial damage, lens removal is indicated. Since this condition is more likely to occur in homocystinuria and Weill-Marchesani syndrome, a thorough workup for systemic disease is indicated.

Causes of Ectopia Lentis

Marfan's Syndrome. Marfan's syndrome is the most common systemic cause of ectopia lentis. The prevalence is approximately 5 per 100,000 population [43]. Marfan's syndrome is an autosomal dominant inherited disease with a high degree of penetrance and variable expressivity that systemically affects connective tissue. Some patients appear to be new, spontaneous mutations.

The systemic manifestations include tall and slender stature, very long extremities, kyphosis, scoliosis, hyperextensibility of the joints, and cardiovascular abnormalities. Associated cardiovascular disorders, including abnormalities of the aortic valves and a greatly increased risk of aortic aneurysms, which may catastrophically dissect, are of major concern. One study has indicated that 93% of all premature deaths in Marfan's syndrome are due to cardiovascular causes [44]. All patients diagnosed with Marfan's syndrome must have a complete cardiovascular workup. Prophylactic surgery is performed to correct these defects.

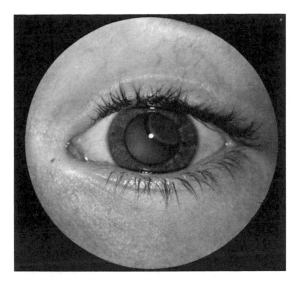

Figure 12.6. Lens dislocation in a supertemporal direction is most common in patients with Marfan's syndrome. (Reprinted with permission from LJ Press, BD Moore. Clinical Pediatric Optometry. Boston: Butterworth–Heinemann, 1993;129.)

The ocular manifestations include congenital megalocornea, microspherophakia, high myopia (up to −30.00 D) and astigmatism, blue sclera, retinal detachment, iridodonesis, and dislocated lenses. Vision may be severely reduced, but amblyopia may be improved with proper refractive correction and occlusion therapy. The high myopia found in some patients may be exacerbated by the marked optical blur present from a very early age, which causes an increase in axial length. The iris often appears abnormal, with a marked decrease in the number and consistency of iris crypts, ridges, and furrows. The pupils tend to be small and are frequently difficult to dilate. The anterior angle may show various abnormalities as well. Ectopia lentis is present in the majority of patients with Marfan's syndrome. It is usually bilateral and somewhat symmetric. The lenses tend to dislocate supertemporally, but this occurrence should not be considered diagnostic (Figure 12.6). Surgery to remove a clear lens should be considered only if the lens subluxates into the anterior chamber, which can lead to compromise of the corneal endothelium and iris bombe glaucoma. There is significant risk of retinal detachment in

Marfan's patients who are left phakic throughout life, but this risk is increased tremendously if lens extraction is performed.

Homocystinuria. Homocystinuria is a metabolic disease with an autosomal recessive hereditary pattern. A deficiency of the cystathionine-synthase enzyme leads to excess levels of homocystine excreted in the urine. Many patients are mentally retarded. The systemic manifestations of patients with homocystinuria appear quite similar to those patients with Marfan's syndrome. In fact, the two conditions have in the past been frequently confused and sometimes lumped together. The major difference other than in the biochemistry is the frequent presence of mental retardation in those patients with homocystinuria. The major cause of premature death in patients with homocystinuria is thrombotic vascular occlusion.

The ocular effects are similar to those in Marfan's syndrome, although lenses tend to displace inferiorly as opposed to superiorly. An increased risk of lens displacement into the anterior chamber is present.

Other Causes of Ectopia Lentis. A few other uncommon conditions also cause ectopia lentis, including Ehlers-Danlos syndrome, Weill-Marchesani syndrome, hyperlysinemia, and sulfite-oxidase deficiency. Patients with aniridia have a high risk of a dislocated lens. The other major cause of ectopia lentis, in addition to Marfan's syndrome, is trauma to the eye [45].

Cataracts

Congenital Cataracts

Congenital cataracts are estimated to occur in approximately 1 in 10,000 live births in the United States [46], approximately 400–500 infants per year. An additional 400–500 cases develop around the first year of life. This is not a high incidence compared with other eye problems, but congenital cataracts are one of the leading causes of serious visual impairment in young children.

Research by Hubel and Wiesel in the 1960s and 1970s showed that the absence of form vision (caused by eyelid suturing or media opacity) in young animals caused a deep type of amblyopia, known as deprivation amblyopia, to occur [47]. They also determined that permanent and severe visual loss occurred if this deprivation of form vision is maintained throughout the critical period of visual development [48]. If the eyelids of animals are sutured after this critical period, less visual loss occurred. Human infants experience a more gradual and less predictable termination of the critical period over the first 4–8 months of age than other primates. From a clinical perspective, treatment of congenital cataracts before 2–3 months of age results in a better outcome than when treatment is initiated later.

Patients with unilateral congenital cataracts always develop amblyopia that must be aggressively treated with patching of the contralateral eye. The nonaffected eye usually develops a relatively normal level of visual acuity, unless the occlusion therapy is so intense that amblyopia results. Care must be exercised during treatment to prevent this occurrence. Frequent monitoring of visual acuity by an objective method (e.g., PL techniques, VEP) is important [49].

Congenital cataracts can be due to many causes; however, the specific etiology is often impossible to identify in individual patients, particularly in those with unilateral congenital cataracts. The causes of congenital cataracts can be divided into several categories:

1. A large number of patients with bilateral cataracts have a hereditary form with no other ocular or systemic manifestations. These patients typically show an autosomal dominant inheritance pattern with mixed penetrance and variable expressivity. The condition may appear in every generation or it may skip one or more generations. It is almost always bilateral. The cataracts are usually quite dense, present at birth, and may produce sensory nystagmus. Early treatment often results in good visual acuity.

2. Cataracts due to maternal infection during pregnancy no longer account for as many cases as before, in large measure due to the development of vaccination for rubella. In the 1960s, before rubella vaccination became available, many infants were born with the congenital rubella syndrome (cataracts, chorioretinitis, mental retardation, deafness, and heart disease). Recently, with a decrease in vaccina-

tion levels, we are again seeing some patients with the congenital rubella syndrome. Other infectious agents such as herpes simplex, cytomegalovirus, and syphilis also cause congenital cataracts as part of a disseminated congenital disease pattern.

3. The incidence of cataracts due to prematurity is on the rise because advances in neonatology have increased the number of very low-birth-weight babies who live. These infants are also at risk for retinopathy of prematurity.

Some infants with unilateral congenital cataracts have persistent hyperplastic primary vitreous. In this condition, the embryonic hyaloid artery extending from the optic disk to the lens does not resorb during fetal development, leaving a glial and sometimes vascular mass retrolentally, along with an opacified lens. This is most often unilateral. Many of these eyes are microphthalmic. Formerly it was believed that the presence of persistent hyperplastic primary vitreous made any attempt at treatment impossible, but it is now apparent that this is not necessarily true [50]. The surgery is more involved than with simple cataract extraction, but in experienced hands may be successful.

4. Many rare metabolic diseases have cataracts as a manifestation of more generalized disease. Galactosemia is important to consider because the cataract may be reversed if promptly diagnosed and treated with a change in diet (Figure 12.7). Other metabolic conditions include Fabry's disease, Refsum's disease, hypoglycemia, and hypocalcemia. There are also many nonmetabolic inherited diseases that have cataracts as a manifestation, most of which are very rare. Included among these are Hallermann-Streiff, Conradi's, Stickler's, Zellweger's, and Lowe's syndromes. All patients with congenital cataracts should have a complete physical examination to screen for metabolic and systemic abnormalities.

5. The majority of congenital cataracts, particularly in patients with unilateral congenital cataracts, are of unknown etiology (Plate 12-1). There is no evidence of previous family history or of systemic disorder, and the child appears otherwise completely normal.

Acquired Cataracts

Acquired cataracts are often less difficult to treat than congenital cataracts because deprivation am-

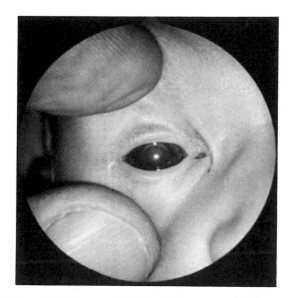

Figure 12.7. The central "oil droplet" appearance in this patient with cataracts secondary to galactosemia is due to a difference in refractive index between the nucleus and the cortex of the lens. Early dietary elimination of galactose can lead to a regression of the opacity of the lens. (Reprinted with permission from LJ Press, BD Moore. Clinical Pediatric Optometry. Boston: Butterworth–Heinemann, 1993;135.)

blyopia does not develop; however, the treatment is still quite complicated. Trauma is by far the most common cause of acquired cataracts in children. Penetrating and concussive trauma to the eye occurs frequently in young children [51] due to injuries from toys (especially broken toys), sports, violence, and accidents. Any patient with a penetrating eye injury is at risk of intraocular infection. The appearance of a traumatic cataract varies greatly, but sometimes it may show a snowflake-like pattern and a Vossius ring of pupillary pigment on the anterior lens surface. Severe trauma may lead to rupture of the capsule and release of lens material into the aqueous or vitreous, causing severe intraocular inflammation.

Chronic uveitis is a frequent cause of acquired cataracts. In particular, the long-term smoldering uveitis associated with pauciarticular juvenile rheumatoid arthritis often leads to cataracts. In addition, topical steroids, the treatment for anterior uveitis, may cause cataracts. It is often impossible

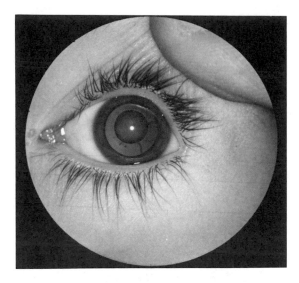

Figure 12.8. This patient has a sharply demarcated zonular cataract. Cursory observation may confuse this cataract with the "oil droplet" galactosemia cataract. (Reprinted with permission from LJ Press, BD Moore. Clinical Pediatric Optometry. Boston: Butterworth–Heinemann, 1993;138.)

to know if the cataracts found in a patient with juvenile rheumatoid arthritis are due to the steroids, inflammation, or a combination of both. Many systemic diseases also require long-term treatment with high dosages of systemic steroids, including asthma, arthritis, lupus, leukemia, and Crohn's disease. These patients need to be examined at approximately 6-month intervals to monitor the development of cataracts or glaucoma secondary to the use of steroids. Patients who have received radiation treatment to the head for neoplastic disease can develop a type of radiation cataract. Atopic diseases may also cause cataracts. Acquired cataracts due to metabolic disorders occur in patients with diabetes mellitus, hypocalcemia, galactokinase deficiency, and hypoglycemia.

Morphology

The shape, position, density, and appearance of cataracts varies considerably. In general, cataracts that are densest and closest to the posterior nodal point of the eye have the most adverse effect on vision. It is necessary to evaluate the cataract's effect on visual acuity before deciding on the efficacy of cataract removal. Many types of cataracts have little if any adverse effect on vision and visual development, particularly those involving only a portion of the anterior lens capsule, which is furthest from the nodal point of the eye. In patients with bilateral congenital cataracts, the presence of early-onset nystagmus is an indication of dense and visually significant cataracts, whereas an absence of early nystagmus may be an indication that vision is less affected. There are, nonetheless, many exceptions to this trend. In addition, a surprising difference in the examiner's estimate of the density of the cataracts by its appearance and the cataract's effect on vision may exist. The objective measurement of visual acuity by PL procedures or by VEP is the only accurate method of assessing vision and should be done routinely in every young patient with cataracts.

Anterior polar cataracts are the most anteriorly positioned cataracts. They appear as a small, white opacity in the pupillary aperture. On slit-lamp examination, it is evident that they are protruding out from the anterior capsule, extending into the cortex minimally. They may be unilateral or bilateral and asymmetric, and generally do not progress. A positive family history is often seen and an association with aniridia, microphthalmus, and pupillary membranes may also be present. Because they lie furthest from the nodal point of the eye, they have the least effect on vision if their size is not greater than that of the pupil. Treatment is not indicated unless they are very large or adversely affect vision, but since progression may occur [52], patients should be monitored. Posterior polar cataracts appear similar in appearance to the anterior polar type. Their effect on vision may be greater because of the proximity to the nodal point of the eye. Vision must be closely monitored in these patients and surgical removal should be considered if vision is significantly affected.

Sutural cataracts occur at the anterior and posterior Y sutures of the fetal nucleus of the lens. They are common, have a variable heredity pattern, and only rarely cause decreased visual acuity. Zonular, or lamellar, cataracts are due to a short-term insult to the developing lens (Figure 12.8). The lens cortex

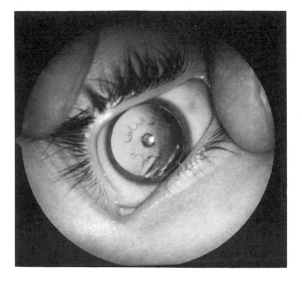

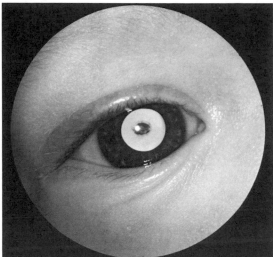

Figure 12.9. Posterior lenticonus cataracts are a common sequelae to radiation therapy to the head when the total exposure to the lens is greater than 800 rads. Subsequent fitting with an aphakic contact lens is complicated by a combination of decreased aqueous tear production and superficial punctate keratitis, which are both common adverse effects of the radiotherapy. (Reprinted with permission from LJ Press, BD Moore. Clinical Pediatric Optometry. Boston: Butterworth–Heinemann, 1993;140.)

Figure 12.10. The long-term use of systemic steroids results in the development of posterior subcapsular cataracts. This patient had a renal transplant and will require the continued use of steroids to prevent rejection, although continued use will lead to a visually disabling cataract necessitating extraction. In other patients, discontinuation of steroids when medically possible at this stage of lens opacification can sometimes allow partial regression of the cataract. (Reprinted with permission from LJ Press, BD Moore. Clinical Pediatric Optometry. Boston: Butterworth–Heinemann, 1993;139.)

surrounding the localized opacity is clear. The effect on vision is dependent on the size, density, and position of the opacity.

Nuclear cataracts are one of the more common visually significant congenital cataracts. They are often bilateral, asymmetric in density, and may be progressive. The progression is sometimes initially slow, but they may suddenly opacify later. Cortical cataracts of many types are also often progressive. They may cause little or no visual problems if they are primarily peripheral, but can be visually significant if central.

Posterior lenticonus cataracts may have surprisingly little effect on visual acuity, at least initially. On the other hand, any difference between the optical clarity of the two eyes may prove strongly amblyogenic. It is difficult to ascertain the specific cause of reduced visual acuity in these patients for this reason. Posterior lenticonus produces outpouchings from the surface of the posterior capsule, appearing somewhat reminiscent of keratoconus

(Figure 12.9). They are often unilateral and have a tendency to progress. It is very important to closely follow these patients with frequent visual acuity testing and to patch as needed to minimize the development of amblyopia before surgical removal.

Posterior subcapsular cataracts are frequently due to chronic uveitis, the use of steroids, or both (Figure 12.10). The degree of visual disturbance is great because of the proximity to the nodal point of the eye. Visual acuity may be more compromised than objective testing indicates, necessitating early removal. However, other patients may be surprisingly unaffected by their posterior subcapsular cataracts. Treatment should be dictated by the level of visual impairment and not solely by the appearance of the opacification.

The Treatment of Pediatric Cataracts

The treatment of congenital cataracts has progressed tremendously in the past 15–20 years. Most experts formerly thought that unilateral congenital cataracts were not worth treatment because of difficulties in surgery and long-term treatment of the aphakia and amblyopia [53]. Other studies have shown that with persistence, the results of treatment can be quite good [54, 55].

The differences between the treatment of young children and adults with cataracts are significant. Adults have had many years of normal vision before the formation of cataracts. The development of amblyopia as a result of the cataract is of no concern in these older patients. However, amblyopia is the main problem in young children with cataracts. The visual system is not fully developed in children with congenital or early-onset cataracts. If the visual system is not properly stimulated by the end of the critical period of visual development, there is essentially no possibility of attaining useful visual acuity. The exact upper age limit of this critical period in humans is not known for certain. It is known that dense congenital cataracts left untreated are almost impossible to treat by 9 months of age. There is still some possibility of a good result until approximately 6 months of age and the rate of success is still better at 3 months of age. Therefore, it is usually best to begin treatment as early as possible.

Older children with acquired cataracts often are able to achieve better levels of vision than children with congenital cataracts. The shorter the period of time that these patients with acquired cataracts have their vision obscured, the better the prognosis of regaining good vision. Cataracts that are very dense have a more adverse effect on vision than cataracts that only partially obscure the retinal image. In general, the greater the density of the opacity and the longer it obscures a clear retinal image, the greater the depth of amblyopia and the more difficult it is to rehabilitate.

Because timing is of such importance in the treatment of pediatric cataracts, rapid treatment is necessary. Surgical removal of the cataract must be completed as soon as it is determined that it is impairing visual acuity. Improvements in the surgical techniques of cataract extraction by aspiration methods and a decrease in the risk of complications from anesthesia and surgery have allowed routine surgery in the first months of life for congenital cataracts. Ensuring the early detection of cataracts has been an ongoing problem. Pediatricians should be the first to see the congenital cataract when looking for a red reflex during the newborn physical examination for hospital discharge, but this is not always the case. Congenital opacities in infants are sometimes not detected for months. If cataracts go undetected, the onset of strabismus may be the first obvious clinical sign of a serious ocular problem.

After surgery is completed and the eye is healed sufficiently, optical correction for the aphakia should be provided. In theory, this can be accomplished in several ways. Glasses work better in bilateral aphakia than in unilateral aphakia. This is due to the enormous difference in the prescription between the lenses, which causes difficulty in getting the glasses to fit properly on the child's face, magnification effects in the aphakic lens compared with the nonaphakic lens, and peripheral vision changes. They may be useful, however, on a temporary basis for children who have lost their contact lens or who are noncompliant with contact lens wear. We have worked with patients with unilateral cataracts that were unsuccessful with contact lenses, but did very well with glasses. An occasional break from contact lens wear may favorably change the child's behavior. It is important that the clinician use whatever means of correction works and not become overly concerned with theory.

Intraocular lens implants (IOLs) have been used by ophthalmologists as an alternative to contact lenses [56] but involve a greater risk of significant complications, including uveitis, improper refractive correction, corneal problems, and glaucoma. Therefore, IOLs are most suitable for those patients who are intolerant of contact lenses. Epikeratophakia had been advocated by some ophthalmologists [57] as an alternative to contact lenses and IOLs. Persistent problems have, however, rendered this procedure obsolete. It is important to remember that the refractive error of young children changes greatly in the first decade of life and that IOLs and epikeratophakia do not allow for changes in power as contact lenses or glasses do.

Contact lenses provide the best optical correction. In general, aphakic neonates can be easily fitted in the office with contact lenses that are especially designed for this purpose [58, 59]. Lenses are chosen based on the age of the patient and the size of the eye [20, 60]. A lens of approximately the correct size, shape, and optical correction is placed on the eye and retinoscopy is performed over the contact lens to minimize the possibility of error by off-axis retinoscopy. The fit and power of the lens are then adjusted until the examiner is satisfied that the parameters are correct. The lens may then either be ordered in the correct parameters or dispensed at this time if in stock. Lens power is often in excess of +35.00 D.

We strongly prefer to use lenses only on a daily-wear basis when possible, in part because of infection and safety concerns, but more importantly because it is much easier for the parent and the child to adapt to daily handling of the lens when the child is very young. This becomes much more difficult when the child is 1–2 years old. Although it does take time and effort to properly instruct parents in the care and handling of the lenses on a daily wear basis, virtually all parents are able to learn the appropriate techniques without too much difficulty. In this way, the parents become daily skilled observers of their child's eye and are able to spot problems early. We have found that the parents of extended-wear patients are usually less able to manage the frequent, minor lens-related problems that invariably occur.

The most difficult aspect of the treatment of children with early-onset unilateral cataracts is patching for amblyopia. In general, most children with unilateral cataracts will require some degree of amblyopia therapy until about 8 years of age. Consistency of patching is the single most critical part of the process of visual rehabilitation. It is easy to ask parents to keep a patch on their child's eye every day, but quite another thing to actually accomplish. We start out by patching the normal eye for approximately three-fourths of waking time. We then titrate this regimen by measuring on each follow-up visit the visual acuity of each eye with PL. As children reach about 1 year of age, patching typically becomes more difficult with adhesive eye patches. We shift to a black occlusive soft contact lens in patients who become intolerant to the patching [61]. This will often work well. It seems that many children object more to the feel of the patch on their face than they do to the effect on their vision that the patching causes. We also encourage the parents to maintain the patching schedule, even if their child is rebelling vigorously to this treatment. If we can get beyond their third birthday with reasonably good patching compli-

ance, we usually are successful in regaining a significant degree of visual acuity. Our own study of a large group of patients with unilateral congenital cataracts [55] shows that one-third end up with acuity worse than 20/200, another third with acuity between 20/80 and 20/200, and the remaining third with acuity better than 20/80. Many of this last group end up with acuity in the 20/30 range. Lenses need to be changed often in order to keep up with the changes in refractive error and the size and shape of the eyes as they grow. In some patients, this may be about every 3–4 months through the first 1–2 years.

Bilateral aphakic patients often do not have significant amblyopia and therefore do not require patching. Many of these patients obtain virtually normal levels of visual acuity, although some will have latent nystagmus. We use both contact lenses and glasses for this group of patients, letting the parents decide which they and their child prefer to use. Parents usually report that children have better gross motor abilities when they wear their contacts than when wearing their glasses. Almost every aphakic child has some problems with photophobia. Hats with long visors and sunglasses work acceptably well, but tinted contact lenses may be a better option. At this point, such lenses are not readily available in the soft lens materials that we prefer. We typically overcorrect the refractive error by about +2.50 D in young children to allow for focusing at near. When the children enter kindergarten, we will usually provide bifocal glasses in polycarbonate material, with an astigmatic correction included if necessary.

A number of potential complications may arise from the treatment of cataracts in young children. The first and most obvious is the inability to obtain good visual acuity. If the parents are able to ensure good patching for a consistent, long period of time, the results are usually quite good. If the patching is not consistent, then the results suffer. If there is no patching in unilateral patients, the results will be as expected, which is very poor (<20/200). Most of these unilateral patients develop strabismus, usually esotropia. This can be treated by surgery at a later time if it is a cosmetic issue. Stereopsis is generally not possible in these patients because of the intensity of the patching. Other problems include nystagmus, glaucoma and retinal detachments due to surgery, and the 20–30% chance of the development of a secondary membrane due to opacification of the posterior lens capsule, which is usually left in place during the cataract removal. If this does occur, either a second surgical procedure or the yttrium-argon-garnet (YAG) laser is required to cut through the membrane.

REFERENCES

1. Singh YP, Gupta SL, Jain IS. Congenital ocular abnormalities of the newborn. J Pediatr Ophthalmol Strabismus 1980;17:162–165.

2. Nelson LB, Ingoglia S, Breinin GM. Sensorimotor disturbances in craniostenosis. J Pediatr Ophthalmol Strabismus 1981;18:32–41.

3. Shillito J, Matson DD. Craniosynostosis: A review of 519 surgical patients. Pediatrics 1968;41:829–853.

4. Robb RM, Boger WP. Vertical strabismus associated with plagiocephaly. J Pediatr Ophthalmol Strabismus 1983;20:58–62.

5. Tessier P. Relationship of craniostenosis to craniofacial dysostoses, and to faciostenosis. Plast Reconstr Surg 1971;48:224–237.

6. Matthews DN. Ophthalmic complications of craniofacial surgery. J R Soc Med 1979;72:19–20.

7. Rosett HL, Weiner L. Alcohol and the Fetus: A Clinical Perspective. New York: Oxford University Press, 1984.

8. Day NL, Richardson GA. Prenatal alcohol exposure: a continuum of effects. Sem Perinatol 1991;15:271–9.

9. Abel EL. An update on incidence of FAS: FAS is not an equal opportunity birth defect. Neurotoxicol Teratol 1995;17:437–43.

10. Miller MT, Epstein RJ, Sugar J, et al. Anterior segment anomalies associated with the fetal alcohol syndrome. J Pediatr Ophthalmol Strabismus 1984;21:8–18.

11. Stafford JR Jr, Rosen TS, Zaider M, Merriam JC. Prenatal cocaine exposure and the development of the human eye. Ophthalmology 1994;101:301–8.

12. Johnson CC. Epicanthus and epiblepharon. Arch Ophthalmol 1978;96:1030–1033.

13. Mulliken JB, Murray JE. Natural History of Vascular Birthmarks. In HB Williams (ed), Symposium on Vascular Malformations and Melanotic Lesions. St. Louis: Mosby, 1982;327.

14. Sjogren H. The lacrimal secretion in newborn premature and fully developed children. Acta Ophthalmol (Copenh) 1955;33:557–560.

15. Liebman SD. Ocular manifestations of Riley–Day syndrome. Arch Ophthalmol 1956;56:719–725.

16. Petersen RA, Robb RM. The natural course of congenital obstruction of the nasolacrimal duct. J Pediatr Ophthalmol Strabismus 1978;15:246–250.

17. Paul TO, Shephard R. Congenital nasolacrimal duct obstruction: natural history and the timing of optimal intervention. J Pediatr Ophthalmol Strabismus 1994; 31:362–327.

18. Robb RM. Probing and irrigation for congenital nasolacrimal duct obstruction. Arch Ophthalmol 1986; 104:378–379.

19. Feingold M, Gellis SS. Ocular abnormalities associated with first and second arch syndromes. Surv Ophthalmol 1968;14:30–42.

20. Moore BD. Mensuration data in infant eyes with unilateral congenital cataracts. Am J Optom Physiol Optic 1987;64:204–210.

21. Skuta GL, Sugar J, Ericson ES. Corneal endothelial cell measurement in megalocornea. Arch Ophthalmol 1983;101:51–53.

22. Angell LK, Robb RM, Berson FG. Visual prognosis in patients with ruptures in Descemet's membrane due to forceps injuries. Arch Ophthalmol 1981;99:2137–2139.

23. Judisch GF, Maumenee IH. Clinical differentiation of recessive congenital hereditary endothelial dystrophy and dominant hereditary endothelial dystrophy. Am J Ophthalmol 1978;85:606–612.

24. Sher NA, Letson RD, Desnick RJ. The ocular manifestations in Fabry's disease. Arch Ophthalmol 1979; 97:671–676.

25. Waring GO, Rodrigues MM, Laibson PR. Anterior chamber cleavage syndrome. A stepladder classification. Survey Ophthalmol 1975;20:3–27.

26. Henkind P, Siegel IM, Carr RE. Mesodermal dysgenesis of the anterior segment: Rieger's anomaly. Arch Ophthalmol 1965;73:810–817.

27 Feingold M, Shiere F, Fogels HR, Donaldson D. Reiger's syndrome. Pediatrics 1969;44:564–569.

28. Riccardi VM, Sujansky E, Smith AC, Francke U. Chromosomal imbalance in the aniridia-Wilm's tumor association: 11p interstitial deletion. Pediatrics 1978;61:604–610.

29. O'Donnell FE, Hambrick GW, Green WR, et al. X-linked ocular albinism: an oculocutaneous macromelanosomal disorder. Arch Ophthalmol 1976;94: 1883–1892.

30. Fulton AB, Albert DM, Craft JL. Human albinism: light and electron microscopy study. Arch Ophthalmol 1978;96:305–310.

31. Taylor WOG. Visual disabilities of oculocutaneous albinism and their alleviation. Trans Ophthalmol Soc UK 1978;98:423–445.

32. Creel D, Witkop CJ, King RA. Asymmetric visually evoked potentials in human albinos: evidence for visual system anomalies. Invest Ophthalmol 1974;13:430–440.

33. Robin AL, Quigley HA, Pollack IP, et al. An analysis of visual acuity, visual fields, and disc cupping in childhood glaucoma. Am J Ophthalmol 1979;88:847–858.

34. Quigley HA. The pathogenesis of reversible cupping in congenital glaucoma. Am J Ophthalmol 1977;84: 358–370.

35. Wright JD, Robb RM, Deuker DK, Boger WP. Congenital glaucoma unresponsive to conventional therapy: a clinicopathological case presentation. J Pediatr Ophthalmol Strabismus 1983;20:172–179.

36. Quigley HA. Childhood glaucoma: results with trabeculotomy and study of reversible cupping. Ophthalmology 1982;89:219–225.

37. Miller SJH. Genetic aspects of glaucoma. Trans Ophthalmol Soc UK 1962;81:425–434.

38. Walton DS. Aniridic glaucoma—the results of goniosurgery to prevent and treat this problem. Trans Am Ophthalmol Soc 1986;84:59–68.

39. Phelps CD. The pathogenesis of glaucoma in Sturge–Weber syndrome. Ophthalmology 1978;85: 276–286.

40. Kanski JJ. Uveitis in juvenile chronic arthritis: incidence, clinical features and prognosis. Eye 1988; 2:641–645.

41. Nelson LB, Maumenee IH. Ectopia lentis. Surv Ophthalmol 1982;27:143–160.

42. Nirankari MS, Chaddah MR. Displaced lens. Am J Ophthalmol 1967;63:1719–1723.

43. Pyeritz RE, McKusick VA. The Marfan syndrome: diagnosis and management. New Engl J Med 1979;300:772–777.

44. Murdoch JL, Walker BA, Halpern BL, et al. Life expectancy and causes of death in the Marfan's syndrome. N Engl J Med 1972;286:804–808.

45. Jarrett WH. Dislocation of the lens: a study of 166 hospitalized cases. Arch Ophthalmol 1967;78:289–296.

46. Edmonds LD, James LM. Temporal Trends in the Incidence of Malformation in the United States, Selected Years, 1970–71, 1982–83. Centers for Disease Control Survey Summary. Atlanta: Centers for Disease Control; 1985;34:1SS–3SS.

47. Weisel TN, Hubel DH. Effects of visual deprivation on morphology and physiology of cells in the cat's lateral geniculate body. J Neurophysiol 1963;26:978–993.

48. Hubel DH, Weisel TN. The period of susceptibility to the physiologic effects of unilateral eye closure in kittens. J Physiol 1970;206:419–436.

49. Mayer DL, Moore BD, Robb RM. Assessment of vision and amblyopia by preferential looking tests after early surgery for unilateral congenital cataracts. J Pediatr Ophthalmol Strabismus 1989;26:61–68.

50. Karr DJ, Scott WE. Visual acuity results following treatment of persistent hyperplastic primary vitreous. Arch Ophthalmol 1986;104:662–667.

51. Nelson LB, Wilson TW, Jeffers JB. Eye injuries in childhood: Demography, etiology, and prevention. Pediatrics 1989;84:438–441.

52. Jaffar MS, Robb RM. Congenital anterior polar cataracts: a review of 63 cases. Ophthalmology 1984; 91:249–252.

53. Costenbader FD, Albert DG. Conservatism in the management of congenital cataract. Arch Ophthalmol 1957;58:426–430.

54. Beller R, Hoyt CS, Marg E, Odom JV. Good visual function after neonatal surgery for congenital monocular cataracts. Am J Ophthalmol 1981;91:559–565.

55. Robb RM. Refractive errors associated with hemangiomas of the eyelids and orbit in infancy. Am J Ophthalmol 1977;83:52–58.

56. Hiles DA. Intraocular lens implantation in children with monocular cataracts. 1974–1983. Ophthalmology 1984;91:1231–1237.

57. Arffa RC, Marvelli TL, Morgan KS. Long-term follow-up of refractive and keratometric results of pediatric epikeratophakia. Arch Ophthalmol 1986;104:668–670.

58. Moore BD. The fitting of contact lenses in aphakic infants. J Am Optom Assoc 1985;56:180–183.

59. Moore BD. Contact Lens Problems and Management in Infants, Toddlers, and Preschool Children. In M Scheiman (ed), Problems in Optometry: Pediatric Optometry. Philadelphia: Lippincott, 1990;365–393.

60. Moore BD. Changes in the aphakic refraction of children with unilateral congenital cataracts. J Pediatr Ophthalmol Strabismus 1989;26:290–295.

61. Moore BD. Contact Lens Therapy for Amblyopia. In R Rutstein (ed), Problems in Optometry: Amblyopia. Philadelpia: Lippincott, 1991;355–368.

Chapter 13
Diseases of the Posterior Segment

Bruce D. Moore

The diagnosis and treatment of chorioretinal disease in children is complex. The first, and sometimes the most difficult, step is the detection of the disorder. Signs of poor vision may be noted by the parents or pediatrician. Adequate examination of the fundus of a young child is not easy, but with persistence, can be accomplished with the use of the indirect ophthalmoscope. Electrophysiologic testing is essential in differentiating many of the conditions affecting the retina. Fundus photography is also very useful. The examiner must perform the evaluation in a systematic manner, using all of diagnostic tools available and required.

CHORIORETINITIS

Congenital Infectious Chorioretinitis

True congenital uveitis is rare, but when it does occur, it is usually associated with disseminated congenital infections. The signs, symptoms, and nature of these congenital infections are often more severe than the acquired infections of these same agents later in life, and the consequences to the child much graver. Many patients with disseminated congenital infections are detected at birth, since these are sick infants with a generally poor prognosis (Figure 13.1).

Congenital toxoplasmosis is transmitted by the mother to the developing fetus during pregnancy as a result of active maternal infection. Toxoplasmosis chorioretinitis is caused by the parasitic organism *Toxoplasma gondii*. The actual mechanism of infection is variable but thought to be caused most often by the mother eating contaminated, poorly cooked meat or cleaning a cat litter box containing cat feces contaminated with the *T. gondii* organism. The earlier the transmission of the organism to the fetus during fetal development, the greater the severity of infection; however, the incidence of transmission is greater with maternal infection during later pregnancy [1]. The mother may manifest few symptoms during her illness, most often appearing to have only a mild flu. Infected infants may not manifest disease at birth. Severely affected infants can have serious neurologic manifestations, including mental retardation, microcephaly, intracranial calcifications, seizure disorder, strabismus, and nystagmus. The child may be born prematurely and have failure to thrive.

The characteristic hyperpigmented chorioretinal lesions are due to recurrent episodes after the initial primary infection occurs. Encysted organisms are released by spontaneous rupture of the cyst, causing a fresh foci of inflammation adjacent to old lesion. The exact mechanism of this recurrence is not well understood at this time. The fresh lesions are surrounded by intense inflammation in the retina, choroid, and vitreous, often completely obscuring the lesion itself. Several antibody tests are used to look for an increasing titer of antibody to the organism in order to confirm the diagnosis of active infection.

Treatment is undertaken when the recurrent lesions threaten the macula or optic disc areas of the

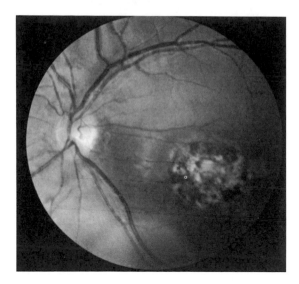

Figure 13.1. This patient exhibits the typical hyperpigmented macular scar resulting from toxoplasmosis chorioretinitis. (Reprinted with permission from LJ Press and BD Moore. Clinical Pediatric Optometry. Boston: Butterworth–Heinemann, 1993;151.)

retina. Peripheral, non–vision-threatening lesions are generally not treated but must be watched closely for flare-up. A combination of oral drugs is used in the treatment of toxoplasmosis, including pyrimethamine, sulfonamides, steroids, and clindamycin. These drugs have significant toxicity and must be closely monitored. One can expect recurrences of toxoplasmosis, and at least yearly follow-up exams are recommended. Patients should be taught to check monocular visual acuity daily for signs of uveitis indicated by decreased acuity.

Congenital cytomegalovirus (CMV) infection is the most common intrauterine infection [2, 3]. Infected neonates may be born prematurely and of low birth weight and have jaundice, hepatitis, hepatosplenomegaly, thrombocytopenic purpura, or pneumonia. Associated neurologic abnormalities include mental retardation, hearing loss, microcephaly, hydrocephalus, seizure disorders, and strabismus. The chorioretinal lesions may be pigmented and similar in appearance to those of toxoplasmosis, or smaller with discrete white foci. Vitreous haze overlying the chorioretinal lesions accompanies acute episodes. These lesions are areas of necrosis in all layers of the retina. There is a

predilection for the macula, with the consequence of dramatic and sudden vision loss. The infection may be passed through the fetal circulation from the mother or may be acquired during transit through the birth canal.

CMV is an opportunistic infection that commonly accompanies acquired immunodeficiency syndrome (AIDS). Retinitis occurs more often in adults than children. Individuals with CD4 T cell counts below 100 per microliter are at greatest risk for the development of retinitis [4]. The initial presentation may be mild and insidious [5], or may be more severe [6]. Retinitis progresses along the blood vessels, leaving large areas of exudates and hemorrhages, necrosis (cotton-wool spots in the nerve fiber layer), and granulation. Vitritis and uveitis are present, although usually less severe than the retinitis. The optic nerve and disc may be involved. This results in chorioretinal scarring, optic atrophy, retinal detachment, and severe vision loss. Treatment with foscarnet and ganciclovir may arrest early ocular inflammation; however, the outlook is bleak, and survival is often less than 2–3 years after retinitis occurs.

Herpes simplex type II can be transmitted to the neonate during passage through the birth canal. Systemic manifestations are similar to that of cytomegalovirus, with the addition of encephalitis. Eye findings include uveitis with hazy media, patches of grayish white chorioretinal focal lesions, and areas of retinal hemorrhage leading to pigmented scarring of the retina. Treatment currently includes vidarabine and acyclovir, with other experimental drugs being actively investigated.

Histoplasmosis

Histoplasma capsulatum is a mycotic organism that is endemic to certain areas of the United States, particularly the Ohio River Valley. It is thought to be a major cause of uveitis in those areas. Eye doctors in other areas of the United States rarely if ever see histoplasmosis in the native population. For example, the disease is virtually unknown in native New Englanders, and is seen only in transplanted patients from the "histo belt" of the Midwest. The organism has not actually been histologically proven, but the evidence is strong enough that experts call the clinical disease "presumed histoplasmosis disease." The lesions appear as large numbers of small, discrete, lightly pigmented lesions over the posterior pole of the eye. If the lesions affect the macula, vision can be seriously affected. There are also a host of significant systemic effects, and it is a cause of considerable morbidity in the geographic areas where it is endemic.

Toxocara

Ocular *Toxocara* infection occurs by ingestion of the ova of the *T. canis* or *cati* parasite by young children, often as a result of playing in a sandbox contaminated by cat or dog feces that harbor the organism. The larvae hatch in the child's digestive tract, pass into the bloodstream, and migrate to the choroid, where they can penetrate into the retina or even into the vitreous. This results in a white mass on the retina, often in the vicinity of the macula, and there is usually a severe inflammatory reaction that may completely obscure any view of the fundus. The inflammation can be so severe that it may appear as a totally white pupil (leukocoria), arousing suspicion of retinoblastoma. Vision is usually completely lost permanently due to the massive inflammation. Cataracts and optic atrophy may ensue. There is no effective treatment, but steroids have been used to quiet the inflammation, and various antiparasitic drugs are used to attempt control of the systemic effects of the parasite. It is almost always unilateral.

Pars Planitis

Pars planitis, also called peripheral or intermediate uveitis, is a type of uveitis affecting the region of the pars plana and the ciliary body. It is a disease prevalent in young boys 4–5 years of age. Onset is insidious and may not be detected until failure on school vision screening or absence of red reflex on ophthalmoscopy by the pediatrician. It is almost always bilateral. There is usually an absence of the typical symptoms of uveitis, such as photophobia or pain, and signs of conjunctival or limbal injection. Posterior synechiae almost never occur. There may be a dense, postlenticular, cyclitic membrane, composed of inflammatory cells and a fibrotic response within the vitreous that is the prime cause of

Table 13.1. Retinal Disorders

Congenital
  Perinatal infection
  Stickler's syndrome
  Choroidal coloboma
  Congenital high myopia
  Medullated nerve fibers
  Retinal dysplasia
  Persistent hyperplastic primary vitreous
  Achromatopsia
Tapetoretinal degenerations
  Leber's congenital amaurosis
  Retinitis pigmentosa
  Usher's syndrome
  Laurence-Moon-Bardet-Biedl syndrome
  Metabolic tapetoretinal degenerations
Juvenile macular degenerations
  X-linked retinoschisis
  Best's vitelliform degeneration
  Fundus flavimaculatus
  Cone degeneration
Exudative retinopathies
  Familial exudative vitreoretinopathy
  Coats' disease

the decreased vision. A "snowbank" of white inflammatory debris and collagen is located in the area of inflammation at the inferior pars plana. There is a three-dimensional quality to this mass. Additionally, there may be retinal edema of the nerve fiber layer and the macula, which can affect vision. The disease tends to be quite chronic, with periods of quiescence and flare, during which the density of the postlenticular cyclitic membrane varies along with the effect on vision. Cataracts may occur from the chronic inflammation. There is an increased risk of late retinal detachments and retinoschises. There may be only minimal residual vision loss due to the membrane and the cataracts. Amblyopia caused by the opacified membrane at earlier ages must be considered, particularly if there is asymmetry in the density of the membranes. Treatment is with the use of the minimal dosage of topical and systemic steroids that decreases the inflammation to a reasonable level. It is usually impossible to completely rid the eye of all signs of inflammation, and one must keep in mind the effects of long-term use of steroids on the patient (Table 13.1).

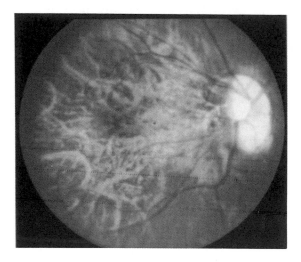

Figure 13.2. This patient with myopic retinal degeneration has conus formation, peripapillary atrophy, tilted disc, posterior staphyloma, macular changes, and choroidal thinning. The best corrected vision is 20/100. (Reprinted with permission from LJ Press and BD Moore. Clinical Pediatric Optometry. Boston: Butterworth–Heinemann, 1993;154.)

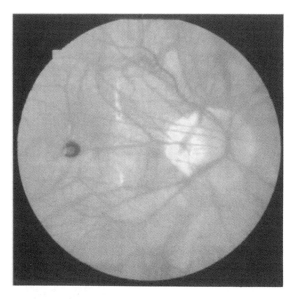

Figure 13.3. This patient with myopia of more than –20 diopters spontaneously developed a Fuchs' spot, resulting in the loss of macular vision.

CONGENITAL ABNORMALITIES

Choroidal Colobomas

Choroidal colobomas typically occur in the inferonasal quadrant off the optic disc, the last area of the fetal fissure to close. The size of the coloboma and its effect on vision vary greatly. Choroidal colobomas involving the disc and macula are likely to have a more adverse effect on vision, resulting in congenital blindness, strabismus, or both [7].

Patients with choroidal coloboma face an increased risk of retinal detachment in areas adjacent to or overlying the choroidal coloboma. The abnormally thin retinal tissue is poorly attached to the underlying scleral tissue [8]. These detachments may be difficult to visualize because of the absence of the typical color patterns and contrasts that one associates with retinal detachments and holes. The presence of posterior staphyloma further reduces the relative visibility of these retinal abnormalities.

Chromosomal abnormalities associated with ocular colobomas include trisomy 13 and 18, incomplete deletions of chromosomes 13 and 18, and Turner's and Klinefelter's syndromes. Other associations include Aicardi's, CHARGE, basal cell nevus, and Goldenhar's syndromes. CHARGE is an acronym for the following signs: *c*oloboma, *h*eart disease, choanal *a*tresia, *r*etarded growth and development, *g*enital hypoplasia, and *e*ar abnormalities [9]. Isolated choroidal colobomas may also occur sporadically.

High Myopia

High myopia is frequently associated with retinopathy (Figures 13.2 and 13.3). Specific structures affected include the vitreous, the disc and peripapillary regions, the macula and fovea, and the retinal periphery.

Vitreous detachment and opacification are encountered less often in children than adults with high myopia. The myopic or scleral crescent or ring, located at the disc margin, is frequently seen even in young patients with moderate to high myopia. The disc may be tilted if the nerve exits eccentrically or if there is a posterior staphyloma.

High myopic patients are more susceptible to the effects of elevated intraocular pressure (or even to "normal" pressures) because of structural compromises to the nerve head. This type of glaucoma is uncommon in young children, however.

Choroidal thinning is evident in most patients with high myopia. The thinning may be severe enough to lead to breaks in Bruch's membrane. Posterior staphyloma, which is an ectasia or outpouching of the eye, is due to weakness in the structure of the eye from excessive stretching. This tends to be progressive and can lead to extreme degrees of myopia. These eyes are at high risk of retinal detachment. There is similarly increased risk of retinal detachment in congenital myopia [10]. Trauma is a frequent predisposing factor in retinal detachment. All high myopic patients and their families must be clearly warned of the signs and symptoms of retinal detachments, and should be strongly cautioned to avoid activities that increase the risk. High myopia may occasionally be seen in neonates, particularly those having strabismus or visual inattentiveness, which leads to very early detection.

Changes to the macula can lead directly to decreased vision. Breaks in Bruch's membrane at the macula cause a Fuchs' spot. This can be sudden and precipitous. Pigmentary abnormalities resulting from high myopia are often visible in the macula of older children, but may go undetected ophthalmoscopically in younger children. Decreased visibility of the foveal reflex may be confused with other retinal abnormalities. The retinal stretching can affect the density and orientation of the photoreceptors and can cause a variable degree of visual loss. Similarly, tilted disc and macula may result in vision loss from the Stiles-Crawford effect.

There are a number of ocular and systemic abnormalities that are associated with high myopia. This includes retinopathy of prematurity (ROP), congenital glaucoma, Marfan's syndrome, Stickler's syndrome, homocystinuria, fetal alcohol syndrome, and Weill-Marchesani syndrome (Figure 13.4).

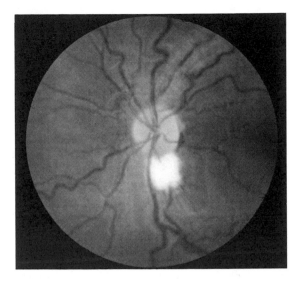

Figure 13.4. The feathered edge of the patch of medullated nerve fibers is starkly visible against the normal fundus coloration. (Reprinted with permission from LJ Press and BD Moore. Clinical Pediatric Optometry. Boston: Butterworth–Heinemann, 1993;156.)

typically seen adjacent to the optic disc, but it is not unusual to see patches of myelination in discontinuous areas of the retina. They may be bilateral, but are more commonly seen as unilateral incidental findings on routine examination. There is a feathery edge to the starkly whitish patches of myelinated fibers. An absolute visual field defect corresponds to the area of myelination. It is uncommon to have significant central visual loss due to isolated cases of medullated nerve fibers. A subgroup of patients have unilateral high myopia, extensive patches of myelinated nerve fibers off the disc sometimes extending to the fovea, and dense amblyopia. Some respond to amblyopia treatment, but others show no improvement, leading to the assumption that the amblyopia is of organic origin related to the myelination [11].

Medullated (Myelinated) Nerve Fibers

This common anomaly of the retinal nerve fiber layer is due to a continuation of the myelination of the ganglion cells beyond its normal termination at the lamina cribrosa. Medullated nerve fibers are

Retinal Dysplasia

Retinal dysplasia is an abnormal development of the retina producing folds, gliosis, and generalized disorganization of the structure of the retina. It may be unilateral or bilateral and may be associated with a host of systemic abnormalities, or it may be an isolated finding [12]. The hallmark of retinal dysplasia is the histopathologic finding of dysplastic retinal rosettes. These rosettes are categorized into several types depending on their degree of organization [13]. This can vary from relatively normal retina that is only partially folded over itself, to completely folded retinal tissue containing only a few layers of retinal cells. Eyes may range in appearance from virtually normal on examination to microphthalmic with leukocoria and blindness. Patients with severe bilateral retinal dysplasia have congenital searching nystagmus. Retinal detachments are common in the more severe forms. There is no treatment. Systemic disorders with ocular manifestations of retinal dysplasia include trisomy 13–15, Norrie's disease, and Meckel's syndrome. Possible prenatal causes include radiation and toxic chemical exposure, trauma, and viral infection.

Persistent Hyperplastic Primary Vitreous

Persistent hyperplastic primary vitreous (PHPV) is due to failure of further embryologic development of the vitreous beyond the earliest primary stage. This results in the continued presence of the fetal hyaloid vasculature and its attendant glial elements within the retrolental space. There are a number of ocular features that may be present, depending on the severity and location of the condition.

The mildest defects within this broad spectrum of abnormalities affecting the hyaloid system are Bergmeister's papilla and Mittendorf dot. Bergmeister's papilla appears as a vessel, often corkscrew in configuration, arising perpendicularly out of the optic disc. The size of this vessel is variable, but usually it results in no visual problems, unless there is attachment to the posterior surface of the lens. There are isolated reports of this vasculature bleeding due to severe trauma. Mittendorf dot is the remnant of the fetal vasculature at its point of attachment on the posterior surface of the lens. It is of no visual importance.

Pruett [14] has described three clinical forms of PHPV—an anterior and a posterior form, and an intermediate form showing characteristics of both. The anterior variety manifests microphthalmia, a whitish glial mass in the retrolental area that is usually vascularized, vascular traction of the ciliary body, and persistent hyaloid artery. The posterior form shows microcornea, vitreous membranes, retinal folds, and the presence of hyaloid artery remnants. The intermediate type may have a combination of anomalies found in each of the other categories of PHPV. Patients with each type are likely to have a shallow anterior chamber, cataracts, increased risk of glaucoma, retinal detachments, and vitreous hemorrhages. The most common presenting sign of patients with PHPV is leukocoria, although milder forms may present only with strabismus. PHPV is usually unilateral, but bilateral cases are seen.

These patients have in the past been considered difficult to treat. With the recent advances in the treatment of congenital cataracts and in neonatal retinal surgery, attempts at treating these patients have been more successful. Early removal of the lens and the retrolental tissue by combined aspiration and vitrectomy, along with aggressive optical and amblyopia treatment, has proven successful in some patients with less severe cases of PHPV [15]. The most severe cases may benefit from open-sky vitrectomy.

Stickler's Syndrome

Stickler's syndrome includes a variety of ophthalmic and skeletal anomalies [16]. There is an autosomal dominant hereditary pattern. The most prominent ocular features are high myopia and retinal detachments, along with cataracts and retinal pigmentary changes. Stickler's syndrome is one of the most common systemic disorders associated with high myopia [17]. Associated systemic findings include flattened facies, skeletal dysplasia, cleft palate, hearing loss, and mental retardation. Cataract surgery and the subsequent management of the aphakia in these patients is greatly complicated by the association of retinal detachments. Close follow-up is required throughout life.

Achromatopsia (Rod Monochromatism)

The normal color vision system is composed of three types of cones, each with visual pigments that absorb light preferentially at different wavelengths.

Color vision defects are caused by either an absence of one or more types of cones, or a shift in the absorption spectrum in one or more of the cone types. The vast majority of patients with color vision anomalies are only mildly affected.

Achromatopsia is an extreme form of color vision defect. It is either the absence of all cones or a deficiency in the functioning of the cone system [18]. The rod system is generally intact. The result is a complete absence of color vision, poor visual acuity, nystagmus, and severe photophobia. These patients, like those with congenital stationary night blindness, may exhibit a paradoxical pupillary constriction to darkness that may prove to be of significant diagnostic usefulness [19]. Patients often have high refractive errors, particularly hyperopic astigmatism. There may be a reduced foveal reflex, but otherwise ophthalmoscopically, the fundus appears relatively normal. The electroretinogram (ERG) produces a minimal or absent photopic response and normal scotopic function. The flicker fusion frequency is reduced. An autosomal recessive hereditary pattern is more frequently noted than an X-linked form, which may show a less severe effect on visual functioning. Achromatopsia is a relatively uncommon condition, with an incidence of about 3 per 10,000 births [20]. These patients may be helped by darkly tinted contact lenses for correction of the high refractive error and reduction in retinal illumination. I have seen dramatic improvements in subjective visual behavior with these contact lenses.

TAPETORETINAL DEGENERATIONS

Leber's Congenital Amaurosis

Leber's congenital amaurosis is a frequent cause of congenital blindness. It usually has an autosomal recessive inheritance pattern. Leber's is a tapetoretinal degeneration consisting of dystrophic and degenerative changes in the ganglion cells, pigment epithelium, and photoreceptor outer segments of the retina [21]. Although Leber's has historically been grouped as a single entity, recent speculation is that it may instead be a much more diverse group of conditions related more by appearance than etiologic features.

At birth, patients are either blind or severely visually impaired and have sensory nystagmus. Pupil-lary reactions are very sluggish or absent, and there may be marked photophobia. Optic atrophy, pigmentary retinopathy, and attenuation of retinal vessels develop by a later age, although the fundus appearance of the infant may look normal. High hyperopic refractive errors are common [22]. Keratoconus secondary to habitual eye rubbing and cataracts also may occur later in the course of the disorder. Mental retardation and a wide range of neurologic problems are frequently associated with a subgroup of Leber's patients, but many patients show relatively normal intelligence levels [23]. The diagnosis is confirmed by absence or severe decrease in the ERG response, which should be obtained in any infant with connatal blindness. There is no treatment. Many of these children have in the past been institutionalized.

Neonates with congenital blindness presumed to be due to Leber's may instead have congenital stationary night blindness [24]. Vision in these infants is quite poor at birth but improves under photopic conditions by 1–2 years of age. The ERG response, which is initially poor under both photopic and scotopic conditions, shows later improvement in photopic response. There is a tendency for myopia. These patients may exhibit a paradoxical pupillary response of constriction to darkness [25]. This can be a useful diagnostic sign in differentiating patients with congenital stationary night blindness from those with Leber's (Figure 13.5).

Retinitis Pigmentosa

Retinitis pigmentosa is a very heterogeneous group of conditions having as a common finding a dystrophy of the retinal pigment epithelium. Most patients with retinitis pigmentosa have a genetically inherited disease, with all types of hereditary patterns noted, but sporadic and presumably noninherited patients are known. Retinitis pigmentosa encompasses a very heterogenous group of abnormalities.

The pigmentary changes are usually present in the first decade of life, but there is much variability as to the time of onset, with changes in some patients becoming evident in the first year of life and others in the second and third decades. The earliest retinal signs are fine spots of pigmentation and depigmentation (the classic "salt and pepper fundus"). The later typical ophthalmoscopic appearance is a

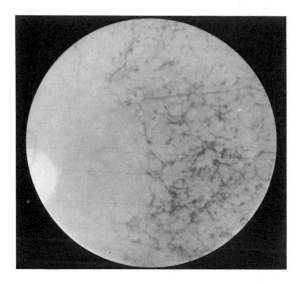

Figure 13.5. The typical bone spicule pigmentary clumping in the midperiphery of the retina and the attenuation of retinal vessels are typical of retinitis pigmentosa. (Reprinted with permission from LJ Press and BD Moore. Clinical Pediatric Optometry. Boston: Butterworth–Heinemann, 1993;159.)

"bone spicule" pigmentary retinopathy, with small areas of dark pigment in stellate patterns, interspersed with whitish areas of depigmentation in the midperipheral areas of the retina. This geographic retinopathy gradually spreads anteriorly and posteriorly, resulting in a widening ring scotoma visual field defect. Choroidal sclerosis develops later. There are in addition many atypical forms of retinitis pigmentosa that may show widely variable ophthalmoscopic changes, even within the same families [26, 27]. It is important to keep in mind that the specific appearance of the fundus is not diagnostic as to the specific etiologic features or classification of the disease.

Histologically, the rods are first affected by the dystrophy of the pigment epithelium, leading to sclerosis of the retinal vasculature. The nerve fiber and ganglion cell layers are unaffected even late in the course of the disease process.

The ERG is an important diagnostic tool in both confirming the diagnosis and predicting the clinical course of patients with retinitis pigmentosa. There is an absent or subnormal ERG response in affected patients, and many female carriers of the X-linked variety may also show a subnormal B-wave. These changes in the ERG generally precede visual function and ophthalmoscopic changes.

There are several important syndromes exhibiting retinal pigment epithelial dystrophy. Usher's syndrome patients have pigmentary dystrophy along with hearing loss. They have an autosomal recessive inheritance pattern. Bardet-Biedl syndrome patients have pigmentary dystrophy along with mental retardation, hypogenitalism, polydactyly, and obesity [28]. Vision tends to be poor in these patients. Laurence-Moon syndrome is similar in ocular appearance but lacks the polydactyly and obesity [29] found in Bardet-Biedl patients.

Metabolic Tapetoretinal Degenerations

There are a large number of rare metabolic diseases that have as an ocular manifestation a pigmentary retinopathy [30]. François has divided these conditions into three primary classifications, based on the general biochemical abnormalities of lipid, carbohydrate, and protein metabolism. Other categorizations exist. These disorders usually follow an autosomal recessive inheritance pattern, although several appear to be X-linked recessive. Severe vision loss may occur early. The only common denominator is the presence of pigmentary retinopathy at some point in the course of the disease. These conditions are discussed in Chapter 15. Readers are directed to the work of François and others for a more detailed description of these generally rare disorders.

Juvenile Macular Degenerations

Although many of the conditions categorized under the general heading of juvenile macular degenerations do not become evident until well past the first or even second decade of life, they are of clinical importance even in much younger children. Therefore, brief descriptions of these conditions are included.

The diagnosis and classification of juvenile macular degenerations has been the source of considerable confusion over the years. The original macular disease described by Stargardt [31] consisted of an atrophic macular lesion and visual loss in several young patients in two families. This became known as Stargardt's disease. Several additional unrelated diseases with somewhat similar appearances were then subsequently included within the category of Stargardt's disease. Fundus flavimaculatus, originally thought to be a completely separate disease from Stargardt's, has a very different initial appearance, consisting of a variable number of white flecks that are visible in the fundus. Krill [32] eventually differentiated the various juvenile macular degenerations into a coherent scheme based on anatomic and electrophysiologic correlates. Krill's classification of the juvenile macular degenerations include X-linked retinoschisis, vitelliform macular degeneration, fundus flavimaculatus, and cone degeneration.

Electrophysiologic testing with the ERG and the electro-oculogram (EOG) is required for proper diagnosis of these conditions. Dark adaptation, visual evoked potentials, color vision assessment, and visual fields are also used in the diagnostic workup.

X-Linked Retinoschisis

X-linked retinoschisis is an X-linked recessive hereditary disease of males that results in a splitting of the nerve fiber layer of the retina [33]. Ophthalmoscopically, it is seen most frequently in the inferotemporal periphery and at the macula. There is a spoke-like pattern of cystoid macular changes that is very characteristic, but its appearance may be difficult to visualize early in the course of the disease. Peripherally, there is a visible splitting of the retina, with vessels present on the outer layer, and retinal holes on the inner layer. Retinal detachments and vitreous hemorrhages may be seen. The ERG shows a reduction in the B-wave with a normal A-wave remaining. Visual acuity is variable, depending on the extent of the retinoschisis, but tends to decrease over time. Retinal detachments occur up to, but not including, the ora serrata and are common in later stages. Progression may be quite slow, with good vision remaining in some patients even during the late adult years. Onset may begin at a very early age, but the condition may go undetected until visual loss occurs.

Best's Vitelliform Degeneration

Best's vitelliform degeneration is an autosomal dominant inherited disease with mixed expressiv-

ity and penetrance. The ophthalmoscopic appearance is a macular lesion that appears like a "sunny-side-up egg yolk" in the early stages. The lesion is sharply defined and cystic in appearance, with a yellow to orange color, which eventually "scrambles," leaving a pigmented macular lesion. It is only rarely unilateral. It is usually first noted between 3 and 15 years of age, often on routine examination, and there may be a complete absence of any symptoms or perhaps only a mild metamorphopsia on examination. The vision is normal or only slightly reduced until the yolk begins to scramble, when the acuity may decrease to the 20/200 level, but it is not unusual to maintain good visual acuity throughout life whether the yolk scrambles or not. Color vision may be affected even before acuity is seriously compromised, with a tritan defect being most commonly noted. ERG, peripheral visual fields, and dark adaptation are normal, but the EOG is abnormal even for phenotypically normal carriers. The EOG is the key diagnostic tool in this disease. There may be a diffuse abnormality of the pigment epithelium in these patients. Treatment is supportive and genetic counseling should be performed.

Fundus Flavimaculatus

Fundus flavimaculatus includes the original disease described by Stargardt. There are actually two forms that have distinctly different appearances in the earlier stages of the disease. These two forms have often been considered to be separate disease entities by some authors but are here treated as one. There is marked variability of the appearance of this disorder, and many authors differentiate the forms based solely on the ophthalmoscopic appearance [34].

The form that is generally called fundus flavimaculatus is an autosomal recessive inherited disease. The characteristic retinal lesions are large numbers of yellowish-white flecks of variable shape, size, and density. The lesions may become confluent over time, with the lesions becoming less distinct in color and border. New lesions continue to appear as old ones fade. They tend to be located mainly in the posterior pole and the equator.

Stargardt's disease is the second and more commonly seen lesion of fundus flavimaculatus. It appears between ages 8 and 14 as an atrophic macular degeneration, first with a decreased foveal reflex, then with a round, pigmented macular degeneration. It is progressive and usually lowers visual acuity to the 20/200 level. Histologically, there is a loss of photoreceptors and pigment epithelium in the perimacular area.

Many patients have both forms of retinal lesions during the course of their disease. Patients with only the retinal flecks may be spared significant visual loss unless a fleck directly affects the fovea. A few of these patients will, in addition, have a diffuse cone degeneration that appears similar to that of primary cone degeneration patients. This group of patients will show a reduced photopic and flicker ERG, as would be expected. Scotopic function is not impaired. Patients without the cone degeneration have normal or only slightly abnormal ERG responses. The EOG is usually, but not always, abnormal, and dark adaptation is slower than normal. Peripheral fields are generally intact. It is now thought that a massive accumulation of an abnormal lipofuscin material within the pigment epithelium is the metabolic cause of the disease [35].

Cone Degeneration

Cone degeneration is an uncommon juvenile macular degeneration that has an autosomal dominant hereditary pattern. The appearance of the macular lesion is usually that of a "bull's-eye," with a central, dark red area surrounded by a sharply defined ring of depigmentation. It appears similar to chloroquine retinopathy. Rarely, the lesion will show only pigment clumping and a diffuse atrophic macula instead of the bull's-eye. Attenuation of the retinal vessels and a peripheral pigmentary retinopathy and optic atrophy may be noted later.

Visual acuity deficits range from mild to severe (20/25–20/200) and there is usually some degree of progression. Photophobia and nystagmus are frequently noted. The level of vision loss is related to the degree of destruction of the photoreceptors. There are two patterns of photoreceptor involvement, one affecting only the cones, the other affecting both the rods and cones. Cone outer segment and pigment epithelial destruction may begin at a young age, with rod involvement, if any, beginning later in most cases. Peripheral fields tend to remain normal unless there is extensive rod involvement. Color vision is affected when visual acuity is still only mildly decreased. There seems to be an early propensity toward protan and deutan color defects, in contrast to many other macular diseases that show a tritan defect, but these patients often progress to severe tritan defects as well. There is an abnormality of the photopic ERG in all cone degeneration patients, with scotopic abnormalities in patients having simultaneous rod involvement. Dark adaptation, even in those with rod involvement, remains unaffected, as does the EOG.

EXUDATIVE RETINOPATHIES

Familial Exudative Vitreoretinopathy

Familial exudative vitreoretinopathy is a rare autosomal dominantly inherited disease that has clinical features that resemble aspects of ROP, Coats' disease, and peripheral uveitis [36]. Individual patients and probands may have clinical signs that vary from minimal occult disease to very severe ocular disease causing major visual loss. Although the disease may be progressive, many patients are asymptomatic and have minimal disease. Onset may occur in infancy or much later in the teenage years.

Fully manifested familial exudative vitreoretinopathy may present as dense vitreous membranes and subretinal and intraretinal exudation, particularly temporal to the ora serrata. A fold of retinal detachment temporally, which may appear very similar to ROP, is generally present when there is significant exudative retinopathy. Neovascular retinopathy may be found in this region beyond the age noted in ROP. Retinal detachment may occur at later stages of progressive disease. Three stages of the familial exudative vitreoretinopathy disease have been described. Treatment consists of laser photocoagulation and cryotherapy for proliferative retinopathy and retinal detachment (Figure 13.6).

Coats' Disease

Coats' disease is a type of retinal telangiectasia that is found most typically in young males. Coats' disease is usually unilateral. It may present at a very young age as a leukocoria. In the past, it was not

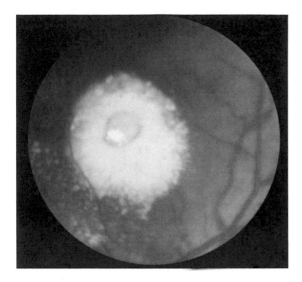

Figure 13.6. This patient with Coats' disease exhibits the typical retinal telangiectasia that is sometimes described as a "light bulb" lesion. These telangiectasias tend to leak subretinal exudates, which may become so massive that the patient first presents with a leukocoria. (Reprinted with permission from LJ Press and BD Moore. Clinical Pediatric Optometry. Boston: Butterworth–Heinemann, 1993;163.)

uncommon that these eyes were removed as a consequence of misdiagnosis of retinoblastoma. This is still an important diagnostic concern.

The primary retinal lesion is a telangiectatic retinal vessel or vessels in the periphery that is highly permeable. Vessels may show aneurysms, beading, anomalous arteriovenous communications, and loss of the surrounding capillary beds. A "light bulb"–appearing lesion may be present. The location of these lesions is often in the superotemporal quadrant of the retina [37]. The resulting exudation may be serous, hemorrhagic, or proteinaceous in nature or may be a combination. Eventually, it turns to a yellowish, subretinal, dense exudate that causes significant visual loss.

Treatment is directed at sealing off the telangiectatic vessels as early as possible with laser photocoagulation and cryotherapy. Retinal detachment is a not infrequent sequela of fulminant disease. Not surprisingly, eyes with less geographic involvement show the best results of treatment. Early, aggressive treatment can prevent serious visual loss.

RETINOPATHY OF PREMATURITY

ROP is a retinal vascular disease that is due to premature birth and very low birth weight. The disease was first recognized in the early 1940s [38], and shortly thereafter an association between the use of supplemental oxygenation and ROP was made [39]. This led to a reduction in the frequency and degree of supplemental oxygenation given to neonates, which decreased the incidence of ROP but led to increased morbidity and mortality. As the subspecialty of neonatology developed in the 1970s, many infants of low and very low birth weight were kept alive by the emerging technologies, which included greatly increased use and levels of supplemental oxygenation. There was, as a result of these advances, a significant increase in the incidence of ROP in these infants. We are today seeing many more infants with ROP than before, and this is likely to continue as neonates of very low birth weight are routinely kept alive. In addition, infants born to mothers that are substance abusers (particularly of crack cocaine) during their pregnancy, are at increased risk of prematurity and therefore more likely to develop ROP. There are recent estimates that up to 40% of infants with birth weights in the range of 1 to 1.5 kilograms and up to 50–80% of neonates under 1 kilogram may develop some degree of ROP [40, 41]. However, only a relatively small percentage of these neonates will experience significant visual loss [42].

The cause of ROP is thought to be due to the effects of high oxygen levels affecting immature retinal vascular tissue. There is an initial vasoconstriction of retinal vessels caused by increased oxygen levels in the blood due to supplemental oxygenation. This constriction leads to occlusion of the vessels if the arterial oxygen levels remain high enough. When this eventually returns to a more normal oxygen level, there is proliferation of vascular endothelium, leading to neovascularization and the typical clinical appearance of ROP [43]. There are also several other theories that have been proposed, but the final mechanism is not as yet certain. The degree of prematurity and the size of the neonate are probably more important factors in the cause and effect of ROP than is the level of supplemental oxygenation. Lighting in neonatal intensive care units has also been implicated as a possible factor in the development of ROP [44]. Regardless of the cause, we can expect to see more ROP in the future as these tiny infants are kept alive.

There have been several systems of classifying the appearance and the extent of retinal involvement of patients with ROP. The classification that is currently used is based on three main parameters—the location, the extent, and the staging of ocular changes brought about by the ROP [45]. The location is divided into three circumferential zones, with the center being the optic disc. Zone 1 extends just beyond the macula with an equal distance in other directions, zone 2 extends almost up to the ora serrata, and zone 3 is beyond that to the most anterior retina. The extent is based on hours of the clock. The staging is based on the severity of the retinal changes, especially at the junction of the temporal avascular retinal zone. Each succeeding stage shows the characteristics of the previous stages in addition to the more severe characteristics of its own. Stage 1 has a flat demarcation line between the vascular and avascular area. Stage 2 has a demarcation line that has mild elevation above the plane of the retina and early neovascular changes posterior to the demarcation line. Stage 3 shows a fibrovascular proliferation posterior to the demarcation line arising into the vitreous. Stage 4 shows partial retinal detachments, and stage 5 shows total retinal detachments. This system allows for a more exacting classification than its predecessors.

The classification described above is based on the appearance of the retinal changes that are visible. In actuality, it is often difficult to perform an adequate examination on a tiny, crying infant. Maximal pupillary dilation with a combination of phenylephrine (Neo-Synephrine) and cyclopentolate is essential. A thorough view of the fundus may then be obtained with indirect ophthalmoscopy. The Multicenter Cryotherapy Group has reported that the onset of ROP is likely to begin 32–42 weeks from the time of conception (median, 37 weeks) [46]. Infants should therefore be examined shortly after this time. It is necessary to follow infants at risk for ROP for 6 months or longer after birth, since the retinal changes are progressive during this period.

As just described, there is a junction or demarcation in the temporal retina between the area of vascularized and nonvascularized tissue. This junction tends to progressively advance until the entire retina becomes completely vascularized, which normally occurs sometime in the months after full-term birth. The vascularized retina appears relatively transparent, whereas the nonvascularized retina appears as a translucent or somewhat opaque whitish color. Milder stages of ROP appear as bud-like tips to the developing retinal vessels at the demarcation line amongst a yellowish band of intraretinal tissue. Larger vessels adjacent to the demarcation line may be tortuous at this point. Somewhat more severe ROP shows an elevation of tissue at the demarcation line, with neovascularization at this ridge beginning to develop. Fibroplasia and retinal detachments are the most severe manifestations and can lead to the classic appearance of the dragged disc in the temporal direction that is seen in severe cases. In addition to the retinal manifestations of ROP, patients tend to be moderately to severely myopic and have a high incidence of amblyopia, strabismus, cataracts, glaucoma, nystagmus, and corneal problems [47, 48].

Vitamin E therapy was suggested as a means of prophylaxis in neonates at risk for the development of ROP. This is based on the ability of vitamin E to neutralize oxygen free radicals that may cause cell damage to the developing retinal vasculature. Premature infants typically have reduced levels of vitamin E. Giving supplemental vitamin E may decrease this level of vascular damage. Several studies indicated that vitamin E supplementation significantly reduces the incidence and the degree of damage from ROP [49], but other studies have been less conclusive. Also, it is known that there are significant risks of toxicity to vitamin E in premature infants [50], including death. This issue is not as yet settled.

Surgical procedures to treat retinal detachment and fibrosis in the most severe forms of cicatricial ROP include closed and open-sky vitrectomy and scleral buckling. Retinal surgeons have advocated these procedures, but the results have been disappointing in many patients.

A promising treatment for ROP has been cryotherapy, which has been shown to significantly decrease the degree of retinal involvement in ROP patients [51, 52]. The specific indications and techniques of cryotherapy are evolving, and improvements in the ultimate outcome for affected patients appear likely.

CHOROIDAL HEMANGIOMA

There are two general categories of choroidal hemangiomas: those that are localized and those that are diffuse. They may present at birth or may not become apparent until later. The diffuse type is most commonly associated with Sturge-Weber disease and rarely with the Klippel-Trenaunay-Weber syndrome. It appears as a large, red lesion underlying or temporal to the macula. It may be stationary or slowly progressive. Visualization is difficult with the direct ophthalmoscope, since the border is quite indistinct. Dilated fundus examination with binocular indirect ophthalmoscopy is necessary for detection and diagnosis. There is an association with developmental glaucoma. A hyperopic shift in refractive error due to displacement of the macula forward may occur, leading to anisometropic amblyopia. Although isolated cases of choroidal hemangioma are seen, the presence of this lesion should arouse a strong suspicion of Sturge-Weber disease.

The localized type of choroidal hemangioma appears as an oval, raised, yellowish-red mass, usually in the posterior pole of the eye. There may be a pigmented rim. The overlying retina may take on a cystic appearance. Due to the risk of retinal detachment and cystoid macular degeneration, these patients should be closely followed.

CHOROIDEREMIA

Choroideremia is an uncommon, bilateral, progressive atrophy of the choroid and the retinal pigment epithelium. There is an X-linked recessive inheritance pattern, with full expression in males and incomplete expression in female carriers. Nyctalopia and visual field loss develops during childhood in males, along with a strikingly white fundus appearance due to a loss of pigmentation. Female carriers may show only a mild pigmentary change in the macular area.

REFERENCES

1. Desmonts G, Couvreur J. Congenital toxoplasmosis. A prospective study of 378 pregnancies. N Engl J Med 1974;290:1110–1116.
2. Hanshaw JB. Congenital cytomegalovirus infection: a fifteen year perspective. J Infect Dis 1971;123:555–561.
3. Stagno S, Pass RF, Alford CA. Perinatal infections and maldevelopment. In AD Bloom, LS James (eds), The Fetus and the Newborn. New York: Alan R. Liss, 1981;31–50.
4. Balfour HH. CMV retinitis in persons with AIDS: selecting therapy for a sight-threatening disease. Postgrad Med 1995;97:109–118.
5. Dennehy PJ, Warman R, Flynn JT, et al. Ocular manifestations in pediatric patients with acquired immunodeficiency syndrome. Arch Ophthalmol 1989;107:978–982.
6. Levin AV, Zeichner S, Duker JS, et al. Cytomegalovirus retinitis in an infant with acquired immunodeficiency syndrome. Pediatrics 1989;84:683–687.
7. Pagan RA. Ocular coloboma. Surv Ophthalmol 1981;25:223–236.
8. Jesberg DO, Schepens CL. Retinal detachment associated with coloboma of the choroid. Arch Ophthalmol 1961;65:163–173.
9. Pagan RA, Graham JM, Zonana J, et al. Coloboma, congenital heart disease, and choanal atresia with multiple anomalies:CHARGE association. J Pediatr 1981;99:223–229.
10. Scott JD. Congenital myopia and retinal detachment. Trans Ophthalmol Soc U K 1980;100:69–71.
11. Straatsma BR, Heckenlively JR, Foos RY, et al. Myelinated retinal nerve fibers associated with ipsilateral myopia, amblyopia, and strabismus. Am J Ophthalmol 1979;88:506–510.
12. Fulton AB, Craft JL, Howard RO, et al. Human retinal dysplasia. Am J Ophthalmol 1978;85:690–698.
13. Lahav M, Albert DM, Wyand S. Clinical and histopathologic classification of retinal dysplasia. Am J Ophthalmol 1973;75:648–6 67.
14. Pruett RC. The pleomorphism and complications of posterior hyperplastic primary vitreous. Am J Ophthalmol 1975;80:625–629.
15. Karr DJ, Scott WE. Visual acuity results following treatment of persistent hyperplastic primary vitreous. Arch Ophthalmol 1986;104:662–667.
16. Stickler GB, Becau PG, Farrel FS, et al. Hereditary progressive ophthalmo-arthropathy. Mayo Clin Proc 1965;40:433–455.
17. Opitz JM. Ocular abnormalities in malformation syndromes. Trans Am Acad Ophthalmol Otol 1972;76:1193–1196.
18. O'Connor PS. Achromatopsia, clinical diagnosis and treatment. J Clin Neuro-Ophthalmol 1982;2:219–226.
19. Price MJ, Thompson HS, Judisch GF, Corbett JJ. Pupillary constriction to darkness. Br J Ophthalmol 1985;69:205–211.
20. Krill AE. Congenital Color Vision Defects. In AE Krill (ed), Krill's Hereditary Retinal and Choroidal Diseases. Hagerstown, MD: Harper & Row, 1977;355–390.

21. Mizuno K, Takei Y, Sears ML, et al. Leber's congenital amaurosis. Am J Ophthalmol 1977;83:32–42.
22. Foxman SG, Heckenlively JR, Bateman JB, Wirtschfter JD. Classification of congenital and early onset retinitis pigmentosa. Arch Ophthalmol 1985;103:1502–1506.
23. Nickel B, Hoty CS. Leber's congenital amaurosis: is mental retardation a frequent associated defect? Arch Ophthalmol 1982;100:1089–1091.
24. Weleber RG, Cibis Tongue A. Congenital stationary night blindness presenting as Leber's congenital amaurosis. Arch Ophthalmol 1987;105:360–365.
25. Barricks ME, Flynn JT, Kushner BJ. Paradoxical pupillary responses in congenital stationary night blindness. Arch Ophthalmol 1977;95:1800–1804.
26. Krill AE, Archer D, Martin D. Sector retinitis pigmentosa. Am J Ophthalmol 1970;69:977–987.
27. Yee RD, Herbert PN, Bergsma DR, et al. Atypical retinitis pigmentosa in familial hypobetalipoproteinemia. Am J Ophthalmol 1976;82:64–71.
28. Lahav M, Albert DM, Buyukmihci N, et al. Ocular Changes in Laurence Moon Bardet Biedl Syndrome: A Clinical and Histopathologic Study of a Case. In MB Landers, ML Wolbarsht, JE Dowling, et al. (eds), Retinitis Pigmentosa. New York. Plenum, 1976;51–84.
29. Green JS, Parfrey PS, Harnett JD, et al. The cardinal manifestations of Bardet-Biedl syndrome, a form of Laurence-Moon-Biedl syndrome. N Engl J Med 1989;321:1002–1009.
30. François J. Metabolic tapetoretinal degenerations. Surv Ophthalmol 1982;26:293–333.
31. Stargardt K. Uber familiare, progressive degeneration in der maculagegend des auges. Graefes Arch Klin Exp Ophthalmol 1909;71:534–550.
32. Krill AE, Deutman AF. The various categories of juvenile macular degeneration. Trans Am Ophthalmol Soc 1972;70:220–245.
33. Yanoff M, Rahn EK, Zimmerman LE. Histopathology of juvenile retinoschises. Arch Ophthalmol 1968;79:49–53.
34. Bither PP, Berns LA. Stargardt's disease: a review of the literature. J Am Optom Assoc 1988;59:106–111.
35. Eagle RC, Lucier AC, Bernardino VB, Yanoff M. Retinal pigment epithelial abnormalities in fundus flavimaculatus. Ophthalmology 1980;87:1189–1200.
36. Criswick VG, Schepens CL. Familial exudative vitreoretinopathy. Am J Ophthalmol 1969;68:578–594.
37. Egerer I, Tasman W, Tomer TL. Coats' disease. Ophthalmology 1974;92:109–112.
38. Terry TL. Extreme prematurity and fibroplastic overgrowth or persistent vascular sheath behind each crystalline lens. I. Preliminary report. Am J Ophthalmol 1942;25:203–205.
39. Campbell K. Intensive oxygen therapy as a possible cause of retrolental fibroplasia: a clinical approach. Med J Aust 1951;2:48–50.
40. Flynn JT. A cohort study of transcutaneous oxygen tension and the incidence and severity of retinopathy of prematurity. Trans Am Ophthalmol Soc 1991;89:77–92.
41. Johnson LH, Quinn GE, Abbasi S, et al. Retinopathy of prematurity prevalence and treatment over a 20 year period at a Pennsylvania hospital. Doc Ophthalmol 1990;74:213–22.
42. Phelps DL. Retinopathy of prematurity: an estimate of vision loss in the U.S.—1979. Pediatrics 1981;67:924–926.
43. Patz A. Current concepts of the effects of oxygen on the developing retina. Curr Eye Res 1984;3:159–163.
44. Sission TRC. Hazards to vision in the nursery [editorial]. New Engl J Med 1985;313:445.
45. Committee for the Classification of Retinopathy of Prematurity. An international classification of retinopathy of prematurity. Arch Ophthalmol 1984;102:1130–1134.
46. Cryotherapy for Retinopathy of Prematurity Cooperative Group. Incidence and early course of retinopathy of prematurity. Ophthalmology 1991;98:1628–1640.
47. McCormick MC, Brooks-Gunn J, Workman DK, et al. The health and developmental status of very low birth weight children at school age. JAMA 1992;267:2204–2208.
48. Robinson R, O'Keefe M. Follow-up study on premature infants with and without retinopathy of prematurity. Br J Ophthalmol 1993;77:91–94.
49. Hittner HM, Godio LB, Rudolph AJ, et al. Retrolental fibroplasia: efficacy of vitamin E in a double-blind clinical study of preterm infants. N Engl J Med 1981;305:1365–1371.
50. Phelps DL. Vitamin E and retrolental fibroplasia in 1982. Pediatrics 1982;70:420–425.
51. Cryotherapy for Retinopathy of Prematurity Cooperative Group. Multicenter trial of cryotherapy for retinopathy of prematurity. Arch Ophthalmol 1989;106:471–479.
52. Cryotherapy for Retinopathy of Prematurity Cooperative Group. Multicenter trial of cryotherapy for retinopathy of prematurity: three-month outcome. Arch Ophthalmol 1990;108:195–204.

Chapter 14

Inflammatory and Traumatic Eye Disease in Children

Bruce D. Moore

ORBITAL DISORDERS

Proptosis

Although relatively uncommon in children, proptosis is an important sign of orbital disease (Table 14.1). The differential diagnosis of proptosis includes hemangioma, lymphangioma, dermoids, orbital cellulitis, hematoma, pseudotumor, craniostenosis, hyperthyroidism, trauma, and neoplasms, such as rhabdomyosarcoma. Enophthalmos of the fellow eye may be mistaken for proptosis. Conditions such as congenital glaucoma, megalocornea, or unilateral high myopia, which increase the anteroposterior diameter of the eye or the corneal diameter, may simulate proptosis. Proptosis may be stationary or progressive. Radiologic and neurologic consult is required if proptosis is suspected. An important consideration in proptotic eyes is the possibility of corneal exposure leading to keratitis and scarring. Lubrication of the eye is important to prevent this from occurring.

Orbital Inflammation

Most causes of orbital and periorbital inflammation are due to inflammation involving the surrounding tissues. The rigorous definition of orbital and periorbital cellulitis is often confused and used imprecisely [1]. The connective tissue membrane of the

orbital septum acts as a porous barrier between the periorbital and orbital tissues. The periosteum is a connective tissue that is contiguous with the dura and overlies the bones of the orbit. This comprises the major portion of the periorbital tissue. The orbital tissue lies within the periosteum and the periorbital tissues and consists of the globe itself and the areolar tissue and orbital fat surrounding the globe.

Periorbital cellulitis may be a precursor to the more serious orbital cellulitis and occurs much more frequently [2]. It may arise from a hordeolum, trauma, or systemic bacterial infection due to *Haemophilus influenzae* or *Streptococcus pneumoniae*. This must vigorously be treated with systemic antibiotics to prevent serious and potentially life-threatening sequelae.

Inflammation of the ethmoid sinus, dental abscess, dacryocystitis, and periorbital cellulitis are common causes of acute orbital cellulitis. *H. influenzae* and *S. pneumoniae* are the most prevalent bacterial agents cultured. The infected tissues must be drained and intensive antibiotic therapy initiated, or there is a serious risk of cavernous sinus thrombosis, meningitis, and brain abscess. These patients require hospitalization.

Cavernous sinus thrombosis presents as a severe orbital cellulitis, with the development of papilledema, decreased visual acuity, ophthalmoplegia, and various serious neurologic signs. This is a life-threatening condition requiring intensive treatment. Pseudotumor is a chronic orbital inflammation of uncertain etiologic features that often presents as a

Table 14.1. Types of Orbital Inflammation

Proptosis
Inflammatory causes
Orbital cellulitis
Periorbital cellulitis
Cavernous sinus thrombosis
Pseudotumor
Vascular causes
Capillary hemangioma
Lymphangioma

unilateral proptosis with limitation of extraocular muscle movement. Although it usually improves spontaneously, resolution is hastened when treated with systemic steroids.

The differentiation of these conditions depends on a combination of careful physical examination, laboratory studies, including blood workup, and imaging studies, including computed tomography and magnetic resonance imaging, along with evidence that the initial therapy is effective [3]. Therapy must be aggressive and follow-up is critical to ascertain resolution of the inflammation.

Vascular Anomalies of the Orbit

Capillary hemangiomas of the orbit are sometimes associated with related conditions of the skin and face. They develop rapidly during the early months of life, sometimes to impressive size, becoming deep red or purplish in color, intensifying in appearance when the child cries. Orbital capillary hemangiomas cause a pulsating proptosis. They generally regress spontaneously by age 4–7 years, but may linger longer in some cases. Management is conservative unless amblyopia occurs from the lid mass deforming the globe resulting in induced astigmatism [4]. Other important sequelae include dense amblyopia from eyelid closure or induced anisometropic refractive error and corneal exposure secondary to proptosis. Surgical intervention is avoided, since there is often direct vascular connection to the carotids, and the lesion may bleed profusely if disturbed. Direct injection with steroids is indicated if amblyopia or proptosis develops [5].

Treatment may be repeated as required, but the possibility of systemic involvement due to growth retardation should be considered.

Lymphangiomas are similar to capillary hemangiomas but are lymphoid in nature. They may cause unilateral proptosis, strabismus, and amblyopia. They tend not to regress and may require surgical intervention in extreme cases. Management is usually restricted to preventing amblyopia and the adverse effects of proptosis.

EYELID DISORDERS

Capillary Lid Hemangioma

These benign vascular tumors of the eyelids develop rapidly after birth. They exhibit abnormally rapid turnover of endothelial cells during the early proliferative stages of development of the hemangioma. They typically become evident during the second to fourth weeks of life and are only rarely present at the time of birth. Hemangiomas usually reach maximum size by 1–1½ years of age and then regress over the next 6–8 years. The size varies from a small patch of a millimeter or two on the upper lid to a massively disfiguring growth covering most of one side of the face. There is a predilection for the upper lid, and they are somewhat more common in females, being rarer in blacks than whites. Hemangiomas become darker red or blue in color when the child cries due to increased blood volume within the abnormal capillary bed. These vascular lesions are of significant ophthalmic concern because of the possible development of amblyopia by occlusion of the pupillary axis (causing deprivation amblyopia), or the effect of the tumor mass pressing against the globe and inducing anisometropic astigmatism, the axis perpendicular to the eyelid tumor mass [4]. The amblyopia is difficult to treat. The anisometropia must be optically corrected and occlusion therapy instituted as quickly as possible. The refractive error induced by the hemangioma is not reduced even after the hemangioma mass regresses.

Treatment is required if the tumor mass causes amblyopia. The current best method of treatment is direct steroid injection into the hemangioma [5]. This may be repeated if the mass does not regress.

In some patients, the results of steroid injection can be dramatic; in others it may be relatively ineffective. There is the potential of systemic steroid side effects, such as adrenal suppression and growth retardation, along with cushingoid effects. There have also been reports of eyelid necrosis following injection [6]. The capillary hemangioma is very fragile and has a propensity to show vascular breakdown and spontaneous massive bleeding. Most patients with lid hemangioma have a nearly complete resolution by age 7–10 years, the only significant ocular sequelae being amblyopia of varying degree. Some patients may exhibit redundancy of the skin overlying the region of the old tumor mass that may be of cosmetic concern to the parents and the child.

Blepharitis

Chronic blepharitis is a common disorder in children. It is typically caused by a combination of bacterial and seborrheic components, and treatment should be directed at both. *Staphylococcus aureus* and *Staphylococcus epidermidis* are the most common pathogens associated with blepharitis. Poor hygiene may predispose the child to chronic staphylococcus blepharitis. Clinical signs of chronic blepharitis include scaling of the eyelids at the base of the lashes, redness of the lid margins, purulent discharge, skin ulceration, and corneal involvement with inferior punctate keratitis. Additional signs found in long-term chronic cases include madarosis and trichiasis of the lashes, entropion and ectropion of the lids, and a thickening of the lid margins. There is often associated an inflammation or infection of the meibomian glands of the upper and lower eyelids.

The most effective treatment is hot compresses applied over the eye with a washcloth and lid scrubs with baby shampoo to loosen the scales and discharge and physically reduce the population of bacteria, along with massage of the eyelids to express any material from inflamed meibomian glands. Alternatively, commercial lid scrub preparations may be used, although they do not appear to be more effective than the simple and inexpensive use of baby shampoo. Topical antibiotic ointments applied several times per day during acute phases may also be considered when there is copious discharge or evidence of significant bacterial infection. Bacitracin and erythromycin ointments are both effective and rarely cause sensitization.

The concomitant use of topical steroids is somewhat controversial. The anti-inflammatory effects of steroids may hasten resolution, but the potential adverse effects of steroids include glaucoma, superinfection with resistant organisms, and the potential exacerbation of herpes simplex keratitis. Steroids should be reserved for those cases in which its use is clearly warranted, and only when very good follow-up is possible. Since blepharitis tends to be of a chronic nature, treatment is often directed at controlling rather than eliminating the disease.

Blepharitis may be due to seborrhea of the eyelids alone or a more generalized condition affecting the face, brow, and scalp. There is often an increase in meibomian secretions resulting in a foamy discharge collecting on the cilia and the lateral canthus. The meibomian glands tend to be full, and an oily discharge is readily expressed with direct pressure on the glands. Cases of pure seborrheic blepharitis will present without any associated keratitis or purulent discharge on the lashes or in the tear film, but there may be a particularly greasy appearance to the lids and lashes. There is usually a bacterial component present in patients with primary seborrheic blepharitis. The treatment for seborrheic blepharitis is similar to bacterial blepharitis, consisting of hot soaks, strenuous lid scrubs, and massage of the meibomian glands. Topical antibiotics are not required. Steroids may be of some benefit, but care must be exercised in their use.

Although blepharitis is usually thought of as a condition affecting patients older than young children, it is in fact relatively common to see affected young patients. Patients with trisomy 21 (Down syndrome) often have a chronic form of seborrheic blepharitis that is very resistant to treatment. This may lead to excessive rubbing of the eyes, which may directly cause the development of keratoconus [7]. As a result, the aggressive treatment of blepharitis in Down syndrome patients is warranted.

There are many less common inflammatory conditions of the eyelids that are seen in children. Patches of impetigo, which are caused by local infection by staphylococcal or streptococcal organisms, may be noted around the eyes. The patches are usually yellowish in color and vesicular and crusty in appearance. Treatment is by scrupulous hygiene, removal of the crusts, and topical antibiotic ointments. Primary herpes simplex blepharitis is usually clinically inapparent, but patients may present with a wet, ulcerative series of vesicles on the eyelids. Antiviral agents may be used to limit the duration of active inflammation. *Molluscum contagiosum* is a viral infection that presents as a nodular, umbilicated series of small lesions, usually at the upper eyelid or brow. They may precipitate a follicular conjunctivitis. Treatment is by incision of the lesions.

Hordeolum

Hordeolum is a common, acute infection (often by *S. aureus*) of the meibomian glands or the glands of Zeis and Moll's glands. Hordeolum presents as a local area of redness, pain, and swelling within the eyelid, often at the lid margin. The most effective treatment is hot soaks repeated several times a day. Topical antibiotics poorly penetrate the lesion and are of little value, unless there is an associated bacterial blepharoconjunctivitis. Hordeolum typically resolves within a week or so, with the lesion spontaneously opening up and draining, but occasionally a chalazion will result if drainage is incomplete. Very rarely, hordeolum will progress to a preseptal cellulitis, which requires aggressive medical intervention.

Chalazia

Chalazia are chronic granulomatous inflammations of the meibomian glands and are usually secondary to a hordeolum. They appear as a hard, mobile mass within the tarsus of the lid and are generally not painful. If they are very large, they may press on the globe, temporarily inducing an astigmatic refractive error with the axis perpendicular to the mass. In a young child, this could be amblyogenic if present for long. Treatment is initially by hot soaks several times per day. If this does not reduce the mass in a reasonable time period, local steroid injection or surgical removal is indicated. Recurrent hordeolum and chalazion occur in patients with poor hygiene and in patients with chronic seborrheic or infectious blepharitis or meibomianitis. Treatment in these patients must be directed at scrupulous daily lid hygiene.

Parasites

The crab lice (*Phthirus pubis*) and body and head lice may infect the eyelids and lashes. Sexual activity and poor hygiene increase the likelihood of infestation, but large-scale infestations have become very common in preschools and elementary schools through casual contact and sharing of articles of clothing by children. Lice cause itching of the lids and sometimes conjunctivitis secondary to metabolic waste products of the organism. Treatment is directed at removal of the nits and the use of ointment to poison the arthropods. Careful disinfection of contaminated bedding, clothes, and cloth toys with commercially available chemical products is required, as well as thorough and repeated shampooing with over-the-counter preparations.

DISORDERS OF THE CONJUNCTIVA (CONJUNCTIVITIS)

Ophthalmia Neonatorum

Neonatal conjunctivitis and keratoconjunctivitis caused by *Neisseria gonorrhoeae* have been significant historical problems. Before the use of Credé's prophylaxis (silver nitrate), which began about 100 years ago, there was widespread visual loss due to corneal infection by *Neisseria*. With routine use of silver nitrate drops at the time of birth, the incidence of neonatal *Neisseria* eye infection has been greatly reduced. Today, the threat of ophthalmia neonatorum by *Neisseria* has been partially overshadowed by the greatly increased incidence of neonatal ocular infection caused by chlamydia.

The prevalence of all types of venereal disease in sexually active individuals has increased greatly in recent years, due to changes in mores and society. In spite of routine ocular prophylaxis at the time of birth, there has been an increase in cases of neonatal conjunctivitis due to infection by both *Neisseria* and chlamydia. This may in some cases be due to improper instillation of medication into the baby's eyes, premature flushing of the medication from the eyes, or the accidental failure to use the medication at all. In many states, alternatives to the use of silver nitrate (which causes frequent but temporary chemical conjunctivitis of the newborn) include erythromycin and tetracycline ointments [8]. These ointments have some effectiveness against chlamydia in the eye, but not systemically, and may have reduced effectiveness against *Neisseria*. Hammerschlag has shown that silver nitrate and both erythromycin and tetracycline ointments are all relatively effective as prophylaxis for *Neisseria* but are not effective prophylaxis for chlamydia [9]. The best method of prevention of neonatal chlamydial conjunctivitis would be universal screening of all women during their prenatal care. However, this is not the case at this time in the United States. Ideally, all infants born of mothers with either *Neisseria* or chlamydia should be treated with a full course of topical and systemic antibiotics; however, many women with venereal disease go undetected, and the eye infection may not appear in the infant until after discharge from the hospital. This is even more true today when many women and newborns are released from the birthing hospital within 24 hours or less of birth. Furthermore, ocular prophylaxis may have the unintended effect of covering up the ocular clinical signs of chlamydial infection, allowing the systemic aspects of this disease to progress to a more serious level before detection and initiation of systemic treatment. To summarize, the issue of the best single dose prophylaxis against neonatal eye infection is not as yet completely settled.

All neonatal infections, both ocular and systemic, must be treated as a serious medical problem. Preliminary diagnosis can be made on the clinical signs, but cultures and sensitivities must be obtained for confirmation. The clinical signs are not always reliable. It is possible that the infant may have two or more agents that are responsible for the keratoconjunctivitis. Neonates have an immature immune system and reduced ability to fight off infection. Any infection can rapidly progress to a life-threatening state. The neonate with an eye infection should be under the care of his or her pediatrician during all phases of treatment.

Neisseria Gonorrhoeae Infection

One study has shown that, in selected populations, up to 10% of women are infected with *Neisseria* [10] at the time of delivery. Many of these women were asymptomatic and did not receive any prenatal or postnatal treatment, and some of these women received little or no prenatal care at all. There is undoubtedly a relationship between babies born infected with *Neisseria* and the use of illegal drugs by the mother, including crack-cocaine, during gestation. It is clear that the best means of prevention of venereal eye diseases in neonates is through much better prenatal care and effective screening and treatment of the mothers at risk [11].

Neisseria usually causes a bilateral (less commonly unilateral), hyperacute, purulent infection with lid edema, membrane or pseudomembrane formation, and the possibility of severe keratitis and corneal scarring leading to visual loss. The infection may in some cases be less severe, leading to misdiagnosis, unless culture results are obtained. *Neisseria* must be treated aggressively, usually in an inpatient hospital setting, with appropriate systemic and local antibiotics and support therapy. The mother must also be treated, and the appropriate public health authorities must be notified to track down the mother's sexual contacts. *Neisseria* infection in a neonate is a medical emergency requiring proper medical treatment. Failure to treat may result in severe corneal scarring and decreased vision or even to overwhelming systemic infection, leading to increased morbidity and mortality of the infant.

Chlamydial Conjunctivitis

The leading cause of neonatal conjunctivitis is now considered to be due to *Chlamydia trachomatis*. It may be responsible for one-third to one-half of all neonatal conjunctivitis [12]. It is the most common sexually transmitted disease in the United States. [13] Various studies have indicated that up to one-half of infants born to women with cervical chlamydial infection will become infected during passage through the birth canal [14].

Chlamydial infection presents as a unilateral or bilateral conjunctivitis of mild to moderate severity, and it is certainly less acute than *Neisseria* infection. There may be lid swelling, redness and chemosis of the bulbar and palpebral conjunctiva, papillary hypertrophy, and mild discharge. Mild corneal pannus and superficial punctate keratitis, usually superiorly, along with mild subepithelial infiltrates, may be seen later in the course of the infection.

Even though the initial presentation may be solely ocular, chlamydial conjunctivitis is properly considered part of a systemic infection. It is a leading cause of pneumonia, pharyngitis, otitis media, and vaginitis in the infected newborns [15]. Infants must be treated with both local and systemic antibiotics (erythromycin is generally used, not tetracycline, which can cause malformations in teeth and bones in infants), and the mother and her sexual contacts must also be treated with systemic antibiotics.

Other Causes of Neonatal Conjunctivitis

Many other bacterial organisms cause eye infections in neonates. Infants with compromised immune systems (due to various types of congenital immunodeficiencies, medications such as steroids, and human immunodeficiency virus [HIV] infection) are at increased risk of serious sequelae from otherwise mild ocular infections. *S. aureus* is a frequent cause of nosocomial infection in newborn nurseries. Although usually fairly mild in severity, immunocompromised infants may have serious complications. *S. pneumoniae* and *viridans*, *Escherichia coli*, and *H. influenzae* also may cause conjunctivitis in newborns [16]. *Pseudomonas aeruginosa* is a rare but serious cause of neonatal conjunctivitis primarily occurring in premature infants. It can rapidly lead to keratitis and a septicemia that may be life threatening. All of these organisms may be associated with serious systemic infection that requires aggressive medical treatment with appropriate local and systemic antibiotics.

Viruses are an infrequent cause of external eye disease in otherwise normal and healthy neonates. Infants, particularly those that are breast-fed, obtain a substantial degree of immunity from their mother for the first few months of life. Infants that are immunocompromised are at greatly increased risk of severe, disseminated, viral infection, which is completely different from the relatively harmless type of viral conjunctivitis commonly seen in normal children. The same is true for external fungal infections.

Conjunctivitis in Children Older Than Infancy

Bacterial Conjunctivitis

Bacterial conjunctivitis in young children is quite common. Most healthy children respond readily to topical antibiotics once the organism has been identified and the appropriate antibiotic agent is used. Cultures and sensitivities ideally should be obtained in all anterior segment ocular infections, but in practice cultures are usually obtained only when the infection proves resistant to the initial antibiotic used. By this time, however, accurate culture results are almost impossible to obtain due to the treatment itself.

The use of antibiotic ointments instead of drops is preferable in younger children because it is more certain that ointments actually get into the eyes of a struggling child than drops. Ointments also have a much longer contact time on the eye before they are flushed away by tears, leading to a higher level of drug reaching the locus of infection than with drops.

S. aureus is the most frequently encountered bacterial conjunctivitis in children. It presents as a mild to moderate conjunctivitis with redness and mucopurulent discharge and crusty lids, especially on awakening. If incompletely treated, it becomes chronic, often causing hordeola, chalazia, keratitis, and blepharitis. Treatment is with bacitracin, erythromycin, gentamicin, or tobramycin ointments 4 or 5 times a day for 1 week, with a follow-up visit to assess the efficacy of treatment. Gentamicin is best not routinely prescribed as a first choice antibiotic agent due to its potential toxicity to the corneal epithelium, causing punctate keratitis. Since sulfacetamide, even in topical instillation [17], has been linked with Stevens-Johnson syndrome (erythema multiforme), it should not be routinely used to treat mild external eye disease. It is also less effective than most standard antibiotics. Since chloramphenicol has been implicated as a cause of aplastic anemia in a few persons, its use should be restricted to those instances in which it is shown by culture and sensitivity to be required. When drops are indicated, polymyxin B sulfate (Polytrim) has become a good alternative due to its very wide spectrum and lack of toxicity. If a conjunctivitis is not resolving after the first course of antibiotics, another antibiotic should be instituted since resistance may have developed. It is also wise to make certain that the parent is using the medication appropriately.

Acute hemorrhagic conjunctivitis is caused by *S. pneumoniae* and *H. influenzae* bacteria and several types of adenoviruses. These occasionally cause epidemics of hemorrhagic conjunctivitis in preschool and school settings and are sometimes associated with important systemic disease. *S. pneumoniae* is said to be a more common cause of hemorrhagic conjunctivitis in northern regions of the United States with *H. influenzae* more common in the south, but there is little actual evidence to support this, and either organism can be a causative agent in hemorrhagic conjunctivitis. *H. influenzae* is an important cause of periorbital cellulitis and meningitis in young children. Vaccination for *H. influenzae* is now available and highly recommended for all young children as part of a complete immunization schedule.

External eye infections are caused by other bacteria, including enteric rods such as *E. coli*, *Serratia marcescens*, *Proteus*, *Klebsiella*, *Moraxella*, and *Pseudomonas*. Differentiation of these organisms is generally impossible without accurate cultures, since the clinical appearance is often nonspecific. The choice of an antibiotic agent should be based on cultures and sensitivities, but patients may initially be placed on a broad-spectrum antibiotic until the results are obtained.

Recurrent, external eye infections in young children should arouse suspicion of nasolacrimal duct obstruction. Evaluation for this by the Jones' test (instillation of fluorescein on the surface of the eye and checking for transit through the ducts into the nostril with a cotton-tipped applicator) should be performed. Broad-spectrum antibiotic ointments are prescribed for acute episodes of conjunctivitis.

Patients with external infectious eye disease that are immunosuppressed, whether from congenital and hereditary causes or acquired due to treatment of underlying disease, must be treated aggressively to guard against superinfection, with potentially catastrophic results. Included in this category are patients undergoing treatment for various neoplastic diseases (especially following bone marrow transplantation), any of the primary immunodeficiency disorders, and HIV infection.

Viral Conjunctivitis

In general, viruses are the most common cause of external eye infections in children beyond the age of infancy. Epidemics of various adenoviruses are often encountered in preschools. Viral conjunctivitis secondary to a systemic viral illness is also common. Less common are primary herpes simplex and *molluscum contagiosum* infection. Treatment for all viral conjunctivitis, except that caused by herpes simplex, is palliative in nature. Immunosuppressed patients can develop both external and internal ocular infections from a host of viruses, especially herpes simplex and zoster. Aggressive viral therapy with topical agents, such as trifluridine (Viroptic) or vidarabine (VIRA-A) and systemically with acyclovir is required. Concomitant use of topical and systemic steroids is advocated by some, but not all, authorities.

Conjunctivitis Caused by Sexually Transmitted Diseases

Particularly in older children, the possibility of sexually transmitted diseases, such as chlamydia [18], *Neisseria*, and herpes, must always be considered. Eliciting a positive history may be nearly impossible, but should be attempted when suspected. The presence of a confirmed, sexually transmitted eye disease in a younger child should arouse a strong suspicion of sexual abuse. This must be carefully followed up and the appropriate social service agency must be contacted. Systemic treatment is essential in all of these diseases. Penicillin is the drug of choice in *Neisseria* infection. Chlamydia is treated with systemic tetracycline in patients older than 8 years who are not pregnant, and with systemic erythromycin in those patients not able to use tetracycline because of the risk of dental and bone defects in young children.

Allergic Conjunctivitis

Vernal conjunctivitis is a relatively severe, usually seasonal allergy that primarily affects young males. It is associated with itching that may be severe, burning and redness of the conjunctiva, and a marked papillary response of the upper tarsus and possibly the limbus. Initial treatment is with vasoconstrictors and systemic and topical antihistamines, with mast cell inhibitors, and topical, nonsteroidal anti-inflammatory agents and topical steroids added as needed for more severe cases. The condition usually subsides during late adolescence, but may prove to be almost incapacitating for some patients.

The milder form of atopic conjunctivitis may occur in up to 20% of the population. This is often associated with other atopic conditions, including eczema, asthma, and hay fever. Treatment is with topical vasoconstrictors, antihistamines, desensitization, and only rarely with topical steroids. Symptoms are often more severe than the clinical appearance of papillae, chemosis, and injection of the conjunctiva would seem to indicate.

DISORDERS OF THE CORNEA (KERATITIS)

Corneal infections may begin as a routine conjunctivitis or blepharitis and spread to the cornea due to compromise of the integrity of the corneal epithelium. Prompt treatment of the blepharitis or conjunctivitis may prevent a more serious infection. The presenting signs of a corneal infection are likely to include discharge, conjunctival injection, tearing, photophobia, and behavioral changes in the young child. There may also be a generalized, systemic illness.

Examination of children, particularly of infants and toddlers, is more difficult than for adults. Adequate slit-lamp examination is important, and, with persistence, is possible on most children, especially if a hand-held, portable slit-lamp is available. A complete set of cultures is mandatory before any treatment is initiated. If the practitioner is unable to manage this in an office setting, referral to an appropriate source is essential. Serious visual loss may be prevented by prompt diagnosis and treatment.

Bacterial Keratitis

S. aureus is the most common cause of bacterial keratitis. There is often associated blepharitis or conjunctivitis, and there may be a history of prior incomplete treatment. It may present in several ways. An inferior, superficial epithelial punctate keratitis is the most common and least severe presentation. Chronic cases may include a marginal corneal ulcer that is mediated by an antigen-antibody type of reaction and is usually sterile, at least initially. There is a clear area of normal corneal tissue between the limbus and the lesion, the so-called lucid interval. These lesions can be quite painful, and there may be considerable injection of the adjacent bulbar conjunctiva. A different hypersensitivity reaction may cause the formation of a phlyctenule at the limbus. Treatment of these staphylococcus infections is with topical antibiotics and possibly steroids. The most serious form of staphylococcal keratitis is a central corneal ulcer. It is associated with a red, painful eye, photophobia, mucopurulent discharge, and sometimes hypopyon. Aggressive treatment with topical or systemic antibiotics, or both, should be started only after cultures and scrapings are obtained. The fluoroquinolones and fortified aminoglycosides are generally the antibiotics of choice.

S. pneumoniae and *H. influenzae* both cause hemorrhagic conjunctivitis and, less commonly, keratitis in children, particularly during the winter months. *P. aeruginosa* keratitis can occur due to the use of contact lenses or contaminated eye drops. Both *Neisseria* and *Pseudomonas* can rapidly destroy the cornea, and must be treated very aggressively in an inpatient hospital setting.

Viral Keratitis

Herpes simplex keratitis is the leading cause of visual acuity loss due to corneal infection. Many cases of mild herpetic keratitis are made much worse by the inappropriate shotgun use of antibiotic-steroid combinations for red eyes by primary care providers. By the time that the child is finally seen by an eye doctor, there is severe dendritic herpes keratitis. Infants have adequate maternal antibody protection for approximately 6 months after birth. Over the next 5 years of life, 90% of children will develop a systemic or ocular primary herpes infection, with only a relatively small percentage going on to develop a secondary ocular infection. Current treatment uses trifluridine and debridement of the ulcer.

Keratitis caused by adenovirus infection is frequently seen in children along with acute follicular conjunctivitis. Systemic involvement commonly includes upper respiratory infection and pharyngitis. Epidemic keratoconjunctivitis causes a punctate keratitis and subepithelial opacities that may linger for months, causing a mild degree of temporarily decreased visual acuity. These lesions may be prolonged by the use of steroids, which should generally be avoided, unless the presence of subepithelial infiltrates is so extensive that visual acuity is severely affected. Varicella keratitis secondary to chickenpox is not uncommon. It may manifest as a mild, superficial punctate keratitis or as limbal vesicles with corneal infiltrates and mild vascularization in adjacent cornea that may progress to a disciform keratitis. There may rarely be an anterior uveitis. Treatment is generally not required, but topical steroids may be used if symptoms warrant.

Other Causes of Keratitis

Mycotic infections are occasionally seen in patients that are immunosuppressed. These infections are usually severe and may result in overwhelming systemic infection and death. The indiscriminate use of topical and systemic steroids may precipitate mycotic infection of the cornea and conjunctiva. Any infection that proves resistant to standard therapy or is clinically difficult to diagnose should arouse some suspicion of mycotic or amebic involvement. *Acanthamoeba* has become a significant concern as a pathogen in patients wearing soft contact lenses, particularly for extended-wear contacts and contacts worn while swimming in fresh water and should be considered in patients presenting with serious keratitis.

DISORDERS OF THE UVEA (UVEITIS)

Uveitis is an inflammation of the uveal tract of the eye (Table 14.2). The uvea is composed of the iris, ciliary body, and the choroid. Uveitis causes a number of pathologic changes in the vasculature of the uvea. These changes include a leakage of protein and inflammatory cells into the aqueous and vitreous, which appear as flare and keratic precipitates (KPs). The degree of flare and KPs is somewhat proportional to the degree and type of inflammation

Table 14.2. Causes of Uveitis

TORCH
Kawasaki's disease
Juvenile rheumatoid arthritis
Lyme disease
Systemic lupus erythematosus
Crohn's disease
Intermediate uveitis
Toxocara infection
Human immunodeficiency virus infection
Histoplasmosis
Trauma

TORCH = *t*oxoplasmosis, *o*ther (including especially syphilis), *r*ubella, *c*ytomegalovirus, and *h*erpes simplex.

of the tissue. KPs are often classified as "fine KPs" or "mutton-fat KPs," depending on their size and appearance. The uveal tissue may also become swollen and thickened. The combination of exudate and swelling can cause adhesions between the iris and cornea (anterior synechia) and the iris and lens (posterior synechia), which can be temporary or permanent. Under certain conditions, a posterior synechia can impair the drainage of aqueous, causing acute glaucoma. Chronic uveitis can lead to the formation of membranes of inflammatory debris that can block the pupillary axis and lead to a reduction in visual acuity. This can also occur at the ciliary body, creating a "snowbank" of inflammatory cells inferiorly, and may lead to detachment of the choroid or pars plana. A similar process in the choroid can lead to necrosis of both the choroid and adjacent retina, causing visible scarring and visual field loss.

The general symptoms of uveitis include pain, tearing, photophobia, and decreased visual acuity. Pain may be surprisingly absent in young patients with even severe uveitis, particularly in peripheral or intermediate uveitis (pars planitis), so it is not as good an indicator of uveitis as in adults. Photophobia may be a more significant symptom in children, even in cases of mild uveitis. Young children with chronic uveitis may exhibit decreased visual acuity due to inflammatory material in the ocular media and to lens and corneal opacification. Amblyopia and strabismus can therefore directly result from this inflammation, particularly if the uveitis is unilateral and chronic.

The signs of uveitis include flare, cells, and KPs in the aqueous and vitreous, anterior and posterior synechiae, chorioretinal lesions, and band keratopathy in chronic (especially from juvenile rheumatoid arthritis [JRA]) uveitis. Cataracts and vitreous membranes develop in response to chronic or severe acute uveitis. Intraocular pressure (IOP) is usually low in juvenile uveitis, except for those with iris bombe or massive anterior chamber membranes that may block the drainage of the aqueous.

The treatment of uveitis includes the use of topical steroids and cycloplegic agents. Dosage is titrated based on the initial severity of the inflammation and the response to the medication. The steroids should be tapered when the uveitis begins to resolve. Care must be exercised to minimize the total amount of steroids because of the potential for cataract formation, the development of glaucoma, and the concern over adrenal suppression and growth retardation. Generally, these are of significant concern only when the medication must be maintained for extended periods of time. Occasionally, systemic steroids may be required, especially in cases of posterior and peripheral uveitis.

Congenital-Onset Uveitis

True congenital uveitis is uncommon, but when it does occur, it is usually associated with disseminated congenital infections that are of a serious nature. The signs, symptoms, and nature of these congenital infections are much more severe than those of the acquired infections of these same agents later in life, and the consequences to the child much graver. These patients are relatively uncommon, however, for these are sick infants with generally poor outlooks. The acronym TORCH (*t*oxoplasmosis, *o*ther [including especially syphilis], *r*ubella, *c*ytomegalovirus [CMV], and *h*erpes simplex) comprises the leading cause of congenital infection and uveitis. Serum antibody titers may be obtained from the mother and neonate when there is suspicion of infection to help confirm the diagnosis.

Congenital toxoplasmosis is first acquired by the mother during pregnancy, often by eating contaminated, poorly cooked meat or during the cleaning of a cat litter box with cat feces that are contaminated

with the *Toxoplasma gondii* organism. The earlier the transmission of the organism to the fetus during fetal development, the greater the severity of infection, but the incidence of transmission is greater with maternal infection during later pregnancy [19]. Most infected infants have no manifest disease. In its most severe form, the infant may have multiple neurologic manifestations, including mental retardation, microcephaly, intracranial calcifications, seizure disorder, strabismus, and nystagmus. The child may be born prematurely and have failure to thrive. The chorioretinal lesions are similar to the more typical late reactivated form, and there may be a severe to mild anterior uveitis.

Congenital CMV infection is among the more common intrauterine infections [20]. The neonate with congenital CMV infection may be born prematurely with low birth weight and may have jaundice, hepatitis, hepatosplenomegaly, thrombocytopenic purpura, and pneumonia. Multiple neurologic manifestations, including mental retardation, microcephaly, hydrocephalus, seizure disorders, and strabismus, are typical. Chorioretinal lesions may appear similar to those of toxoplasmosis, but more likely appear as small, discrete white foci with overlying vitreous haze that lead to small, pigmented chorioretinal scars. The infection can be passed through the fetal circulation from the mother or may be acquired during transit through the birth canal. The drug ganciclovir has proven useful in treating the retinopathy resulting from CMV infection. Infants born with manifestations of congenital CMV infection invariably have more fulminant disease than those initially asymptomatic.

Herpes simplex type II is transmitted to the neonate during passage through the birth canal. Systemic manifestations are similar to that of CMV, with the addition of encephalitis. Within the eye, a hazy media with patches of grayish white chorioretinal focal lesions and areas of retinal hemorrhage are seen. These lesions cause pigmented scarring of the retina. Treatments currently include ganciclovir for CMV and acyclovir for herpes, with other experimental drugs being actively investigated.

Congenital rubella infection results in uveitis, retinal pigment abnormalities, cataracts, deafness, microcephaly, and mental retardation. Congenital syphilis causes interstitial keratitis, chorioretinitis, and a variety of neurologic abnormalities, but has become rather rare.

Acquired Uveitis

Kawasaki's Disease

See Chapter 15 for a discussion of Kawasaki's disease.

Juvenile Rheumatoid Arthritis

JRA is a fairly common inflammatory disease of the joints that can have serious ocular manifestations in children. There are estimates of about 200,000 children with JRA in the United States [21]. The prevalence in another study was estimated at 64 to 113 per 100,000 [22]. Uveitis may occur in 14–34% of patients with JRA [23]. Onset of the disease can occur in infancy, with the diagnosis often difficult to make. The initial presentation often appears as a skin rash with fever of undetermined origin. Joint disease may not be evident in some patients during pediatric examinations for the rash and fever. The first sign may be noted when the child shows increasing difficulty with movement, possibly to the extent that the child suddenly is unable to move at all. The degree of joint swelling ranges from minimal to severe. Histocompatibility antigens and antinuclear antibody (ANA) testing may help in the diagnosis, but a thorough pediatric physical examination should allow for clinical diagnosis. The etiologic cause is uncertain, but is thought to have an autoimmune component.

Clinically, JRA is divided into three groups based on the number of joints that are involved. Patients with pauciarticular JRA have five or fewer joints involved and are the least likely to have serious, systemic manifestations. This condition is more common in females by a ratio of approximately 3 to 1. Patients with polyarticular JRA have more than five but less than most joints involved. Patients with systemic JRA have almost all joints involved and are most likely to develop systemic manifestations in addition to their joint disease [24]. Ocular involvement is most common in the pauciarticular form with the very highest incidence of ocular involvement in young girls with pauciarticular JRA and positive ANA titers.

Ocular involvement does not necessarily follow a time course similar to systemic involvement. The ocular inflammation can be unilateral or bilateral, although not necessarily at the same time. Ocular symptoms may be surprisingly absent. Patients with acute inflammation often present without any complaints. The uveitis tends to show more flare than cells, but this is not pathognomonic. The ocular inflammation may, in some cases, precede the onset of joint or systemic disease by years. Acute or chronic anterior uveitis usually precedes the secondary effects of chronic inflammation, such as synechiae, cataracts, and band keratopathy [25]. Posterior synechiae can occur quickly in the course of the uveitis and may even occur in the absence of significant cells and flare. Cataracts form due to a combination of the chronic inflammation and the treatment with steroids. The cataracts require surgical removal when visual acuity drops below functionally useful levels. There may be vitreous haze or a pupillary membrane, or both, that arises from the inflammatory cells within the anterior chamber. Both can have an effect on vision similar to that of secondary membranes after cataract extraction. Band keratopathy is a frequent result of the uncontrolled, long-term uveitis that these patients manifest. In unilateral or asymmetric bilateral cases, the threat of amblyopia must always be considered in young children.

The uveitis in JRA is invariably difficult to control with topical agents. It is routine to require steroids for years to minimize the inflammation to a "tolerable" level, since complete control of the uveitis may be impossible during childhood. Steroid-induced glaucoma must be considered during treatment. The goal of the treatment is to taper the dosage to the minimal level possible without encountering a flare-up of the inflammation. Concomitant use of cycloplegic agents is usually required. The refractive effects of the long-term use of these cycloplegic agents must be considered; near adds should be prescribed when appropriate. Constant attention to amblyopia must always be kept in mind.

Systemic treatment is initially by the use of high doses of nonsteroidal anti-inflammatory drugs. In a small number of patients, gold therapy and hydroxychloroquine (Plaquenil) are added. Hydroxychloroquine has significant toxicity to the retina; patients must be closely followed for color vision and Amsler's grid changes along with pigmentary changes to the retina, cornea, and lens.

All patients with the pauciarticular form of JRA must be followed for ocular involvement at 3- to 6-month intervals to monitor for silent flare-up of ocular disease. Patients with the other forms of JRA should be followed about every 6–9 months.

Lyme Disease

Lyme disease has been occasionally confused with JRA. The disease is caused by a spirochete and is spread by ticks. It was first described in 1975 in Lyme, Connecticut, but appears to now be widely distributed around the United States and Europe. Lyme disease is a multisystem disorder that includes a bull's-eye–appearing skin rash, flu-like symptoms, arthralgia, and, late in its course, cardiac and neurologic disease. There are also a number of eye findings, including conjunctivitis, anterior and posterior uveitis, retinal vasculitis, pseudotumor and optic neuritis, and keratitis [26]. The ocular complications are quite variable, except for the conjunctivitis, which is a common sign of the disease. Any patient with acute arthritic symptoms should be evaluated for Lyme disease.

Systemic Lupus Erythematosus

Systemic lupus erythematosus (SLE) is a multisystem disease that primarily affects females. Like JRA, the specific etiologic cause of SLE is uncertain, but is also thought to be an autoimmune disease. Most patients exhibit the presence of ANAs. The major systemic effects include joint inflammation; various skin problems; and necrosis of the heart and peripheral vasculature, kidneys, and brain. Death may result due to these causes. The ocular manifestations include retinal vascular disease, cotton-wool spots, papilledema, and, less commonly, chronic anterior uveitis. Systemic treatment is similar to that of JRA patients, with the frequent use of antimalarial agents such as hydroxychloroquine and steroids. These patients should be followed at least yearly, even in the absence of eye disease, particularly if they are taking steroids or hydroxychloroquine. Although onset is typically in adolescence or later, earlier onset is occasionally seen.

Crohn's Disease and Ulcerative Colitis

Crohn's disease and ulcerative colitis are inflammatory diseases of the lower gastrointestinal tract that may include acute anterior uveitis. These conditions are occasionally associated with JRA. Episcleritis, corneal ulcers, and scleritis have also been reported [27]. These patients often require long-term use of systemic steroids to control their gastrointestinal disease. They need to be followed about every 6–9 months for the potential ocular sequelae of the steroid treatment and the possibility of occult uveitis.

Intermediate Uveitis

Intermediate uveitis, also called pars planitis or peripheral uveitis, affects the region of the pars plana and the ciliary body. It is most prevalent in young boys 4–5 years of age. Its onset is insidious, and it may not become apparent until the child fails a school vision screening, with badly decreased visual acuity, or on examination by a pediatrician unable to find a red reflex. It is almost always bilateral.

There is usually a paucity of symptoms, such as photophobia or pain, and absence of signs of conjunctival or limbal injection. Posterior synechiae almost never occur. There may be a dense, postlenticular cyclitic membrane composed of inflammatory cells and a fibrotic response within the vitreous, which is the prime cause of the decreased vision. A "snowbank" of white inflammatory debris and collagen is located in the area of inflammation at the inferior pars plana. There is a definite three-dimensional quality to this mass. Additionally, there may be retinal edema of the nerve fiber layer and the macula, which can affect vision.

The disease tends to be chronic, with periods of quiescence and flare, during which the density of the postlenticular cyclitic membrane varies along with its effect on vision. Cataracts may occur from the chronic inflammation. There is an increased risk of late retinal detachments and retinoschises. There is a tendency for the disease to lessen in intensity by around age 10–15 years. There may be only minimal residual vision loss due to the membrane and the cataracts. Amblyopia caused by the opacified membrane at earlier ages must be considered, particularly if there is asymmetry in the density of the membranes.

Treatment is with the use of the minimal dosage of topical and systemic steroids that decreases the inflammation to a tolerable level. It is usually impossible to completely rid the eye of all signs of inflammation, and one must consider the effects of long-term use of steroids on the patient.

Uveitis Due to Trauma

By far the most common cause of anterior uveitis in the pediatric population is trauma. This can be due to accident or to abuse. Most eyes that have received mild to moderate degrees of concussive force develop a low-grade and self-limited anterior uveitis. These eyes will improve rapidly with or without treatment by topical steroids and cycloplegics. Care must be exercised to be certain that there is no further ocular damage (e.g., angle recession and microscopic hyphema) that is inapparent on initial examination.

Band Keratopathy

Band keratopathy is a calcific degeneration of the cornea that occurs after chronic anterior uveitis or as a sequela of an alkaline burn to the cornea. It appears as a grayish to milky-white opacification at about Bowman's layer and initially is concentrated at the nasal and temporal limbus. There may be a lucid interval at the limbus due to the absence of Bowman's layer at the limbus. It eventually may extend centrally, but is almost always less dense centrally than peripherally, and is clearer superiorly and inferiorly. It occurs most commonly secondary to chronic anterior uveitis due to JRA. Band keratopathy may cause reduced visual acuity when the opacification becomes centrally located. Treatment is by chelation with ethylenediaminetetraacetic acid (EDTA), which can dramatically clear the cornea. Patients with uncontrolled, long-term, anterior uveitis may require repeated treatments by chelation.

Uveitis Due to Acquired Cytomegalovirus and Acquired Immunodeficiency Syndrome

The severe congenital form of CMV disease is discussed in "Congenital-Onset Uveitis." The acquired form of CMV ocular disease previously was only rarely seen. It appears as discrete, usually white, chorioretinal lesions that may be pigmented and that are smaller than those of toxoplasmosis. These are areas of necrosis of all layers of the retina. There may be considerable vitreous haze adjacent to the chorioretinal lesions. CMV disease is seen primarily in immunosuppressed patients, especially in conjunction with acquired immunodeficiency syndrome (AIDS). The appearance of the disease in these patients, both young children and adults, is much more severe than those without AIDS [28]. Instead of the relatively discrete lesions that are seen in non-AIDS patients, the eyes of some pediatric AIDS patients have been described as looking like "pizza," with enormous amounts of exudates and hemorrhage covering large areas of the fundus. Other patients, at least initially, show a milder form of eye disease, with smaller areas of retinal thickening, cotton-wool spots, and hemorrhage and vitritis [29]. CMV ocular disease is the leading cause of blindness in AIDS patients, and the systemic effects of CMV have become a major factor of death in these patients. Death within 2–3 years appears likely in patients having developed CMV retinitis. Ganciclovir and foscarnet are currently the primary treatments for CMV retinitis, but since this is a rapidly developing area of treatment, considerable change in treatment protocols is to be expected.

Glaucoma Secondary to Uveitis

Glaucoma is an important consideration in children with chronic or acute uveitis. Glaucoma can occur as a result of blockage of the trabecula by inflammatory cells and debris or by neovascularization of the angle. Iris bombe and angle closure due to inflammation may also cause secondary glaucoma. JRA is a relatively frequent cause of this type of glaucoma [30]. It must be remembered that the primary treatment for most forms of uveitis is topical or systemic steroids, which by themselves can cause glaucoma, making it somewhat unclear if it is the uveitis, the treatment, or more likely a combination of both that precipitates the glaucoma. Regardless of the cause, the treatment consists initially of medical therapy followed when needed by surgical intervention.

TRAUMA

Epidemiology of Eye Injuries

Ocular trauma is the most common cause of acquired blindness in children. Eye injuries are reported two to four times as often in boys than girls, probably due to the greater statistical likelihood of boys being involved in rougher sports and play than girls. In a study by Nelson [31], the most frequent cause of eye injury was accidental or intentional trauma by another child, followed by sports-related injuries. Injuries were more frequent during the spring. Nonperforating anterior globe injuries, such as corneal abrasions and foreign bodies, and anterior segment contusion injuries were the most common category of injuries, followed by extraocular injuries such as lid lacerations, ecchymosis, and orbital fractures. Perforating injuries to the globe and posterior segment injuries were less frequently noted.

Assessment of the Traumatized Eye

The major difference in the assessment of a child's traumatized eye compared with that of an adult revolves around the difficulty in examining a child crying, scared, and in pain. A complete evaluation is imperative in order to arrive at the proper diagnosis; an incomplete examination may lead the examiner to a dangerously misleading conclusion.

The first step in the assessment should always be to obtain a thorough history from the parent or person who is accompanying the child. If there is any indication of head or systemic injury in addition to the eye trauma, first aid should be applied and the child transported to a hospital for complete neurologic and systemic evaluation. Details of the history must be carefully recorded for medico-legal purposes. A history that is not consistent with the physical findings must arouse a suspicion of child abuse, and should be dealt with appropriately.

An attempt should always be made to assess visual acuity in each eye by an age-appropriate procedure. Infants can be assessed by subjective techniques such as fixation preference, ability to fix and follow, or simply by pupillary responses. Objective techniques, such as preferential looking, optokinetic nystagmus, and visual evoked potentials, may be too time consuming or impossible to undertake on a crying child but should be attempted if feasible. The child's general mental and physical state should be assessed. A careful evaluation of pupillary responses, eye movements and position, the integrity of the globe and adnexa, and a slit-lamp examination of the anterior segment should follow. Pupils should not be dilated during the initial phase of the evaluation because this renders a thorough neurologic evaluation impossible. Only after neurologic assessment has been performed can the pupils be dilated by, preferably, a short-acting agent. Examination by binocular, indirect ophthalmoscope and slit-lamp should then be performed through the dilated pupil. IOP can be measured by slit-lamp mounted tonometer or a hand-held applanation tonometer. If this proves impossible, a comparison of ocular rigidity by palpation should be done. If it proves impossible to perform a complete examination on a screaming child, a consideration of referral to a hospital and examination under anesthesia should be made.

Types of Ocular Trauma

Birth Trauma

Estimates of the frequency of ocular injury due to the process of birth range up to 25% of all births and up to 50% of difficult births [32]. Only a small percent of these injuries are apparent, and an even smaller percentage have any lasting significance, but some of these injuries may lead to ocular complications and visual loss that may prove difficult to diagnose later.

The most commonly noted ocular sequelae of birth is a chemical conjunctivitis that is secondary to the instillation of silver nitrate drops for ocular prophylaxis at birth. Silver nitrate may cause ecchymosis of the eyelids and chemical conjunctivitis, occasionally severe enough to swell the lids shut. This clears within a few days of birth. Conjunctival hemorrhages are frequently noted at birth, more often in difficult deliveries, but they are seen even in easy deliveries. They are of no significance.

Mild edema and ecchymosis of the eyelids is seen fairly often just after birth, particularly in difficult deliveries. Rarely, traumatic ptosis of the upper lid occurs after difficult delivery or as a result of the use of forceps. If ptosis is severe enough to cause closure of the eyelid, deprivation amblyopia and induced axial myopia should be considered [33]. Eversion of the lids at birth has been reported. This may resolve spontaneously, or may require surgical intervention.

Corneal injury from forceps delivery can lead to serious ocular complications. This type of corneal trauma may appear as faint vertical striae or ruptures in Descemet's membrane or as a more generalized, denser corneal opacity of large size. This resemblance to congenital glaucoma may complicate the diagnosis. The density of the opacity usually decreases over a period of several weeks, but some degree of scarring and striae usually remain. These opacities can lead to large degrees of corneal astigmatism, myopia, and amblyopia [34]. Infants with corneal birth trauma most be closely monitored for these refractive problems and should be treated aggressively for amblyopia.

Retinal hemorrhages occur frequently, even in uncomplicated deliveries. The incidence is lowest in cesarean sections and greatest in long, traumatic vaginal births. In most cases, the hemorrhages resolve completely within 1–2 weeks of birth. Rarely, a macular hemorrhage in the foveal area may cause amblyopia [35]. Vitreous hemorrhages have also been reported. The effect of these hemorrhages may mimic that of a congenital cataract if they do not spontaneously resorb soon after birth. Dense vitreous hemorrhages may require early surgical intervention.

Blow-Out Fracture of the Orbit

Blow-out fractures of the orbit result from serious ocular trauma to the bony areas surrounding the globe. The area most commonly affected is the ethmoidal plate and the area of the infraorbital groove, but any of the surrounding bony structures can be affected as well. Symptoms include pain at the point of injury; pain on eye movement; loss of sensation over the cheek; and diplopia, blurred vision, or both. Signs include ecchymosis, enophthalmos, limitation of ocular movement, especially on attempted up-gaze, and ptosis. Nausea and vomiting may occur. It is important to note that there is great variability in the presentation of patients with a blow-out fracture, with some having an essentially occult presentation.

Many patients experience apparent weakness of the inferior rectus muscle due to the mechanical effects of the orbital fractures, including complete incarceration of the muscle. Elevation and depression of the eye is impaired, and strabismus and ptosis may occur. Radiologic evaluations are helpful in confirming the diagnosis and deciding on the most appropriate treatment. Surgical intervention may be required, but determination of the proper treatment is best left to the surgeon.

Ocular Trauma Caused by Superficial Foreign Bodies

Superficial foreign bodies are a common acute pediatric problem. The child presents with epiphora, blepharospasm, and crying. Assessment of visual acuity is expedited by the use of an anesthetic eyedrop, but a measurement of visual acuity without an anesthetic should be attempted first for medicolegal reasons. Either slit-lamp examination or inspection of the anterior segment with loupes will allow a visualization of the superficial foreign body or a corneal abrasion. Complete eversion of both eyelids is important. Be certain that there is no visible penetration of the globe.

Foreign bodies can be removed by irrigation, cotton swabs, fine gauge needles, or a spud. Extreme care must be exercised to prevent further ocular trauma to the eye during removal with a sharp instrument. If the child is not controllable, the foreign body removal may need to be performed while the child is under anesthesia, but most children can be steadied by the parents or ancillary help. A broad-spectrum antibiotic ointment should be applied for prophylaxis against bacterial infection. Pressure patching may reduce the symptoms and increase the rate of epithelialization, but many children object more to the patch than the eye discomfort. The eye should be rechecked the following day. Scarring is unlikely to occur, unless the foreign body penetrates deep into the stroma.

Ocular Trauma Caused by Chemical Burns

Chemical burns are a true ocular emergency requiring immediate first aid in order to minimize the potentially catastrophic results. Regardless of the type of chemical that has gotten on the eye, the initial treatment is the same, namely copious flushing of the eye with water. Acids tend to precipitate out corneal proteins on contact, which actually limits the amount of damage that they cause, due to both a buffering effect and a physical barrier to further penetration into the corneal tissue.

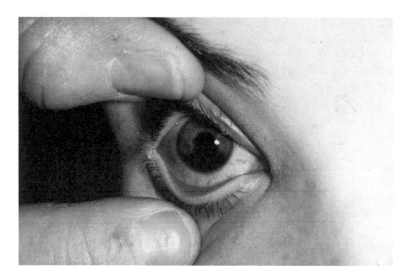

Figure 14.1. Blood in this patient's anterior chamber is easily visible. Contusion injuries severe enough to cause hyphema place the eye at future risk for angle recession glaucoma. Hyphema may also result in bloodstaining of the cornea, leading to impairment of corneal functioning. (Reprinted with permission from LJ Press, BD Moore. Clinical Pediatric Optometry. Boston: Butterworth–Heinemann, 1993;205.)

Alkalies, on the other hand, tend to penetrate very deeply and can cause necrosis of tissue even days after the initial burn. In general, alkalies cause far more damage than acids to the eye. The degree of damage is related to the strength of the alkali and the length of time before the alkali is completely neutralized or flushed from the eye. There are four levels of alkali injury to the anterior segment of the eye: Level 1 shows generalized epithelial involvement and a red eye; level 2 shows a white eye with blanching of vessels in the conjunctiva; level 3 shows a glassy cornea with stromal involvement; and level 4 shows a white, ground-glass appearance. There is a likelihood of an IOP rise shortly after the injury. The use of topical steroids is very controversial because they may increase the activity of corneal collagenase, increasing the level of corneal damage, and also may decrease resistance to secondary infection. Steroids, however, do decrease inflammation and corneal pannus. Citrate solution has recently been recommended in the initial stages as a means of increasing collagen development. Extreme care must be taken to avoid secondary infections due to the massively disrupted ocular surface.

Ocular Contusion Injuries

Traumatic Uveitis.   Mild ocular contusion can lead to a conjunctival hemorrhage or a traumatic iritis. Both of these tend to resolve spontaneously, with few symptoms and no sequelae. Occasionally, the iritis may be more severe, with considerable photophobia as a presenting symptom. The pupil may be either miotic or mydriatic and sluggish, cells and flare present to varying degrees, and the IOP is usually lower than the nonaffected eye. The examination should include gonioscopy if there is any evidence of an angle recession or if the IOP is increased. The presence of an angle recession raises the prospect of the development of glaucoma at some point in the future. Treatment of uncomplicated traumatic iritis is with a combination of cycloplegic agents and topical steroids, with frequent rechecks for hyphema, IOP increases, and secondary infections from corneal abrasions.

Hyphema.   More severe contusion to the eye can lead to angle recession and hyphema, along with retinal contusion (Figure 14.1). Hyphema is usually caused by a tear in the iris root or the iris stroma and is often associated with angle recession. The anterior chamber fills with blood, either partially or completely, obscuring the view of the iris. In general, the greater the height of blood in the anterior chamber, the greater the risk of long-term visual acuity loss. Rebleeding after initial partial or complete resolution of the hyphema also makes the prognosis for full recovery poorer. In the past, children with hyphemas were invariably hospitalized on complete bed rest, with both eyes patched, but many children are now sent home with bed rest alone. These patients must be followed very closely, as often as daily, until the risk of rebleeding is past (at least 1–2 weeks). The use of cold compresses in the immediate post-trauma period have been advocated by some, but studies have not confirmed its efficacy.

The use of aspirin has been found to greatly increase the risk of rebleeding and is no longer used as part of the treatment [36]. Aminocaproic acid has been advocated, but there are significant side effects from the drug, and its routine use in the treatment of hyphema is still uncertain [37]. The major complications of hyphema are blood staining of the cornea, with a reduction in visual acuity and corneal health, and sharp rises in IOP, which can be very difficult to control. This is greatly complicated by the presence of significant degrees of angle recession. The trauma may also be severe enough to cause anterior and posterior synechiae. Less commonly, the lens may become subluxated, leading to severe visual acuity loss from optical causes and iris bombe-type glaucoma. Cataracts are a fairly frequent sequela of trauma to the eye that may not become significant until long after the injury. This is perhaps the most common type of acquired cataract in children.

Traumatic Glaucoma.   Trauma is the leading cause of all glaucomas in children, with hyphema being the single most important predisposing event. Several specific factors increase the risk of development of secondary glaucoma: the size of the hyphema, the occurrence of rebleeding, and the presence of significant angle recession. Treatment includes paracentesis of the anterior chamber and trabeculectomy along with medical treatment. Angle recession without hyphema may cause glaucoma soon after the injury or many years later. The greater circumference of angle that is recessed, the greater the risk of glaucoma. If three-fourths of the angle is involved, glaucoma at some point in the future is almost assured.

Retinal Trauma.   The most frequently seen retinal disorder resulting from ocular contusion injury is Berlin's edema, or commotio retinae. This typically appears in the posterior pole region, particularly at the macula, and can result in a significant decrease in visual acuity. The retina in the affected area becomes cloudy, with a whitish haze, except at the fovea, which usually retains its reddish col-

oration. This change in fundus appearance is thought to be due to a disruption in the architecture of the outer segments of the photoreceptors, and is not due to actual extracellular retinal edema. It is usually easiest to observe the borders of the injury, with the surrounding tissue maintaining its normal appearance. Commotio retinae is almost always self-limited, with resolution over a period of days or weeks, but there can be retinal pigmentary changes and a loss of vision if the macula is affected. More severe injury to the retina can cause flame-shaped hemorrhage in the nerve fiber layer, rupture of Bruch's membrane leading to large atrophic scars, and rhegmatogenous retinal detachments and its typical sequelae. Occasionally in young children, the visual acuity of the traumatized eye may be affected by the retinal edema, leading to strabismus and amblyopia. The retina may subsequently heal, leaving no visible evidence of the cause of the amblyopia and strabismus.

Penetrating Ocular Injury.   Penetrating injury to the eye is a true ocular emergency. The major risk, in addition to the direct effects of the injury itself, is that of secondary endophthalmitis. Penetrating intraocular foreign bodies may be seen with a slit-lamp or binocular indirect ophthalmoscope, but special imaging techniques may be required for a complete diagnosis. Depending on the material and the location of the foreign body, surgery to remove it may or may not be necessary. Rupture of the globe can be caused by a severe contusion injury. There may be a hyphema in addition to the rupture, significantly worsening the prognosis. Penetration by sharp objects can lead to a variety of injuries, including corneal and scleral lacerations, hyphema, puncture of the lens and a leakage of lens material into the aqueous and vitreous, and retinal damage. Endophthalmitis is a serious risk in this situation. First aid can be applied, but these patients need to be admitted to a tertiary care facility for evaluation and treatment.

Prevention of Ocular Injury

The best method of improving the prognosis in all types of ocular trauma is by prevention of the injury itself. Many pediatric eye injuries are easily preventable by the use of adequate eye protection during any activity that puts the eye, and the child, at risk. For example, in the 1960s, many children in the United States and Canada experienced serious eye injuries while playing ice hockey. Through the efforts of eye doctors, such as Dr. Paul Vinger [38, 39], protective face masks were made mandatory for all players, resulting in an enormous decrease in the incidence of eye injuries. Similar results in racquet ball sports have occurred more recently. There is no excuse for not recommending proper eye protection when it is warranted. It is our responsibility as eye doctors to continue to urge all patients to wear proper protection during both work and play. Excellent-fitting sports and work eye wear is now readily available in all sizes, and lenses of polycarbonate plastic, which is extremely resistant to breakage, are in common use. Patients should be clearly informed of the availability and importance of proper protective eye wear. Furthermore, any monocular patient should wear such protection at all times. It is important for both legal and ethical reasons that all monocular patients be so informed!

Child Abuse

Any inexplicable or improbable eye injury to a child should lead the examining eye doctor to consider child abuse as a potential cause. The incidence of physical child abuse is now recognized as being much higher than previously thought. It has been estimated that as many as 40% of all children that are physically abused may show ocular signs [40]. The specific types of ocular injuries run the gamut from periorbital ecchymosis (black eye), corneal abrasions and lacerations, hyphema and angle recession, cataracts and dislocated lenses, to all sorts of retinal injuries, including total detachments. Suspicion should be aroused when the history does not agree with the physical findings or when the history is inconsistent or illogical. A frequent history of ocular or systemic injuries should also arouse suspicion of abuse. An additional and very important sign of child abuse lies in the child's behavior itself. As one who comes in contact with large numbers of children, the pediatric optometrist learns through experience when a child's behavior seems questionable. Child abuse may also take the form of sexual and emotional abuse. Unusual behavior patterns are likely to be evident in abused children [41]. It is

very important to pursue your suspicions by carefully questioning the child and parent. You have a legal and moral responsibility to immediately report those suspicions to the appropriate state or local authorities. Rapid reporting of all suspected child abuse is mandatory, and the reporter is protected by law in all states from any liability (see Chapter 18 for a thorough discussion of this important topic).

REFERENCES

1. Shapiro ED, Wald ER, Brozanski BS. Periorbital cellulitis and paranasal sinusitis: a reappraisal. Ped Infect Dis 1982;1:91–94.
2. Gellady AM, Shulman ST, Ayoub EM. Periorbital and orbital cellulitis in children. Pediatrics 1978;61:272–277.
3. Gold SC, Arrigg PG, Hedges TR. Computerized tomography in the management of acute orbital cellulitis. Ophthalmic Surg 1987;18:753–756.
4. Robb RM. Refractive errors associated with hemangiomas of the eyelids and orbit in infancy. Am J Ophthalmol 1977;83:52–58.
5. Kushner BJ. Local steroid therapy in adnexal hemangioma. Ann Ophthalmol 1979;11:1005–1009.
6. Sutula FC, Glover AT. Eyelid necrosis following intralesional corticosteroid injection for capillary hemangioma. Ophthalmic Surg 1987;18:103–105.
7. Pierse D, Eustace P. Acute keratoconus in mongols. Br J Ophthalmol 1971;55:50–54.
8. American Academy of Pediatrics. Prophylaxis and treatment of neonatal gonococcal infections. Pediatrics 1980;65:1047–1048.
9. Hammerschlag MR, Cummings C, Roblin PM, et. al. Efficacy of neonatal ocular prophylaxis for the prevention of chlamydial and gonococcal conjunctivitis. N Engl J Med 1989;320:769–772.
10. Armstrong, JH, Zacarias F, Rein MF. Ophthalmia neonatorum: a chart review. Pediatrics 1976;57:884–892.
11. Schachter J. Why we need a program for the control of chlamydia trachomatis [editorial]. N Engl J Med 1989;320:802–803.
12. Rapoza PA, Quinn TTC, Kiessling A, Taylor HR. Epidemiology of neonatal conjunctivitis. Ophthalmology 1986;93:456–461.
13. Centers of Disease Control. Chlamydia trachomatis infections: policy guidelines for prevention and control. MMWR CDC Surveill Summ 1985;34(Suppl)3S:53S–74S.
14. Hammerschlag MR, Anderka M, Semine DZ, et al. Prospective study of maternal and infantile infection with chlamydia trachomatis. Pediatrics 1979;64:142–148.
15. Schachter J, Grossman M. Chlamydial infections. Ann Rev Med 1981;32:45–61.

16. Sandstrom I. Treatment of neonatal conjunctivitis. Arch Ophthalmol 1987;105:925–928.

17. Genvert GI, Cohen EJ, Donnenfeld ED, Blecher MH. Erythema multiforme after the use of topical sulfacetamide. Am J Ophthalmol 1985;99:465–468.

18. Greydanus DE, McAnarney ER. Chlamydia trachomatis: an important sexually transmitted disease in adolescents and young adults. J Fam Pract 1980;10:611–615.

19. Desmonts G, Couvreur J. Congenital toxoplasmosis. A prospective study of 378 pregnancies. N Engl J Med 1974;290:1110–1116.

20. Hanshaw JB. Congenital cytomegalovirus infection: a fifteen year perspective. J Infect Dis 1971;123:555–561.

21. Baum J. Epidemiology of juvenile rheumatoid arthritis. Arthritis Rheum 1977;20:158–160.

22. Andersson Gare B, Fasth A. Epidemiology of juvenile chronic arthritis in southwestern Sweden: a 5-year population study. Pediatrics 1992;90:950–958.

23. Arnason JA, Bell CL. Juvenile rheumatoid arthritis: current concepts and practice. J Pediatr Ophthalmol Strabismus 1995;32:383–385.

24. Spiera H. Rheumatic diseases in children. J Pediatr Ophthalmol Strabismus 1982;19:103–107.

25. Wolfe MD, Lichter PR, Ragsdale CG. Prognostic factors in the uveitis of juvenile rheumatoid arthritis. Ophthalmology 1987;94:1242–1248.

26. Aaberg TM. The expanding ophthalmologic spectrum of Lyme disease. Am J Ophthalmol 1989;107:77–80.

27. Petrelli EA, McKinley M, Troncale FJ. Ocular manifestations of inflammatory bowel disease. Ann Ophthalmol 1982;14:356–360.

28. Levin AV, Zeichner S, Duker JS, et al. Cytomegalovirus retinitis in an infant with acquired immunodeficiency syndrome. Pediatrics 1989;84:683–687.

29. Dennehy PJ, Warman R, Flynn JT, et. al. Ocular manifestations in pediatric patients with acquired immunodeficiency syndrome. Arch Ophthalmol 1989;107:978–982.

30. Kanski JJ. Uveitis in juvenile chronic arthritis: incidence, clinical features and prognosis. Eye 1988;2:641–645.

31. Nelson LB, Wilson TW, Jeffers JB. Eye injuries in childhood: demography, etiology, and prevention. Pediatrics 1989;84:438–441.

32. Duke-Elder S. System of Ophthalmology (Vol 14). St. Louis: Mosby, 1972;9–17.

33. Hoyt CS, Stone RD, Fromer C, et al. Monocular axial myopia associated with neonatal eyelid closure in human infants. Am J Ophthalmol 1981;91:197–200.

34. Angell LK, Robb RM, Berson FG. Visual prognosis in patients with ruptures on Descemet's membrane due to forceps injury. Arch Ophthalmol 1981;99:2137–2139.

35. Isenberg SJ. The Eye in Infancy. Chicago: Year Book, 1989;381.

36. Crawford JS, Lewandowski RL, Chan W. The effect of aspirin on rebleeding in traumatic hyphema. Am J Ophthalmol 1975;80:543–545.

37. Kraft SP, Christianson MD, Crawford JS, et al. Traumatic hyphema in children. Ophthalmology 1987;94:1232–1237.

38. Vinger PF. Sports injuries, a preventable disease. Ophthalmol 1981;88:108–113.

39. Vinger PF. The Eye and Sports Medicine. In TD Duane, EA Jaeger (eds), Clinical Ophthalmology. Philadelphia: Lippincott, 1987;1–39.

40. Harley RD. Ocular manifestations of child abuse. J Pediatr Ophthalmol Strabismus 1980;17:5–13.

41. Smith SK. Child abuse and neglect: a diagnostic guide for the optometrist. J Am Optom Assoc 1988;59:760–765.

Chapter 15

Ocular Manifestations
of Systemic Disorders

Bruce D. Moore

This chapter describes systemic disorders of young children that have important ocular manifestations. Many of the more commonly seen conditions are discussed elsewhere in the text. A number of conditions that are quite rare and unlikely to be seen in a general practice are also discussed in this chapter because they are important for the clinician to be aware of. Finally, several relatively common systemic conditions that have not been discussed elsewhere in this text are presented here.

CYSTIC FIBROSIS

This autosomal recessive disease is considered to be the most common serious genetically based disorder in white patients. The disease occurs in about 1 in 2,000 whites, and the gene is present in approximately 5% of individuals. It is less common in black and Asian populations.

Many organ systems are affected. Pancreatic insufficiency leads to widespread endocrine and exocrine dysfunction, resulting in malabsorption and malnutrition in some individuals. The mucous glands are grossly affected, causing severe chronic pulmonary problems. Abnormal sweat glands hyperexcrete various minerals, providing a simple clinical method of diagnosis. Patients with cystic fibrosis require constant antibiotic and respiratory therapy to reduce the greatly increased risk of pneumonia, a significant cause of early mortality. The life expectancy of cystic fibrosis patients has in-

creased in the past few decades through the use of prophylactic measures such as antibiotics, pancreatic enzymes, and vitamins, allowing patients to survive into adulthood and occasionally middle age. The specific gene locus has been identified, bringing new hope of a definitive cure using genetic engineering techniques. Lung transplantation is also being developed as an endstage therapy.

Cystic fibrosis can affect the eyes and visual system in several ways. Malabsorption of vitamin A can lead to xerophthalmia [1] and night blindness [2], which is both preventable and reversible with vitamin A supplementation. Retinal edema, retinal vascular changes, macular cystic changes, and papilledema have been reported. Because of the abnormal mucus, lipid, and sweat excretions [3], the composition of the tears may be abnormal as well. Cystic fibrosis patients wearing contact lenses tend to have increased levels of deposits on their lenses that appear to be both mucoid and mineral in nature. Vigorous cleaning with an alcohol-based cleaner is helpful in extending the useful life of lenses.

INFLAMMATORY COLLAGEN AND CONNECTIVE TISSUE DISEASES

The most common of these conditions in the pediatric population is juvenile rheumatoid arthritis (JRA). The incidence is estimated at 9.2–19.6 per 100,000 [4]. JRA is a major cause of anterior uveitis in children. Onset may be in infancy, and diagnosis may be difficult. It is not unusual to see patients with acute uveitis whose pediatrician has not considered the diagnosis of JRA. The uveitis, which is difficult to control, is treated initially with topical steroids and cycloplegic agents. Medications are tapered and titrated until the minimal dosage that reduces the wheal-and-flare reaction to an acceptable level is found. It is likely that the medications will need to be used over many years. The cumulative effects of this long-term steroid use are glaucoma and cataracts in a significant number of patients. Because of the potential for insidious late onset of eye disease, it is important that all patients with JRA, particularly the pauciarticular form (affecting five or fewer joints), be followed periodically (at least every 3–6 months), even in the absence of ocular disease.

Ankylosing spondylitis causes inflammatory disease of the sacroiliac joints. A more disseminated arthritis may also be present. Ankylosing spondylitis most commonly affects males in the second decade of life, but the disorder can appear earlier. The human leukocyte antigen (HLA)-B27 is usually present and is very helpful in making the correct diagnosis. Uveitis is the primary manifestation of ocular involvement.

Lupus erythematosus is a necrotic condition affecting various organ systems. Antinuclear antibodies are likely to be present, indicating that lupus is an autoimmune disease. Females are affected much more frequently than males. Ocular manifestations include retinal vascular disease, uveitis, and dry eyes.

Reiter's syndrome mostly affects adolescent and young adult males; it is rare in younger children and in females. The cause is uncertain, but may be autoimmune. A relationship to a history of severe diarrhea and to venereal diseases, particularly chlamydial and gonococcal diseases, may exist. HLA-B27 is often present. The major manifestations of the syndrome include pauciarticular arthritis, urethritis, and conjunctivitis. Uveitis and keratitis may also be associated with this syndrome.

Kawasaki's Disease

Kawasaki's disease is also known as mucocutaneous lymph node syndrome. It was originally described in Japan, where it has been diagnosed quite frequently. Evidence indicates that it is distributed more widely around the world than previously thought, but is often misdiagnosed. The condition most commonly affects young children.

Kawasaki's disease is characterized by a persistent high fever, maculopapular truncal rash, "strawberry tongue," desquamation of the skin at the fingertips, and lymphadenopathy [5]. The most serious complication is a form of coronary vasculitis that may lead to death in approximately 2% of patients. The primary ocular effects are an occasionally severe conjunctivitis without mucopurulent discharge, without anterior uveitis, and, in a few cases, without a mild vitritis.

The etiology of the disease is mysterious. Environmental contaminants have statistically been implicated, particularly those related to carpet cleaning. A retrovirus has been tentatively identified as a possible causative agent [6], but much uncertainty surrounds this idea. A form of toxic shock syndrome has also been theorized as a possible cause. Steroids, gamma globulin, and aspirin are widely used in the treatment of Kawasaki's disease. Any young child presenting with fever, rash, reddened tongue, and severe conjunctivitis should be strongly suspected of having Kawasaki's disease and should have an immediate workup by his or her pediatrician.

Ehlers-Danlos Syndrome

Ehlers-Danlos syndrome is an autosomal recessive disorder characterized by hyperextensibility of skin and joints and kyphoscoliosis. Patients may exhibit a number of urogenital and vascular abnormalities. The ocular manifestations include epicanthal folds, blue sclera, keratoconus, ectopia lentis, angioid streaks, choroidal hemorrhages, and disciform macular degeneration.

Pseudoxanthoma Elasticum

This autosomal recessive disease features a yellowish, thickened discoloration of the skin of the neck, orbit, limbs, and abdomen. Vascular complications, including telangiectasias, hypertension, and peripheral vascular insufficiency, may occur. Typical ocular manifestations include angioid streaks and chorioretinal degenerations.

Marfan's Syndrome

This autosomal dominant condition quite commonly is seen in clinical practice and has significant ocular effects. Patients are generally of tall and thin stature, with frequent and severe kyphoscoliosis and hyperextensibility of the joints. Patients may have aortic aneurysms, which can spontaneously dissect, leading to early sudden death. All patients suspected of having Marfan's syndrome (including any patient with ectopia lentis) should have a cardiovascular evaluation for this potential problem. The major ocular manifestations include ectopia lentis, high to extreme myopia and astigmatism, retinal detachments, cataracts, megalocornea, amblyopia, and strabismus.

Weill-Marchesani Syndrome

Ectopia lentis and high myopia are the most common ocular defects in this autosomal recessive disorder. Patients tend to be of short stature, in contrast to patients with Marfan's syndrome. The likelihood of an anteriorly displaced lens causing pupillary block glaucoma is greater in Weill-Marchesani than in Marfan's syndrome.

SKIN DISORDERS

Ichthyosis

This condition has been classified into several categories based on the hereditary pattern [7]. All subtypes present with dry, scaly skin. The scaling may be very extensive and appear similar to the scales of fish, giving the condition its name. Ectropion, chronic conjunctivitis, keratinization and papillary hypertrophy of the conjunctiva, corneal stromal opacities, and corneal epithelial opacities have been reported. An extreme form of ichthyosis noted at birth has been called the "collodion baby condition" [8]. In this condition, a parchment-like membrane completely covers the neonate. This then desquamates over a period of weeks or months. Visual acuity is usually unaffected in patients with ichthyosis.

Juvenile Xanthogranuloma

Patients with juvenile xanthogranuloma develop yellowish or reddish-brown papules on the skin of the scalp and face during infancy. The ocular manifestations include infiltrates of the uveal tract leading to recurrent hyphemas in some patients.

Erythema Multiforme

Erythema multiforme (Stevens-Johnson syndrome) is a disease of uncertain origin that causes a severe, occasionally fatal inflammatory process, primarily affecting the skin and mucous membranes. The condition may be triggered by infection or the use of drugs and is probably immune-complex mediated. Various sulfa drugs have been specifically implicated and several cases have been traced to the use of topical sulfacetamide for mild external eye disease [9]. The disease may cause severe ocular complications [10], including ulcerative conjunctival lesions, symblepharon and cicatricial scarring of the conjunctiva, entropion and trichiasis of the lids, and corneal ulceration and opacification. Marked visual loss is not uncommon in severe cases. Treatment is by topical and systemic steroids.

Eczema and Atopic Dermatitis

These important dermatologic conditions have been associated with several types of ocular complications. Itching of the periorbital areas is a common symptom of both conditions. The itching can lead to vigorous rubbing of the eyes, lids, and periorbita, which can lead over time to keratoconus. A particular type of atopic cataract may also occur.

SKELETAL DISORDERS

Craniofacial Abnormalities

For information on this diverse group of craniosynostoses, see Chapter 12.

Osteogenesis Imperfecta

Osteogenesis imperfecta is one of the more common of the fragile bone diseases. Patients experience frequent and sometimes spontaneous fractures of their fragile bones, progressive loss of hearing due to conduction abnormalities, and blue sclera. The blue sclera is due to ectasias of the sclera itself and is not a result of the visible scleral vasculature that is often seen in normal patients or the bluish cast due to the thinness of the sclera seen frequently in infants. Other ocular manifestations include anterior embryotoxon, cataracts, keratoconus, and megalocornea.

Other Skeletal Conditions

The Arnold-Chiari malformation is a central nervous system malformation that often results in hydrocephalus and spina bifida and a "bull-neck" appearance. Downbeat nystagmus and diplopia are among the more common ocular manifestations.

Klippel-Feil syndrome involves abnormalities of the cervical vertebrae and a "bull-neck" appearance. Strabismus, nystagmus, and marked disorders of ocular motility are the primary ocular manifestations.

Hallermann-Streiff syndrome results in short stature and marked anomalies of the facies. Bilateral microphthalmus and congenital cataracts are the most severe of the ocular manifestations, with nystagmus and strabismus also occasionally present.

METABOLIC DISORDERS

Many uncommon metabolic disorders have important ocular manifestations. Some of these disorders are discussed in Chapters 12 and 13.

Mucopolysaccharidoses

This very diverse group of inherited metabolic diseases is characterized by an abnormal accumulation of mucopolysaccharides, primarily in connective tissue. The etiology lies in a specific defect in a lyosomal enzyme that is responsible for degradation of the particular mucopolysaccharide in each of these disorders. There are currently seven major disorders that have been characterized as mucopolysaccharidoses (MPS), all of which are autosomal recessive in their heredity patterns. They are classified as follows: MPS IH (Hurler's syndrome), MPS IS (Scheie's syndrome), MPS I H/S (Hurler-Scheie syndrome), MPS II (Hunter's syndrome), MPS III (Sanfilippo's syndrome), MPS IV (Morquio's syndrome), MPS VI (Maroteaux-Lamy syndrome), and MPS VII (Sly syndrome). No syndrome has been classified as MPS V.

The systemic manifestations of these disorders are variable, including cardiovascular problems, dwarfism, mental retardation, skeletal abnormalities, and, in some cases, premature death. The ocular manifestations include progressive corneal clouding, glaucoma, and retinal degenerations in a few.

Mucolipidoses

This diverse group of inherited metabolic disorders affects the storage of both mucopolysaccharides and either sphingolipids or glycolipids. The systemic manifestations include facial and skeletal abnormalities and mental retardation. Ocular manifestations include corneal stromal opacities and a cherry-red spot in the macula.

Fabry's Disease

A storage abnormality of ceramide trihexoside caused by a deficiency in the breakdown enzyme ceramide trihexosidase is responsible for this condition. Fabry's is an X-linked recessive disease. Female carriers often present only with the ocular characteristics of the disease, but affected males may experience serious or fatal renal and cardiovascular problems. The most apparent ocular abnormality is a striking whorl-like opacity of the cornea at the level of Bowman's membrane [11]. A propeller-like lenticular opacity or a spoke-like deposit on the posterior lens capsule may also be seen. Retinal vascular changes in the form of tortuosities and dilatations of the veins and, rarely, central retinal artery occlusion have also been reported.

Wilson's Disease

This hepatolenticular disorder results in abnormal deposition of copper in the brain, liver, kidneys, cornea, and lens. It is inherited in an autosomal recessive pattern, with greater expressivity in males than females. It typically presents in the second decade of life, but early signs may appear in childhood.

The characteristic ocular sign of Wilson's disease is a Kayser-Fleischer ring, a bluish- or greenish-brown ring of copper deposits at the limbus. It is easily seen on slit-lamp examination in most cases. A few patients may also develop cataracts. Early diagnosis is important because the disease can be effectively treated with a variety of drugs. Any patient that presents with a blueish or greenish limbal ring should be referred to a pediatrician for evaluation.

Refsum's Disease

Refsum's disease is a disorder of fatty acid metabolism characterized by an accumulation of phytanic acid in various tissues. The disease manifests several abnormalities, including a pigmentary retinopathy, cerebellar ataxia, peripheral polyneuritis, and proteinemia of the cerebrospinal fluid. Dermatologic problems and cardiomyopathy may also occur. It is transmitted in an autosomal recessive pattern.

Ocular signs are distinctive and helpful in making the correct diagnosis. The pigmentary retinopathy is initially located peripherally with typical bone spicule formation and a salt-and-pepper appearance. The macula may eventually show involvement. Visual fields show peripheral constrictions, and night blindness will develop. The clinical appearance in general may be quite similar to classic retinitis pigmentosa. A few patients will develop an atypical retinal appearance, also similar to cases of retinitis pigmentosa. In addition, cataracts, glaucoma, and pupillary anomalies may be found. Abnormalities are usually seen on the electroretinogram.

Aminoacidurias

Aminoacidurias include a diverse group of abnormalities of amino acid metabolism. These abnormalities are generally due to an aberrant enzyme or pathway. Most are autosomal recessive, with the exception of Lowe's syndrome, which is X-linked recessive. All have significant ocular manifestations. Several of the more commonly seen aminoacidurias are discussed here.

Cystinosis

This disease of amino acid metabolism results in deposition of the amino acid cystine in the tissues of the body. It often leads to early death. A characteristic deposition of refractile crystals of cystine in the cornea occurs. Centrally, the opacities are located only in the anterior stroma. Full-thickness opacities occur in the periphery. These opacities are virtually pathognomonic of cystinosis. There is also a peripheral pigmentary retinopathy that gives a salt-and-pepper appearance.

Lowe's Syndrome

Lowe's syndrome is also known as oculocerebrorenal syndrome. Congenital cataracts are almost a universal finding, and many patients have congenital glaucoma. Strabismus, microphakia, nystagmus, miosis, and iris atrophy are also noted. Mental and growth retardation is common, and early death occurs often.

Homocystinuria

This disorder of methionine metabolism is due to a lack of the enzyme responsible for its breakdown and a concomitant increase in the level of homocystine and methionine in the body. Among the important systemic manifestations of homocystinuria are abnormalities of the vascular system and mental retardation. Ectopia lentis, often with inferior displacement of the lens, is the most important ocular abnormality. Anterior displacement is more likely in homocystinuria than in the other common causes of ectopia lentis. Secondary glaucoma, myopia, cataracts, cystoid retinal degeneration, and optic atrophy may also occur.

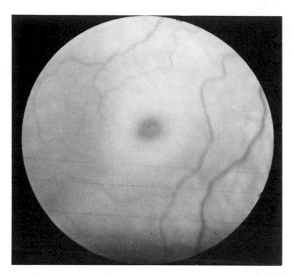

Figure 15.1. The fundus of a patient with Tay-Sachs disease. The cherry-red spot of the macula is easily differentiated from the rest of the pale fundus, which is obscured by abnormal deposition of ganglioside material in the ganglion cell layer of the retina. The normal appearance of the macula is spared because of the absence of ganglion cells in the macula. The rest of the retina is full of whitish material in the ganglion cell layer, making the macula stand out in appearance, but the problem is in the rest of the retina. (Reprinted with permission from LJ Press, BD Moore. Clinical Pediatric Optometry. Boston: Butterworth–Heinemann, 1993;217.)

Galactosemia

Galactosemia is due to a defect in the metabolism of the sugar galactose. It can be caused either by a deficiency in the activity of the breakdown enzymes galactose kinase or galactose-1-phosphate uridyl transferase. A deficiency of the latter causes a more severe form of the disease. This disorder results in the development of cataracts, hepatosplenomegaly, and mental retardation. Early diagnosis is important because prompt treatment can lead to a reversal of the cataract and prevention of further systemic progression. This is one of the few forms of cataracts that is treatable through nonsurgical means.

Sphingolipidoses

This diverse group of disorders of sphingolipid metabolism leads to premature death. They are sometimes called the amaurotic familial idiocy disorders,

indicating their degenerative nature. A generalized accumulation of lipids within the nerve cells gradually affects their functioning. Tay-Sachs disease, one of the most well-known of the sphingolipidoses, is characterized ocularly by the appearance of a cherry-red spot at the macula (Figure 15.1). This is caused by a whitening of the retina at the ganglion cell layer, with the macula being spared by the anatomic absence of ganglion cells in the area. Optic atrophy eventually develops. Tay-Sachs disease has the earliest onset of this group of disorders and leads to death by 2–4 years of age. The disease affects primarily people of Jewish and French-Canadian descent. Bielschowsky-Jansky, Batten-Mayou, Spielmeyer-Vogt, and Kufs' diseases appear progressively later in life. They do not produce the cherry-red spot characteristic of Tay-Sachs disease, but they do cause progressive neurologic degeneration. Other causes of cherry-red spots include gangliosidosis, Niemann-Pick disease, Farber's disease, and Gaucher's disease.

CHROMOSOMAL ABNORMALITIES

Major chromosomal deletions and trisomies that have important ocular affects are discussed in this section. A more comprehensive discussion of hereditary factors within the area of pediatric optometry is found in Chapter 16.

Trisomy 13 (Patau's Syndrome)

This chromosomal abnormality generally results in the death of the infant in the first few months of life. Affected infants manifest a large number of ocular and systemic anomalies. Most infants have a normal or near-normal birth weight but fail to thrive. Major cardiovascular, urogenital, and neurologic abnormalities are present. Infants are mentally retarded and deaf. The ocular defects include microphthalmus, uveal colobomas, cataracts, retinal dysplasia, intraocular cartilage formation, corneal opacities, and optic nerve hypoplasia. The incidence is equal in males and females.

Trisomy 18 (Edwards' Syndrome)

Most infants with Edwards' syndrome who survive birth are female, whereas spontaneous abortion oc-

Figure 15.2. Brushfield's spots are seen frequently in patients with trisomy 21 and occasionally in normal patients. They are areas of normal iris tissue surrounded by hypoplastic iris stroma that do not affect vision. (Reprinted with permission from LJ Press, BD Moore. Clinical Pediatric Optometry. Boston: Butterworth–Heinemann, 1993;219.)

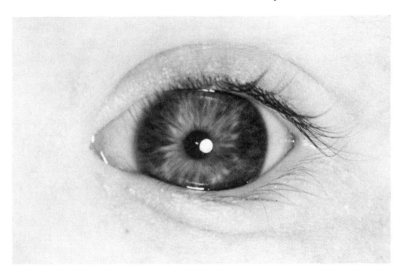

curs in most pregnancies in which the affected fetus is male. Most affected neonates will not survive past the first year of life. They exhibit low birth weight; hypertonicity; and a characteristic facial appearance consisting of micrognathia, microstomia, narrow palatal arch, low-set ears, and a narrow occiput. The hands and feet are malformed. Severe cardiac and renal defects are present. Infants are mentally retarded. The ocular anomalies include epicanthal folds, blepharophimosis, ptosis, hypertelorism, corneal opacities, microphthalmia, glaucoma, and uveal colobomas.

Trisomy 21 (Down Syndrome)

Down syndrome is considered to be the most common of all of the chromosomal abnormalities. The incidence is estimated to be approximately 1 in 600 live births [12]. Incidence increases with increasing maternal age. Patients may have virtually normal lifespans, but premature death is not uncommon. The major systemic abnormalities include mental retardation, characteristic facies, low-set ears, dental hypoplasia, thickened tongue, anomalies of the hands and feet, congenital heart defects, and gastrointestinal abnormalities. The ocular defects include epicanthus, mongoloid slant, Brushfield's spots, strabismus, cataracts, keratoconus, nystagmus, blepharitis, and high refractive errors (Figure

15.2). All patients with trisomy 21 should have eye examinations at an early age.

Deletion 5p– (Cri Du Chat Syndrome)

Cri du chat syndrome is due to a partial deletion of the short arm of chromosome 5. These infants typically have low birth weight and are hypotonic. They have a very characteristic cry that resembles a cat's cry. Infants are mentally retarded and have characteristic facies and neurologic and cardiovascular abnormalities. Ocular abnormalities include myopia, strabismus, epicanthal folds, and hypertelorism.

Deletion 11p–

This deletion is strongly associated with aniridia and Wilms' tumor. It may also lead to urogenital abnormalities and mental retardation.

Deletion 13q–

These patients manifest characteristic facies, neurologic abnormalities, and mental retardation. A strong association with retinoblastoma [13] has been noted and evidence of the specific location of the "retinoblastoma" gene on chromosome 13 has been found [14]. Additional ocular defects include hypertelorism, microphthalmus, epicanthus, ptosis, colobomas, and cataract.

Deletions 18p– and 18q–

Patients with an 18p– deletion may present with mild to severe systemic abnormalities, probably depending on the extent of deletion of the chromosome arm. These may include microcephaly, mental retardation, short stature, and neurologic defects. The ocular manifestations include hypertelorism, epicanthal folds, ptosis, strabismus, and microphthalmia.

The 18q– deletion is also known as DeGrouchy's syndrome. These low-birth-weight infants exhibit failure to thrive, characteristic facies, and mental retardation. The ocular manifestations include antimongoloid slant, epicanthus, ptosis, strabismus, blue sclera, corectopia, cataracts, color vision defects, colobomas, and various retinal abnormalities.

NEOPLASTIC EYE DISEASE

Ocular neoplasms are rare in young children, with the significant exception of retinoblastoma. Their prompt diagnosis and treatment is critical to the survival of the child. Although the treatment of ocular tumors is beyond the scope of optometry, the detection and initial diagnosis is an important responsibility of the pediatric optometrist. This section emphasizes the diagnostic signs and typical presentations of these disorders. The treatments are mentioned only briefly in the discussion of the specific disease.

Retinoblastoma

Heredity and Genetics

Retinoblastoma is the most common and most significant pediatric tumor encountered by the optometrist. The incidence of the tumor is estimated at approximately 1 in 15,000 births [15] in the United States, but there is considerable variability in different ethnic populations both within and outside the country. Without treatment, it is invariably fatal. Early detection and treatment before the tumor spreads beyond the eye yields a high survival rate [16].

A "two-hit hypothesis" model has been postulated to describe the hereditary basis of retinoblastoma [17]. Cases of retinoblastoma arise when two independent mutations occur. When the first mutation occurs in a prezygotic cell, the tendency for the tumor is transmissible. The second mutation allows the tumor to arise. This tumor would then be hereditary. Since a cell line having the first mutation is now present, a greatly increased likelihood of multiple unilateral or bilateral tumors being caused by multiple second-stage mutations exists. If the first mutation is postzygotic, the second mutation would then not lead to a hereditary-type tumor, reducing the likelihood of multiple unilateral or bilateral tumors. The hereditary types may have been passed on by a parent or may be a new mutation that will then be transmissible to the patient's offspring. It is currently assumed that the prezygotic retinoblastoma cells in some way either disappear or become inactive after 3–4 years of age, explaining why new retinoblastomas rarely develop after this time. Considerable evidence indicates that the locus of the retinoblastoma gene is on chromosome 13q14. A small number of cases of retinoblastoma appear to be due to deletions of the long arm of chromosome 13 [13]. Yandell et al. [14] have identified the approximate location on the gene that is responsible for retinoblastoma. This may have great importance in distinguishing hereditary from nonhereditary types of retinoblastoma.

A determination of the hereditary-versus-nonhereditary nature of retinoblastoma can usually be made based on the clinical characteristics and family history. Almost all bilateral cases and cases having four or more independent tumors in one eye are assumed to be hereditary, since the likelihood of multiple unilateral or bilateral tumors in a postzygotic cell line is remote. Approximately 8–15% of unilateral cases are due to the hereditary form, which tends to appear at a younger age (about 1 year versus 2 years in nonhereditary tumors) [17]. It is important to keep in mind that a second tumor in the other eye may develop at a later age, thus indicating that a tumor previously thought to be nonhereditary was hereditary.

Genetic counseling for the family is important and should focus in particular on the likelihood of the parents having another child with retinoblastoma and of that child subsequently having children of his or her own with the tumor. If the child has a unilateral tumor without prior family history, there is about a 1% chance of another child of those parents having retinoblastoma. The sibling of a child with bilateral tumors with no additional family history has an 8% risk of having retinoblastoma. If there is another sibling with retinoblastoma, the risk to a third child increases to approximately 40%. A child with a nonhereditary unilateral tumor has about a 10% risk of later having a child with retinoblastoma. A child having bilateral tumors has about a 50% chance of later having a child with retinoblastoma. There should be a degree of skepticism about these risk estimates, since it cannot be stated with certainty that a particular tumor is either hereditary or nonhereditary in origin, at least until chromosome analysis is clinically perfected. It is also important to keep in mind that not all carriers of the retinoblastoma gene manifest the disease (reduced penetrance) and that the form that the disease assumes may vary considerably (variable expressivity).

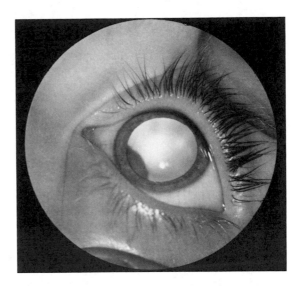

Figure 15.3. Dense leukocoria resulting from retinoblastoma. (Reprinted with permission from LJ Press, BD Moore. Clinical Pediatric Optometry. Boston: Butterworth–Heinemann, 1993;170.)

Presentation

From the optometric point of view, the issue of detection of patients with retinoblastoma is of critical importance. Patients with retinoblastoma have a relatively small number of typical presenting signs and symptoms. A study by Ellsworth showed that leukocoria (Figure 15.3) was by far the most common presenting sign of retinoblastoma (seen in 56% of patients) [18], followed by strabismus (20%), red, painful eyes with glaucoma (7%), and poor vision (5%). A number of relatively less common presentations include orbital cellulitis, pupillary and iris anomalies, and hyphema. A few patients had no signs or symptoms of retinoblastoma and were identified on routine examination.

Although leukocoria is the most common presenting sign of retinoblastoma, it does not always indicate an intraocular tumor. Other conditions presenting with leukocoria include persistent hyperplastic primary vitreous, retinopathy of prematurity, cataract, colobomas of the choroid or disk, uveitis, toxocara or other parasitic infections of the eye, congenital retinal folds, Coats' disease, and other rarer conditions. In general, any child presenting with a white pupil, strabismus, or amblyopia must

be thoroughly evaluated. Evaluation should include a dilated fundus examination by binocular indirect ophthalmoscopy to look for retinoblastoma or other serious types of eye disease. Diagnostic imaging should be performed to aid in the diagnosis. The presence of calcifications on computed tomography scan is highly suggestive of retinoblastoma.

A retinoblastoma may appear as a whitish, almost pearly iridescent mass, either on the surface or adjacent to the retina and extending into the vitreous, or as discrete small or large masses in the vitreous itself. The tumors may be necrotic and calcified or may take on a form known as a rosette, which is a cluster of tumor cells around a central lumen. The diagnostic criterion that is most predictable concerning patient morbidity and mortality is the extent of tumor growth at the time of diagnosis [19]. Large, multiple tumors are worse than small, singular tumors. The presence of tumor anterior to the equator carries a less favorable prognosis than tumor restricted to the posterior pole. Choroidal involvement also indicates a less favorable prognosis than if the tumor is limited to the retina and vitreous. This choroidal spread makes possible the metastasis through the vasculature to the rest of the body. Spread through the optic nerve is the most common route of metastases. Spontaneous regression of the tumor has been reported. A small percentage of patients will develop a nonmalignant form of the tumor known as a retinoma.

Treatment

The treatment of retinoblastoma has changed greatly in the past decade or so. Formerly, eyes affected by unilateral tumors were enucleated, and the most affected eye of bilateral patients was enucleated. Now, there is an emphasis on treating eyes that have visual potential with a combination of irradiation, cryotherapy, and chemotherapy. Enucleation is usually restricted to those eyes with massive involvement, when there is thought to be little if any potential of retaining useful levels of vision. The appropriate treatment decision is based on the size and location of the tumors. Chemotherapy and radiation are given to patients that exhibit spread beyond the eye, but the prognosis remains poor in these patients. It is important to note that the use of radiation may involve significant risk to the patient from the treatment itself. It is now recognized that some patients who survive the treatment of the retinoblastoma will later develop other malignancies, in particular osteogenic sarcoma. It is unclear if this is related to the radiation or if it is another tumor that is related to the underlying genetic disorder that results in the retinoblastoma itself [20]. Other types of orbital tumors and cataracts have also been attributed to the use of radiation therapy.

Gliomas

Gliomas can occur in the eye or in the anterior or posterior visual pathways. Several different clinical types of gliomas exist, each with a very different prognosis. Histologically, gliomas are astrocytic tumors that arise from the optic nerve.

Most gliomas affecting children are considered to be benign tumors that are fibrous in nature, growing slowly by extension and not metastasis. They can affect the visual system primarily by extension and compression of adjacent neurologic structures. There may be proptosis if the tumor is anterior in location. Reduced visual acuity, optic atrophy, and papilledema are often seen in these patients, depending on the location and size of the tumor [21]. Visual field deficits corresponding to the location of the tumor are present [22]. An afferent pupillary defect may also occur. Many of these tumors will stop their progression at some point, making treatment necessary only in those patients who experience progressive vision loss. This variety of optic nerve glioma is associated with neurofibromatosis (NF) and may be classified as a hamartoma [23].

The other type of optic nerve glioma, a posterior glioma, is a much more threatening disease that may be rapidly progressive and fatal. These gliomas tend to be located in the posterior chiasm and the hypothalamic or third ventricular area [24]. They require aggressive treatment. The optometrist may have the opportunity to follow patients with the slowly progressive form of anterior optic nerve glioma. Very careful visual field testing is an important component in the long-term follow-up care of these patients.

Leukemia

Enormous improvements in the treatment of many types of pediatric leukemia have been made during the past 20 years. Survival rates for the most common type of pediatric leukemia, acute lymphoblastic leukemia, have increased from virtually 0% to greater than 80% and are still rising [24]. Several of the other types of leukemia are still difficult to treat. In general, progress has been made in understanding the disease and developing appropriate treatments.

The clinical picture that we now see in children with leukemia is very different from the picture of 20 years ago. Previously, these patients presented with massive leukemic infiltrates that were visible in the fundus as whitish exudates, reminiscent of the appearance one sees in Coats' disease. Retinal hemorrhage; leukemic infiltration of the optic nerve, iris, and orbit; hyphema; and hypopyon were also routinely seen in the eyes of patients with leukemia. Because the central nervous system is separated from the rest of the body by the blood-brain barrier, leukemia patients who have infiltrates in their retinas (a part of the central nervous system) are occasionally seen, even when the leukemia is under control elsewhere in their body. Most patients today, however, show no ocular evidence of the disease.

The effects of the treatment itself can be seen in patients years after the disease is considered to be in remission. The current primary treatment is a combination of chemotherapy and radiation [25]. Bone marrow transplantation may be used when required. The radiation and chemotherapy combination causes posterior subcapsular cataracts in approximately 50% of patients [26]. It is also now recognized that patients who receive radiation may experience reduced tear production as a result of damage to the lacrimal gland and may develop a particular form of punctate keratitis that extends superficially over the entire cornea. These corneal complications may affect the success of patients in wearing contact lenses, particularly in those patients who become surgically aphakic as a result of secondary cataract formation.

Rhabdomyosarcoma

Rhabdomyosarcoma is an uncommon soft tumor of children, with an annual incidence in young white patients of about four cases per million and a slightly higher incidence in blacks [27]. The average age at onset is 2–5 years [28]. The primary site of the tumor may be around the eyes or in adjacent areas of the head, especially the nasopharynx. The typical ocular presentation is unilateral proptosis, ptosis, or a lid mass that rapidly progresses. It may initially appear somewhat similar to an orbital or periorbital cellulitis or even to a chalazion or hordeolum. The effect of local trauma around the eye can be confused with the presence of an active tumor, significantly delaying treatment in one patient that the authors have seen. Since the hallmark of rhabdomyosarcoma is rapid progression, any lid mass or proptosis that either becomes worse or does not resolve in the anticipated manner should arouse suspicion. Included in the differential diagnosis are chalazion, hordeola, orbital cellulitis, ocular trauma, dermoids, hemangioma, and neurofibroma. The diagnosis is aided by imaging studies and biopsy. The prognosis is dependent on the size and location of the tumor at the time of diagnosis. The current methods of treatment involve a combination of surgery, radiation, and chemotherapy. Cataracts secondary to radiation often occur.

NEURO-OPHTHALMIC DISORDERS

This section on pediatric neuro-ophthalmic disorders includes only a few of the conditions that are commonly encountered in clinical pediatric optometric practice. Consult a suitable text for further information on these subjects.

Pediatric neuro-optometry is an exceedingly complex specialty. The complete diagnosis and treatment of many of these entities may be beyond the scope of office-based optometric practice. The diagnosis of neuro-ophthalmic problems can often be made only tentatively when based on the apparent clinical signs and symptoms. Diagnostic imaging and complete pediatric neurologic testing is generally required whenever significant disease is present or suspected. Prompt referral to a pediatric ophthalmologist or neurologist at a tertiary care center should be made, since these conditions may be life threatening. The pediatric optometrist is an excellent resource for the detection of neurologic disorders that affect the eyes and visual system.

Congenital and Early Acquired Nystagmus

Congenital and early acquired nystagmus have been classified using varying systems. Some classify nystagmus into "normal" physiologic and "abnormal" pathologic varieties. The normal types include optokinetic, vestibular, and endpoint nystagmus, each of which can be elicited in most normal infants under appropriate testing conditions. The two more commonly used classifications of abnormal or pathologic types are based on the suspected etiology (sensory and motor nystagmus) and the appearance (pendular and jerky nystagmus).

Additional classifications depend on motor characteristics, such as the direction of motion of the eyes, the speed of motion, the extent of the motion, and the specific testing conditions under which the nystagmus is active, as opposed to the underlying etiology. No universal definitions or standardizations of the various categories of nystagmus exist, making the appearance of a particular patient's nystagmus difficult to describe. Furthermore, the particular etiology of the nystagmus—for example that caused by solely ocular defects as opposed to defects in the brain itself—has a significant effect on the appearance and the classification of the nystagmus. Aspects of all of these classification systems are used in the following discussions of the more clinically important congenital and early acquired types of nystagmus.

*Sensory Nystagmus Secondary
to Decreased Vision*

Sensory nystagmus is usually thought of as being due to bilaterally reduced visual acuity present either at birth or at an early age [29]. This reduced visual acuity can be due to problems within the eye, along the optic nerve pathways, or in the cortical areas of the brain responsible for the processing of visual information. Clinically, sensory nystagmus is seen in patients with such varying conditions as congenital media opacities of the cornea and lens; geographic retinal problems such as macular colobomas and lesions; generalized retinal disorders such as albinism, aniridia, Leber's congenital amaurosis, and achromatopsia; and optic nerve disorders such as optic nerve hypoplasia [30].

Patients with sensory nystagmus usually have significant bilateral vision loss (20/200 or worse), but others with less severe vision loss from conditions characterized by foveal hypoplasia (such as ocular albinism) may also have sensory nystagmus. The nystagmus is usually of a pendular nature, implying equal amplitude and speed from the midpoint of the ocular motion, but it can be of a jerky character. It is also usually horizontal in orientation, even on vertical gaze, with an infrequent vertical or rotatory component. The amplitude tends to be larger and coarser when the vision is more severely affected at an early age. The amplitude and speed of the nystagmus tends to decrease over time, even when the visual acuity does not improve significantly. Patients often have a null point, where the nystagmus is minimized and visual acuity maximized. The eye with better vision assumes a fully adducted position with the head turned in the opposite direction.

Although sensory nystagmus occurs most often when vision of both eyes is compromised, patients with unilateral vision loss may also develop sensory nystagmus. The amplitude of this type of nystagmus is usually less than in bilateral patients and the likelihood of a vertical or rotatory component may be increased.

Hereditary Pendular Nystagmus

Congenital hereditary pendular nystagmus occurs in the absence of visible ocular disease or abnormality. The family history is consistent with a dominant or X-linked hereditary pattern. A horizontal pendular nystagmus similar in appearance to sensory nystagmus results from reduced vision without apparent ocular abnormalities and essentially normal visual acuity. The amplitude of this nystagmus tends to decrease over time. It is possible that some of these patients may actually have a mild ocular albinism known as the albinoid form. The foveal light reflex may be only slightly attenuated in these individuals, making ophthalmoscopic identification difficult. For this reason, it is important to carefully look for iris transillumination in any patient with nystagmus.

Latent Nystagmus

Latent nystagmus is a jerky nystagmus commonly found in patients with strabismus and amblyopia and made more apparent when one eye is occluded [31]. Both the fast phase and the greatest amplitude are toward the fixating eye. The nystagmus is often present only when one eye is occluded. When both eyes are open, there is usually no evidence of nystagmus. This nystagmus is associated with strabismus and amblyopia. A reduction in measurable visual acuity invariably occurs during occlusion and in the presence of the active latent nystagmus. To accurately assess monocular visual acuity in patients with latent nystagmus, the use of a high plus lens (about +6.00 D) or a neutral density lens in front of the fellow eye will usually minimize the latent nystagmus. The nystagmus is generally noted in each eye when occluded; however, the amplitude is often greater in the eye that is more strabismic or amblyopic. This condition may interfere with the treatment of amblyopia by reducing the level of visual acuity beyond that of the amblyopia itself. The author has found that occlusion with neutral density filters or occlusive soft contact lenses that are not totally opaque may facilitate the treatment of amblyopia by minimizing the potential for latent nystagmus.

Spasmus Nutans

Spasmus nutans is a relatively common form of an early acquired pendular nystagmus that is associated with head nodding and head turn or torticollis [32]. It is not present at birth, but develops during the first year of life, often quite suddenly. The child will begin turning or tilting the head, often while nodding the head, and will show a pendular nystagmus simultaneously with the head movements. Parents may assume that this is a type of seizure activity. The frequency of these episodes varies greatly. The nystagmus tends to be fine in amplitude and rapid in speed. It is often unilateral or asymmetric if bilateral. The condition is usually much reduced in frequency by 5 years of age or less. Some patients manifest only the nystagmoid eye movements, without the head turning or nodding. The specific etiology is unknown, but there are apparently no long-term sequelae. There have been reports of significant neurologic disease that is unrelated to the condition itself occurring coincidentally in patients with spasmus nutans. It is important not to make too hasty a diagnosis of spasmus nutans, since more serious neurologic disorders may on occasion mimic the much more benign and isolated spasmus nutans. It is wise to have patients undergo a full neurologic workup to rule out this possibility.

Congenital Jerky Nystagmus

This is a jerky nystagmus with the fast phase toward the position of gaze. Generally, no identifiable ocular abnormalities are present other than the nystagmus and a secondary form of mild to moderate amblyopia that is due to the nystagmus itself. The nystagmus is present at a very young age, occasionally even at birth, and the amplitude and the speed tend to diminish somewhat over time. Most patients with jerky nystagmus will have a null point, which is a combination of a head and eye position that minimizes the nystagmus and maximizes the vision. This usually entails the eye with better visual acuity assuming a fully adducted position with the head turned to the opposite direction. Patients may not assume this null point during normal activities, but

when maximum visual acuity is required (e.g., for looking at the blackboard in school or at an eye chart in the optometrist's office) the child will assume the compensatory posture. Prisms in various combinations are sometimes prescribed to reposition the null point. Patients who require an extreme null point position may be aided by a complex extraocular muscle operation called a Kestenbaum procedure, in which the position of both eyes is changed equally to reposition the null point to a more straight-ahead position. Some patients may also use bilateral convergence to minimize the amplitude of the nystagmus. This may lead to esotropia in a few patients. It is relatively common to see patients with strabismus and amblyopia have both latent nystagmus and a null point for a jerky nystagmus component.

Contact lenses have been used in patients with nystagmus and significant refractive errors to improve visual acuity [33]. The mechanism for this improvement in acuity is uncertain, but it may result from improved optical correction of the refractive error as the contact lenses move with the eye, which reduces optical aberrations and prismatic effects in comparison to spectacles, and the increased vergence and accommodative effort through the contact lenses.

"Neurologic," or Pathologic, Nystagmus

Jerky, or pendular, nystagmus may also be caused by a variety of neurologic disorders that often affect the posterior fossa. Jerky nystagmus takes a myriad of appearances, resulting in a difficult diagnostic problem. Since the clinical appearance of neurologic forms of nystagmus may be very similar if not identical to the nonpathologic ocular forms, thorough evaluation by a pediatric ophthalmologist or neurologist should always be considered in patients with nystagmus, unless the optometrist is completely certain of its etiology. Even then, referral should be at least considered, since the early diagnosis of significant neurologic disease usually improves the prognosis and lessens morbidity and mortality.

Optic Nerve Head Abnormalities

The appearance of the optic nerve head is important in the proper diagnosis of both ocular and sys-

Table 15.1. Optic Nerve Head Abnormalities

Abnormality	Appearance and Effects
Optic nerve pit	Mini coloboma; vertically oval; gray, yellow, or black; risk of central serous retinal detachment
Optic nerve coloboma	Incomplete closure of fetal fissure, variable size, usually inferonasal
Optic nerve hypoplasia	Maldevelopment of ganglion cells, pigmented double-ring sign, afferent pupillary defect
Optic atrophy	Degeneration of optic nerve fibers, loss of vascularity and cupping, pale nerve head
Optic neuritis	Inflammation of the optic nerve, reduced visual acuity, visible or invisible ophthalmoscopically
Papilledema	Swelling of disk resulting from increased intracranial pressure, blurred margins
Pseudopapilledema	Apparent swelling of disk margins; may be due to glial tissue, refractive error, or drusen
Optic nerve drusen	Hyalin material within the disk causes elevation and indistinct appearance

temic disease (Table 15.1). The normal appearance of the optic disk is quite variable, making detection of subtle abnormalities difficult. Careful study of the nerve head by slit-lamp examination and direct and indirect ophthalmoscopy are luxuries often not possible except under anesthesia in a young, uncooperative child. The optic disk in young infants is pale and without the typical coloration of the adult disk. Cupping is usually not present. To the inexperienced examiner, all infant disks may look atrophic.

Optic nerve head abnormalities often result in functional as well as structural deficits, including decreased vision and field defects (see Table 15.1). Because of the difficulty in detecting these structural abnormalities in young children, decreased vision may be incorrectly attributed to amblyopia. If the examiner recognizes correctly that decreased vision is due to optic nerve head abnormalities, an inappropriate trial of occlusion therapy may be precluded.

This section describes some of the more clinically significant optic nerve head abnormalities and

the clinical signs and symptoms of those conditions. Additional ocular and systemic testing may be necessary for a thorough diagnosis of conditions affecting the optic nerve head.

Optic Nerve Head Coloboma

Like other colobomas of the eye, optic nerve head colobomas are the result of incomplete closure of the fetal fissure (Figure 15.4). The defect may be isolated in the optic nerve head only, but more commonly includes colobomas of the adjacent choroid, retina, and sclera. The degree of the defect varies greatly, from relatively minor and occult to quite extensive with involvement of adjacent structures. Likewise, the extent of visual loss varies greatly from mild to complete blindness. Central visual acuity and visual field may be compromised, depending on the location and extent of the coloboma. Although optic nerve head colobomas are usually unilateral, they can be bilateral. A family history of the problem is rare. Optic nerve head colobomas are usually isolated events, not generally associated with other systemic or neurologic disorders. They are, however, seen as part of the CHARGE association (*c*oloboma, *h*eart defects, *a*tresia choanae, *r*etarded growth, *g*enital hypoplasia, and *e*ar anomalies) and Aicardi's and Waardenburg's syndromes [34, 35]. An increased long-term risk of serous macular detachment accompanies colobomas [36]. The morning glory anomaly, often categorized as an optic nerve head coloboma, is actually a funnel-shaped dilatation of the optic stalk. The retinal vasculature is abnormal, and often peripapillary pigmentary changes are more significant than in true coloboma [37].

Optic Nerve Pits

Optic nerve pits are small, deep holes in the lower temporal quadrant of the optic disk (Figure 15.5). The color and shape are variable. Most are unilateral. They are considered by some to be a minimal coloboma of the optic nerve head, but the fact that they are typically located temporally instead of inferonasally like colobomas raises questions about their etiology. Deficits of both visual acuity and visual fields may occur depending on the size and location of the pit. Most are unilateral. An important consequence of optic nerve pits is the association

Figure 15.4. Extensive coloboma of the optic disk resulting in severe vision loss.

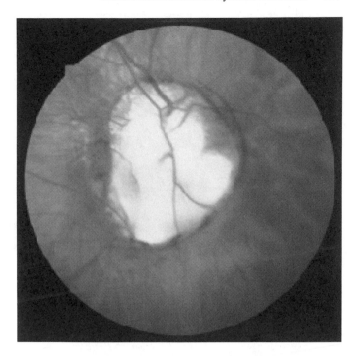

with serous macular detachments during the second and third decades of life. Patients with optic pits located temporally are at increased risk of serous retinal detachments [38]. Prophylactic laser photocoagulation may be advisable before the onset of actual serous detachment.

Optic Nerve Hypoplasia

Optic nerve hypoplasia was formerly thought to be rare, but now its role as a frequent cause of vision loss is appreciated [39]. The condition is due to a reduced number of retinal ganglion cells and optic nerve fibers. Optic nerve hypoplasia is characterized by a smaller than normal optic nerve head surrounded by a pigmented ring of sclera that occupies the space between the nerve head and the retina and choroid.

The ophthalmoscopic picture is often described as a double-ring sign, with a whitish, atrophic, small disk surrounded by a pigmented ring extending to the edge of chorioretinal tissue, which appears normal (Figure 15.6). Mild cases may be difficult to diagnose in young children who do not tolerate prolonged examination with the direct ophthalmoscope, which is the preferred method of examination due to the larger image size of the disk in comparison to the binocular indirect ophthalmoscope.

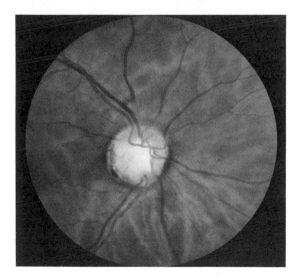

Figure 15.5. Optic pits located inferotemporally within the optic disk. The depth of the pit is best visualized by slit-lamp examination with a Hruby lens. (Reprinted with permission from LJ Press, BD Moore. Clinical Pediatric Optometry. Boston: Butterworth–Heinemann, 1993;177.)

The extent of the optic nerve hypoplasia is variable, as is the effect on vision, which ranges from minimal visual loss to complete blindness. An afferent pupillary defect matches in degree to the relative

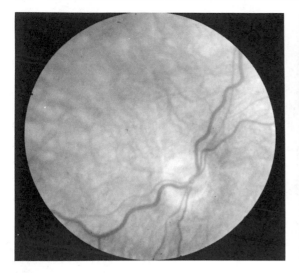

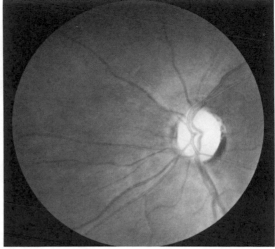

Figure 15.6. The double-ring sign in a patient with optic nerve hypoplasia. The disk itself is small and pale (less than one-half the normal size) and is surrounded by a pigmented ring and a whitish area that is scleral in nature. This patient has a hypopigmented fundus as well. (Reprinted with permission from LJ Press, BD Moore. Clinical Pediatric Optometry. Boston: Butterworth–Heinemann, 1993;179.)

Figure 15.7. The pale appearance of the disk in eyes with optic nerve atrophy is due to a loss of the vasculature and substance and structure of the optic nerve fibers. Both visual acuity and pupillary function are compromised due to the loss of the nerve fibers. (Reprinted with permission from LJ Press, BD Moore. Clinical Pediatric Optometry. Boston: Butterworth–Heinemann, 1993;180.)

number of remaining optic nerve fibers. Optic nerve hypoplasia can be unilateral or bilateral, and it may occur as part of septo-optic dysplasia and a host of other neurologic disorders. Other associations have been made with maternal diabetes [40] in a partial form of optic nerve hypoplasia, fetal alcohol syndrome, and maternal substance abuse. No treatment has been found for this condition.

Optic Atrophy

Optic atrophy results from the destruction of the optic nerve fibers from any one of a number of causes (Figure 15.7). Optic atrophy in young children may be difficult to visualize during the examination, however, because an infant's optic disk normally appears pale and without the definition of the adult disk. Therefore, simply getting an adequate view of the disk may be difficult or impossible in an active child. Optic atrophy in older children appears similar to that of adults, consisting of pallor of the nerve head, a reduction in the capillary content of the disk and adjacent tissue, attenuation of the retinal vasculature, a loss of cupping

and a flat appearance to the disk, and glial proliferation, which often occurs at a later stage. Visual acuity is compromised, nystagmus may be present if the optic atrophy is bilateral (and sometimes if it is unilateral), and an afferent pupillary defect is present in the affected eye. The electroretinogram response is severely reduced in patients with optic atrophy. Since optic atrophy is only a sign of a serious neurologic disorder, a complete neurologic evaluation is mandatory in order to assess the child's condition.

Optic Neuritis

Optic neuritis in infants and young children has a similar appearance to that of adults, but its detection and diagnosis is more difficult (Figure 15.8). The primary signs of optic neuritis are acute visual acuity loss, usually unilateral and painless, and visual field loss, depending on the cause and location of the optic neuritis. If the lesion occurs far enough behind the orbit, visible change in the appearance of the optic nerve head is unlikely. If the lesion is more anterior, evidence of disk edema,

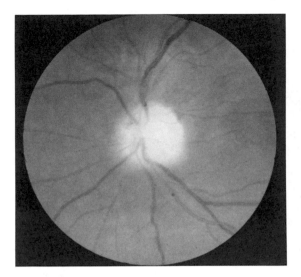

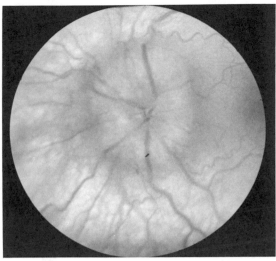

Figure 15.8. The white or pale appearance of the optic nerve head affected by optic neuritis is accompanied by a loss of visible ophthalmoscopic detail. The disk margins may be slightly blurred. Patients will have decreased visual acuity and afferent pupillary defects. (Reprinted with permission from LJ Press, BD Moore. Clinical Pediatric Optometry. Boston: Butterworth–Heinemann, 1993;181.)

Figure 15.9. This patient has florid papilledema secondary to a posterior fossa tumor. (Reprinted with permission from LJ Press, BD Moore. Clinical Pediatric Optometry. Boston: Butterworth–Heinemann, 1993;182.)

with or without hemorrhages and exudates, may be seen. Unilateral acute visual acuity loss secondary to optic neuritis in young children is unlikely to be detected early unless it leads to strabismus or some other neurologic or systemic manifestation becomes apparent. Visual field testing [41] may aid in the diagnosis of this and other pediatric neuro-ophthalmic disease. Many potential causes of optic neuritis exist and a discussion of the specific etiologies is beyond the scope of this text.

Papilledema and Pseudopapilledema

Papilledema is a swelling of the optic disk that occurs due to an increase in intracranial pressure (Figure 15.9). An ophthalmoscopically visible elevation of the optic nerve head with a loss of clarity of the disk margin is associated with hemorrhages, exudates, and venous congestion adjacent to the disk margin. Patients will not have spontaneous retinal vein pulsation, which is a valuable clinical sign in the differentiation of papilledema from pseudopapilledema. Vision is usually unaffected

until later in the course of the disease. Most children presenting with papilledema appear quite ill.

Papilledema must be distinguished from the more common pseudopapilledema. Pseudopapilledema is any condition that looks like papilledema but is not. The most common causes of pseudopapilledema are high hyperopia, hyperplastic glial tissue overlying the surface of the disk, and optic nerve drusen (Figure 15.10). Gliosis is associated with other anomalies of the hyaloid system such as Bergmeister's papilla, in which no signs of hemorrhage or exudate in the areas adjacent to the disk are present (unless the gliosis is instead associated with pseudopapilledema). Optic nerve drusen are usually not visible in young children since the hyaloid bodies are buried within the matrix of the nerve head. Their appearance becomes more distinct later [42]. A familial pattern of optic disk drusen has been noted, making an examination of all family members very helpful. The degree of disk elevation is variable, as is the ophthalmoscopic appearance. An enlarged blind spot on visual field testing is often present. Optic nerve drusen may be a diagnosis of exclusion in certain

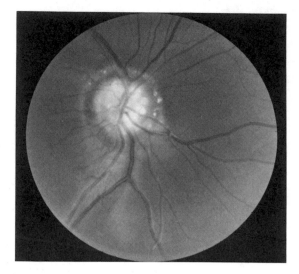

Figure 15.10. This pseudopapilledema is due to optic nerve drusen, which cause an indistinct ophthalmoscopic appearance of the disk. The optic nerve drusen seen in this patient are more readily apparent than in most. Details of this disk are mildly obscured by the drusen. Numerous, discrete drusen in the peripapillary area make this diagnosis straightforward. (Reprinted with permission from LJ Press, BD Moore. Clinical Pediatric Optometry. Boston: Butterworth–Heinemann, 1993;183.)

patients who do not show any evidence of intracranial swelling but have optic disks that appear somewhat elevated. An examination under anesthesia and complete neurologic examination may be required for adequate diagnosis of patients suspected of having disk elevation. Diagnostic imaging is essential.

Phakomatoses

The phakomatoses (from the Greek word for birthmark) are a group of neurologic disorders that are related by the presence of hamartomas, which are benign overgrowths of mature cells and tissues normally present in the affected part (Table 15.2). These conditions may be of a hereditary nature or sporadic. Each has important and distinctive effects on the eyes and the visual system, as well as more generalized neurologic manifestations.

Table 15.2. The Phakomatoses

Type	Appearance and Effects
Tuberous sclerosis (Bourneville's disease)	Glial hamartomas, "butterfly" facial lesion, shagreen patches, café au lait spots, "clumps of tapioca" in retina
Neurofibromatosis (von Recklinghausen's disease)	Neurofibromas, café au lait spots, plexiform neuromas, Lisch nodules, glaucoma, optic nerve glioma Angiomatosis of the cerebellum and retina
(von Hippel-Lindau disease)	Hemangioblastomas of the cerebellum and retina
Encephalofacial angiomatosis (Sturge-Weber syndrome)	Port-wine stain, leptomeningeal angiomas, glaucoma, choroidal hemangioma

von Recklinghausen's Disease

von Recklinghausen's disease, or NF, is a relatively common hereditary disease that has important ocular manifestations. Two major categories of NF—NF1 and NF2—are recognized. Other types probably exist that have yet to be fully described. The dominantly inherited NF1 is by far more common. It has a prevalence of about 1 in 3,000 births [43] in whites and is less common in blacks and Asians. Many patients appear to have new mutations without previous family history. The gene for NF1 is located on chromosome 17. Considerable variation occurs in the phenotypic appearance of the disease in different families, ranging from virtually no significant physical effects to severe neurologic disease.

The diagnosis of NF is made when the affected individual has two or more of the following characteristics: at least six café au lait spots of more than 5 mm in diameter in young children; two or more neurofibromas or one or more plexiform neurofibromas; freckling in the axillary or inguinal regions; optic glioma; two or more Lisch nodules; certain types of bony lesions; or a parent, sibling, or child with confirmed NF [44].

The typical hamartoma is the neurofibroma, a proliferation of Schwann cells within nerves that may greatly affect the function of involved tissue. These hamartomas develop in virtually any organ of the body, leading to variable clinical manifestations. A variety of other tumor types are associated with NF, including optic nerve gliomas, neurofibrosarcomas, astrocytomas, meningiomas, ependymomas, and pheochromocytomas. Neurofibromas and plexiform neuromas may cause significant disfigurement. Neurofibromas develop within nerve tissue throughout the body, causing disturbance of normal neurologic functioning. Serious neurologic problems resulting from NF include seizures, mental retardation, and various tumors of the central nervous system. Of particular ophthalmic importance are gliomas of the optic nerve. A number of skeletal abnormalities, many of which are developmental, may also occur. Once the diagnosis of NF is made, all patients require periodic neurologic and ophthalmic examination, generally every 6–12 months.

NF has many ocular manifestations. The characteristic sigmoid lid sign is due to a plexiform neuroma of the upper eyelid that produces an S-shaped form of ptosis. Other hamartomas can produce extensive deformation of the face and proptosis. Local involvement of the various nerves innervating the ocular tissue may be visible. Of diagnostic importance is the presence of Lisch nodules, which are typically small, discrete, hyperpigmented neurofibromas of the iris stroma (Plate 15.1). These tend to develop over time and may not be visible in young children with NF. They occur in approximately 50% of 5-year-olds, 75% of 15-year-olds, and 95–100% of adults with NF [45]. The presence of Lisch nodules may prove essential to the neurologist in confirming the diagnosis of NF. The nerve fibers in the anterior segment sometimes become more visible. Optic nerve gliomas may cause optic atrophy, optic neuritis, papilledema, visual field defects, or visual acuity loss depending on the site of the tumor. The risk of glaucoma from a number of different etiologies is increased. In general, this is a progressive disease. It is not uncommon for children who have had minimal effects from the disease for many years to suddenly develop much more serious neurologic and ophthalmic complications. These patients must be followed closely for life.

Encephalofacial Angiomatosis (Sturge-Weber Syndrome)

The hamartoma in Sturge-Weber is a vascular anomaly that can affect the skin, the eyes, and the brain. The classic cutaneous lesion is a port-wine stain that typically follows the distribution of the trigeminal nerve on only one side of the face; however, variable distributions have been seen. The vascular lesion contains an extensive series of channels that are present at birth and are flat, as opposed to the strawberry hemangioma that develops after birth and is quite elevated. The color of the nevus flammeus tends to be a dark reddish purple that does not darken with crying, unlike the strawberry hemangiomas that darken considerably with crying. Many patients with Sturge-Weber syndrome also have choroidal hemangiomas that may lie under the macula and are difficult if not impossible to see without the aid of the binocular indirect ophthalmoscope [46]. This choroidal lesion may cause an elevation of the macula above the plane of the retina, leading to an increase in hyperopia. This induced anisometropia can lead to amblyopia if not identified early and treated with appropriate refractive correction and patching.

The most significant ophthalmic manifestation of Sturge-Weber syndrome is a form of congenital, or early-onset, glaucoma that is particularly difficult to treat. This is found in the eye with the port-wine stain and results from the abnormal vasculature caused by the lesion. It is thought that the drainage mechanism is disrupted by the vascular lesion and the anatomy of the drainage angle itself is also affected [47]. An increase in the volume of aqueous production may occur. Some patients develop a form of glaucoma similar to the typical adult-onset, open-angle variety. Treatment is usually difficult and ultimately unsuccessful with blindness resulting. Heterochromia irides (darker on the affected side), retinal vascular changes, and colobomas have also been reported.

A variety of neurologic problems occur in Sturge-Weber syndrome in addition to the ophthalmic manifestations. Leptomeningeal angiomas, which lead to atrophy, gliosis, and calcification of adjacent cerebral cortex, are hallmarks of the disease. Seizure disorders, mental retardation, and hemiplegia are among the more common neuro-

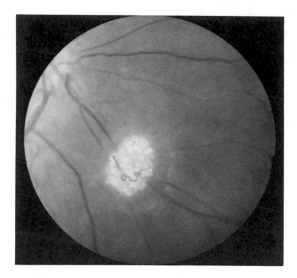

Figure 15.11. The hamartoma of tuberous sclerosis is often described as resembling clumps of tapioca. They appear as whitish, refractile bodies that are usually elevated. This patient has a tortuous vessel traversing the tumor, but other hamartomas may appear avascular. (Reprinted with permission from LJ Press, BD Moore. Clinical Pediatric Optometry. Boston: Butterworth–Heinemann, 1993;187.)

logic manifestations. The hereditary pattern, if any, is unknown.

von Hippel-Lindau Disease

The hamartomas of von Hippel-Lindau disease are hemangioblastomas of the retina and cerebellum. The hemangioblastomas are tumors composed of masses of thin-walled capillaries and endothelial cells, often associated with dilated blood vessels. von Hippel-Lindau disease may be an autosomally dominant inherited disorder with mixed penetrance and expressivity, but most cases appear to be sporadic. The disorder may not become evident until the second or third decade of life, and it is unusual to see significant clinical signs in young children.

The primary neurologic manifestations of the disorder are cerebellar hemangioblastomas composed of a large cystic mass with numerous large feeder vessels. This cyst impinges on adjacent structures within the nervous system, causing ataxia, nystagmus, and increased intracranial pressure.

Retinal hemangioblastomas have a variable appearance, but usually have a large, dilated vessel passing through the lesion and tend to be reddish in color. They may be unilateral or bilateral and may be multiple. Their size is quite variable. Their effect on vision varies depending on the size, position, and progression of the lesions. They can lead to retinal hemorrhage, retinal detachment, and glaucoma. The optic disk is sometimes affected. Current treatment is prophylactic ablation by laser photocoagulation or cryotherapy.

Tuberous Sclerosis

Tuberous sclerosis is also known as Bourneville's disease. It may be inherited in an autosomally dominant pattern. The hamartoma is called a tuber and is a proliferation of glial tissue (Figure 15.11). These lesions occur in the cerebrum and the retina, along with many other organ systems.

The cutaneous signs of tuberous sclerosis are café au lait spots and the adenoma sebaceum, or butterfly rash, of the face. Shagreen patches, which are irregularly pigmented patches that appear on the trunk, face, and extremities, are another characteristic cutaneous sign.

The neurologic consequences of tuberous sclerosis are quite severe. The tubers develop in the cerebrum, cerebellum, midbrain, and spine and undergo cystic degeneration and calcification. This leads to a host of neurologic signs, including increased intracranial pressure, seizure disorders, mental retardation, and behavioral abnormalities that may present in early childhood and be rapidly progressive.

The hamartomas present within the eye as nodular, cystic masses in the fundus that are described as clumps of tapioca or mulberries, but their appearance is quite variable. They occur in about half of patients with tuberous sclerosis [48]. The ocular lesions are generally of much less importance than the neurologic manifestations and treatment is usually not necessary. The lesions are, however, of distinct diagnostic importance.

REFERENCES

1. Poppell S, Poirier RH. Xerophthalmia in an infant with cystic fibrosis. Metabol Ophthalmol 1978;2:41–43.
2. Petersen RA, Petersen VS, Robb RM. Vitamin A deficiency with xerophthalmia and night blindness in cystic fibrosis. Am J Dis Child 1968;116:662–665.

3. Sheppard JD, Orenstein DM, Chao CC, et al. The ocular surface in cystic fibrosis. Ophthalmology 1989;96: 1624–1630.

4. Gare BA, Fasth A. Epidemiology of juvenile chronic arthritis in southwestern Sweden: a 5-year population study. Pediatrics 1992;90:950–8.

5. Rauch AM. Kawasaki syndrome: issues in etiology and treatment. Adv Pediatr Infect Dis 1989;4:163–182.

6. Marchette NJ, Ho D, Kihara S, et al. Search for retrovirus etiology of Kawasaki syndrome. Prog Clin Biol Res 1987;250:31–39.

7. Katowitz JA, Yolles EA, Yanoff M. Ichthyosis congenita. Arch Ophthalmol 1974;91:208–210.

8. Orth DH, Fretzin DF, Abramson V. Collodion baby with transient bilateral upper lid entropion. Arch Ophthalmol 1974;91:206–207.

9. Genvert GI, Cohen EJ, Donnenfeld ED, Blecher MH. Erythema multiforme after the use of topical sulfacetamide. Am J Ophthalmol 1985;99:465–468.

10. Arstikaitis MJ. Ocular aftermath of Stevens-Johnson syndrome. Arch Ophthalmol 1973;90:376–379.

11. Sher NA, Letson RD, Desnick RJ. The ocular manifestations in Fabry's disease. Arch Ophthalmol 1979; 97:671–676.

12. Frynes JP. Chromosomal anomalies and autosomal syndromes. Birth Defects 1987;23:7–32.

13. Sparkes RS, Muller H, Klisak I, Abram JA. Retinoblastoma with 13q– chromosomal deletion associated with maternal paracentric inversion of 13q. Science 1979;203:1027–1029.

14. Yandell DW, Campbell TA, Dayton SH, et al. Oncogenic point mutations in the human retinoblastoma gene: their application to genetic counseling. N Engl J Med 1989;321:1689–1695.

15. Devessa SS. The incidence of retinoblastoma. Am J Ophthalmol 1975;80:263–265.

16. Abramson DH, Ellsworth RM, Grumbach N, et al. Retinoblastoma: survival, age at detection and comparison 1914–1958, 1958–1983. J Pediatr Ophthalmol Strabismus 1985;22:246–250.

17. Knudson AG, Hethcote HW, Brown BW. Mutation and childhood cancer: a probabilistic model for the incidence of retinoblastoma. Proc Natl Acad Sci U S A 1975;72:5116–5120.

18. Ellsworth RM. The practical management of retinoblastoma. Trans Am Ophthalmol Soc 1969;67:463–534.

19. Redler LD, Ellsworth RM. Prognostic importance of choroidal invasion in retinoblastoma. Arch Ophthalmol 1973;90:294–296.

20. Abramson DH, Ronner HJ, Ellsworth RM. Second tumors in nonirradiated bilateral retinoblastoma. Am J Ophthalmol 1979;87:624–627.

21. Hoyt WF, Baghdassarian SA. Optic glioma of childhood. Br J Ophthalmol 1969;53:793–798.

22. Glaser JS, Hoyt WF, Corbett J. Visual morbidity with chiasmal glioma. Arch Ophthalmol 1971;85:3–12.

23. Gass JDM. The Phakomatoses. In JL Smith (ed), Neuro-Ophthalmology (Vol 2). St. Louis: Mosby, 1965;223–268.

24. Miller NR, Iliff WJ, Green WR. Evaluation and management of gliomas of the anterior visual pathways. Brain 1974;97:743–754.

25. Clavell LA, Gelber RD, Cohen HJ, et al. Four-agent induction and intensive asparaginase therapy for treatment of childhood acute lymphoblastic leukemia. N Engl J Med 1986;315:657–663.

26. Hoover DL, Smith LEH, Turner SJ, et al. Ophthalmic evaluation of survivors of acute lymphoblastic leukemia. Ophthalmology 1988;95:151–155.

27. Weichselbaum RR, Cassady JR, Albert DM, Gonder JR. Multimodality management of orbital rhabdomyosarcoma. Int Ophthalmol Clin 1980;20: 247–59.

28. Anderson GJ, Tom LWC, Womer RB, et al. Rhabdomyosarcoma of the head and neck in children. Arch Otolaryngol Head Neck Surg 1990;116:428–31.

29. Cogan DG. Neurology of the Ocular Muscles. Springfield, IL: Thomas, 1956; 189–192.

30. Cogan DG. Congenital nystagmus. Can J Ophthalmol 1967;2:4–10.

31. Dell'Osso LF, Schmidt D, Daroff RB. Latent, manifest latent, and congenital nystagmus. Arch Ophthalmol 1979;97:1877–1885.

32. Norton EWD, Cogan DG. Spasmus nutans: a clinical study of twenty cases followed two years or more since onset. Arch Ophthalmol 1954;52:442–446.

33. Allen ED, Davies PD. Role of contact lenses in the management of congenital nystagmus. Br J Ophthalmol 1983;67:834–836.

34. Pagan RA, Graham JM, Zonana J, et al. Coloboma, congenital heart disease, and choanal atresia with multiple anomalies: CHARGE association. J Pediatr 1981;99:223–229.

35. Pagan RA. Ocular coloboma. Surv Ophthalmol 1981;25:223–236.

36. Lin CCL, Tso MOM, Vygantas CM. Coloboma of the optic nerve associated with serous maculopathy: A clinicopathologic correlative study. Arch Ophthalmol 1984;102:1651–1654.

37. Brodsky MC. Congenital optic disk anomalies. Surv Ophthalmol 1994;39:89–112.

38. Brown GC, Shields JA, Goldberg RE. Congenital pits of the optic nerve head. II. Clinical studies in humans. Ophthalmology 1980;87:51–65.

39. Walton DS, Robb RM. Optic nerve hypoplasia. Arch Ophthalmol 1970;84:572–578.

40. Petersen RA, Walton DS. Optic nerve hypoplasia with good visual acuity and visual field defects. Arch Ophthalmol 1977;95:254–258.

41. Mayer DL, Fulton AB, Cummings MF. Visual fields of infants assessed with a new perimetric technique. Invest Ophthalmol Vis Sci 1988;29:452–459.

42. Hoover DL, Robb RM, Petersen RA. Optic disc drusen in children. J Pediatr Ophthalmol Strabismus 1988; 25:192–195.

43. Riccardi VM. Von Recklinghausen neurofibromatosis. N Engl J Med 1981;305:1617–1627.

44. Ragge NK. Clinical and genetic patterns of neurofibromatosis 1 and 2. Br J Ophthalmol 1993;77:662–672.

45. Ragge NK, Falk RE, Cohen WE, Murphree AL. Images of Lisch nodules across the spectrum. Eye 1993;7:95–101.

46. Susac JO, Smith JL, Scelfo RJ. The "tomato catsup" fundus in Sturge-Weber syndrome. Arch Ophthalmol 1974;92:69–70.

47. Phelps CD. The pathogenesis of glaucoma in Sturge–Weber syndrome. Ophthalmology 1978;85:276–286.

48. Lagos JC, Gomez MR. Tuberous sclerosis: reappraisal of a clinical entity. Mayo Clin Proc 1967;42:26–33.

Chapter 16

The Young Child with Developmental Disabilities: An Introduction to Mental Retardation and Genetic Syndromes

Dominick M. Maino

On June 26, 1994, the American Optometric Association House of Delegates adopted the following resolution:

Whereas, the Americans with Disabilities Act provides a federal mandate which recognizes the need to accommodate persons with disabilities; and

Whereas, Doctors of Optometry must continue to be sensitive to and accessible for persons with disabilities; now therefore be it

Resolved, that the American Optometric Association urges schools and colleges of optometry, as well as affiliates of the American Optometric Association, to provide educational programs relating to the Americans with Disabilities Act for both students and Doctors of Optometry; and be it further

Resolved, that the American Optometric Association urges Doctors of Optometry to continue providing appropriate access to optometric care for persons with disabilities, as mandated by the Americans with Disabilities Act.

"… be it further resolved, that the American Optometric Association urges Doctors of Optometry to continue providing appropriate access to optometric care for persons with disabilities." This access to care is of primary importance to those who are the most vulnerable and adversely affected by deleterious exogenous and endogenous factors: the infant, toddler, and preschool child. The provision of this care requires the expertise and skills the primary care pediatric optometrist provides [1].

It is estimated that more than five million individuals may demonstrate a cognitive or motor dysfunction and up to two million would qualify under the Americans with Disabilities Act as requiring lifelong medical, social, and psychoeducational services [2, 3]. Only recently has optometry taken a renewed interest in the diagnosis and management of the ocular, visual, and visual perceptual abnormalities associated with children at risk for and diagnosed as having disability [4–6]. This renewed interest is primarily due to the ever-expanding scope of the optometric profession into primary care health care and the recent federal and state legislative support given for both infant early intervention (0–3 years) and preschool programs (e.g., Head Start).

FACTORS THAT CONTRIBUTE TO DEVELOPMENTAL DISABILITIES

Genetics

Each year, more than 250,000 infants are born with developmental disabilities due to chromosomal abnormalities that result in structural or metabolic disorders [7–11]. Approximately 4,000 discrete, distinct, and separate genetic problems have been identified within the human race [12]. Those families at risk for inherited disorders should have access to genetic counseling and screening if desired.

Genetic counseling and screening [13] may be appropriate for any parent who already has an identified child with an inherited disease or defect. Those with family members who have been diagnosed with a genetic disease, any pregnant woman older than 35 years, and those who belong to ethnic groups that are prone to genetic anomalies should also consider an appropriate workup for possible genetic problems. Others who have a history of substance abuse; who have entered into a consanguineous marriage; or who have a history of repeated stillbirths, miscarriages, and sudden infant death should be informed of the possible genetic consequences as well.

As noted, there are thousands of mendelian disorders. These are usually classified as autosomal dominant, autosomal recessive, X-linked dominant, and X-linked recessive. In autosomal dominant disorders, there is a 50% chance that the infant will be affected, with both males and females being equally at risk. Many autosomal dominant disorders, however, cannot be diagnosed prenatally. Relatively common autosomal dominant anomalies include achondroplasia, Huntington's disease, myotonic dystrophy, and Marfan's syndrome.

Autosomal recessive disorders also affect the sexes equally, but a person must have a pair (two) of the abnormal genes before displaying the phenotype. Twenty-five percent of all offspring will be affected. There is a 50% chance that any future child will be a carrier and a 25% chance that a child will be an unaffected noncarrier. Autosomal recessive disorders that can be diagnosed before birth include Tay-Sachs disease, phenylketonuria (PKU), and cystic fibrosis (the most frequently encountered autosomal recessive disorder in whites).

Since males are hemizygous for genes on the X chromosome, any X-linked disorder will result in its phenotype being expressed. Females may be affected as well, but usually to a lesser degree depending on unfavorable lyonization and inactivation of major portions of the nonaffected X chromosome. Many of the more frequently encountered X-linked recessive problems include hemophilia (50% risk for having affected sons, 50% risk for having carrier daughters), fragile X syndrome, and Lesch-Nyhan syndrome [7, 14].

If multiple genes and the environment are involved in a disorder, it is most often referred to as being multifactorial in nature. These abnormalities have a typical recurrence risk of 2–5%. With each affected first-degree relative, however, the risk of occurrence can be up to three times greater. Other factors affecting risk include gender, severity of the condition, and whether the affected person is the mother or the father (e.g., affected mothers present a greater risk of having an affected child). Frequently encountered multifactorial disorders include refractive error, various cardiac defects, and cleft palate [7].

Prenatal Care

All mothers-to-be must have appropriate prenatal care, which should start with a comprehensive medical history and physical examination. Adequate nutrition that results in a weight gain of up to 30 pounds (approximately 14 kg) should be noted as well. All pregnant women should be screened for alloimmunization anomalies (Rh antibody and other blood group antigens), anemia (hemoglobin value of less than 10 g/dl) [15], hypertension, and diabetes mellitus. The presence of congenital infections (e.g., cytomegalovirus), sexually transmitted diseases, and genetic anomalies should be assessed as needed. Those with a greater likelihood of having a multifetal pregnancy (which could result in intrauterine growth retardation) should be informed of the associated risks to the newborn [16]. It cannot be overemphasized that insufficient or absent prenatal care, including proper medical supervision, adequate nutrition, and healthy lifestyle, is associated with increased maternal and neonatal morbidity.

Labor and Delivery Complications

Various labor and delivery complications are routinely associated with the infant being at risk for developmental delay, disability, or both. For instance, newborns presenting as a breach delivery are more likely to have cerebral palsy (CP). Breach birth may also be associated with de Lange syndrome, Potter syndrome, and Prader-Willi syndrome [17]. Intrauterine hypoxia as a result of mothers with abruptio, placenta previa, or a prolapsed cord may result in a child's being at risk for disability and even death.

Several studies have noted that newborns exposed to anesthesia or analgesia during birth had adversely affected attention span and habituation patterns. On the other hand, physiologic stress may affect the mother so that the fetal pH and oxygen saturation falls. It is possible, then, that not administering an appropriate anesthetic or analgesic could also cause fetal distress. In most instances, medication given judiciously will aid both mother and child [18].

Neonatal Intensive Care

With the advent of improved neonatal intensive care techniques, the mortality for medically fragile infants has drastically decreased [19]. For instance, the mortality for children with birth weights of 1,000–1,500 g fell from 50% in the 1960s to below 10% in the 1980s. If the infant was born weighing less than 1,000 g, the mortality rate decreased from 90% to 50% during this same time period. The trend in improved neonatal care, however, has increased the prevalence of various disabilities, with CP showing an approximate increase of 20% between 1960 and 1986 [20]. As mortality decreases, the optometrist will be called on to evaluate, diagnose, and manage an ever increasing scope of functional, pathologic, optical, developmental, and perceptual anomalies.

These abnormalities may include children with respiratory distress syndrome (RDS) and bronchopulmonary dysplasia. RDS is the primary cause of death in premature infants, with bronchopulmonary dysplasia occurring in one-third of those young children who have been mechanically ventilated. If either RDS or bronchopulmonary dysplasia have been diagnosed for your patient, you should also suspect the presence of retinopathy of prematurity (ROP). As a major etiology of long-term disability, ROP must be diagnosed and treated as soon as possible. The classification of ROP involves four stages [21]. Stages I and II are frequently seen but will often resolve without major sequelae. Stages III and IV, however, often result in characteristic retinal scarring and eventually moderate to severe visual impairment [22, 23].

Hyperbilirubinemia

The sensitivity of the newborn's central nervous system to the toxicity of bilirubin has been known for some time. The child with severe hyperbilirubinemia may develop opisthotonos, a high piercing cry, hypertonicity, a decreased suck response, and seizures soon after birth. Long-term neurologic deficits include choreoathetosis, hearing loss, poor gait and balance, oculomotor deficits, and possible mental retardation (MR). Although the pathogenic mechanism of bilirubin toxicity is not known, it has been demonstrated that newborns of low birth weight or who have a very high birth weight with asphyxia, sepsis, or respiratory distress are more likely to exhibit the consequences of increased sensitivity to higher levels of bilirubin. The treatment for severely elevated levels of bilirubin is a whole blood exchange transfusion. If lower levels are detected, phototherapy is often used [24].

Periventricular-Intraventricular Hemorrhage

The most frequently encountered serious neurologic event in the neonatal period is periventricular-intraventricular hemorrhage (PIH) [25], with up to 45% of all infants with birth weights of less than 1,500 g or of less than 35 weeks' gestation, or both, affected by this disorder. Various anatomic and physiologic factors may determine if the newborn is prone to PIH. These factors include asphyxia, hypoxic cardiac failure, hypertension, hyaline membrane disease, and anomalies of the anatomic structure concerning the vasculature of the germinal matrix (all of which affects cerebral blood flow and pressure).

Since up to 50% of children at risk will exhibit PIH within the first 24 hours of birth, diagnosis of this disorder (ultrasound and computerized tomographic scanning) should be instituted in a timely manner. If diagnosis and treatment appropriately occur, mild to moderate lesions usually result in very low rates of mortality. More severe involvement, however, has been associated with significantly decreased motor and intellectual abilities and death.

PIH frequently presents as one of two basic clinical syndromes. The first of these includes the catastrophic classic presentation of a major hemorrhage that results in deep stupor or coma, nonreactive pupils, tonic seizures, abnormal respiration, absent oculomotor ability, and flaccid quadriparesis. Other associated anomalies that may accompany this catastrophic event include hypotension, bradycardia, temperature fluctuations, metabolic acidosis, poor water and glucose homeostasis, hydrocephalus, and even death. The more subtle, second clinical syndrome develops over several hours to days and is characterized by variable levels of alertness, hypotonia, eye movement anomalies (downward drifting of the eyes), and a decreased response to the doll's head maneuver. This more subtle form of PIH can easily be overlooked in a child with numerous other systemic and neurologic abnormalities [26].

Metabolic Disorders

Several metabolic disorders can result in a newborn's being at significant risk for disability, including phenylketonuria (PKU), congenital hypothyroidism, galactosemia, maple syrup urine disease, and homocystinuria [27]. Undiagnosed and untreated PKU results in severe MR and emotional or behavioral disorders. This autosomal recessive disorder occurs when the body cannot convert phenylalanine into tyrosine. General PKU characteristics include oligophrenia, partial albinism, and muscle hypertonicity. Other findings are epilepsy, microcephaly, and hyperreflexia of the tendons. Blue sclera, photophobia, cataracts, corneal opacities, and macular atrophy are frequently encountered oculovisual findings characteristic of this metabolic anomaly.

If managed early with proper diet control, affected children will develop normal cognitive function. Even with treatment, however, many learning-related vision problems (developmental or visual-perceptual dysfunctions) may persist, with substantial academic disabilities being present [28]. It is now recommended that all patients with PKU continue dietary treatment of this disorder well into adulthood. Another important issue with PKU is that of maternal effects on the newborn. If a mother with PKU does not follow a phenylalanine-restricted diet, her offspring have a greater chance of being born with a low birth weight, heart disease, and microcephaly.

Congenital hypothyroidism (sporadic cretinism) is seen three times more frequently than PKU in the general population. If appropriately diagnosed and treated, these children will also develop normal intelligence quotients (IQs.) The pediatric optometrist, however, should be aware that many of these cognitively normal children will develop learning disabilities, emotional or behavioral problems, nystagmus, and visual-perceptual-motor deficits similar to those seen in children with PKU.

Newborn screening programs have noted the frequency of galactosemia to be as prevalent as 1 in 30,000 children. Once again, dietary intervention (milk restriction) has saved thousands of lives. Delayed growth and speech and language problems frequently occur within this population, even with treatment. The oculovisual abnormalities found are nystagmus and bilateral cataracts (i.e., nuclear, cortical oil droplet, and zonular with punctate opacities in the periphery).

Approximately 1 in 225,000 infants have maple syrup urine disease. This autosomal recessive disorder is characterized by elevated levels of valine, leucine, isoleucine, and their analogue branched-chained amino acids. The child shows hypotonia or hypertonia, lethargy, seizures and, if not treated, death. Neonatal management includes peritoneal dialyses or hemodialysis, intravenous fluid support, and antiseizure medication. Later, a special diet that restricts leucine (and other branched-chain ketoacid analogues) is used to control this disease. With prompt initial and long-term treatment, many of these children go on to lead productive lives. The eye and vision problems include ptosis, hypertelorism, and cataract. Other abnormalities noted are strabismus, poor pupillary response to light, nystagmus, and optic atrophy.

Children who have homocystinuria exhibit orthopedic or skeletal anomalies, reduced cognitive function, and an increased incidence of thromboembolism. This inherited autosomal recessive abnormality produces a disorder of methionine metabolism that results in increased levels of homocystine and methionine in both the blood and urine and a reduced level of cystathionine in the brain. If homocystinuria is managed through early dietary treatment, MR and many of the skeletal anomalies can be prevented. Of particular interest to the eye care provider is that even with treatment ectopia lentis frequently occurs and should be monitored and managed as needed. Additional visual anomalies seen are cataract, retinal detachment, optic and iris atrophy, keratitis, and uveitis, as well as high myopia, strabismus, and pupillary block glaucoma.

Table 16.1. Online Resources for Information Regarding Children and Disability

Resource	Online Address	Description
Online Mendelian Inheritance in Man	http://www3.ncbi.nlm.nih.gov/omim/	Contains information on all known human genetic syndromes and is updated weekly
Centers for Disease Control Atlanta	http://www.cdc.gov	—
Occupational Safety and Health Administration	http://www.osha.gov	—
Infants	http://galaxy.einet.net/galaxy/community/the-family/infants.html	—
National Library of Medicine	http://www.nlm.nih.gov	Contains information regarding young children and disability for the pediatric optometrist
Fragile X Research Foundation	http://www.worx.net/fraxa@seacoast.com	—
Advocacy for Persons with Developmental Disabilities: The ARC	http://www.metronet.com/thearc/welcome.html	—
Multimedia Virtual Hospital	http://indy.radiology.uiowa.edu/virtualhospital.html	—
Genome Research	http://www-genome.wi.mit.edu/	—
Florida MENTAL Health Institute	http://hal.fmhi.usf.edu/	—
The World Health Organization (WHO)	http://www.who.ch	—
AltaVista	http://altavista.digital.com	Outstanding World Wide Web search engine
Dominick Maino, O.D., M.Ed., F.A.A.O.	http://www.webcom.com/~optcom/maino.html icomaino@minna.acc.iit.edu dmaino@juno.com	—
College of Optometrists in Vision Development (COVD)	http://www.optom3.com/covd	Contains up-to-date information about pediatric vision dysfunction

Infections

Numerous congenital infections, such as rubella [27], toxoplasmosis [29], tuberculosis [30], cytomegalic inclusion disease [27], human immunodeficiency virus infection/acquired immunodeficiency syndrome [31], and herpes simplex infection [32], can cause significant mortality and morbidity during the pre-, peri-, and postnatal period. Specific recommendations for controlling these communicable diseases have been published by the Centers for Disease Control, and the Occupational Safety and Health Administration (Table 16.1) has mandated workplace regulations that are designed to stop infection [33]. However, many mothers are exposed to these infections during the prenatal period despite these guidelines.

TORCH Syndrome

TORCH syndrome [34] (i.e., *t*oxoplasmosis, *o*ther, *r*ubella, *c*ytomegalovirus, *h*erpes simplex) consists of several infections contracted in utero, with the primary clinical symptoms being petechiae, purpura, jaundice, anemia, thrombocytopenia, hepatomegaly, and splenomegaly. These children are typically small for gestational age and have several oculovisual problems, including chorioretinitis.

This syndrome is also referred to as STORCH when it includes syphilis [35].

Infections included in TORCH syndrome are the following:

Toxoplasmosis   A parasitic infestation caused by *Toxoplasma gondii* that results in cysts being noted in numerous organs (i.e., brain or muscle). The ocular manifestations include keratitis, uveitis, optic atrophy, and papillitis. The optometrist will also find anisocoria, scleritis, cataract, and microphthalmos, as well as esotropia, nystagmus, and myopia [27].

Rubella   An infection that results in a child exhibiting low birth weight, hepatosplenomegaly, petechia, and osteitis. Other signs and symptoms noted are heart defects, microcephaly, deafness, thyroid abnormalities, diabetes, autisticlike behaviors, and MR. Ocular sequelae include cataracts and micro-ophthalmia.

Cytomegalovirus   A viral infection with systemic anomalies that include anemia, thrombocytopenia, enlarged spleen, jaundice, and encephalitis, with deafness, psychomotor retardation, and microcephaly being noted as well. Expected eye problems are micro-ophthalmia and retinopathy [36].

Herpes simplex   A disseminated disease that affects multiple organs (i.e., liver, central nervous system, and lungs). Microcephaly, intracranial anomalies, retinopathy, and neurologic deficits are frequently seen.

An exhaustive review of infectious agents cannot be adequately addressed in this single chapter. Other sources concerning this issue should be consulted for a more complete review of the subject [37].

Teratogens

If, during the embryonic or fetal period, a drug, chemical, infectious, or environmental agent alters the morphology or function of the organism in the postnatal period, it is considered a teratogen [38]. These teratogens include various infectious agents (noted previously), as well as socially promoted behaviors such as the ingestion of alcohol and cigarette smoking [39]. Other teratogens and descriptions of their effects on the very young are noted in Table 16.2.

MENTAL RETARDATION AND GENETIC SYNDROMES

Fragile X Syndrome

During the past two decades, the most significant discovery in the area of MR research was that of an X-linked disorder now known as fragile X syndrome (fra X). Fra X is one of the most frequently encountered etiologies of X-linked MR (1 per 1,000 males and 1 per 2,000 females, with a gene frequency as high as 1 per 625 in the general population) and among children with chromosomal abnormalities is second only to Down syndrome (DS) in prevalence. Besides being the most common heritable cause of MR, fra X is one of the first-known genetic etiologies of learning disabilities. It is the first genetic disease discovered to be caused by a repeated deoxyribonucleic acid (DNA) nucleotide sequence (cytosine, guanine, and guanine) [14, 40]. This genetic disorder is also responsible for almost 7% of moderate and 4% of mild MR among males and 2.5% of moderate and 3% of mild MR among females [41]. Although there are thousands of articles, monographs, texts, and newsletters readily available to the health care practitioner, surprisingly little has been published concerning the ocular, visual, and visual-perceptual anomalies commonly associated with this condition

The young child with fra X is usually brought to the family physician when the parents note hypotonia (and the resultant dysfunctional fine and gross motor control), delayed speech and language development, or various behavioral abnormalities (gaze avoidance, hyperactivity, and autisticlike mannerisms). The correct diagnosis is often delayed, however, because few professionals recommend that the appropriate cytogenetic and DNA studies be conducted (Table 16.3).

The differential diagnosis should begin with a careful case history [42]. If, during this case history, it is reported that MR, learning problems, and emotional and psychological anomalies are common within the patient's family and the child exhibits one or more typical fra X behaviors (i.e., hand biting, preservative speech, or short attention span), there exists a strong possibility for the presence of this syndrome [43]. The pediatric optometrist may

Table 16.2. Teratogens and a Brief Description of the Medical Sequelae

Teratogen	Description
Alcohol	Fetal alcohol syndrome and fetal alcohol effect; 1 in 300 to 1 in 2,000 live births; 30–40% of infants born to alcoholic mothers; growth deficiency, developmental delay, CNS deficits, mental retardation, delayed motor skills, hyperactivity, attention deficits, short palpebral fissures, flat nasal bridge, evident epicanthal folds, short nose, indistinct philtrum, thin upper lip, hypoplastic midface, and congenital heart abnormalities (30% of the population)
Heroin and methadone	Anatomic defects, intrauterine growth retardation, prematurity, microcephaly, emotional and behavioral anomalies, perceptual and learning deficits
Cocaine	Weak or aberrant cry, poor sleeping, tremors, poor temperature regulation of extremities, yawning, fluctuating respiration, excessive sucking, poor feeding, gaze averting (setting sun sign), auditory averting, and irritability
Smoking	Decreased birth weight, intrauterine growth retardation, possible decreased academic performance (reading, mathematics, and other cognitive skills) and various behavioral anomalies
Aminopterin and methotrexate	Potent abortifacient, folic acid antagonist, anatomic and structural deficits, intrauterine growth retardation
Diethylstilbestrol	Risk of clear cell adenocarcinoma of the vagina, anatomic defects of the genital tract
Diphenylhydantoin	Phenytoin (Dilantin) (fetal hydantoin syndrome): prenatal growth deficiency, mental deficiency, wide anterior fontanel, ocular hypertelorism, metopic ridge, depressed nasal bridge, short nose, bowed upper lip, cleft lip or palate, hypoplasia of distal phalanges, nail hypoplasia, low arch dermal ridge patterns, and developmental delay
Isotretinoin or etretinate	Vitamin A or derivatives; isotretinoin (Accutane) use during first trimester; craniofacial, cardiac, and CNS anomalies; hydrocephalus; microcephaly; and spontaneous abortions
Lithium	Various congenital heart defects
Methyl mercury	Neurologic dysfunction, mental retardation, microcephaly, spasticity, and cerebral palsy
Radiation	At doses of >10 rads, fetal loss, microcephaly, and mental retardation
Tetracycline	Brown stain on teeth, susceptibility to caries, hypoplastic teeth enamel
Thalidomide	Phocomelia, polydactyly, syndactyly, facial capillary hemangiomata, hydrocephaly, renal anomalies, cardiovascular anomalies, ear and eye defects, intestinal anomalies
Trimethadione	Mental retardation, prenatal growth deficiency, midfacial hypoplasia, short nose, flat nasal bridge, upslanted eyebrows, strabismus, ptosis, cleft lip or palate, unusual pinnae, cardiovascular defects, genital abnormalities
Valproic acid	Meningomyelocele fetal valproate syndrome: prominent forehead, flat nasal bridge, short nose with anteverted nares, ocular hypertelorism, small, down-turned mouth, thin upper lip
Warfarin	Fetal warfarin syndrome: prenatal growth deficiency, seizures, marked nasal hypoplasia, chondrodysplasia punctata, CNS anomalies

CNS = central nervous system; rads = radiation absorbed doses.
Source: Adapted from HE Hoyme. Teratogenic Causes of Developmental Disabilities. In SM Pueschel, JA Mulick (eds), Prevention of Developmental Disabilities. Baltimore: Paul H. Brooks Publishing, 1990;105–121; JR West, AC Wei-Jung, NJ Pantazis. Fetal alcohol syndrome: the vulnerability of the developing brain and possible mechanisms of damage. Metab Brain Dis 1994;9(4):291–322; and JG Cole. Intervention strategies for infants with prenatal drug exposure. Inf Young Child 1996;8(3):35–39.

want to use a Butler's checklist (Figure 16.1) to ascertain the child's risk of having fra X.

Males with fra X exhibit phenotypic features that include a long face, large, elongated ears, and macro-orchidism (enlarged testes). Other less common features are musculoskeletal manifestations (pes planus [flat feet], excessive joint laxity, scoliosis, and double-jointed thumbs), cardiac anomalies (mitral valve prolapse), and numerous speech and language problems. Children with fra x exhibit frequent ear infections, seizures, and a large body size for chronologic age.

Females with fra X present with many of the anomalies noted above, but usually to a lesser degree. They will also show reduced IQ on completion of standardized testing, learning disabilities

Table 16.3. Fragile X Syndrome Resource Centers

Name	Mailing Address
Elizabeth Berry-Kravis, M.D., Ph.D. (Fragile X Clinic/Research Group includes Elizabeth Berry-Kravis, M.D., Ph.D.; Rush-Presbyterian-St. Lukes Medical Center; Dominick M. Maino, O.D., M.Ed.; and Sandra Block, O.D., M.Ed.; Illinois College of Optometry; William Pizzi, Ph.D. and Rita Brusca, Ed.D.; Northeastern Illinois University; Terry Treitman, Fragile X Association of America; Peter D'Aloia, D.D.S.; Sue Ellen Krause, Ph.D.; Speech and Language Services.)	Fragile X Clinic/Research Group Professional Building Rush-Presbyterian-St. Lukes Medical Center 1725 W. Harrison St., Suite #710 Chicago, IL 60612 phone: (312) 942-4036
The National Fragile X Foundation	1441 York St., Suite 303 Denver, CO 80206 phone: (800) 698-8765 fax: (303) 353-4369
FRAXA Research Foundation, Inc.	PO Box 935 West Newbury, MA 01985 phone: (508) 462-1990 e-mail: fraxa@seacoast.com
John Michael Jones, Ph.D.	Lincoln Center 248 W. 64th St., #1B New York, NY 10023 phone: (212) 875-0632
Leeanne and David Clayton	6203 W. 35th S. Court Wichita, KS 67215 phone: (316) 522-1880
Dr. Herbert Gabriel	1203 Leonard Ave. Oceanside, CA 92054 phone: (619) 722-8821 fax: (619) 722-3121
Fragile X Resource Center of Missouri	2 Valley View Pl. St. Louis, MO 63124 phone: (314) 997-0431
Kevin and Peggy Kourajian	2212 9th Ave. SE Mandan, ND 58554 phone: (701) 663-4115 fax: (701) 221-2338
Terry Treitman	Fragile X Association of America 206 Shermer Rd. Glenview, IL 60025 phone: (708) 724-8626
Stephanie Jacob	Northern California Fra X Association PO Box 3812 Walnut Creek, CA 94598 phone: (510) 938-3150

Condition	Score*
Mental retardation	
Large ears	
Large testes	
Plantar crease	
Hyperactivity	
Family history of mental retardation and autism	
Short attention span	
Tactile defensiveness	
Hyperextensible finger joints	
Preservative speech	
Hand flapping	
Pale blue eyes	
Hand biting	
Gaze avoidance	
Simian crease/Sydney line	

*Scoring: Score two points for each item definitely present. Score one point if the item was present in the past, questionable, or borderline. Score no points if item was never present. A score of 16 or greater means a high probability of having fragile X syndrome [14].

Figure 16.1. Butler's modified 15-item checklist for screening mentally retarded males for fragile X syndrome.

(i.e., decreased math, and speech and language skills), and sensory integration anomalies. Attention and psychiatric problems may be present, including excessive shyness. Girls with fra X tend to show a greater variability of ability and disability than males. This variability ranges from those who have severe dysfunctions to those with no noticeable abnormalities being present [44].

Several commonly associated ocular, visual, and visual-perceptual abnormalities have been reported in children and adults with fra X. Maino et al. [45–47], Storm et al. [48], Maino and King [49], and Amin and Maino [50] have noted that up to 50% of the fra X population studied may exhibit a strabismus (with esotropia being noted more frequently than exotropia). Uncorrected refractive errors are seen, with up to 60% of the population studied showing at least 1.00 D of hyperopia. Myopia and astigmatism are present as well. Nystagmus, oculomotor dysfunction, vergence anomalies, and disorders of accommodation have also been reported.

Developmental and visual-perceptual abnormalities are now being investigated. Individual case reports (and a limited number of studies) have reported information processing problems in the areas of laterality and directionality, visual figure ground, visual closure, visual form constancy, visual memory, visual sequential memory, and other cognitive deficits [50–53]. Block et al. [51] have reported a significant correlation between the perceptual and cognitive deficits present and the number of CGG repeats found for women with fra X.

Table 16.4. Characteristics of Down Syndrome

Neurologic
  Moderate mental retardation
  Delayed motor skills
  Delayed speech
  Hearing loss
Behavioral
  Mouth breathing
Craniofacial
  Small, brachycephalic skull
  Frontal or perinasal sinus hypoplasia
  Flat occiput
  Flat, protruding tongue
  Dental hypoplasia
  Flat nasal bridge
  Skin elasticity around neck
  Small, low-set ears
Musculoskeletal
  Hypotonia
  Joint hyperextensibility
  Pelvic hypoplasia
  Short, broad, stubby hands
  Incurving fifth finger
  Feet abnormalities
Dermatologic
  Simian palmar crease
  Fingerprints with ulnar deviated loops
  Dry skin
Cardiac
  Ventricular and atrial septal defects
  Endocardial cushion defects
  Tetralogy of Fallot
  Patent ductus arteriosus
  Aortic regurgitation
  Mitral valve prolapse
Demonstrated genetic predisposition
  Leukemia
  Alzheimer's disease
  Hypothyroidism
  Diabetes mellitus
Decreased immunologic function
  Chronic hepatitis
  Alopecia areata
  Chronic infections

Down Syndrome

DS [54–63] is the most frequently encountered chromosomal anomaly in children, with up to 1 in 600 live births being affected. Three modes of genetic transmission are involved. The first of these, trisomy 21 (an extra twenty-first chromosome), is the etiology for up to 95% of all patients with DS.

The translocation mode of transmission may occur when a normal number of chromosomes are present but a portion of a chromosome (a g group, numbers 21 or 22) attaches to another chromosome (usually numbers 13, 14, or 15). The final method of transmission is referred to as mosaicism (approximately 1% of the DS population). This occurs when some of the cells are normal while others express the trisomy condition. Patients with mosaicism tend to function at a mildly MR to low-normal range of intelligence.

Characteristic physical, neurologic, cognitive, and ocular abnormalities are present (Tables 16.4 and 16.5). The physical features include a short stature, brachycephalic skull, flat occiput, and low-set ears. A flat nasal bridge, large protruding tongue, dental problems, and dry skin are also noted. Delays in development of visual processing and motor function (i.e., hypotonia, and speech and language development) are frequently present with attention, recognition, and memory deficits evident. The ability to process auditory information appears to be affected as well [54].

The most common cause of decreased visual acuity in patients with developmental disabilities is uncorrected refractive error. This is also true for those with DS. Moderate to high refractive errors, strabismus, and amblyopia are frequently encountered. Wesson and Maino have noted that although there are more hyperopic patients than myopic patients in the DS population, those with myopia tend to display greater magnitudes. They also characterize the young child having DS and strabismus as showing less than 20 prism diopters of constant unilateral esotropia, with the etiology of this deviation being related to a high accommodative-convergence/accommodation ratio (AC/A) [55].

Other specific ocular anomalies noted include delayed visual acuity development [56], deficits in color vision [57], keratoconus [58], optic nerve anomalies, lens opacities, and nystagmus [59–61]. Children with DS will also demonstrate prominent epicanthal folds, infantile glaucoma, iris abnormalities (i.e., Brushfield's spots), and other systemic and functional abnormalities [62].

Concern has been expressed that using topical diagnostic pharmaceutical agents (such as atropine and its various derivatives) may cause unwanted side effects that can lead to cardiac and respiratory complications. Although caution should be used with all patients who may be medically fragile and although the benefits versus the risks of any procedure should always be weighed, in general, most patients with DS do not show any higher risk of adverse effects to these agents than the nondisabled population [63].

Cerebral Palsy

CP is a nonprogressive disorder that results in a constellation of signs and symptoms, usually without a genetic etiology, and that results in major disruptions and abnormalities affecting the motor centers of the central nervous system. Its etiology arises from disease, injury, or defect of the nervous tissue. It is estimated that more than 700,000 people are affected. CP may be classified by the extent and nature of brain damage (i.e., spastic, athetoid, ataxic, or mixed), the level of involvement (i.e., paraplegia; di-, tri-, quadriplegia; or hemiplegia), or time of onset (pre-, peri-, postnatal). Many individuals with CP will exhibit normal to superior intelligence [41, 64].

Oculovisual-perceptual findings include significant refractive error, accommodative dysfunction, strabismus, and amblyopia. There are more individuals with hyperopia, but those with myopia demonstrate greater magnitudes and ranges [55]. Optic atrophy, nystagmus, delayed visual development or cortical blindness, and lenticular anomalies are also seen. All perceptual areas involving a motor component typically show delay as well. Improvement in visual function can be expected with the judicious application of lenses, prisms, and vision therapy. Due to the neurologic etiology of the strabismus, however, neither vision therapy nor surgical intervention has a particularly high cosmetic or functional cure rate [65–68].

Mental Retardation Without Specific Etiology (Nonspecific Mental Retardation)

Individuals with MR without a known etiology make up the majority of those exhibiting cognitive

Table 16.5. Oculovisual Findings of Down Syndrome

Anterior
  Narrow interpupillary distance
  Upward and outward slanting palpebral fissures
  Prominent epicanthal folds
  Blepharitis (33%)
  Eyelid eversion
  Keratoconus (1–8%)
  Iris
    Brushfield's spots (85%)
    Iris hypoplasia (95%)
    Iridoschisis
Lens
  Flake-like lens opacities (2%)
  Punctate opacities
  Senile cataracts at young age
  Congenital cataracts
Fundus
  Blond coloration of fundus
  Retinoblastoma
  Retinal folds
  Retinal dysplasia
  Retinal pigment epithelial disturbances at disk
    margins (30%)
  Myopiclike fundus changes
    Temporal crescents
    Choroidal thinning
  Optic nerve
    Increased number of vessels at disk margin
    Spoked pattern of vessels
    Hyperemic appearance
    Hypoplasia (?)
    Glioma (?)
Oculomotor
  Strabismus (23–44%)
    Esotropia
    Exotropia (occasionally)
  Nystagmus
    Fine, rapid, pendular
    Rotary (occasionally)
Amblyopia (10–12%)
Refractive anomalies
  Hyperopia usually seen
  High myopia >−8.00 D
  Astigmatism >2.50 D

impairments. Up to 3% of the general population (6 million people) are considered to have mild to severe MR. The American Association on Mental Retardation defines a person with MR as a person who exhibits substantial limitations in present functioning. It is characterized by significantly subaverage intellectual functioning, existing concurrently with related limitations in two or more of the following applicable adaptive skill areas: communications, self-care, home living, social skills, community use, self-direction, health and safety, functional academics, leisure, and work. MR manifests before the age of 18 [69].

Substantial limitations in present functioning means exhibiting a basic difficulty in daily living skills and general learning aptitude; *subaverage intellectual functioning* is defined as a standardized IQ score of less than 75. At the same time (*concurrently*), two or more limitations in adaptive skills (e.g., communications and self-care) must be present before the age of 18 years.

It is important to note what this definition does not address. This definition does not discuss issues concerning etiology. It is not a group of medical, psychological, or educational classification codes (i.e., International Classification of Diseases–Clinical Modification-9 [ICD–CM-9] or the Diagnostic and Statistical Manual of Mental Disorders IV [DSM IV]). It also does not predict the future abilities or disabilities, strengths or weaknesses, or eventual life outcomes for any single person. It is, however, a temporal description of a specific state of adaptive, cognitive, behavioral, and intellectual functioning [70].

Infants, toddlers, and preschool children with nonspecific MR generally are not brought to the attention of the pediatrician or other professionals until the child starts school. Once the child begins an academic program, however, any cognitive deficits become apparent. Although no studies assessing the oculovisual status have been conducted on very young children with nonspecific MR, Wesson and Maino [55] found that, for older children (median age 45 months), visual acuities can be determined using standard assessment techniques, that refractive errors are comparable to what would be found in a general optometric practice population, and that ocular health abnormalities were typically not seen. They did note, however, that a higher than expected incidence of strabismus (up to 38% of the subjects) should be expected.

Syndrome of Nonverbal Learning Disabilities

A relatively new but potentially important syndrome has been described by Rourke [71]. He has developed a white matter model to explain the deficits seen in children with the syndrome of nonverbal learning disabilities (NLDs). This model depends on the number of destroyed or dysfunctional white brain matter fibers, the developmental stage and type of destruction or dysfunction, and the development (i.e., right or left hemispheric) and maintenance of behaviors that are learned. As the basis of NLDs, this white matter model theory clarifies why such a wide variety of abnormalities are within its definitional scope.

Children with NLDs demonstrate several strengths and weaknesses. Deficits include bilateral tactile-perceptual anomalies, retarded psychomotor skills, impaired visual discrimination, poor recognition of detail, and inappropriate visual spatial organizational abilities. These patients also find it difficult to tolerate novel stimuli. NLDs are an all-encompassing anomaly that includes Asperger, Williams, and de Lange syndromes; hydrocephalus; hypothyroidism; and callosal agenesis. Traumatic brain injury; toxicant-induced encephalopathy; as well as Sotos, Turner, and fetal alcohol syndromes are all within its scope [71–73].

There are several levels within the NLD hierarchy that denote decreasing phenotypic similarity and that describe the manifestations of this syndrome. Patients with level I of NLDs demonstrate almost all of the strengths and weaknesses associated with NLDs, whereas patients with level II are considered to show a considerable number of these manifestations. Patients with level III, however, will show many, although not all, of the signs and symptoms of this disorder (Table 16.6) [74].

NLDs are of importance to the optometrist because many of these children have the signs and symptoms most likely to be diagnosed and treated by the optometrist (i.e., poor prereading skills). Rourke [75] notes, however, that many of these children begin remediation or therapy and then improve quite suddenly. Although the special education specialist, occupational or physical therapist, tutor, or optometric vision therapist may take credit for the child's rapid progress, these children would have improved *without* therapy or remediation. No specific optometric research has been conducted with patients diagnosed as having NLDs at this time. It is uncertain if Rourke's hypothesis concerning therapeutic intervention for poor prereading skills is correct.

IMPORTANCE OF EARLY INTERVENTION

Early intervention is vital if very young children with disabilities are to develop and become productive members of their family, school, and community. These early services may include enrolling these children in nationally known programs (such as Head Start) or other similar programs at the local level. Infants, toddlers, and young children in early intervention programs have a high prevalence of oculovisual disorders. These may include significant refractive error, strabismus, ocular disease, and nystagmus [76].

Optometrists must develop and use all the appropriate diagnostic and therapeutic tools available to meet the many challenges this unique population offers the practicing pediatric specialist. These diagnostic and therapeutic modalities have been fully described in detail in other texts and should be reviewed and mastered by the student clinician and seasoned practitioner [77–79].

CONCLUSION

Young children with developmental disabilities require many of the services offered by the optometrist. We diagnose and treat the prevalent oculovisual, perceptual, and ocular diseases [80] frequently encountered within this population [81]. The primary care optometrist will also act as the gatekeeper and then conduit through which appropriate nonoptometric, therapeutic, remedial, and related medical and psychoeducational services are provided for these special patients [1, 82, 83]. We also have the appropriate knowledge, clinical skills and primary care acumen to provide the quality eye and vision care these patients require [34, 77, 84].

REFERENCES

1. Maino DM, Block SS. Diagnosis and management of special populations: the role of the developmental optometrist. J Optom Vis Dev 1994;25:219–221.
2. Ingalls RP. Mental Retardation: The Changing Outlook. New York: Wiley, 1978.
3. Baroff GS. Predicting the prevalence of mental retardation in individual catchment areas. Ment Retard 1982;20:133–135
4. Bartlett J. Toward Better eye and vision care. J Am Optom Assoc 1987;1:6–7.
5. Maino D. What's So Special? In D Maino (ed), Diagnosis and Management of Special Populations. St. Louis: Mosby, 1995;ix.
6. Maino D. The mentally handicapped patient: a perspective. J Am Optom Assoc 1987;58:14–17.

Table 16.6. Nonverbal Learning Disabilities: Levels of Neurologic Disease, Disorder, and Dysfunction

Level I
  Callosal agenesis (uncomplicated)
  Asperger syndrome
  Velocardiofacial syndrome
  Williams syndrome
  de Lange syndrome
  Hydrocephalus (early and shunted)
  Congenital hypothyroidism
Level II
  Sotos syndrome [72]
  Prophylactic treatment for acute lymphocytic leukemia (long-term survivors)
  Metachromatic leukodystrophy (early in disease progression)
  Turner syndrome
  Fetal alcohol syndrome
Level III
  Multiple sclerosis (early to middle stages)
  Traumatic brain injury (diffuse white matter perturbations)
  Toxicant-induced encephalopathies (affecting white matter)
  Autism (high functioning)
Suggestive of NLDs
  Fragile X syndrome [14, 40, 43–52]
  Haemophilus influenzae meningitis
  Neurofibromatosis (early to middle stages)
  Early treatment for phenylketonuria
  Intracranial hemorrhage (early)
  Congenital adrenal hyperplasia
  Prader-Willi syndrome [17]
  Insulin-dependent diabetes mellitus (very early onset)
Difficult to classify
  Cerebral palsy of perinatal origin
Similar
  Tourette syndrome

NLDs = nonverbal learning disabilities.
Source: Reprinted with permission from KD Tsatsanis, BP Rourke. Conclusions and Future Directions. In BP Rourke (ed), Syndrome of Nonverbal Learning Disabilities Neurodevelopmental Manifestations. New York: Guilford Publications 1995;476–496.

7. Fatt H, Griffin J, Lyle W. Genetics for Primary Eye Care Practitioners (2nd ed). Boston: Butterworth–Heinemann, 1992.

8. Lyle W. Genetic Risks: A Reference for Eye Care Practitioners. Waterloo, Ontario Canada: University of Waterloo Press, 1990.

9. Jones RN, Richards GK. Practical Genetics. Philadelphia: Open University Press, 1991.

10. Klug WS, Cummings MR. Concepts of Genetics (3rd ed). New York: Macmillan, 1991.

11. The National Foundation March of Dimes. Birth Defects: Tragedy and Hope. White Plains, NY: The National Foundation March of Dimes, 1977.

12. McKusick VA. Mendelian Inheritance in Man: Catalogs of Autosomal Dominant, Autosomal Recessive, and X-Linked Phenotypes (Vols 1 and 2). Baltimore: Johns Hopkins University Press, 1992.

13. SR Applewhite, DL Busbee, DS Borgaonka (eds). Genetic Screening and Counseling: A Multidisciplinary Perspective. Springfield, IL: Thomas, 1981.

14. Martinez S, Maino D. A comprehensive review of the fragile X syndrome: oculo-visual, developmental, and physical characteristics. J Behav Optom 1993;4:59–64.

15. Prichard JA, Scott DE. Iron Demands During Pregnancy. In L Hallberg, HG Harwerth, A Vanotti (eds), Iron Deficiency: Pathogenesis, Clinical Aspects, Therapy. New York: Academic, 1970.

16. Scholl GT. Growth and Development. In AA Rosenbloom, MW Morgan (eds), Principles and Practice of Pediatric Optometry. Philadelphia: Lippincott, 1990;3–30.

17. Libov A, Maino D. Prader-Willi syndrome. J Am Optom Assoc 1994;65:355–359.

18. Coustan DR. Prevention of Complications During Labor and Delivery. In SM Pueschel, JA Mulick (eds), Prevention of Developmental Disabilities. Baltimore: Paul H. Brooks Publishing Co., 1990;157–177.

19. Hansen NB, McClead RE. Advances in Neonatal Intensive Care to Improve Long-Term Outcome. In SM Pueschel, JA Mulick (eds), Prevention of Developmental Disabilities. Baltimore: Paul H. Brooks Publishing, 1990;179–188.

20. Bhusan V, Paneth N, Kiely J. Impact of improved survival of very-low-birth-weight infants on recent secular trends in the prevalence of cerebral palsy. Pediatrics 1993;91:1094–1100.

21. Silverman WA, Flynn JJ. Contemporary Issues in Fetal and Neonatal Medicine: Retinopathy of Prematurity (Vol II). Boston: Blackwell, 1985.

22. Page JM, Schneeweiss S, Whyte HE, et al. Ocular sequelae in premature infants. Pediatrics 1993;92:787–790.

23. Vieth J, Scharre J. Retinopathy of prematurity: review of the pathophysiology and classification. J Am Optom Assoc 1992;63:496–499.

24. Cashore WJ. Contribution of Hyperbilirubinemia to Developmental Disabilities. In SM Pueschel, JA Mulick (eds), Prevention of Developmental Disabilities. Baltimore: Paul H. Brooks Publishing, 1990;189–196.

25. Volpe JJ. Neurology of the Newborn. Philadelphia: Saunders, 1981.

26. Volpe JJ. Intraventricular hemorrhage in the premature infant—current concepts. II. Ann Neurol 1989;25:109–116.

27. Roy FH. Ocular Syndromes and Systemic Diseases (2nd ed). Philadelphia: Saunders, 1989;61–62, 120, 161, 205, 384, 409, 451.

28. Strupp B. PKU: learning and models of mental retardation. Dev Psychobio 1984;17(2):109–120.

29. Meenken C, Assies J, Van Nieuwenhuizen O, et al. Long term ocular and neurological involvement in severe congenital toxoplasmosis. Br J Ophthalmol 1995;79(6):581–584.

30. Conrad V. Ocular and systemic manifestations of tuberculosis. Clin Eye Vis Care 1994;6(2):71–75.

31. Conrad V. Ocular manifestations of acquired immunodeficiency syndrome. Clin Eye Vis Care 1994;6(2):53–61.

32. Beigi B, Algawi K, Foley-Nolan A, O'Keefe M. Herpes simplex keratitis in children. Br J Ophthalmol 1994;78(6):458–460.

33. Conrad V. Transmission of human immunodeficiency virus, hepatitis B, and tuberculosis: infection control protocol. Clin Eye Vis Care 1994;6(2):80–83.

34. Maino DM, Maino JH, Cibis GW, Hecht F. Ocular Health Anomalies in Patients with Developmental Disabilities. In D Maino (ed), Diagnosis and Management of Special Populations. St. Louis: Mosby, 1995;189–206.

35. Fine JD, Arndt KA. The TORCH syndrome: a clinical review. J Am Academ Derm 1985;12:697–706.

36. Grose C, Itani O, Weiner CP. Perinatal diagnosis of fetal infections: advances from amniocentesis to cordocentesis—congenital toxoplasmosis, rubella, cytomegalovirus, varicella virus, parvovirus, and human immunodeficiency virus. Ped Infect Dis J 1989;8:459.

37. Behrman RE, Kliegman RM, Nelson WE, Vaughan VC (eds). Textbook of Pediatrics (14th ed). Philadelphia: Saunders, 1992;495–500.

38. Shepard TH. Teratogenicity of therapeutic agents. Curr Probl Pediatr 1979;10:5–42.

39. Rojahn J, Aman MG, Marshburn E, et al. Biological and environmental risk for poor developmental outcome of young children. Am J Ment Retard 1993;97:702–708.

40. Hagerman RJ, Silverman AC (eds). Fragile X Syndrome Diagnosis, Treatment, and Research. Baltimore: Johns Hopkins University Press, 1991.

41. Thapar A, Gottesman II, Owen MJ, et al. The genetics of mental retardation. Br J Psychiatry 1994;164:747–758.

42. Cotter S, Scharre JE. Optometric Assessment: Case History. In M Scheiman, M Rouse (eds), Optometric Management of Learning-Related Vision Problems. St. Louis: Mosby, 1994;226–266.

43. Dibler LB, Maino DM. Martin-Bell phenotype, fragile X syndrome, and the very low birth weight child: the differential diagnosis. J Optom Vis Dev 1994;25:233–246.

44. Schopmeyer BB, Lowe F. The Fragile X Child. San Diego: Singular Publishing Group Inc., 1992.

45. Maino D. Wesson M, Schlange D, et al. Optometric findings in the fragile X syndrome. Optom Vis Sci 1991;68:634–640.

46. Maino D. Schlange D, Maino J, Caden B. Ocular anomalies in fragile X syndrome. J Am Optom Assoc 1990;61:316–323.

47. Maino D. Oculo-visual abnormalities associated with fragile X syndrome. Natl Fragile X Found Newsletter 1990;Summer:4–5.

48. Storm RL, Pebenito R, Ferretti C. Ophthalmologic findings in the fragile X syndrome. Arch Ophthalmol 1987;105:1099–1102.

49. Maino D. King R. Oculo-Visual Dysfunction in the Fragile X Syndrome. In R Hagerman, P McKenzie (eds), 1992 International Fragile X Conference Proceedings. Dillon, CO: Spectra Publishing, 1992; 71–78.

50. Amin V, Maino D. The fragile X female: visual, visual perceptual, and ocular health anomalies. J Am Optom Assoc 1995;66(5):290–295.

51. Block SS, Brusca-Vega R, Pizzi WJ, et al. Comparison of performance of mothers of fragile X children exhibiting full versus premutation on tests of visual information processing and cognitive skills. Presented at the American Academy of Optometry annual meeting. New Orleans, December, 1995.

52. Smith SE. Cognitive deficits associated with fragile X syndrome. Ment Retard 1993;31:279–283.

53. Kail R. General slowing of information-processing by persons with mental retardation. Am J Ment Retard 1992;97:333–341.

54. Karrer R, Wojtascek Z, Davis MG. Event-related potentials and information processing in infants with and without Down syndrome. Am J Ment Retard 1995; 100(2):146–159.

55. Wesson M, Maino D. Oculo-Visual Findings in Down Syndrome, Cerebral Palsy, and Mental Retardation with Non-Specific Etiology. In D Maino (ed), Diagnosis and Management of Special Populations. St. Louis: Mosby, 1995;17–54.

56. Courage ML, Adams RJ, Reyno S, Poh-Gin K. Visual acuity in infants and children with Down syndrome. Dev Med Child Neurol 1994;36:586–593.

57. Perez-Carpinell J, de Fez MD, Climent V. Vision evaluation in people with Down's syndrome. Ophthal Physiol Optics 1994;14:115–121.

58. Haugen OH. Keratoconus in the mentally retarded. Acta Ophthalmol (Copenh)1992;70:111–114.

59. VanDyke DC. Medical problems in infants and young children with Down syndrome: implications for early services. Inf Young Child 1991;1:39–50.

60. Wagner RS, Caputo AR, Reynolds RD. Nystagmus in Down's syndrome. Ophthalmology 1990;97:1439–1444.

61. Catalono RA, Simon JW. Optic disk elevation in Down's syndrome. Am J Ophthalmol 1990;110:28–32.

62. Catalono RA. Down syndrome. Surv Ophthalmol 1990;34:385–398.

63. North RV, Kelly ME. A review of the uses and adverse effects of topical administration of atropine. Ophthal Physiol Optics 1987;7:109–114.

64. Maino J. Ocular defects associated with cerebral palsy: a review. Rev Optom 1979;710:69–70, 72.

65. Scheiman M. Optometric findings in children with cerebral palsy. Am J Optom Physiol Opt 1984;61: 321–323.

66. Duckman R. The incidence of visual anomalies in a population of cerebral palsied children. J Am Optom Assoc 1979;9:1013–1016.

67. Duckman R. Accommodation in cerebral palsy: function and remediation. J Am Optom Assoc 1984;4: 281–283.

68. Maino D, Maino J, Maino S. Mental retardation syndromes with associated ocular defects. J Am Optom Assoc 1990;61:707–716.

69. Luckasson R (ed). Mental Retardation Definition, Classification and Systems of Supports (9th ed). Washington, DC: American Association on Mental Retardation, 1992.

70. Maino DM, Rado ME, Pizzi WJ. Ocular anomalies of individuals with mental illness and dual diagnosis. J Am Optom Assoc 1996;67:740–748.

71. Rourke BP. Nonverbal Learning Disabilities: The Syndrome and the Model. New York: Guilford Press, 1989.

72. Maino DM, Kofman J, Flynn MF, Lai L. Ocular manifestations of Sotos syndrome. J Am Optom Assoc 1994:65:339–346.

73. Castane M, Peris E, Sanchez E. Ocular dysfunction associated mental handicap. Ophthal Physiol Optics 1995;15:489–492.

74. Tsatsanis KD, Rourke BP. Conclusions and Future Directions. In BP Rourke (ed), Syndrome of Nonverbal Learning Disabilities Neurodevelopmental Manifestations. New York: Guilford Publications, 1995;476–496.

75. Rourke BP. Introduction: The NLD Syndrome and the White Matter Model. In BP Rourke (ed), Syndrome of Nonverbal Learning Disabilities Neurodevelopmental Manifestations. New York: Guilford Publications, 1995;1–26.

76. Hatch S. The Role of Optometry in Early Intervention. In D Maino (ed), Diagnosis and Management of Special Populations. St. Louis: Mosby, 1995;283–295.

77. Schlange D, Maino D. Clinical Behavioral Objectives: Assessment Techniques for Special Populations. In D Maino (ed), Diagnosis and Management of Special Populations. St. Louis: Mosby, 1995;151–188.

78. Duckman R. Management of Functional and Perceptual Disorders in Special Populations. In D Maino (ed), Diagnosis and Management of Special Populations. St. Louis: Mosby, 1995;227–264.

79. Rouse M, Borsting E. Vision Therapy Procedures for Developmental Visual Information Processing Disorders. In M Scheiman, M Rouse (eds), Optometric Man-

agement of Learning-Related Vision Problems. St. Louis: Mosby, 1994;494–543.

80. Frantz K, Caden B. Diagnosis and Management of Common Eye Disease in Infants, Toddlers, and Preschool Children. In M Scheiman, R London (eds), Pediatric Optometry Problems in Optometry Series (Vol 3). Philadelphia: Lippincott, 1990;3:420–437.

81. Geering J, Maino D. The patient with mental handicaps: a primary care perspective. South J Optom 1992;10:23–27.

82. Block S. Identification and treatment of amblyopia in infants and young children. Pract Optom 1993;4: 31–38.

83. Haegerstrom-Portnoy G. New procedures for evaluating vision function of special populations. Optom Vis Sci 1993;70:306–314.

84. Scharre JE, Marciniak M. Pediatric clinical decision making. J Am Optom Assoc 1994;65:305–310.

Chapter 17
Pediatric Contact Lenses

Bruce D. Moore

CONDITIONS SUITABLE FOR CONTACT LENS CORRECTION

Contact lenses are a useful treatment modality for young children [1]. High refractive errors and aphakia are the two most frequently encountered ocular conditions in children that benefit from the use of contact lenses. Patients with amblyopia, congenital structural and functional abnormalities, and corneal trauma may be helped as well.

Refractive Error

Myopia

Preschool-age children with low degrees of myopia generally do not require refractive correction unless their myopia is associated with anisometropia or amblyopia. Children with higher degrees of myopia (>2.00 D) do require optical correction. Glasses are usually prescribed, but some children may benefit from the use of contact lenses. Some parents may experience difficulty keeping glasses on their child's face because of the child's activity or intolerance of the glasses. Children with craniofacial abnormalities may be difficult to fit with glasses, necessitating contact lens correction. Contact lenses provide peripheral vision enhancement and image size stabilization, an advantage that glasses do not have. These factors can improve the child's visual perceptual and motor skills. Improved cosmesis may be an important issue for some families. Stud-

ies have indicated that rigid gas-permeable (RGP) contact lenses may help limit the rate of progression of myopia [2].

Hyperopia

Young children with high degrees of hyperopia (3.00–5.00 D) require correction at a young age to prevent or treat the development of accommodative esotropia or refractive amblyopia. These children are usually fit with glasses initially but may not tolerate wearing them on a consistent basis. Contact lenses may be substituted to reduce the risk of amblyopia, strabismus, or both. Their use has proven especially effective in those children with nanophthalmus, a condition in which the globe is much smaller than normal and a very high degree of hyperopia is present.

Contact lenses provide additional benefits for young patients with accommodative esotropia and moderate to high degrees of hyperopia by decreasing the angle of deviation more than glasses [3]. Correction with contact lenses decreases the convergence demand by eliminating the induced base-out prismatic effect caused by plus lenses of glasses. Contact lenses also decrease the accommodative demand below that measured through glasses. In patients with a high ratio of accommodative convergence to accommodation (AC/A) and accommodative esotropia, contact lenses cause an apparent decrease in the AC/A ratio. Bifocal contact lenses have been shown to be of even greater benefit than glasses in controlling accommodative esotropia in young patients with residual deviations at near [4].

Astigmatism

The power and axis of astigmatism in children ages 6–36 months varies considerably [5, 6]. This variability generally does not cause visual problems unless associated with high spherical refractive errors. In these cases, correction is indicated when strabismus or amblyopia is associated with the astigmatism. Since the astigmatism is often so variable, a repeat refraction should be performed before prescribing the correction. Prescribing inappropriate cylindrical correction may actually cause more harm than good by interfering with the process of emmetropization and potentially inducing high refractive errors and refractive or anisometropic amblyopia.

When correction with contact lenses is indicated, custom-made gas-permeable or soft toric lenses can be designed. Aspheric-design RGP lenses correct considerable degrees of hyperopic astigmatism and can be fit empirically without the benefit of keratometric measurements. With improvements in manufacturing technology, custom-made soft toric lenses can now be obtained in virtually any parameter required.

Anisometropia

Anisometropia is a significant cause of amblyopia in young children. Strabismus may be the first sign of anisometropic amblyopia, but often no visible deviation is present. The child often develops a microtropia and amblyopia that will go undiagnosed until a complete eye examination at a later age, when treatment will be more difficult. Detection of anisometropic amblyopia is one of the most important reasons that all children should be screened at 3–4 years of age.

Contact lenses may be useful in correcting the optical component of anisometropic amblyopia because they can be designed to correct almost any refractive error. Compliance with contact lens wear may be better than with glasses in some patients. The optical correction is, however, only the first step in the treatment of anisometropia. Patching of the fellow eye to treat amblyopia is almost always

more difficult than maintaining proper refractive correction. Due to the changing nature of refractive error in young children, contact lenses power must be carefully monitored.

Unequal refractive error creates retinal images of unequal clarity. This may lead to suppression of the less clear image, the first step in the development of amblyopia. When this unequal refractive error is later optically corrected, aniseikonia, or unequal image size, is created at the retinal plane, further compromising the potential for fusion.

Knapp's law states that there is no magnification change in axial ametropes corrected with glasses and that there is no image size change in refractive ametropes corrected with contact lenses. This law has formed the theoretical basis of the treatment of aniseikonia for some time. Evidence indicates that additional factors may influence treatment. Contact lens correction of axial myopia has been shown to improve both visual performance and optical correction more than would be expected solely on the basis of Knapp's law. Romano [7] suggests that stretching of the retinal elements in unilateral high myopes produces a relative micropsia that induces increased aniseikonia. This is best compensated for with contact lenses. Lin's experiments with birds [8] confirm Romano's hypothesis. Moreover, the reduction in vertical prismatic imbalance with contact lenses may be a greater contribution to fusion than the theoretical impediment of aniseikonia in axial ametropias. The use of contact lenses in this situation offers the greatest efficacy for most patients, especially those with unilateral high myopia, and should therefore be the treatment of choice.

Aniseikonic correction with both contact lenses and glasses may prove very beneficial in patients with unilateral aphakia or high myopia, especially in the presence of diplopia that is due to the induced aniseikonia. A regular or reverse Galilean telescope can help to equalize the image sizes and promote fusion. A reverse Galilean telescope uses an overcorrection of a plus power (or less minus power) contact lens and a resultant overcorrection with minus-powered glasses to reduce the image size. A regular Galilean telescope incorporates the use of less plus or more minus in a contact lens and a resulting increase in plus power (or less minus) in the glasses to increase image size [9, 10].

Aphakia

Although cataracts are uncommon in young children, their treatment is a large and important part of any pediatric contact lens practice. Pediatric cataracts may be unilateral or bilateral and congenital or acquired. In the past, congenital cataracts were considered very difficult to treat, particularly when they were unilateral. Cataracts of later onset were thought to be only somewhat more amenable to treatment. Difficulties with surgical techniques, contact lens fitting in young children, and the treatment of amblyopia all played a role in the generally pessimistic outlook in these patients. Techniques to address these difficulties were developed in the 1980s and are now used routinely [11, 12].

The prognosis for good vision in young children with cataracts depends on the time of onset and density of the cataracts, whether early surgical intervention is performed, whether optical correction is appropriate, and whether the cataracts are unilateral or bilateral. Cataract extraction, contact lens correction, and aggressive amblyopia treatment are required before the end of the critical period of visual development (4–6 months of age) in order to attain good visual acuity in the affected eye [13]. Cataracts that develop after the critical period seem to have a less severe impact on visual acuity unless they become dense and persistent.

Children with bilateral aphakia may be fit with either contact lenses or glasses. Although some patients perform better with one method of optical correction than the other, the use of contact lenses has distinct advantages. The magnification produced by glasses is about 20–30% and only 8–12% with typical pediatric aphakic-powered contact lenses. This allows the child to experience a more natural visual perceptual environment so that the child's general development may progress at a more normal rate. The child's appearance may be better with contact lenses than with glasses, thus enhancing his or her psychosocial development due to enhanced cosmesis. In addition, it is difficult to keep heavy glasses on a child's face, particularly if the child has craniofacial abnormalities.

Although contact lenses have advantage over glasses, they may prove difficult for the parent or child to deal with. Their cost may be prohibitively greater than glasses, especially for those patients

who replace their lenses frequently [14]. The author has found that many children with bilateral cataracts do best with both contacts and glasses, with the parent and the child deciding which is best under various conditions.

In unilateral aphakia patients, contact lenses provide superior treatment. Although glasses may work for the small number of patients who do not tolerate contact lenses, contact lenses should be tried initially. Intraocular lens implants are reserved for those patients unable to wear contact lenses or glasses who nonetheless tolerate amblyopia therapy.

Pediatric aphakic contact lens fitting is an ongoing process. As the eye grows, the prescription and (therefore the lenses) change. Diligent and continual attention to amblyopia therapy is the single most important but difficult aspect of the treatment of aphakia. These patients require very intensive levels of care.

The treatment of acquired aphakia in children older than 7 years of age is usually less difficult because deprivation amblyopia is not a factor. However, some degree of refractive, anisometropic, or strabismic amblyopia invariably results from any childhood cataract.

Older aphakic children are best fit with daily wear lenses in either soft or RGP materials. The Silsoft (Bausch & Lomb; Rochester, NY) silicone elastomer lens is tolerated poorly by older children due to discomfort. Its poor edge design and hydrophobic surface cause an uncomfortable lipid buildup on the surface of the lens. In the case of corneal trauma resulting in an irregular corneal surface, rigid lenses provide better levels of visual acuity and may reduce the risk of amblyopia. Soft lenses cannot achieve these optical effects.

Amblyopia is always a prime consideration in any aphakic child. Treatment may be with either orthoptic eye patches or occlusion soft lenses, depending on the patient and the circumstances. It is very important to consider the effects of aniseikonia in monocular aphakic patients. These effects are described in the section on anisometropia.

Amblyopia

Contact lenses may be used in the treatment of amblyopia in two different ways. High plus lenses can

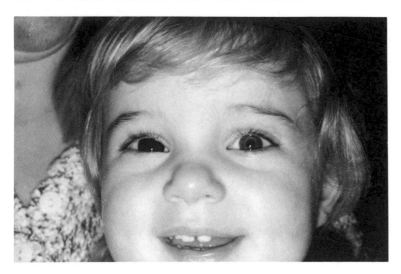

Figure 17.1. This patient with a unilateral congenital cataract is wearing an aphakic soft contact lens on the left eye and an occluder soft contact lens on the right eye in lieu of an eye patch. (Reprinted with permission from LJ Press, BD Moore. Clinical Pediatric Optometry. Boston: Butterworth–Heinemann, 1993;224.)

be worn over the normal eye to blur or fog the image quality to a level below that of the amblyopic eye. Surprisingly, the author has found that in patients treated for early-onset cataracts and dense amblyopia, the degree of optical blur achieved with even a + 30.00 D contact lens over the normal eye may not be sufficient to induce the child to use the amblyopic eye. The esotropic and amblyopic aphakic eye will not pick up fixation even when a very high-power plus contact lens is applied to the non-amblyopic eye. The child will actually prefer fixing with the now severely fogged but otherwise normal eye instead of the appropriately optically corrected amblyopic eye. High plus lenses may be more useful in patients with milder strabismic or refractive amblyopia.

Black occlusion soft contact lenses have been used in a wide variety of amblyopic patients, including those with congenital and acquired cataracts and strabismic and refractive amblyopia [15, 16] (Figure 17.1). These occlusion lenses are most effective in patients already using a contact lens for optical purposes because the family will already understand handling and care techniques for lenses. Patients without previous contact lens experience may also benefit when parental motivation is high. Many young patients object more to the sensation of the patch on their face than to the effect of the patch on their vision. These young patients may accept an occlusion lens without behavioral problems, yet object strenuously when a patch is applied

over the eye with an occluder lens in place. However, behavioral problems can arise with contact lens wear. For example, children may become adept at manipulating the lens off the cornea by hand or by blinking, reducing its effectiveness.

The most important concern in the use of an occlusion contact lens is the risk of complications from the lens itself. A risk of developing a vision-threatening corneal ulcer exists whenever a contact lens is used, regardless of the individual or the condition being treated. This risk must be carefully considered by the parents and clinician before using an occlusion contact lens.

Corneal Masking and Nystagmus

Contact lenses have several uses in corneal masking. A lens can be used to cover a disfigured eye with no useful vision (e.g., an eye that has sustained corneal insult leading to blindness and poor cosmesis). A blind, disfigured eye can become a serious impediment to the normal socialization of the child and may result in behavioral and psychological problems. Although this is likely to be more of an issue with older children, it may be just as important for younger children and their families. Contact lenses used to mask disfigured eyes may provide dramatic improvements in these patients and should be strongly considered as a treatment option. These lenses may be obtained from various sources in a variety of colors and patterns. Photographs of the normal and damaged eyes may be sent to several manufacturers to aid in the optimal design of the lens. A good cosmetic match to the normal fellow eye is easier to obtain when the patient has dark irides. These lenses tend to be quite expensive and may take a considerable period of time to obtain, but the results can be very gratifying for the patient, the family, and the practitioner.

Wesley-Jessen manufactures a modified line of its Durasoft Colors lenses for corneal masking. They are relatively expensive but are readily available and highly reproducible. The normal eye can be fit with a standard Durasoft Colors or Fresh Look (also by Wesley-Jessen) lens to provide a near-perfect match. It is also possible to take close-up photographs of both of the patient's eyes and send them to the custom manufacturers (Adventures in Color, Kontur, and the Narcissus Foundation) for color matching. Trial lenses should first be fit to the eye to be certain of a stable fit and position. This may be difficult because many of these eyes will show the effects of trauma, phthisis, or both, making it impossible to achieve normal fitting relationships on these irregularly shaped eyes. Generally, these cosmetic lenses are fit tighter than usual to prevent anomalous positioning and dislodging of the lenses. It is usually necessary to have the appearance or fit of the first lens ordered modified at least once before a satisfactory result is obtained. The parent's and patient's expectation of exact matching of appearance between the lens and the normal eye must be tempered before fitting, as it is almost impossible to obtain an exact match. It has been the author's experience that patients may be critical of small differences in appearance that the practitioner finds acceptable. The patient and family must understand that the eye will not look identical to the normal eye.

Patients with severe photophobia, nystagmus, or both also benefit from clear or tinted contact lenses. In some cases, patients with iris coloboma, aniridia, albinism, or achromatopsia may experience significantly improved vision and comfort with a darkly tinted contact lens. These patients often have high refractive errors and nystagmus and obtain better optics from contact lenses than glasses because the optical center of the contact lenses remains in a more precise alignment with the pupillary axis than the optical center of glasses does. In cases of sen-

sory nystagmus, contact lenses may reduce the optical blur sufficiently to improve visual acuity and decrease the magnitude of the nystagmus [17]. This is especially true in achromatopsia, in which tinted contact lenses reduce the retinal illumination to mesopic levels, under which they are less impaired than at photopic levels.

PEDIATRIC LENS WEAR VERSUS ADULT LENS WEAR

Adults and children do not necessarily use their contact lenses under the same conditions and in the same ways. Differences in pediatric ocular physiology and children's activities dictate lens selection in this population. Lens selection should take into account the activities the child participates in.

Although there are little data concerning the oxygen requirements of the pediatric cornea, the much faster rate of metabolism in children indicates that pediatric corneas generally need higher levels of oxygen than do adult corneas. In young children that nap, contact lenses must have a sufficiently high oxygen permeability so that they can be worn under occasional closed-eye conditions. Lenses tend to dry out and become dislodged after naps. Careful lens lubrication before and immediately after naps may avoid loss.

Since children are usually more physically active than adults, contact lenses must maintain a stable position on the eye. Decentration of the lens is more problematic in children than adults, requiring a tighter lens fit. This tight fit should generally be avoided in adults because of the possibility of inducing corneal hypoxia and "tight lens syndrome." Lenses can be safely fit more tightly in children than adults because of the greater moisture level in children's eyes. The increased aqueous component of the tear film prevents further tightening of the lens as eyes become drier later in the day or under dry environmental conditions.

Pediatric lenses should be quite durable and easy to handle. They require even sturdier lens materials than usual because of the rougher handling and wear they will undergo. Very active children who participate in sports benefit from lens diameter that is larger than normal. The lenses need to stay in place and resist popping out or decentering off the cornea during play. Because RGP lenses may dislodge easily, soft lenses are a better option for some active patients.

CHARACTERISTICS OF THE EYES OF YOUNG CHILDREN

Mensuration

The eyes of young children are not simply a smaller version of adult eyes. Both the configuration of the eye and the physiology of the ocular surface differ significantly from those of adults. The ideal contact lens design for children should take this into account. Unfortunately, all of the currently available pediatric contact lenses were designed initially for use on adults and are simply modified in power. Most of the lenses intended for pediatric use simply do not fit the small eyes of infants or are not available in appropriate powers. Various ocular parameters should be taken into consideration when designing a lens for a particular category of patient. Although studies have provided data [18–20] on the configuration and physiology of the child's eye, contact lens manufacturers have not yet applied this information to appropriate lens design.

Lacrimation

Infants do not begin reflexive tearing until at least several weeks of age. However, contact lens wear during this very early stage is only rarely complicated by this lack of tearing. Once normal tearing begins, infants appear to have a reduced protein, lipid, mucous, and mineral composition and an increased aqueous composition of their tears compared with adults. Infants and young children rarely have problems with protein, lipid, or mineral deposits on their hydrophilic contact lenses. On the other hand, silicone elastomer lenses, because of their unique properties, are prone to lipid buildup, which compromises visual acuity and comfort. The high aqueous content of the tear film of young patients enhances the oxygen supply to the cornea via tear interchange and pumping under the contact lens. This results in a lower incidence of corneal infections and hypoxia in children than in older patients. Even during napping, infant eyes rarely become dry enough to lead to contact lens–related complications. Lens loss, however, does tend to occur around nap time.

Young patients who receive radiation therapy to the head for various types of cancers have a potential for serious dry eye complications. The radiation decreases lacrimal gland function and affects the ability of the corneal epithelium to resist drying and may cause surface irregularity. Because these patients are at high risk for the development of cataracts, long-term aphakic contact lens wear success is decreased. Supplemental ocular lubrication is often necessary in these patients. Children born with Riley-Day syndrome, a rare neurologic disorder, have severely reduced aqueous tear production leading to compromise of the ocular surface.

Eyelids and Palpebral Aperture

The small palpebral aperture of the young child makes insertion and removal of contact lenses more difficult than in adults. Lid tension is greater while the child is awake and less while asleep. Lids clamp tightly shut when children cry, making the process of lens insertion and removal exceedingly difficult. Attempts to forcibly pry the eyelids open to insert or remove a contact lens on a screaming child frequently cause the lids to evert, making insertion or removal nearly impossible. Initially, parents may find it easier to insert or remove lenses when the child is sleeping (if the child sleeps deeply enough).

Pupils

The pupillary diameter of a normal, awake infant is quite small (approximately 1.5–3.0 mm). Surgery, trauma to the eye, or anatomic abnormalities often cause the pupil to become irregular or eccentric. This irregular or eccentric character of the pupil affects the positioning of the optical center of a contact lens over the pupillary aperture.

The small pupillary aperture may provide one important benefit. The greatly increased depth of focus of a small pupil may reduce the apparent necessity of optimal refractive correction with the contact lens. For example, the residual spherical or cylindrical refractive error in an infant wearing a contact lens may be adequately compensated for by the increased depth of focus of the eye as a result of the small pupil. In addition, the short axial length of the eye (17–19 mm in infants) leads to a further increase in the depth of focus. As a result, residual refractive error may be more tolerable in infants than in older patients.

Corneal Diameter

The corneal diameter of normal full-term neonates ranges from 9.25 mm to 10.50 mm. Premature infants have smaller corneal diameters. This diameter increases rapidly in the first year of life and then at a slower rate over the next few years, reaching an adult diameter of approximately 11.5–12.0 mm by 3–4 years of age.

Smaller corneal diameters may either indicate a generalized microphthalmia or may be restricted to the cornea only. Infants with congenital cataracts usually have smaller corneal diameters than normal in the affected eye(s). Infants with persistent hyperplastic primary vitreous often have both markedly reduced corneal diameters and generalized microphthalmia, with corneal diameter sometimes as small as 6–7 mm. In addition, the rate of growth of these eyes is usually less than normal eyes. Thus, the relative difference in corneal diameters becomes greater as the child grows. This can become a significant cosmetic issue later. The visual prognosis for patients with microcornea or microphthalmia is worse than for those patients with eyes of normal size. This trend does not necessarily hold true for all infants, however [21]. It is likely that very small eyes have other ocular abnormalities, including retinal abnormalities and developmental glaucoma, that worsen the long-term prognosis for successful visual rehabilitation. Small eyes usually require smaller-diameter contact lenses than do normal-size eyes.

A corneal diameter that is larger than normal at birth should immediately arouse a suspicion of congenital glaucoma, although there are other, less serious causes of increased corneal diameter. Patients with Marfan's syndrome may have megalocorneas (up to 14–15 mm in diameter) and very high degrees of myopia. These patients may particularly benefit from the use of contact lenses. The large corneal diameter requires large-diameter contact lenses.

Corneal Curvature

The central corneal curvature of neonates is quite steep. Studies have indicated that it may be as steep as 49.50 D in healthy premature infants and 47.00 D in the first 1–2 months of life in full-term infants. These values flatten to normal adult values of 43.00–44.00 D by 4 years of age. Studies of infant aphakic eyes show similar results [20], with most of the flattening taking place in the first 6 months of life. Lightman and Marshall [22] have also noted that the flattening of the infant cornea necessitates appropriate changes in the base curve of the contact lens to maintain proper fit.

Very little is actually known about the configuration of the peripheral cornea in young children. There are indications that it is very flat during early infancy and begins to steepen by 1 year of age. This greatly affects the corneal vault, or sagitta, and is a significant factor in the way contact lenses fit on these young eyes [23]. The author has seen a lens become looser fitting on an infant eye between 4–8 months of age, a period in which the lens would be expected to become tighter fitting because of the rapid flattening of the cornea that occurs at this time [20]. My assumption, based on the experience of Enoch, is that the increasing corneal vault, which effectively causes the lens to fit in a less stable manner on the eye, has a greater effect on the fit of the contact lens than the decrease in central corneal curvature. Often the practitioner will need to refit a contact lens so that it is tighter and steeper than the one previously worn in order to counteract the tendency of lenses to fit more loosely during this period.

Refractive Error

Refractive error in young children can change quite rapidly. This is particularly true in astigmatism. High hyperopes may appear to have a large increase in refractive error after wearing an optical correction for even a short period of time because the correction results in a relaxation of accommodation. Careful and repeated retinoscopic refractions are critical to the accurate determination of refractive error in these young patients.

Young children who are aphakic experience dramatic changes in refractive error during the first years of life. Studies have shown the average refractive error at the corneal plane in aphakic infants to decrease from about +31.00 D at 1 month to +21.00 D at 4 years [24], with two-thirds of the change occurring by 1.5 years of age. Lightman and Marshall [22] have confirmed these findings. It is essential to carefully monitor these changes in refractive error and make changes in the contact lens prescription so that the patient will not be overcorrected.

LENS MATERIALS

Contact lenses are currently available in three types: soft, RGP, and silicone elastomer. Each material has advantages and disadvantages that may be different for infants and young children than for adults.

Soft Lenses

Soft lenses currently comprise approximately 80–90% of the total contact lens market in the United States and are widely used in children. The oxygen permeability of lenses must be carefully considered in young contact lens wearers. Since many of the young children who wear contact lenses require strong prescriptions, the lenses tend to be much thicker than those typically used in the general population of contact lens wearers. Low-water-content soft lenses for young children are only marginally permeable to oxygen. High-water-content lenses are more permeable but are also more fragile and not as suitable for daily wear. Although children are less prone to deposits on their lenses because of the higher aqueous composition of their tears, giant papillary conjunctivitis does occur more commonly with high-water than low-water-content materials. Extended-wear soft lenses must have excellent oxygen permeability. However, the subject of the overall safety of extended-wear lenses remains quite controversial.

Soft lenses for children offer advantages over other materials. They are generally easy to fit and do not require special equipment or procedures. Their excellent comfort minimizes the adjustment period. The cost of these lenses varies greatly depending on the materials used. The risk of injury to the infant's eye by improper handling is minimal with soft lenses.

The major disadvantage of soft contact lenses is their handling difficulties. These difficulties depend on the lens material and parameters, the dexterity of the parent, and cooperation of the child. Soft lenses are more fragile than other types and are rubbed out of the eye fairly easily. Protein and lipid deposits can become problematic for some patients. The risk of infection from poor hygiene and disinfection compliance is greater than with other materials. Availability of soft lenses in pediatric parameters is limited. Many are available only on a custom-made basis, entailing delays in dispensing. The optical and general quality of hydrophilic lenses is also sometimes not as good as those made of other materials.

Rigid Lenses

Polymethylmethacrylate material is obsolete and should not be used as a contact lens material for children because of its complete lack of oxygen permeability. RGP contact lenses have been used with excellent results in many children. In the relatively thick parameters required for aphakic patients, they are quite durable. However, some fluorosilicone acrylate materials are known for chipping at their edges. RGP lenses are easy for parents to handle and care for. Cleaning and disinfection is simple and the risk of lens-induced ocular infection is low. RGPs are both the least costly and the most readily available lens material in a wide spectrum of lens designs and parameters. Lens quality is generally quite good and easy to verify in the office. Although oxygen permeability is excellent (usually higher than that of soft lenses), it is still not as high as that of silicone elastomer lenses.

The major disadvantage of RGP lenses is the difficulty in fitting them to a child's eye. RGP lens fit is highly individualized, requiring a custom design for each patient. This usually prevents lens dispensing at the time of fitting. RGP lens are also more likely to eject or decenter than lenses of other materials, increasing the frequency of replacement and therefore the expense. The initial comfort of RGP lenses may be poorer than other lens materials, requiring a longer adaptation period. There is also a theoretically greater likelihood of corneal insult resulting from eye rubbing, insertion, or removal. In spite of these concerns, many practitioners prefer

RGPs for their young patients and obtain excellent results with their use.

Silicone Elastomer Lenses

The Bausch & Lomb Silsoft lens is currently the only silicone elastomer lens available for the correction of pediatric aphakia. The Silsoft lens is made of a silicone rubber material with many properties that make it particularly useful in young aphakic children. It has the best oxygen permeability of any contact lens material; studies have shown that the amount of oxygen available to the cornea may actually be greater with the lens on the eye than with no lens on at all. The oxygen permeability of the Silsoft lens far exceeds that of any other extended-wear material. Its durability is much better than that of soft lenses and nearly as good as RGP lenses. In addition, the lenses are readily available in a series of stock aphakic parameters, making Silsoft fairly easy to fit. Another advantage is that fluorescein can and should be used to help in the fitting and the evaluation of the lenses and the eye on follow-up visits. The lenses tend to stay on the young child's eye better than other lenses, even with vigorous rubbing by the child.

Several significant problems exist with these lenses, however. When fit too tightly, they adhere tenaciously, becoming immobile on the eye and potentially leading to corneal complications. Inherent wettability problems plague its use. Silicone is a highly hydrophobic material that must have a surface treatment applied in order to be wettable on the eye. When the surface treatment is compromised due to the lens drying out or inappropriate cleaning, the surface becomes highly hydrophobic, thereby increasing the likelihood of corneal complications. Silicone has a strong affinity for surface lipid deposits, causing the lens to cloud over and adversely affect vision, comfort, and corneal health. The use of hand creams and soaps containing lanolin or other similar greasy ingredients can literally "poison" the lens surface—that is, make the lens hydrophobic. Parental hygiene must be scrupulous. An alcohol-based cleaner such as CIBA Vision (Duluth, GA) Miraflow must be used to minimize these problems of lipid deposition. It is worth noting that the Food and Drug Administration–approved lens care systems that Bausch & Lomb recommends in the Silsoft package insert are not the best systems possible and may actually cause problems for patients and practitioners. A better care system includes the Miraflow cleaner and a rigid-lens soaking solution, such as Boston Conditioning Solution (Bausch & Lomb), for storage of the lens. Because of cleaning problems, the life expectancy of the lens may be very short in certain patients. Silsoft lenses are the most expensive commercially available stock contact lens currently on the market. They tend to be relatively uncomfortable due to the edge design and the coating and wetting problems. Children become less tolerant of the lens by the end of the first decade, making the lens suitable only for young aphakic children. Silsoft is currently available only in aphakic parameters. It has been said for the past 20 years that silicone elastomer is the "lens material of the future." In my opinion, it still is.

CONTACT LENS FITTING PROCEDURES

Fitting Under Anesthesia

Some pediatric contact lens practitioners prefer to fit infants and young children while the child is under general anesthesia. This is the easiest method of obtaining measurements of corneal configuration and refractive power. A lens may be inserted and its fit evaluated without the child's behavior interfering with the process.

There are, however, several problems with examination under anesthesia. Most significant is the risk that anesthesia will precipitate a potentially serious medical emergency. Because of efforts at cost containment in health care, the cost of anesthesia must be considered as well. The measurements and information obtained under anesthesia may not be identical to those obtained in the conscious state. In the operating room, the child is lying on his or her back, lid forces are reduced, lacrimation is virtually absent, and the cornea is completely desensitized. This environment is hardly a realistic one for fitting contact lenses.

The intraocular pressure may be greatly decreased from normal levels by the anesthesia drugs. This reduction in intraocular pressure may cause the shape of the anterior segment of the eye, including the cornea, to be quite different under anesthesia. This change, therefore, is not only a confounding factor in the care of infantile glaucoma, but also in the relationship of the cornea and lens. A lens that appears to fit well in the operating room may fit completely differently in the office later the same day. Thus, the accuracy of lens fitting under anesthesia is questionable. I prefer to restrict examination and fitting of contact lenses under anesthesia to situations in which anesthesia is indicated for other reasons, such as the need for additional ocular or systemic procedures or for an extensive examination in a child who would be impossible to examine for medical or behavioral reasons.

When an examination and fitting under anesthesia have been deemed necessary, keratometry, refraction with trial lenses, and measurement by calipers of the corneal diameters should be performed after the induction of the anesthesia [25]. Contact lenses of appropriate design and material should then be inserted in the eye. The lens is evaluated for proper fit by observing the retinoscopic reflex; fluorescein pattern (if possible); and the position and movement of the lens, both spontaneously and by attempting to move the lens by manipulating the child's eyelid with the practitioner's finger. The base curve and diameter are then modified based on this fit. Once the optimal fit has been achieved, careful refraction is performed. When high powers are involved, the trial lens should be close to the target spectacle prescription. Vertex distance compensation should be taken into consideration to minimize induced error from off-axis retinoscopy and improper vertex distance effects. The eye should then be thoroughly examined by gonioscopy and binocular indirect ophthalmoscopy for ocular health assessment. The intraocular pressure should also be measured. The fit and power of the lens must then be verified on the awake child before dispensing.

Fitting Without Anesthesia

It is generally preferable to fit lenses to young children in the office setting without use of anesthesia [26]. The results will likely be at least as satisfactory as those achieved with use of anesthesia, but without the risk and cost. If the initial fit or prescription requires change, it will be detected on subsequent visits and the lenses changed before any permanent adverse effect develops. Measurements of corneal curvature by keratometry are not absolutely necessary, but hand-held autokeratometry (with the Alcon autokeratometer) (Alcon) is useful if available. Retinoscopy with a contact lens on the eye confirms proper refractive correction.

There are six main steps for the fitting of pediatric contact lenses without anesthesia:

1. A thorough eye examination should be completed to ensure that the eye is ready to be fit with a contact lens. This should be performed in conjunction with the child's ophthalmologist or pediatrician, when appropriate. Most aphakic eyes are healed and ready for lens fitting 1 or 2 weeks after surgery. If the lens is for nonaphakic correction, a general examination should be performed before fitting.

2. An initial set of lens parameters for the trial lens should be determined. An estimate of corneal diameter of both eyes should be obtained and a determination of the initial lens diameter made. Often, the practitioner will select the initial base curve of a soft or silicone elastomer trial lens by choosing a lens that is one step flatter than the steepest lens available in that design. RGP lens base curves can be estimated from keratometry readings or trial lens fitting, as described in the fourth step listed in this section.

3. The initial lens power used in aphakic children is estimated by adding approximately 2.00–3.00 D more plus than the refractive error indicated for the child's age in Figure 17.2 [24]. If the child is nonaphakic, retinoscopy should be performed with trial lenses and an initial lens power obtained by converting for the vertex distance at the corneal plane.

4. The fitting characteristics of this first trial lens are evaluated by inserting a lens of appropriate power and base curve for that design. The position and movement of the lens is then evaluated after a few minutes, when the lens has stabilized on the eye. Soft or silicone elastomer lenses should position centrally over the cornea and exhibit slightly less movement than would be preferred for adults. The lens should not decenter more than slightly on the blink or after manipulation by the practitioner's finger on the child's eyelid. If it does, choose a steeper base curve, different diameter, or a lens configuration with a larger corneal vault or sagitta. If there is inadequate movement, choose a flatter base curve or a lens configuration with a smaller sagitta.

Figure 17.2. The mean spherical refractive error obtained longitudinally from a group of 14 infants with unilateral congenital cataracts who were followed from birth to 4 years of age. (Reprinted with permission from Slack Inc. BD Moore. Changes in the aphakic refraction of children with unilateral congenital cataracts. J Pediatr Ophthalmol Strabismus 1989;26:290–295.)

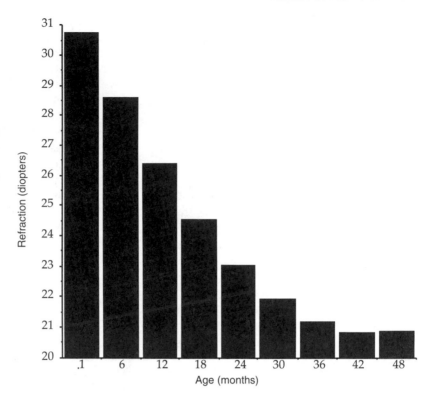

A completely different lens design or material may be required if this lens design does not fit properly. Careful attention must be given to the fitting characteristics of the periphery of the lens. It is not unusual for a lens to appear to fit well centrally, but exhibit edge fluting or lift peripherally. If this occurs, a change in lens design is required. This may include a change in diameter, thickness, base curve, edge design, or material. RGP lenses should position slightly superiorly and demonstrate an acceptable fluorescein pattern.

5. The final lens power is then determined. After the correct material and base curve have been established, careful retinoscopy should be performed with hand-held lenses over a contact lens as close to the correct power and configuration as possible. In aphakics, the power of the contact lens should be approximately +2.50 D to +3.00 D greater than the actual refractive error to provide for focusing at the near and intermediate distances, which are most important to young children. The power of a nonaphakic lens should be determined in the usual manner.

6. Finally, the correct fit of the lens should be confirmed. The lens should be rechecked several times to be certain that it fits properly and the power is correct. Changes in lens design or parameter should be made, if necessary, to achieve the ideal fit. The child should be encouraged to rub the eyes to be certain that the lens does not decenter or pop out easily. Pediatric lenses are fit more tightly to minimize the risk of ejection. Finally, parents must demonstrate the ability to remove the lens without too much difficulty before leaving the office and must thoroughly understand the techniques of lens handling, care, and disinfection.

Material-Specific Fitting Characteristics

Silicone Elastomer Lenses

Silicone elastomer is an excellent material for aphakic extended-wear lenses and is undoubtedly the most frequently used material for pediatric aphakes. The Bausch & Lomb Silsoft lens is currently the only silicone elastomer lens on the market. The fitting of these lenses is quite straightforward [27]. A high plus power lens with a 7.7-mm base curve is inserted if the child is less than 2 years old. These lenses are only available in the 11.3-mm diameter in powers over +20.00 D. Evaluate the centration and movement. The lens should center well and have at least 1.0 mm of movement. If there is less movement, select a flatter base curve; if there is too much movement, select a steeper base curve. It is very important to check the fluorescein pattern. There must be adequate flow of fluorescein under the lens; if there is a sealing off of the fluorescein flow, the lens is too tight. The lens edge is much thinner than the optic zone and should show several (2–4) "flutes," or small areas of peripheral edge lift, to guarantee tear flow under the lens. If there are no flutes, the lens is too tight and should be flattened. If the flutes are either too large or too numerous, the lens is too flat and should be steepened. Using retinoscopy, adjust the power as required. The Silsoft lens is available in a diameter of 11.3 mm in 3.00 D steps between +20.00 and +32.00 D. In both the 11.3-mm and 12.5-mm diameters, the lens is available in powers from +12.00 D to +20.00. Available base curves range from 7.7 mm to 8.3 mm.

Soft Contact Lenses

The method of fitting soft contact lenses depends on the age of the child and the underlying diagnosis [28]. Children older than 4–5 years of age are fit in the same manner as adults, using refraction, keratometry, and slit-lamp examination. An appropriate lens is inserted and evaluated in the usual manner for position, movement, refractive correction, visual acuity, and comfort. Several manufacturers sell stock lenses with a base curve steep enough and a diameter small enough for children ages 4–5 years and older. Custom-design lenses in spheres and cylinders are available from several sources. Aphakic lenses in sufficiently steep base curves may be obtained in powers up to +20.00 D from several manufacturers [29].

Aphakic lenses for younger children can be much more difficult to obtain in the very steep base curves (7.0–7.9 mm) and higher plus powers (+20.00 D to +40.00 D) often required. Generally these must be custom ordered.

Basic fitting of soft lenses for aphakic children begins with careful trial lens retinoscopy, giving

particular attention to correct vertex distance and on-axis retinoscopy. A trial contact lens is then inserted in a 12.5- to 13.0-mm diameter and a 7.5- to 7.9-mm base curve in a power that is as close as possible to that required, taking into account the vertex distance. After settling, the position and movement of the lens are assessed. It should center well and show little lag on movement. The lens should be fit slightly tighter than the normal fit for an adult. Next, retinoscopy is performed with close observation of the refractive error and the quality of the retinoscopic reflex. The appearance of the retinoscopic reflex is the most accurate indicator of whether the lens fits properly. A steep-fitting lens appears as a dark, fluctuating central retinoscopic reflex with momentary sharpening of the reflex immediately after the blink. A flat-fitting lens appears as a less-than-sharp retinoscopic reflex, especially toward the periphery, and may look sharpest centrally just before the beginning of the blink.

It may be difficult to observe these reflexes in some children because of the child's behavior or the effects of the surgery itself. A diminished or absent retinoscopic reflex may indicate increased intraocular pressure resulting in a cloudy cornea, retinal detachment, or opacification of the vitreous face or posterior lens capsule. A contact lens that is so decentered that the optic zone no longer coincides with the pupillary aperture or a required lens power that is so different than that of the cornea that it causes high residual refractive error may also cause the retinoscopic reflex to be difficult to assess.

The lens should be changed until the lens is well centered with a minimal but finite amount of movement and a sharp retinoscopic reflex is displayed. The lenticular portion of a well-fitting soft lens may show some mild fluting of the edge of the lens. If this appears excessive, a different base curve or edge design is required or the lens may be "kicked" by the eyelids and dislodged from the eye. Ideally, the power of the lens should be about +2.50 D to +3.00 D above neutrality. If a lens fits reasonably well but is of insufficient power, dispense that lens and order the correct power lens. It is better to have a +20.00 D lens on an eye needing a +35.00 D than no lens at all. In addition, the parent and child can begin learning insertion and removal and wear of the lens immediately.

The fitting process for phakic patients is similar. Proper power is estimated by cycloplegic retinoscopy.

Rigid Gas-Permeable Lenses

The technique of fitting RGP lenses to children 4–5 years and older is similar to that used in adults. Refraction, slit-lamp examination, and keratometry are performed to arrive at a starting point for lens fitting. Depending on the design and diameter of the lens used, a trial lens can be placed on the eye and evaluated for position, movement, power, and fluorescein pattern. The lens is changed as required, and a final set of lens parameters is determined. The lens is then ordered in the desired material and dispensed after the parents and child are instructed on proper lens care and handling.

In younger and less cooperative patients [30, 31], it may not be possible to perform keratometry to provide a starting point for selection of the base curve. The hand-held autokeratometer from Alcon has proven useful in these young patients. A lens design is chosen based largely on a combination of experience and intuition and inserted and assessed for position, movement, and fluorescein pattern. Additional lenses are then inserted as required to obtain the optimal lens fit. Careful refraction determines the final lens power to be ordered. A drop of topical anesthetic may be instilled prior to insertion of the lens.

CHOOSING EXTENDED-WEAR OR DAILY-WEAR LENSES

Considerable controversy continues over the safety of extended-wear contact lenses in all age groups, including infants and young children. Data in adults show that changes occur in all layers of the cornea in response to extended wear for even short periods of time [32]. Studies sponsored by the contact lens industry and the Harvard Medical School [33, 34] have clearly shown an increased risk of serious complications with extended wear. Numerous other studies have estimated the increased relative risk with extended wear to 1.5–15.0 times that of daily wear. This risk may be exacerbated by the thick-parameter lenses required for aphakic children (with the exception of the silicone elastomer lenses). It is also possible that constant wear of contact lenses over soft, young corneas may have some lasting effect on the development of the size, shape, and refraction of the growing eye.

Taking into account these disadvantages, why do some practitioners consider extended wear acceptable for their young patients? Proponents of extended wear contend that it is easier for parents and children to manage than daily wear and is relatively safe, in spite of the concerns. Opponents argue that its safety is uncertain and that extended wear may actually be more difficult to manage over time. Extended wear in children should be considered only in instances of aphakia and high refractive error or when daily wear proves too difficult for the parents and child to manage successfully. It is certainly easier to train parents and condition the child to manage daily insertion and removal of lenses when the child is very young. Even if extended wear works well in the first few years, there is no guarantee that it will continue to do so in the future. The child may be unable to maintain wear of the original lens design and may require a switch to a lens that cannot be used for extended wear.

It has been argued that the major cause of treatment failure in aphakic infants is the inability to maintain contact lens wear. The use of extended-wear lenses is supposed to make the continuation of contact lens wear easier. However, visual rehabilitation in pediatric aphakia fails due to the lack of compliance with amblyopia therapy. Over the long term, it is this aspect of treatment, rather than any contact lens–related problem, that leads to submaximal vision [35].

The option of extended-wear lenses should be reserved for those patients with such small, tight palpebral apertures that daily insertion and removal is simply impossible or for children who fight so vigorously that even the practitioner finds it impossible to insert and remove the lens. Even in these situations, extended-wear lenses should be considered only a temporary measure.

PARENTAL INSTRUCTION

Communication with the parents of a young child is probably the most critical element in the process of contact lens fitting and aftercare. Parents and caregivers must fully understand the goals and objectives of the proposed treatment and its potential benefits and risks. They need to anticipate the common day-to-day problems, the long duration of care and use of lenses, and the considerable expenses involved. They must also understand that only through their own efforts is there any likelihood that their child will be able to see better. Their confidence must be enhanced and their expectations made realistic.

The psychosocial implications of the child's underlying eye problem must be fully explored. The parents, particularly the mother, may possess hidden feelings of guilt about being the cause of the child's eye problem. The mother may believe that something she did wrong (e.g., from use of alcohol, prescribed or illegal drugs, ultrasound) during her pregnancy may have precipitated the child's ocular abnormality. It is best to confront these issues as early as possible during the treatment process to preclude problems later. Discuss the effects on other siblings of spending extra time with the child needing therapy. Relatives such as grandparents may also play an important role in the treatment and should be considered as important assets in the treatment.

Parents are often initially apprehensive about inserting and removing lenses from their child's eyes. With proper instruction, much encouragement, and patience, most do well. Many parents find lens removal easier than insertion when they begin. They must be adept at these procedures before they leave the office on the day of dispensing. Proper cleaning and disinfection are critical to the long-term safety and success of lens wear. Parents must be familiar with the correct cleaning procedures and must understand the rationale for each component of the system that is dispensed for their child's lenses. It is important for parents to have an emergency phone number to call if problems occur during non-office hours.

FOLLOW-UP VISITS

Frequent follow-up visits are needed to ensure that the lenses are performing well and the amblyopia therapy is proceeding in the desired manner. This frequency is determined by the child's underlying diagnosis, age, the level of competency of the parents, the distance the family lives from the practitioner's office, and the rate of progress of the treatment.

Visual acuity must be assessed at each follow-up visit. The visual acuity of young children can be measured using visual evoked potentials, the preferential looking procedure, or a behavioral test. Teller acuity cards are useful in the younger age groups. Older children can be tested by recognition acuity procedures such as LEA symbols, HOTV cards, Broken Wheel test, or Snellen's test. An assessment of monocular visual acuity is essential for evaluating the efficacy of amblyopia treatment. These measurements provide valuable feedback for the parents. They can easily see the improvement in their child's vision from visit to visit if recommended patching therapy is being adhered to or will see the decrease in visual acuity if compliance is low. Patching for amblyopia is achieved with orthoptic eye patches or with occlusive soft contact lenses if patches are not tolerated.

The lens fit should be evaluated on each follow-up visit. Changes in the shape of the eye and the refractive error occur rapidly in infants, affecting the efficacy and fit of the lens. Lenses must be changed as required in order to maintain optimal fit and optical correction. This may need to be done a number of times in the first year. Ocular health must also be assessed on each visit. A hand-held slit-lamp, biooptic loupes, or ophthalmoscope may be used to inspect the anterior segment.

The combination of contact lens wear and amblyopia therapy must be continued until the possibility of acuity regression is past. This varies in individual patients and will occur between the ages of 6–9 years. The amount of patching is usually decreased after 5 years of age to a level that allows for maintenance of the acuity level. Patching time should be increased if acuity drops.

COMPLICATIONS

Although most young patients who are fit with contact lenses will have a very good experience with them, complications may arise. These problems will range from the trivial to serious and could potentially even result in loss of vision. Education and comprehensive follow-up care are the best way to avoid problems. However, even in the best of circumstances, unintended sequelae are to be expected and should be prepared for. During the fitting of the contact lenses, the optometrist must warn patients and parents of the potential for lens-related problems. This is important for professional, ethical, and legal reasons. Failure to adequately explain these problems and risks may constitute malpractice.

Many of the problems seen in follow-up examinations are related to the patient's or parents' lack of understanding about the correct handling and care procedures. Problems related to handling and proper care of the lenses are encountered most frequently. Usually, clear explanations to the parents, along with written instructions and audiovisual aids, will minimize the potential for these problems. Sometimes, the problem is related to lenses that are not performing as anticipated or are simply fitting poorly. A change in lens design may solve the problem.

Lenses that have caused a physiologic or pathologic ocular response that requires treatment and may result in permanent sequelae are of greatest concern. Problems of this type range from corneal hypoxia to severe ocular inflammation or infection. The first step in remediation is correct diagnosis of the underlying problem, which may not be easy. If the problem is severe enough and the diagnosis is unclear, the patient should be referred to a corneal specialist. In any event, lens wear should not be attempted again until the problem is completely resolved. These patients must then be monitored very closely to be certain that the lenses and the eye are performing correctly.

Corneal ulceration is the most severe contact lens–related complication. Any treatment must be preceded by complete culturing of the cornea, including aerobic and anaerobic culture media and Gram's stain. Initial treatment should be appropriate to the clinical appearance and should be modified when culture and Gram's stain reports are available or if the initial treatment appears ineffective. Fluoroquinolones are the antibiotics of choice for treatment of corneal ulceration. Gentamycin or tobramycin drops (at least every other hour) may also be used alone or in combination with fluoroquinolones. Ointments should be instilled frequently overnight. An agent effective against gram-positive bacteria such as bacitracin ointment should be included if indicated by laboratory tests or clinical appearance indicates that *Staphylococcus* or *Streptococcus* is a likely cause. Steroids should not be used initially, particularly if there is any possibility of herpes simplex keratitis infection. Patients must be seen again the following day. Under certain circumstances the patient may even require hospitalization to ensure that the medications are used correctly and the infection is resolving. Referral to a corneal specialist or a pediatric ophthalmologist is indicated.

A variety of other problems may also be encountered on follow-up. Sensitivities to various components of the cleaning and disinfecting systems occur despite improvement in care systems. Patients or parents will report conjunctival injection, a foreign body sensation, and an increasing level of contact lens intolerance. The child usually develops decreased tolerance to lens wear, manifested by frequent rubbing of the eyes and lenses, chronic redness, lens ejection, and behavioral changes when the lenses are worn for variable lengths of time. Lens wear should be discontinued until the inflammation has abated and a different set of solutions should be used. A new pair of lenses may also be helpful. Giant papillary conjunctivitis can occur even in young contact lens wearers. It should be treated initially with discontinuation of lens wear and the use of mast-cell inhibitor or steroidal anti-inflammatory eyedrops until the papillae reduce in size and the eye becomes quiescent. Lens wear can then be attempted with new lenses. Concomitant treatment with mast-cell inhibitors should be continued until most signs of the giant papillary conjunctivitis have resolved. A switch to either RGP lenses or disposable daily-wear lenses may prove very helpful although these patients will remain vulnerable to the recurrence of giant papillary conjunctivitis.

Lens management problems are also significant. Abrasion of the cornea from rough handling or wear and recurrent corneal erosion are more likely caused by a condition unrelated to contact lens wear. Repeated lens loss and tearing are the most common problems. A change in lens design may alleviate the frequent lens loss. The proper handling techniques should be reviewed with parents. Lenses may develop deposits that affect vision or comfort. Rigid lenses may solve this problem. In addition, the patient's behavior may be the cause of any of these lens-related problems.

REFERENCES

1. Halberg GP. Contact Lenses for Infants and Children. In RD Harley (ed), Pediatric Ophthalmology. Philadelphia: Saunders, 1983;1280–1288.

2. Grosvenor T, Perrigin J, Perrigin D, Quintero S. The use of silicone-acrylate contact lenses for the control of myopia: results after two years of lens wear. Am J Optom Physiol Opt 1989;66:41–47.

3. Sampson WG. Correction of refractive errors: effect on accommodation and convergence. Trans Am Acad Ophthamol Otolaryngol 1971;75:124–132.

4. Moore BD, Olivares GE. Treatment of accommodative esotropia with Unilens RGP Aspheric Multifocal contact lenses. Optom Vis Sci 1994;71(12S):127.

5. Mohindra I, Held R, Gwiazda J, Brill S. Astigmatism in infants. Science 1978;202:329–331.

6. Fulton AB, Dobson V, Salem D, Marg C, et al. Cycloplegic refractions in infants and young children. Am J Ophthalmol 1980;90:239–247.

7. Romano PE. An exception to Knapp's law: unilateral axial high myopia. Binocular Vision 1985;1:166–170.

8. Lin T, Grimes PA, Stone RA. Expansion of retinal pigment epithelium in avian myopia. Invest Ophthalmol Vis Sci 1990;31:253–225 .

9. Enoch JM. Use of inverted telescopic corrections incorporating soft contact lens in the (partial) correction of aniseikonia in cases of unilateral aphakia. Adv Ophthamol 1976;32:54–66.

10. Enoch JM, Hamer RD. Image size correction of the unilateral aphakic infant. Ophthalmic Pediatr Genet 1983;2:153–165.

11. Robb RM, Mayer DL, Moore BD. Results of early treatment of unilateral congenital cataracts. J Pediatr Ophthalmol Strabismus 1987;24:178–181.

12. Mayer DL, Moore BD, Robb RM. Assessment of vision and amblyopia by preferential looking tests after early surgery for unilateral congenital cataracts. J Pediatr Ophthalmol Strabismus 1989;26:61–68.

13. Beller R, Hoyt CS, Marg E, Odom JV. Good visual function after neonatal surgery for congenital monocular cataracts. Am J Ophthalmol 1981;91:559–565.

14. Lightman JM, Marshall D. Analysis of annual quantities of contact lenses needed to correct pediatric aphakia. Poster presented at Annual Meeting of American Academy Optometry 1994. Optom Vis Sci 1994;71(12S):153.

15. Moore BD, Smith L. Occluder soft contact lenses in the treatment of amblyopia in young children. Presented at the Annual Meeting of the American Academy of Optometry; December 7, 1984; St. Louis.

16. Moore BD. Contact Lens Therapy for Amblyopia. In R Rutstein (ed), Problems in Optometry; Amblyopia. Philadelphia: Lippincott, 1991;355–368.

17. Allen ED, Davies PD. Role of contact lenses in the management of congenital nystagmus. Br J Ophthalmol 1983;67:834–836.

18. Chase WW, Fronk SJ, Micheals BA. A theoretical infant schematic eye. Presented at the Annual Meeting of American Academy of Optometry; December 8, 1984; St. Louis.

19. Enoch JM. The fitting of hydrophylic (soft) contact lenses to infants and young children. I. Mensuration data on aphakic eyes of children born with congenital cataracts. Contact Lens Med Bull 1972;5:36–40.

20. Moore BD. Mensuration data in infant eyes with unilateral congenital cataracts. Am J Optom Physiol Optic 1987;64:204–210.

21. Karr DJ, Scott WE. Visual acuity results following treatment of persistent hyperplastic primary vitreous. Arch Ophthalmol 1986;104:662–667.

22. Lightman JM, Marshall D. Clinical evaluation of back optic radius and power determination by age in pediatric aphakia due to congenital cataract fitted with a silicone elaster contact lens. Optom Vis Sci 1996;73:22–27.

23. Enoch JM. Techniques for evaluating scleral curvature and corneal vault. Contact Lens J 1979;8:19–31.

24. Moore BD. Changes in the aphakic refraction of children with unilateral congenital cararacts. J Pediatr Ophthalmol Strabismus 1989;26:290–295.

25. Enoch JM. The fitting of hydrophylic (soft) contact lenses to infants and young children. II. Fitting techniques and initial results on aphakic children. Contact Lens Med Bull 1972;5:41–47.

26. Moore BD. The fitting of contact lenses in aphakic infants. J Am Optom Assoc 1985;56:180–183.

27. Cutler SI, Nelson LB, Calhoun JH. Extended wear contact lenses in pediatric aphakia. J Pediatr Ophthalmol Strabismus 1985;22:86–91.

28. Weissman BA, Donzis PB. Contact Lens Application After Infantile Cataract Surgery. In SJ Isenberg (ed), The Eye in Infancy. Chicago: Year Book, 1989;320–326.

29. Moore BD. Contact Lens Problems and Management in Infants, Toddlers, and Preschool Children. In M Scheiman (ed), Problems in Optometry; Pediatric Optometry. Philadelphia: Lippincott, 1990;365–393.

30. Pratt-Johnson JA, Tillson G. Hard contact lenses in the management of congenital cataracts. J Pediatr Ophthalmol Strabismus 1985;22:94–96.

31. Saunders RA, Ellis FD. Empirical fitting of hard contact lenses in infants and young children. Ophthalmology 1981;88:127–130.

32. Holden BA, Sweeney DF, Vannas A, et al. Effects of long-term extended contact lens wear on the human cornea. Invest Ophthalmol Vis Sci 1985;26:1489–1501.

33. Schein OD, Glynn RJ, Poggio EC, et al. The relative risk of ulcerative keratitis among users of daily-wear and extended-wear soft contact lenses. N Engl J Med 1989;321:773–778.

34. Poggio EC, Glynn RJ, Schein OD, et al. The incidence of ulcerative keratitis among users of daily-wear and extended-wear soft contact lenses. N Engl J Med 1989;321:779–783.

35. Moore BD. Pediatric contact lens wear, rates of successful wear. J Pediatr Ophthalmol Strabismus 1993; 30:221–230.

Chapter 18
Child Abuse

Ruth E. Manny

Poor shaken babe, guileless tyke,
Rocked by love and hate alike,
Your mother's tongue locked in silence,
Hush untold tales of guilty violence,
But when we flood your flesh with radiant streams,
Bruised bones shine through the truthful gleams,
It's stretch, squeeze, stretch; not bash, hit, batter,
Which bloody your bones and dura mater.

—John Caffey. The parent-infant traumatic stress syndrome (Caffey-Kempe syndrome) (battered babe syndrome). *American Journal of Roentgenology, Radium Therapy and Nuclear Medicine* 1972;114(2):218–229.

Hark ye good parents, to my words true and plain,
When you are shaking your baby, you could be bruising his brain.
So, save the limbs, the brain, even the life of your tot;
By shaking him never; never and not.

—John Caffey. On the theory and practice of shaking infants: its potential residual effects of permanent brain damage and mental retardation. *American Journal of Diseases of Children* 1972;124(2):161–169.

Guard well your baby's precious head,
Shake, jerk and slap it never,
Lest you bruise his brain and twist his mind,
Or whiplash him dead, forever.

—John Caffey. The whiplash shaken infant syndrome: manual shaking by the extremities with whiplash-induced intracranial and intraocular bleedings, linked with residual permanent brain damage and mental retardation. *Pediatrics* 1974;54(4):396–403.

Perhaps one of the things that makes child abuse so frightening is that any one of us who has spent time around children can recall at least one occasion in which we, or someone close to us, came very near to losing control and injuring a child in a moment of uncontrolled frustration or anger. Helfer [1], a noted author in the field of child abuse, relates one such personal incident that occurred after the birth of his sixth child. The child weighed 5 pounds and was born 6 weeks early. Because his wife was suffering from hepatitis, Dr. Helfer assumed the responsibilities of caring for the newborn. The child was a difficult, sick baby. The baby screamed and cried and kept them awake at night. Dr. Helfer recalled one particular night about 3 AM when he was awakened by the crying newborn after getting the infant to sleep only 1½ hours earlier. His wife, despite her own nausea and pain, offered to hold the baby for a few minutes when she observed that her husband was very distressed and was handling the baby with "much too much vigor." He asked, "What would have happened if she had not offered help at that time?"

This scenario highlights some of the complex interactions that have been posited as factors in abuse. The social interaction model [2] suggests that the potential for abuse increases as various child and parental characteristics interact with environmental situations. The previous vignette also demonstrates that within this setting, not only were there potentiating factors that increased the risk of abuse (i.e., a difficult, inconsolable child; and a stressed, sleep-deprived parent), there were also compensatory factors (i.e., a spouse who recognized the problem and intervened to relieve stress) that can reduce the risk of abuse. These compensatory factors have become important components of many models of child abuse—the ecological model [2, 3], the transactional model [2], and the transitional model [2]. It is also important to remember that less than 10% of those who abuse children are seriously mentally ill (psychopathology model) [2, 4, 5] and that anyone can potentially abuse a child [6, 7].

Although a detailed review of the various theories of child abuse is beyond the scope of this chapter, it is important to realize that child abuse is a multifaceted, complex, interactive problem. This chapter explores some of the more common potentiating components of the problem (the parent, the child, and environmental triggers or crises) that have been associated with the physical abuse of young children. In addition, the ocular and physical signs of physical abuse that may be encountered by eye care professionals are reviewed. The responsibilities of eye care professionals to report suspected cases of child abuse, and the long-term consequences of physical abuse are also discussed. The chapter ends with a few strategies that the eye care professional may implement in an attempt to prevent child abuse.

DEFINITIONS

Child maltreatment includes physical, emotional, or sexual abuse; and physical, educational, or medical neglect [8]. *Physical neglect*, or *deprivation of necessities*, refers to the failure to provide needed, age-appropriate care [8]. *Medical neglect* refers to a specific form of neglect—that is, "the failure to provide for appropriate health care of the child, though financially able or offered financial or other means, except when a parent or other person responsible for the child's welfare is legitimately practicing religious beliefs and by reason thereof does not provide specified medical treatment for a child" [8]. The American Medical Association Council on Scientific Affairs includes failure to provide necessary prosthetics, including eyeglasses and hearing aids, in its description of medical neglect [9]. Neglect accounted for 49% of the substantiated cases of abuse in 1994 (based on reports from 36 states); physical abuse was second, representing 21% of substantiated cases [10]. Although neglect is more frequent, physical abuse may be more dramatic, easier to recognize [7, 9], and more frequently encountered by eye care professionals. Therefore, this chapter focuses on physical abuse.

PHYSICAL ABUSE

The Federal Child Abuse Prevention and Treatment Act (Public Law 93-247), enacted in 1974, established the National Center for Child Abuse and Neglect (NCCAN, an agency within the U.S. Department of Health, Education and Welfare, currently the Department of Health and Human Services) and set standards for identification and management of child maltreatment. However, the federal law (Public Law 93-247) left the definition of maltreatment, the investigation of suspected abuse, and the services available to families and victims to the discretion of each state [8, 11]. In an attempt to provide a working definition of abuse, the U.S. Department of Health and Human Services NCCAN defines physical abuse as "physical acts that caused or could have caused physical injury to a child" [8]. However, this broad definition, which includes both abuse and the potential for abuse, makes it difficult to estimate the actual incidence of physical abuse. Therefore, the Third National Incidence and Prevalence Study of Child Abuse and Neglect (conducted in 1993; the First National Incidence Study was conducted in 1980; the Second National Incidence Study was conducted in 1986) required the child to suffer a physical injury as a result of actions by a parent or caretaker to be recognized as abuse (the Harm Standard definition) [12]. Using the Harm Standard definition, the incident rate of physical abuse in the United States in 1993 was estimated to be 5.7 per 1,000 children [12]. Statistics from the 1994 annual survey of states conducted by the National Committee to Prevent Child Abuse, which uses a different sampling procedure, estimates the incident rate of substantiated cases to be 16 per 1,000 children [10].

Despite these definitions of physical abuse, there is still considerable disagreement about what constitutes appropriate discipline and what constitutes physical abuse. This is particularly germane, as physical abuse most frequently occurs when a parent is attempting to discipline or modify a child's behavior [13]. Hitting a child has been an accepted form of physical punishment [3, 6, 14] and is still allowed in many schools in the country [15]; however, many Americans consider physical punishment a form of physical abuse, and many groups are working to change parents' attitudes about physical punishment. Physicians also disagree on what constitutes appropriate discipline and what constitutes abuse that should be reported [16]. Thus, it is important to have some guidelines to help delineate physical abuse from "reasonable" physical punishment or legal corporal punishment. Most state laws consider corporal punishment that results in physical injury to be physical abuse. Needleman [17] suggests that physical abuse be considered if the punishment (1) results in bruises; (2) requires medical treatment; (3) is delivered by kicking, a closed fist, or a blunt instrument; (4) is not delivered to the buttocks, legs, or hands; (5) results in multiple, repeated blows; (6) is administered more than three times per day; or (7) is administered to a child who is not yet walking. In addition, the vigorous shaking of a young infant is considered a form of physical abuse. It is important to identify children suffering from physical abuse or those at risk for physical abuse early, as the maximum incidence for physical abuse occurs within the first year of life [18, 19]. Eighty-eight percent of fatalities attributed to abuse between 1992 and 1994 occurred in children less than 5 years of age, and 46% of these fatalities were infants less than 1 year of age [10]. These figures are similar to those reported by McClain et al. [20]. Nonaccidental injury has been cited as the leading cause of death in infants 1 month to 1 year of age in North America [21].

IDENTIFYING ABUSE

Fifty to 60% of physical injuries resulting from nonaccidental trauma are considered moderate rather than severe [13, 22]. However, one report suggests that the proportion of severe injuries increased significantly between the early 1970s and the early 1980s (from 32% to 54%) without a significant increase in the incidence of hospitalized cases [23]. Although several factors are proposed to explain this disturbing trend, one conjecture, an improved awareness of abuse that has resulted in minor injuries being identified earlier, offers some encouragement. In the following sections, the more common types of physical abuse occurring in young children are reviewed. Minor trauma characteristic of nonaccidental trauma (bruises and burns), as well

as severe trauma often resulting from the shaken baby syndrome and its associated ocular findings, are presented. A brief discussion of failure to thrive and Munchausen syndrome by proxy is also included due to their propensity for affecting the young child.

Case History

Regardless of the presenting or observed injuries, a careful and complete history remains one of the most useful tools for unraveling cases of suspected abuse [7, 13, 16, 18, 19, 24]. Parents of children injured accidentally typically seek immediate care for their child and usually provide a detailed and accurate account of the trauma that is consistent with the extent of the injury. When the history is vague or is not compatible with the observed injury [16, 19, 25, 26] or the child's developmental abilities [19, 27], the possibility of nonaccidental injury should be pursued through additional history, examination, or referral. Young children who are not yet mobile cannot create situations that place them at risk for physical injury. Falls have been reported to be the most common mechanism of accidental injury in children less than 3 months of age [28]; however, it is important to note that falls from a bed, couch, or changing table are not likely to result in serious injury [28–34]. Similarly, when a child accidentally falls down stairs severe, multiple, truncal, and proximal extremity injuries are rarely seen [35]. The more typical injury resulting from a fall down stairs is a single injury to the head in a child younger than 4 years old. The head injuries are not usually severe and typically do not require neurologic intervention [35]. Thus, a child who presents with moderate or severe head trauma reportedly resulting from a fall from a short distance should arouse suspicion [31, 36].

Bruises to the Skin and Subcutaneous Tissues

It is estimated that injuries to the skin and underlying tissues are present in 90% of abused children [7, 19]. Compared with the infant, who is unlikely to injure himself accidentally, however, nonaccidental injury may be more difficult to identify in preschool children who are adventurous, inquisitive, and fearless, but often lack sound judgment and a sense of danger [19, 28]. Lacerations in children are typically more common in accidental trauma than in nonaccidental trauma [22], whereas bruises are seen in both inflicted and accidental injury. Clues to physical abuse may be found by noting the location and pattern of soft-tissue injury.

Location

When a child falls in an accident, the bruising is most often confined to the overlying bony prominences (e.g., forehead, cheek bone, chin, elbows, knees, and shins) [37]. Inflicted injuries, however, frequently involve the soft, fatty areas such as cheeks, mouth, abdomen, thighs, and upper arms [7, 19, 22]. Symmetric or bilateral injuries are also much more common in nonaccidental trauma than in accidental trauma [19]. The head is the most common site of serious injury in children younger than 1 year of age [30]. Approximately 25% of all head injuries in children younger than 2 years of age are inflicted [32]. Looking at cases of physical abuse, trauma to the head has been reported in more than 50% of children, with soft-tissue injuries to the head and face being the single most common injury sustained in child abuse [17].

Since many of these inflicted injuries involve the face and head, the eye care practitioner may observe suspicious injuries suggestive of abuse during the course of a routine pediatric patient encounter. Lacerations to the palate, mouth, gums, or lips [9] may result from attempts to force feed a child [17]. Fractured teeth may also be present. Bruises to the corner of the mouth occur when the child had been gagged and are not likely to result from accidental trauma. However, burns that involve the corner of the mouth may occur accidentally when a young child bites into an electrical cord. Injuries to the nose, nostrils, or nasal septum may also be observed in cases of physical abuse.

The ears are also unlikely sites of accidental injury but may be involved in cases of physical abuse. The earlobes may be pinched or pulled, resulting in residual bruising [37]. Subtle petechial bruising may also be observed on the top of the pinna of the ear, or more obvious bruising on the inside and outside of the ear may be present [38]. The underlying scalp or the skin below the ear may be bruised by a blow to the side of the head [38, 39].

Bruises to the cheek are also common in inflicted injury but uncommon in accidental injury, since the cheeks are protected by the bony or cartilaginous protuberances of the cheekbones, chin, forehead, and nose. A high-velocity injury resulting from a slap often leaves a negative unbruised image of the hand or fingers delineated by small petechiae. The small petechiae outline the object of the injury (in this case, a hand) when the underlying capillaries are stretched and torn [38]. Another common bruise seen in nonaccidental injury to the cheek is characterized by a single bruise to one side of the face caused by a thumb and two to four bruises on the other cheek from the fingers. These grab or squeeze marks may occur in force feeding or when a caretaker grabs the child's face and shakes his or her head from side to side in an effort to gain attention, often while screaming or yelling at the child.

Bruises to the neck, wrists, and ankles are not often the result of an accident. Hand prints, grab marks, and linear marks encircling or partially encircling the neck are typically the result of choking or grabbing, or pulling on the child's bib or shirt. Circumferential blistering, edema, abrasions, or bruises around the ankles and wrists are seen when a child is bound by the hands or feet. These types of bruises should arouse suspicion of the possibility of physical abuse.

Bruises to the scalp may be hard to observe on casual inspection [15, 40, 41], but traumatic alopecia (bald patches) where the hair has been pulled out of the scalp is usually apparent [7]. Often, there is a tender subgaleal hematoma underlying the bald patch or any place on the scalp where the hair has been pulled. Hemorrhaging in the subaponeurotic space may be large enough to result in hypovolemic shock and cardiorespiratory arrest in young children [41]. Occasionally, severe subaponeurotic bleeding may present as bilateral black eyes as the blood gravitates to the upper and lower eyelids [41].

Pattern of Trauma

Injury on multiple body surfaces or evidence of multiple injuries in various stages of healing may be suggestive of nonaccidental trauma [7, 19, 41]. The time required for a bruise to fade will depend on the extent and depth of the injury [41] and depend on the person [15]. The color of a bruise, however, can provide a crude estimate of the time that has elapsed since the injury. If the bruise is red, the injury probably occurred less than 48 hours earlier. A blue/purple color suggests the bruise is more than 24 hours old. A blue/yellow appearance implies the injury occurred within 1 week of the presentation. A yellow/green bruise is suggestive of an injury that is 1–2 weeks old, whereas a brown bruise is suggestive of an injury more than 2 weeks old [41]. Numerous bruises in various stages of healing should arouse suspicion of possible physical abuse, particularly if reported to have occurred in a single incident or the location of the bruise is not suggestive of accidental injury.

Bruises with distinct patterns resembling the shape of the article that inflicted the injury are typically the result of nonaccidental trauma [27, 38]. Belts or straps often leave a pair of linear marks separated by 1–2 inches, the width of the strap. Loop bruises result when a cord is doubled or folded and used to hit a child. Bruises may also take on the form of the outline of a blunt instrument used to strike a child such as a comb, hairbrush, or boot or shoe imprint if the child is kicked. Small, paired, crescent-shaped bruises facing each other are the result of pinching. Similarly shaped bruises, but much larger, appear from human bite marks. These paired, crescent-shaped bruises have recognizable teeth marks, and when the distance between the canines is greater than 3 cm, the bite is from an adult [7].

Burns

Ten to 20% of all physical abuse cases involve burns [17, 23, 25]. Nonaccidental burns are more common in infants and toddlers, with a peak age range of 13–24 months of age. The average age for inflicted burns is approximately 3 years of age [25, 26, 42]. Burns from abuse are often inflicted by submersion of the infant or toddler into hot water. Frequently, the injury is triggered by a toilet training incident [7], with submersion serving as punishment and cleansing. Unlike accidental burns, in which the depth of the burn and the tissue damage varies, inflicted immersion burns are of uniform depth and have a sharp demarcation line between the burned and the uninvolved tissue [7, 25]. Due to their characteristic appearance, these burns have been referred to as glove (hand immersed and held in a hot liquid) or stocking (foot immersed and held

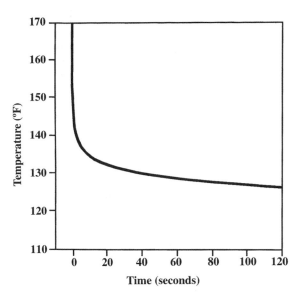

Figure 18.1. Hot water temperature in degrees Fahrenheit as a function of duration of exposure in seconds required to produce a full-thickness (third-degree) burn to the skin of an adult. (Adapted from KW Feldman, RT Schaller, JA Feldman, M McMillon. Tap water scald burns in children. Pediatrics 1978;62(1):1–7.)

in a hot liquid) burns. Another characteristic immersion burn is the doughnut pattern. This burn occurs when a young child's lower torso is lowered and then held in hot water, typically in a bathtub. The areas of skin (usually a portion of the buttocks) forced against the bottom of the cooler tub are not burned. The skin protected by folds or flexion of the knees (back of the thigh and the calf) may also escape the burn.

One approach to reduce both accidental and inflicted burns is to lower the temperature setting on home hot water heaters [7, 43]. Figure 18.1 shows the temperature of water as a function of time required to produce a full-thickness (third-degree) burn to the skin of an adult. It should be noted that a child's thinner skin burns in a shorter amount of time. Estimates suggest that burns in children occur in about one-fourth the time required to produce a burn in an adult [42]. When water heaters are set to 140°F, a full-thickness burn to an adult occurs in just 6 seconds; if set to 150°F, only 2 seconds is required for a full-thickness burn [43]. Lowering the temperature of a water heater to 120°F would reduce the chances of accidental burns, since 10 minutes are required to produce a full-thickness burn

Table 18.1. Possible Ocular Manifestations of Child Abuse

Condition	Reference
Periorbital	
Lid lacerations	19, 45, 112
Periorbital swelling and ecchymosis	19, 45, 46, 113
Phthirus pubis eyelash infestation	112
Proptosis	19, 45, 112
Ptosis	19, 112
Ruptured globe	112
Anterior segment	
Angle recession	112
Anisocoria	46
Conjunctival hemorrhage	112
Corneal scars	19, 112, 113
Glaucoma	104
Hyphema	46
Hypopyon	112
Iris tears, iris dialysis	19, 112, 114
Pupil abnormalities	19, 46, 104, 112, 113
Subconjunctival hemorrhages	45, 46, 113
Posterior segment	
Cataracts	19, 45, 113, 114
Chorioretinal atrophy	113
Optic atrophy	45, 104, 112, 113, 115
Papilledema	19, 45, 46, 112, 113, 115
Preretinal hemorrhage	112
Retinal hemorrhage	19, 45, 46, 112, 113, 115
Retinal detachment	19, 45, 104, 113, 114
Retinal folds	40, 70, 116
Retinal dialysis	112
Subluxated lens	19, 45, 104, 112, 113
Vitreous hemorrhage	19, 40, 45, 112
Extraocular muscles	
Nystagmus	19, 112–114
Palsies	46
Strabismus	19, 45, 104, 112, 113

to the skin of an adult. Inflicted burns would also be more difficult to induce in a rage of uncontrolled anger if the temperature of the water coming from the hot water faucet were reduced. By reducing the temperature setting on hot water heaters, there is an added energy savings, particularly for electric water heaters. It has been estimated that a 4% energy savings occurs with each 10°F of reduction from 150°F [43].

Contact burns induced by hot appliances or cigarettes are another form of burn injury that may or may not be the result of an accident. Hot appliances create pattern burns that resemble the shape of the hot implement, such as an iron, curling iron, or grate. Contact burns to the finger or palm of the hand are often accidental. Patterned burns to the feet, back of the hand, or buttocks, however, are less likely to occur in an accident. Small circular burns approximately 7 mm in diameter are frequently generated by holding a lit cigar or cigarette against the child's soles, palms, back, or buttocks. The appearance of this circular burn will vary depending on the time the cigarette is held in contact with the skin. Cigarette burns to the cornea, conjunctiva, and eyelids in children younger than the age of 2 years should also arouse suspicion of child abuse [44]. However, preschool children who are walking may occasionally accidentally sustain cigarette burns to the cornea or ocular adnexa when they walk too close to an adult holding a cigarette [44].

Ocular Injuries

Several small retrospective studies on the prevalence of ocular involvement in physical abuse suggest that approximately 40% of abused children manifest ocular trauma [45, 46], with 4% [46] to 6% [45] of the patients presenting initially to the ophthalmologist. However, approximately 20% of the cases [45] involve direct trauma to the eye; thus, a significant number of children suffering from nonaccidental trauma could present to the eye care practitioner. The types of injuries observed vary widely and are presented in Table 18.1. One of the most common manifestations, retinal hemorrhages [45], is discussed in the following section, as it has important implications in the identification of abuse [19, 40, 47–51] when no other external signs of trauma are apparent.

Shaken Baby Syndrome

Shaken baby syndrome is also known as the whiplash shaken infant syndrome, the battered child syndrome, the battered baby syndrome, the parent-infant traumatic stress syndrome, and Caffey-Kempe syndrome.

History

Although all of these terms were initially used somewhat interchangeably, the features of this syndrome have evolved as our understanding of child abuse has grown. The term *battered child syndrome* first appeared in a publication by Kempe, Silverman, Steele, Droegemueller, and Silver in the *Journal of the American Medical Association* in 1962 [18]. This paper, considered a landmark in the field of child abuse, was the first to bring the issue to the attention of the medical profession and the public in a way that could no longer be ignored [52]. The paper, along with the conference that preceded it, served as the impetus for the first federal legislation on child abuse in the United States. Kempe [18] defined the features of this syndrome to include most of the common forms of physical abuse in children younger than 3 years of age: bone fracture, subdural hematoma, failure to thrive, soft-tissue swelling, skin bruising, or the sudden, unexplained death of a child. He also noted that the history of the injury was often inconsistent with the degree of injury.

The term *whiplash shaken infant syndrome* appeared in 1974 [53] after a description of 27 cases in 1972 [54] in which shaking rather than beating was believed to be the source of injury. This more narrowly defined syndrome had its roots in observations made by other physicians in the United States in the early 1940s. Ingraham and Matson [55] described a series of infant patients with subdural hematoma frequently associated with retinal hemorrhages. They suspected the etiology was some form of trauma despite an inadequate history or no history of trauma. In 1946, Caffey [56] noted a puzzling association of fresh, healing, and healed multiple fractures in the long bones of infants with chronic subdural hematoma. At least two of the six patients presented had associated retinal hemorrhages.

*Characteristics of Whiplash
Shaken Baby Syndrome*

The primary features of whiplash shaken infant syndrome, or shaken baby syndrome, include subdural hematoma (about 80% bilateral [53]), intraocular hemorrhage (typically bilateral), and multiple changes in the long bones (induced by traction,

stretching, or shearing stresses rather than direct impact) without external evidence of trauma to the head [53]. The trauma is believed to be induced when a caregiver grabs the infant or young child by the shoulders or around the thorax and violently shakes the child. In this case, bruises in the shape of the assailant's finger pads may occasionally be seen on the shoulders or chest, or rib fractures may be apparent on x-ray. The injuries may also be induced by grabbing a child by an extremity (handles for mishandling [52]) and shaking or swinging the child around the caregiver's head. Norton [15] described a potential scenario of a child grasped by the ankles, arched over the adult's head, and accelerated in an arc in which the child's head becomes the end of a whip consisting of his or her own body and the arms of the caretaker.

The frequency of shaking a child and the potential for injury as a result of shaking varies inversely with the age of the child [54]—the younger the child the greater the risk. Violent shaking is generally used by caregivers during uncontrolled anger, rage, or frustration to stop an infant's crying or to discipline an infant, as spanking is uncommon before about 7 months of age [54]. Thus, whiplash shaken infant syndrome, or shaken baby syndrome, is a limited form of physical abuse occurring in young children. Its unique features include subdural hematoma, frequently associated with intraocular hemorrhage, and skeletal abnormalities, with the absence of any external signs of trauma to the head or neck and no history of trauma or with a history of mild trauma not compatible with the seriousness of the injury. Due to their relevance to the eye care practitioner, the remainder of this section focuses on subdural hematoma and intraocular hemorrhage rather than radiologic skeletal findings. The importance of a case history is discussed in "Identifying Abuse, Case History."

Subdural Hematoma. Subdural hematoma secondary to child abuse is most common in infants younger than 24 months of age, with a peak incidence occurring during the sixth month of life [54]. The reported incidence of subdural hematoma in shaken baby syndrome ranges from 38% to 100% [57]; however, the two reports of 100% contained only three patients each. The next highest incidence was 61% (17 of 28 patients). The mechanism of injury is still debated, with some authors suggesting that shaking alone is not sufficient to generate the forces required to produce a subdural hematoma [32, 40]. They suggest that some type of blunt head trauma by itself or in combination with shaking is required to produce the magnitude of the injuries attributed to shaking alone. However, whiplash injuries produced in an animal model are consistent with the notion that shaking alone, particularly if rotational forces are involved, is sufficient to produce a subdural hematoma [58]. Other authors support Caffey's [54] suggestion that shaking without cranial impact can result in subdural hematoma and retinal hemorrhages [48, 50].

It is hypothesized that the heavy infant head with its soft brain and blood vessels is inadequately supported by weak cervical muscles in the early natal period. The heavy head and weak neck make the infant vulnerable to translational and rotational whiplash stress [54], which occur when the infant is shaken. As the infant is shaken, the neck flexes, and the chin strikes the chest, followed by an extension of the neck with the head striking the back. This sequence is often repeated, and the acceleration and deceleration exerts shearing forces and bleeding from the veins bridging the brain and the dural venous sinuses [32, 49, 53].

Generalized symptoms often associated with a subdural hematoma in a young child include failure to feed well, failure to gain weight, fever, lethargy, vomiting, irritability, excessive crying or restlessness, increased head size, bulging fontanelle, hypertonicity, or decreased muscle tone [55, 59]. Other more obvious signs of a central nervous system disorder include coma, convulsions and seizures, paralysis, and pupil abnormalities [55, 59]. The most common symptoms in a series of 98 infants with subdural hematoma from a variety of etiologies were convulsions, vomiting, and irritability [55]. The eye care practitioner should be alert to these often subtle signs and symptoms of occult child abuse, particularly if coupled with retinal hemorrhages and a vague or inconsistent history.

Retinal Hemorrhage. Retinal hemorrhages are present in 34–80% of children who suffer from abuse [32, 59–61]. Hence, the presence of retinal hemorrhages has become a significant diagnostic aid when a caregiver presents with an injured child who on examination shows no significant signs of trauma and only a vague or suspicious history is obtained. Due to its frequent association with abuse, some authors have suggested that the presence of retinal hemorrhage is pathognomonic for child abuse [47, 51, 62]. However, retinal hemorrhages have been associated with other accidental forms of trauma, including from birth [63–68] (which disappear by 1 month of age) [57], from cardiopulmonary resuscitation [69] (see Kanter [62] and Gilliland [51] for an opposing view), from automobile accidents [32, 49], and occasionally from falls [32]. Thus, some authorities think that the presence of retinal hemorrhages is not diagnostic for child abuse [32, 70].

In a review of 169 randomly selected child deaths referred to the medical examiner for study, Gilliland, Luckenbach, and Chenier [51] concluded, "In the absence of a verifiable history of a severe head injury or life-threatening central nervous system disease, retinal and ocular hemorrhages were diagnostic of child abuse." Thus, although retinal hemorrhages are not pathognomonic of child abuse in and of themselves, when coupled with a significant head trauma or central nervous system dysfunction and a history not compatible with the extent of the injury, retinal hemorrhages can aid in the diagnosis of occult child abuse.

The mechanism by which retinal hemorrhages are induced in the shaken baby syndrome remains unresolved [70]. Some theories are that the hemorrhages result from hemodynamic forces elicited by compression of the infants thorax or abdomen (Purtscher's retinopathy); from central retinal vein obstruction from disk edema; from vitreoretinal traction, causing retinoschisis; from retinal venous hypertension, resulting from an increase in intracranial pressure due to cerebral edema or hemorrhage (Terson's syndrome); or from direct head trauma [40, 51]. When retinal hemorrhages are associated with shaken baby syndrome, they are frequently located in the superficial layers of the retina, but deeper hemorrhages have also been reported [50, 70]. Munger [70] also reported that the hemorrhages were more often located posterior to the equator than anterior in his sample of autopsied eyes.

Although not pathognomonic for inflicted injuries, retinal hemorrhages are highly associated with inflicted injuries in children younger than 2 years of age and are almost never seen in trivial, accidental head injuries [32]. Thus, the presence of retinal hemorrhages in any child older than 1 month of age with a history of a trivial, accidental injury should arouse the suspicion of the eye care practitioner. Immediate referral for additional diagnostic workup and for the safety of the child, along with a report of suspected child abuse to the proper authorities (see "Reporting Abuse"), is warranted.

Failure to Thrive

Failure to thrive is a term that has been used to describe a child who fails to grow according to the norms expected for the child's age [71]. Failure to thrive that extends or occurs beyond the neonatal period is only rarely the result of an organic problem [27]. Growth failure in the absence of other disease is an early symptom of a disturbed parent-child relationship and is frequently associated with other signs of neglect and abuse [71].

A malnourished child often appears pale and weak, with a decreased muscle mass and little subcutaneous fat. These children are often listless, apathetic, and sleep for long periods of time [71]. Failure to thrive typically occurs in infants and young children (younger than 2 years of age) during the time of rapid growth but may occur in older children (3–12 years of age) as well. If these children are hospitalized for 7–10 days and given caloric intake sufficient for nutritional recovery, they gain weight. However, this approach is often not possible in today's managed care and cost-containment environment.

Although failure to thrive is the result of inadequate intake of calories, the problem typically stems from difficulties in parenting, home environment, and disturbed parent-child relationships. Treatment must extend beyond that provided to the child by the initial weight gain obtained through adequate nutrition. Treatment must include the family as relapses are common and these children often remain physically and developmentally delayed as they enter school [71].

Munchausen Syndrome and Munchausen By Proxy

Munchausen syndrome describes a condition in which a patient consciously attempts to deceive the medical care practitioner by inventing or creating symptoms that will arouse the practitioner's interest [72]. The typical, clinical presentation is an adult 30–40 years of age [72] who fabricates or induces symptoms in himself or herself and therefore would not appear to be related to child abuse. However, there has been one report of a 12-year-old child instilling various chemicals into her eyes and perforating her eye with a safety pin [73]. This child was treated in two university hospitals for a total of 151 days associated with 10 different treatment periods in less than 2 years. It was later learned that this child's psychiatric disturbances were related to sexual abuse by her father [73]. She viewed her hospitalizations as a respite and escape from the abusive family environment. The other reports of self-inflicted ocular injury described in the literature do not appear to be directly related to child abuse but associated with schizophrenia or other psychological disturbances [74, 75]. However, abuse and incest are frequently encountered in the histories of patients with Munchausen syndrome [72].

Munchausen by proxy, however, is a form of child abuse that occurs when a caregiver either presents with a false history of symptoms of a physical illness in a child or induces physical illness in a child (e.g., seizures by blocking respiration or diarrhea and dehydration through laxatives). It is believed that the caregiver has a need for the attention and the atmosphere and urgency of a medical setting [72]. Occasionally, the parent or caregiver may possess professional experience in the health care system. The symptoms induced are often even life-threatening in nature [72], and therefore Munchausen by proxy involving ocular structures is very rare and not likely to be encountered in a general eye care practice. In cases of Munchausen by proxy, the child is subjected to prolonged, complex, often painful medical procedures in addition to enduring the frequently induced anomalies. In many cases, the children suddenly die by unexplained circumstances [72].

FACTORS THAT MAY INCREASE THE RISK FOR ABUSE

A considerable literature has accumulated on the adults who abuse children, the children they abuse, and the circumstances around which abuse occurs.

The rationale behind this approach has been to identify specific conditions or factors that place children at risk for abuse in an effort to first recognize abuse and then to stop ongoing abuse or prevent abuse from ever occurring [76]. As the understanding of child abuse has increased, however, the limitations of this approach have become apparent [76]. The relationships that have been derived from investigations of abused populations have been primarily retrospective in design and often without control groups. Furthermore, it has become increasingly clear that each characteristic alone is a poor indication of abuse [2, 77]. Abuse results from a complex combination and interaction of people and circumstances. Thus, it is important to remember that these characteristics are only associations; causal relationships cannot typically be derived from most of the literature. Since these relationships may not be causal, their usefulness in prevention may be limited [76]. However, it is still useful to review the characteristics often associated with abuse, since a complete history and understanding of the family dynamics may lead to identification and intervention strategies for those at greatest risk.

Adults

Relationship of the Perpetrator and Victim

There are mixed reports concerning which adults are frequent perpetrators of physical abuse. Starling, Holden, and Jenny [78] conducted a retrospective review of medical records and identified 151 children 3 weeks to 24 months of age who had sustained abusive head trauma. In 127 of these cases, the perpetrators were identified by admission or court conviction, charged with the offense, or suspected of the offense. Of those identified or suspected of abuse, 68.5% were men, with fathers (37%) and boyfriends of the mothers (20.5%) comprising the vast majority. Another significant group of perpetrators were baby-sitters, suspected or charged with abuse in 21.2% of the cases (17.3% female sitters, 3.1% male sitters). Thus, the possibility that the perpetrator of abuse may extend beyond the immediate family should not be ignored, and prevention strategies should include all groups identified with abuse in significant numbers.

Age

Another group that is over-represented in the population of abusive parents is young, single mothers, adolescents [9], and those younger than 20 years of age [76, 79]. Using a survey in which abusive behaviors were identified by self-report, Connelly and Straus [80] found that the younger the mother the greater the risk of physical abuse when the mother's age was measured as the age at the time of birth of the abused child.

Misconceptions About Child Development and Poor Parenting Skills

Failure of caretakers to understand the expected child developmental sequence has also been associated with abuse [1, 9]. Misconceptions and unmet expectations can disrupt appropriate parent-child interactions and may result in violence. Young, first-time parents and inexperienced baby-sitters or caregivers may lack the knowledge necessary to provide appropriate parenting. These associations are supported by the observations of Lynch and Roberts [79], who found that many mothers who are at risk for abusing their children could be identified retrospectively by notes of concern in the hospital chart regarding the mother's inability to cope with the child's physical or emotional needs. Frequently, these parents grew up in families without appropriate parental role models or were exposed to abnormal child-rearing practices as children [9].

Emotional Disturbances

A variety of emotional and psychological disturbances have been associated with abusive behavior [76, 79]. One disturbance is an abnormal, dependent nature of a caregiver. If this need for dependency is not fulfilled by another adult, the adult often turns to the child. In these circumstances, there is often a role reversal, with the child assuming the role of the parent and attempting to care for and comfort the adult [5]. Those who abuse children have also been identified as having inadequate coping skills [18, 77] and low self-esteem [1]. There may also be a history of breakdowns and suicide attempts.

Social Isolation

People isolated from social contacts are at an increased risk of inflicting abuse [1, 6]. Lack of close contacts with friends, family, extended family, or organizations have all been associated with a greater frequency of child abuse [3]. These individuals have no one in the household, neighborhood, or in their social sphere to call and ask for help when they are in a moment of crisis with their children.

Substance Abuse

Drug or alcohol misuse has been frequently associated with child abuse [9, 10, 18, 79]. Parental substance abuse was identified in 4–65% of cases of child abuse in 1994 [10]. Data reported from 11 states suggest that an average of 35% of all confirmed cases of abuse and neglect involve some form of substance abuse [10]. Twenty-nine of 38 states (76%) providing data for the 1994 National Committee to Prevent Child Abuse for the Results of the 1994 Annual Fifty-State Survey named substance abuse as one of the top two problems associated with child maltreatment [10].

Abused as a Child

Not all children who are abused end up abusing their own children; however, in the population of those who do abuse their children, there is a much higher proportion who were maltreated as children than found in the general population [1, 5, 81]. Here is where the phrase "breaking the cycle of abuse" heard in radio and television public service announcements arises [81]. The hope is that preventing abuse in one generation will lessen abuse in future generations. Estimates of intergenerational transmission vary in the literature from 18% to 70% [81]. However, Kaufman and Zigler [81], based on a critical analysis of the literature, estimate the rate of intergenerational transmission to be 30% ± 5%. As with all the associations described, it is important to recall that abusive behavior results from a complex interaction of parent, child, and environmental circumstances.

Children

Many theories of child abuse suggest that the child plays a significant role in the complex interactions that culminate in abuse [1, 4, 82]. The role the child plays may be passive or active. Passive roles center around the child's age and the parent's perceptions or expectations of the child, whereas active roles involve the child's behaviors.

Age

Although abuse can occur at any age, younger children are at greater risk of injury from abuse and neglect [19, 80]. The incidence of abuse in children younger than 6 years of age in the United States is estimated to be 10–15%, with the majority of these children younger than 2 years of age [83]. Younger children are also significantly more likely to die of their injuries than older children. It has been estimated that between three and four children die each day from abuse or neglect and that 88% of these children are younger than 5 years of age and 46% are younger than 1 year of age [8, 10]. The fatality rate for children younger than the age of 5 years in 1994 was 6.6 per 100,000 children [10].

The tantrums that are frequently associated with the "terrible twos" and the anxiety surrounding feeding and toilet training have been documented as incidents that can trigger physical abuse [7]. Here, the child's age and the parent's lack of understanding of normal development may interact as potentiating factors.

Prematurity and Low Birth Weight

Premature and low-birth-weight children are more highly represented in the population of abused children [2, 4, 79, 82, 84, 85]. Although there are many theories about what may place the pre-term infant at greater risk for abuse compared with the full-term infant, the specific characteristics that increase the risk of abuse in pre-term infants have not been sufficiently identified. In addition, the significance of these individual infant characteristics compared to the complex interactions between the infant, an adult, and the environment are not adequately understood.

Several individual characteristics of pre-term infants that have been proposed to contribute to nonaccidental trauma center on the pre-term infant's behavior. Premature children are more likely to be restless, distractible, and difficult to care for during the newborn period [4, 82]. They are more prone to colic and sleep disturbances, may be hypersensitive [4], and have an especially aversive cry [82]. Difficulties in attachment may also be a contributing factor [2].

Special Needs Children

Children with disabling conditions, such as neurologic or physical dysfunctions, hearing impairments, and mental retardation, are also over-represented in the population of abused children [2, 4, 86–88]. Again, it is not clear what factors are responsible for this association, but the association cannot be accounted for on the basis that the impairments are the result of abuse rather than a condition that existed before the abuse [4]. Several factors that have been suggested are (1) disruptions in the formation of the mother-infant attachment, (2) increased levels of parental stress associated with the increased caregiver demands, (3) difficult behavior characteristics often exhibited by these challenged children, and (4) unrealistic and unmet parental expectations [2, 87, 88].

Child Perceived as Different

Children whose caregivers perceive them as different or difficult, even though there may be no corroborating evidence for these perceptions, are often selected as scapegoats and targeted for physical abuse [1, 82, 86]. Oates [89] found that mothers of abused children rated their children as having more deviant behaviors than did the teachers of these children. Although parents of children who were not abused also rated their children's behavior more negatively than did their teachers, the difference between the abused and control group was significant and therefore consistent with the notion that abusive parents perceive these children differently.

Environmental Factors

Stress, induced by environmental circumstances, has been suggested as a trigger mechanism in abuse. However, it is important to make a distinc-tion between environmental circumstances and a person's reaction to these circumstances. Although associations between a person's environment and his or her propensity for abuse have been reported, it is the personalities of the adult and child that interact with the surrounding circumstances to either increase the likelihood or mitigate the possibility of abuse. Stress is just one of many reactions that may occur as a result of an event or a series of events or circumstances. The person and the environment determine whether the circumstances result in stress [3] and how the stress is managed. When environmental circumstances result in stress, however, the adequacy of child care frequently declines [90], and the probability of abuse increases.

Violence and Corporal Punishment

When violence is accepted as a way to manage stress, the potential for abuse increases. Thus, one environmental factor that has been implicated in causing abuse is society's acceptance of violence as a method of settling family disagreements [91]. When physical punishment is used to control a child's behavior, Straus and Kantor [91] suggest that a child learns not only to extinguish the behavior that brings on the physical punishment but also several other unintentional lessons. First, the child associates violence with love: Those that hit are the ones that also love. The second association is a moral justification for hitting other members of the family, since physical punishment is used to teach the child to stop dangerous behaviors. The third association is that of importance: If something is very important, it justifies the use of physical force. The last unintended association is that if one is angry or stressed, physical violence may be comprehensible. Thus, society's sanction of violence and physical punishment contributes to an atmosphere in which abuse is an accepted, or at least a tolerated, reaction for families in crisis.

Poverty

Although abuse occurs at all socioeconomic levels, those living in poverty are over-represented in the population of families who abuse children when compared to the general population [9, 11, 12, 23, 77, 79]. The lack of adequate financial resources associated with inadequate housing, food, clothing, medical care, and child care, frequently stress the family dynamics. When poverty is coupled with other potentiating characteristics of the caregiver or the child, or both, the opportunity for abuse escalates.

*Large Number of Stair-Step Children
or Unwanted Children*

An unwanted pregnancy [90] or a family with multiple children born in close succession can also stress the family both financially and emotionally. In a study reviewed by Connelly and Straus [80], mothers 25 years of age with five or more children at home were almost twice as likely to physically abuse one or more of the children than mothers with only one child at home.

Support Structure

Social isolation has been mentioned as a characteristic associated with adults who abuse children [3, 9, 10]. A support structure or social network is reiterated here, since it has been identified as an important environmental factor that can either mitigate or increase the likelihood of abuse. Abusive parents are often socially isolated. They have few friends and often no support from, or contact with, their extended family. This lack of emotional and social support can increase the possibility of abuse when a crisis occurs and there is no one to turn to for help or stability. It is important to note that if abuse occurs due to stress induced by circumstances surrounding a person prone to abuse, the abuse is typically a reaction to a variety of circumstances and events over a period of time [2] rather than a single, isolated event.

Parents Anonymous, a self-help support group patterned after Alcoholics Anonymous, has been useful in creating a support network for parents who abuse their children. The importance of such a social network for these parents is made apparent by the lower incidence of recidivism [1, 92] in parents who participate in this group.

REPORTING ABUSE

All 50 states, the District of Columbia, Puerto Rico, and the Virgin Islands have statutes that require professionals who work with children to report suspected cases of child abuse and neglect [9, 93, 94]. A review of the state statutes published in 1982 [94] lists 17 states that specifically name optometrists as professionals who are required to report cases of suspected abuse. An additional 15 states mandate the reporting of suspected abuse by any person suspecting abuse [94]. These same laws typically provide immunity from civil and criminal liability if the reports are made in good faith and without malicious intent [93, 94]. In addition, most states impose civil or criminal penalty for failure to report suspected cases of child abuse [93–97]. If a physician fails to report a case of suspected child abuse and the child is subsequently reinjured, failure to report the abuse can be the basis for a medical malpractice action. The physician is liable for damages caused by his or her failure to report suspected abuse [96, 97]. Despite these legal requirements, very few reports of abuse (8–11%) come from health care professionals [7, 98, 99]. Reasons physicians give for not reporting suspected cases of abuse include lack of information on assessing abuse, drain on time and finances, fear of litigation, and perceived inadequacy of the community service system designed to help children and families [7, 100]. Although many of these reasons also appeared in the survey of physicians conducted by Saulsbury and Campbell [101], the two most frequently cited reasons for not reporting suspected abuse in their survey were a feeling that the physician could work with the family to solve the problem without outside intervention and a reluctance to report unless certain of the diagnosis of abuse or neglect. It is important to remember that the law only requires reporting a suspicion of child abuse [94, 96, 97]. It is not the responsibility of those referring a person to the department of social services to accuse, judge, or even discover who the perpetrator of the abuse may be [16, 30, 45]. One way of viewing a report of suspected abuse is that it is not an accusation but a request for intervention by a multidisciplinary team of professionals [19, 102].

The name of the agency responsible for receiving and investigating reports of suspected child abuse differs among the individual states. Typically, the agency is part of the state's public department of human or social services (or resources) [11]. The appropriate reporting agency for your area may be located by checking the government pages in your local phone book. These agencies are mandated by federal law to investigate or assess reports of abuse or neglect and to determine the need for protective services. Reports may be assigned a priority based on the severity of harm or threatened harm, with those given highest priority investigated first. Other reports are investigated as soon as possible but typically no later than 10 days from the receipt of the report.

When making a report of suspected abuse to the appropriate agency, accurate information will expedite the investigation. Relevant demographic information, which should be available from your patient records, including the child's name, child's age or date of birth, the name of the parent or guardian, child's current address, school or day-care facility the child attends, and information about siblings and other adults living with the child, will all be important. Information about the particular signs of the observed physical abuse, including the specific injuries observed (e.g., type of injuries, location of the injuries, and the overall physical condition of the child), and the history provided by the child or parent will be very useful to the agency receiving the report. Based on the information provided, the agency will determine if there is a sufficient basis to investigate the report, and if investigated, under what priority or time frame [100]. Although a report may be made anonymously, greater significance is attached to reports by health care professionals [13, 98] and by those who identify themselves. However, the agency is forbidden from disclosing the source of the report to those under investigation. Therefore, it is the professional's choice to inform the family about his or her intentions to report suspicions.

If the report is investigated and substantiated, several possible interventions may be instituted, including counseling, parenting training, mental health services, physical health services, protective day care, ordered supervision of the child in his or her home, foster placement, emergency shelter services, placement in a public or private agency or in an institution, or criminal charges, depending on the circumstances [9, 103]. If the report is investigated but could not be substantiated, the case is closed and no further action is taken. If the agency fails to contact the person reporting a case of suspected abuse with the disposition of the case, the reporter should contact the agency to receive the case disposition.

CONSEQUENCES OF ABUSE

The consequences of continued abuse without intervention are severe and may even result in death. When a child survives a severe, inflicted head injury, neurologic complications are frequent. These complications may include hydrocephalus, mental retardation, epilepsy, and cerebral palsy [41]. Persistent visual abnormalities and blindness are also a frequent consequence of abusive head trauma [59, 104].

When the abuse is less severe, psychological, behavioral, and social consequences often remain long after the physical injuries are healed. Eighty-seven 8- to 12-year-olds identified from the New York State child abuse register were compared with age-, race-, and classroom-matched controls by Salzinger et al. [105]. The abused children were viewed more negatively by their peers and were less likely to be identified as popular. They were more likely to seek attention and to fight and less likely to be identified for leadership. Oates [89] found that physically abused children were shy with poor self-esteem. They also had fewer friends, more disturbed behavior, and lower ambitions for the future. Cohn [92] has reported similar problems of poor socialization skills, difficulty dealing with frustration, and poor attention span. Hoffman-Plotkin and Twentyman [106] found that children 3–6 years of age with a history of physical abuse scored lower on all their measures of cognitive functioning compared with a group of matched children who had no history of abuse. The abused children were observed to be more aggressive, less mature, and less ready to learn. Daro, as reported by the American Humane Association [11], in a national clinical evaluation of a sample of abused children under 13 years of age, found that (1) approximately 30% had some type of cognitive or language disorder; (2) approximately 14% exhibited self-mutilative or other self-destructive behaviors; (3) approximately one-half had difficulty in school, including poor attendance and misconduct; (4) more than 22% had learning disorders requiring special education service; and (5) approximately 30% had chronic health problems.

An abusive childhood often exerts its influence beyond childhood. A history of abuse in childhood has been associated with school problems, failed marriages, and emotional disturbances. Many people who abuse children were victims of abuse themselves [81].

PREVENTING ABUSE

A review of 11 federal demonstration projects designed to evaluate the effects of treatment of substantiated abusers reported a 30% rate of severe reincidence while undergoing treatment [92]. Thus, prevention of abuse before it occurs appears to be an important tool to address this complex problem. Research on the efficacy of various federal, state, and local programs designed to prevent child abuse is limited and controversial [92, 107] and not the focus of this chapter. At present, the child abuse system is largely remedial. It becomes operational only after the child has been abused and reported. Most resources that are available are used to alleviate the damage after the fact [93]. However, eye care professionals who serve young children have a unique opportunity to implement strategies directed at preventing child abuse through education and advocacy. Medical expenses for each baby hospitalized as a result of shaken baby syndrome were reported at the 1996 National Conference on Shaken Baby Syndrome to be between $75,000 and $95,000 [108]. Thus, it behooves professionals who serve this at-risk population to become proactive and involved in prevention by becoming advocates for children and families.

Most of us have witnessed a stressed parent losing control and physically or verbally mistreating a child in a store, restaurant, or other public place. Although our natural tendency is to avoid the situation and not become involved, the National Committee to Prevent Child Abuse suggests four simple strategies that may be helpful in defusing this awkward situation [109]. Your actions could be the mitigating factor that prevents that incident of abuse.

The first strategy is to direct the adult's attention away from the child by saying something empathetic. Examples include "Your child's behavior seems to be really trying your patience," or "Children can really wear you out." Another strategy is to divert the attention of the misbehaving child. Young preschool children are typically easily distracted, and this may be effective in changing the child's behavior that has set off the adult. A third al-

ternative is to try to get the adult in a positive mood by praising the parent or child at the first appropriate opportunity. Negative remarks, reactions, or body language could escalate the situation, and therefore should be avoided. The fourth option is to offer assistance if you see the child is in danger (e.g., stand by a child who is left alone and is standing in a grocery cart until the caregiver returns). All of these approaches are designed to give the adult a brief moment to regain control of themselves and the situation, which may be all that is needed to defuse the immediate crisis. Although these techniques may defuse an immediate crisis, such brief encounters will not change underlying patterns of abusive behavior that may or may not be present. It is important to remember that the problem is complex and other incidences of abuse may occur in another situation when your mitigating influence is no longer present. However, preventing even just one incident is worth the small amount of effort.

Education offers the potential for more lasting intervention. Prevention is often described at three different levels: primary, secondary, and tertiary [7, 107, 110]. Primary prevention is directed at preventing the occurrence of abuse. It may be directed toward persons or a structure of the society (e.g., eliminating poverty). Educating the general public and parents about the stresses of child rearing and the resources available to assist them is another example of a primary prevention strategy. Secondary prevention targets specific populations thought to be at high risk for child abuse (see "Factors That May Increase the Risk for Abuse"). For example, a child or young adult who has been abused and thus is at greater risk of abusing his or her children, may receive education and training to prevent the occurrence of abuse in the next generation. Attempts to prevent recurrent abuse in families in which abuse has already transpired is the focus of tertiary prevention. While tertiary prevention is typically coordinated by the local social service agency, eye care professionals can easily engage in both primary and secondary prevention strategies.

Our reception rooms provide a unique opportunity to distribute educational materials useful for primary intervention. Materials should be directed at increasing parents' knowledge of child development and the demands of parenting [9]. The "Never Shake A Baby" campaign [111], developed in Ohio and approved by the American Academy of Pediatrics, is one example. Materials (most available in Spanish as well as English) include posters, bookmarks, bumper stickers, pencils, educational cards describing ways to handle a crying baby, and a video tape. The poster is particularly appropriate for the eye care practitioner's office as it mentions blindness as one of the consequences of this form of abuse. Chapter Appendix 18A lists the sources of these and other educational materials. April has been designated as Child Abuse Prevention Month. It is a logical sequel to Save Your Vision Week, which is in March. Consider having materials available in your office in April or all year.

Secondary prevention may be exercised by providing specific educational materials, counseling, and referral sources for patients falling into one of the high-risk groups mentioned in the section titled "Factors That May Increase the Risk for Abuse."

Chapter Appendix 18B lists several national organizations dedicated to protecting children and assisting families under stress. Most of these national organizations have local affiliates. Keep these numbers and those of the contacts in your area readily available to pass along to patients and their families whenever appropriate. Increasing access to health and social services is a prevention strategy that has been recommended by the American Medical Association Council on Scientific Affairs [9] and has been demonstrated to be effective, at least in some cases [107].

Remember, it is estimated that three to four children die each day in the United States and 86% of these children are under the age of 5 years [8]. As primary eye care professionals who examine children and interact with families, preventing, identifying, and reporting suspected cases of child abuse is one of our important responsibilities. We must become proactive advocates of children and their families as society and its members continue to struggle to understand and prevent this pervasive problem.

REFERENCES

1. Helfer RE. The etiology of child abuse. Pediatrics 1973;51(4):777–779.
2. Ammerman RT. The role of the child in physical abuse: a reappraisal. Violence Vict 1991;6(2):87–101.
3. Howze DC, Kotch JB. Disentangling life events, stress and social support: implications for the primary pre-

vention of child abuse and neglect. Child Abuse Negl 1984;8:401–409.
4. Friedrich WN, Boriskin JA. The role of the child in abuse: a review of the literature. Am J Orthopsychiatry 1976;46(4):580–590.
5. Steele B. Psychodynamic Factors in Child Abuse. In RE Helfer, RS Kempe (eds), The Battered Child (4th ed). Chicago: The University of Chicago Press, 1987; 82–83, 85–86.
6. Garbarino J. The human ecology of child maltreatment: a conceptual model for research. J Marriage Fam 1977;39:721–735.
7. Kessler DB, Hyden P. Physical, sexual, and emotional abuse of children. Clin Symp 1991;43(1):1–32.
8. Lewit EM. Reported child abuse and neglect. Future of Children 1994;4(2):233–242.
9. American Medical Association Council on Scientific Affairs. AMA Diagnostic and treatment guidelines concerning child abuse and neglect. JAMA 1985;254(6): 796–800.
10. Wiese D, Daro D. Current trends in child abuse reporting and fatalities: the results of the 1994 annual fifty state survey. National Committee to Prevent Child Abuse (NCPCA) Working Paper 808. April, 1995.
11. Farestad KJ, Winterfield A, England T, et al. Twenty Years After CAPTA: A Portrait of the Child Protective Services System. Englewood, CO: American Humane Association, May 27, 1994.
12. Sedlak AJ, Broadhurst DD. Third National Incidence Study of Child Abuse and Neglect. Washington DC: Department of Health and Human Services (Contract # 105-91-1800). September 1996.
13. Warner JE, Hansen DJ. The identification and reporting of physical abuse by physicians: a review and implications for research. Child Abuse Negl 1994; 18(1):11–25.
14. Straus MA, Gelles RJ. Societal change and change in family violence from 1975 to 1985 as revealed by two national surveys. J Marriage Fam 1986;48:465–479.
15. Norton LE. Child abuse. Clin Lab Med 1983;3(2): 321–342.
16. Morris JL, Johnson CF, Clasen M. To report or not to report. Physicians' attitudes toward discipline and child abuse. Am J Dis Children 1985;139:194–197.
17. Needleman HL. Child abuse and neglect—recognition and reporting. J Am Coll Dent 1994;61(1):30–37.
18. Kempe CH, Silverman FN, Steele BF, et al. The battered-child syndrome. JAMA 1962;181(1):105–112.
19. Quinn KL, Gammon JA. Children's eyes as indicators of physical abuse. Am Orthoptic J 1983;33:99–104.
20. McClain PW, Sacks JJ, Froehlke RG, Ewigman BG. Estimates of fatal child abuse and neglect, United States, 1979 through 1988. Pediatrics 1993;91(2): 338–343.
21. Luerssen TG, Bruce DA, Humphreys RP. Position statement on identifying the infant with nonaccidental central nervous system injury (the whiplash-shake syn-

drome). The American Society of Pediatric Neurosurgeons. Pediatr Neurosurg 1993;19(4):170.

22. Pascoe JM, Hildebrandt HM, Tarrier A, Murphy M. Patterns of skin injury in nonaccidental and accidental injury. Pediatrics 1979;64(2):245–247.

23. Bergman AB, Larsen RM, Mueller BA. Changing spectrum of serious child abuse. Pediatrics 1986;77(1):113–116.

24. Caffey J. Significance of the history in the diagnosis of traumatic injury to children. J Pediatr 1965;67(5):1008–1014.

25. Hight DW, Bakalar HR, Lloyd JR. Inflicted burns in children. JAMA 1979;242(6):517–520.

26. Hammond J, Perez-Stable A, Ward CG. Predictive value of historical and physical characteristics for the diagnosis of child abuse. South Med J 1991;84(2):166–168.

27. Ellerstein NS. The cutaneous manifestations of child abuse and neglect. Am J Dis Children 1979;133:906–909.

28. Stewart G, Meert K, Rosenberg N. Trauma in infants less than three months of age. Pediatr Emerg Care 1993;9(4):199–201.

29. Helfer RE, Slovis TL, Black M. Injuries resulting when small children fall out of bed. Pediatrics 1977;60(4):533–535.

30. Billmire ME, Myers PA. Serious head injury in infants: accident or abuse? Pediatrics 1985;75(2):340–342.

31. Nimityongskul P, Anderson LD. The likelihood of injuries when children fall out of bed. J Pediatr Orthop 1987;7:184–186.

32. Duhaime AC, Alario AJ, Lewander WJ, et al. Head injury in very young children: mechanisms, injury types, and ophthalmologic findings in 100 hospitalized patients younger than 2 years of age. Pediatrics 1992;90(2):179–185.

33. Lyons TJ, Oates RK. Falling out of bed: a relatively benign occurrence. Pediatrics 1993;92(1):125–127.

34. Swalwell C. Head injuries from short distance falls. Am J Forensic Med Pathol 1993;14(2):171–172.

35. Joffe M, Ludwig S. Stairway injuries in children. Pediatrics 1988;82(3):457–461.

36. Chadwick DL, Chin S, Salerno C, et al. Deaths from falls in children: how far is fatal? J Trauma 1991;31(10):1353–1355.

37. Schmitt BD. The Child with Nonaccidental Trauma. In RE Helfer, RS Kempe (eds), The Battered Child (4th ed). Chicago: The University of Chicago Press, 1987;186.

38. Feldman KW. Patterned abusive bruises of the buttocks and the pinnae. Pediatrics 1992;90(4):633–636.

39. Hanigan WC, Peterson RA, Njus G. Tin ear syndrome: rotational acceleration in pediatric head injuries. Pediatrics 1987;80(5):618–622.

40. Elner SG, Elner VM, Arnall M, Albert DM. Ocular and associated systemic findings in suspected child abuse. A necropsy study. Arch Ophthalmol 1990;108:1094–1101.

41. Brown JK, Minns RA. Non-accidental head injury, with particular reference to whiplash shaking injury and medico-legal aspects. Dev Med Child Neurol 1993;35(10):849–869.

42. Feldman KW. Child Abuse by Burning. In RE Helfer, RS Kempe (eds), The Battered Child (4th ed). Chicago: The University of Chicago Press, 1987;198–199.

43. Feldman KW, Schaller RT, Feldman JA, McMillon M. Tap water scald burns in children. Pediatrics 1978;62(1):1–7.

44. Nelson LB, Wilson TW, Jeffers JB. Eye injuries in childhood: demography, etiology, and prevention. Pediatrics 1989;84(3):438–441.

45. Friendly DS. Ocular manifestations of physical child abuse. Trans Am Acad Ophthalmol Otolaryngol 1971;75:318–332.

46. Jensen AD, Smith RE, Olson MI. Ocular clues to child abuse. J Pediatr Ophthalmol Strabismus 1971;8(4):270–272.

47. Eisenbrey AB. Retinal hemorrhage in the battered child. Child's Brain 1979;5:40–44.

48. Riffenburgh RS, Sathyavagiswaran L. The eyes of child abuse victims: autopsy findings. J Forensic Sci 1991;36(3):741–747.

49. Johnson DL, Braun D, Friendly D. Accidental head trauma and retinal hemorrhage. Neurosurgery 1993;33(2):231–235.

50. Budenz DL, Farber MG, Mirchandani HG, et al. Ocular and optic nerve hemorrhages in abused infants with intracranial injuries. Ophthalmology 1994;101(8):559–565.

51. Gilliland MGF, Luckenbach MW, Chenier TC. Systemic and ocular findings in 169 prospectively studied child deaths: retinal hemorrhages usually mean child abuse. Forensic Sci Int 1994;68(2):117–132.

52. Caffey J. The parent-infant traumatic stress syndrome; (Caffey-Kempe syndrome), (battered babe syndrome). Am J Roentgenol Radium Ther Nucl Med 1972;114(2):218–229.

53. Caffey J. The whiplash shaken infant syndrome: manual shaking by the extremities with whiplash-induced intracranial and intraocular bleedings, linked with residual permanent brain damage and mental retardation. Pediatrics 1974;54(4):396–403.

54. Caffey J. On the theory and practice of shaking infants: its potential residual effects of permanent brain damage and mental retardation. Am J Dis Children 1972;124(2):161–169.

55. Ingraham FD, Matson DD. Subdural hematoma in infancy. J Pediatr 1944;24(1):1–37.

56. Caffey J. Multiple fractures in the long bones of infants suffering from chronic subdural hematoma. Am J Roentgenol Radium Ther Nucl Med 1946;56(2):163–173.

57. Dykes LJ. The whiplash shaken infant syndrome: what has been learned? Child Abuse Negl 1986;10(2):211–221.

58. Ommaya AK, Faas F, Yarnell P. Whiplash injury and brain damage. An experimental study. JAMA 1968;204(4):285–289.

59. Ludwig S, Warman M. Shaken baby syndrome: a review of 20 cases. Ann Emerg Med 1984;13(2):104–107.

60. Harcourt B, Hopkins D. Ophthalmic manifestations of the battered-baby syndrome. BMJ 1971;3:398–401.

61. Hahn YS, Raimondi AJ, McLone DG, Yamanouchi Y. Traumatic mechanisms of head injury in child abuse. Child's Brain 1983;10:229–241.

62. Kanter RK. Retinal hemorrhage after cardiopulmonary resuscitation or child abuse. J Pediatr 1986;108(3):430–432.

63. McKeown HS. Retinal hemorrhages in the newborn. Trans Am Ophthalmol Soc 1940;38:510–519.

64. Chace RR, Merritt KK, Bellows M. Ocular findings in the newborn infant. A preliminary report. Arch Ophthalmol 1950;44:236–242.

65. Giles CL. Retinal hemorrhages in the newborn. Am J Ophthalmol 1960;49:1005–1011.

66. Sezen F. Retinal haemorrhages in newborn infants. Br J Ophthalmol 1970;55:248–253.

67. Bergen R, Margolis S. Retinal hemorrhages in the newborn. Ann Ophthalmol 1976;8:53–56.

68. Jain IS, Singh YP, Grupta SL, Gupta A. Ocular hazards during birth. J Pediatr Ophthalmol Strabismus 1980;17(1):14–16.

69. Goetting MG, Sowa B. Retinal hemorrhage after cardiopulmonary resuscitation in children: an etiologic reevaluation. Pediatrics 1990;85(4):585–588.

70. Munger CE, Peiffer RL, Bouldin TW, et al. Ocular and associated neuropathologic observations in suspected whiplash shaken infant syndrome. Am J Forensic Med Pathol 1993;14(3):193–200.

71. Kempe RS, Goldbloom RB. Malnutrition and Growth Retardation ("Failure to Thrive") in the Context of Child Abuse and Neglect. In RE Helfer, RS Kempe (eds), The Battered Child (4th ed). Chicago: The University of Chicago Press, 1987;313, 318, 330–331.

72. Plassmann R. Münchhausen syndromes and factitious diseases. Psychother Psychosom 1994;62(1–2):7–26.

73. Voutilainen R, Tuppurainen K. Ocular Münchhausen syndrome induced by incest. Acta Ophthalmologica 1989;67:319–321.

74. Winams JM, House LR, Robinson HE. Self-induced orbital emphysema as a presenting sign of Munchausen's syndrome. Laryngoscope 1983;93:1209–1211.

75. Rosenberg PN, Krohel GB, Webb RM, Hepler RS. Ocular Munchausen's syndrome. Ophthalmology 1986;93(8):1120–1123.

76. Lealman GT, Haigh D, Phillips JM, et al. Prediction and prevention of child abuse—an empty hope? Lancet 1983;1(8339):1423–1424.

77. Egeland B, Breitenbucher M, Rosenberg D. Prospective study of the significance of life stress in the etiology of child abuse. J Consult Clin Psychol 1980;48(2):195–205.

78. Starling SP, Holden JR, Jenny C. Abusive head trauma: the relationship of perpetrators to their victims. Pediatrics 1995;95(2):259–262.

79. Lynch MA, Roberts J. Predicting child abuse: signs of bonding failure in the maternity hospital. BMJ 1977;1:624–626.

80. Connelly CD, Straus MA. Mother's age and risk for physical abuse. Child Abuse Negl 1992;16(5):709–718.

81. Kaufman J, Zigler E. Do abused children become abusive parents? Am J Orthopsychiatry 1987;57(2):186–192.

82. Frodi AM. Contribution of infant characteristics to child abuse. Am J Ment Deficiency 1981;85(4):341–349.

83. Mazurek AJ. Epidemiology of paediatric injury. J Accid Emerg Med 1994;11(1):9–16.

84. Elmer E, Gregg GS. Developmental characteristics of abused children. Pediatrics 1967;40(4):596–602.

85. Goldson E, Fitch MJ, Wendell TA, Knapp G. Child abuse. Its relationship to birthweight, Apgar score and developmental testing. Am J Dis Children 1978;132:790–793.

86. Morse CW, Sahler OJZ, Friedman SB. A three-year follow-up study of abused and neglected children. Am J Dis Children 1970;120:439–446.

87. Ammerman RT, Van Hasselt VB, Hersen M. Maltreatment of handicapped children: a critical review. J Fam Violence 1988;3(1):53–72.

88. Sullivan PM, Brookhouser PE, Scanlan JM, et al. Patterns of physical and sexual abuse of communicatively handicapped children. Ann Otol Rhinol Laryngol 1991;100(3):188–194.

89. Oates RK. Personality development after physical abuse. Arch Dis Child 1984;59(2):147–150.

90. Elmer E. Hazards in determining child abuse. Child Welfare 1966;45:28–33.

91. Straus MA, Kantor GK. Stress and Child Abuse. In RE Helfer, RS Kempe (eds), The Battered Child (4th ed). Chicago: The University of Chicago Press, 1987;43–45.

92. Cohn AH. Effective treatment of child abuse and neglect. Soc Work 1979;24:513–519.

93. Fraser BG. A glance at the past, a gaze at the present, a glimpse at the future: a critical analysis of the development of child abuse reporting statutes. Chicago-Kent Law Rev 1978;54:641–686.

94. Tinkham T. Child abuse revisited. Med Trial Technique Q 1982;29(1):33–43.

95. Gerber PC. Child abuse: the O.D.'s role in prevention. Optom Manage 1988;24:31–34.

96. Moore TA. Physician liability for failing to report child abuse: part I. N Y Law J January 7, 1992;3, 5.

97. Moore TA. Physician liability in child abuse—II. N Y Law J February 4, 1992;3–5.

98. Saulsbury FT, Hyden GF. Child abuse reporting by physicians. South Med J 1986;79(5):585–587.

99. U.S. Department of Health and Human Services. Child Maltreatment 1993. Reports from the States to the National Center on Child Abuse and Neglect. Washington, DC: U.S. Government Printing Office, 1995.

100. Zellman GL, Antler S. Mandated reporters and CPS: a study in frustration. Misunderstanding and miscommunication threaten the system. Public Welfare 1990;48:30–37.

101. Saulsbury FT, Campbell RE. Evaluation of child abuse

reporting by physicians. Am J Dis Children 1985; 139:393–395.

102. National Center on Child Abuse and Neglect. Study of National Incidence and Prevalence of Child Abuse and Neglect: 1988. Washington, DC: U.S. Department of Health and Human Services (Contract # 105-85-1702, GOVDOC #: HE 23.1210: in 2/2 445-L-1), 1988.

103. Thomas MP. Child abuse and neglect. I. Historical overview, legal matrix, and social perspectives. N C Law Rev 1972;50:293–349.

104. Mushin AS. Ocular damage in the battered-baby syndrome. BMJ 1971;3:402–404.

105. Salzinger S, Feldman RS, Hammer M, Rosario M. The effects of physical abuse on children's social relationships. Child Dev 1993;64(1):169–187.

106. Hoffman-Plotkin D, Twentyman CT. A multimodal assessment of behavioral and cognitive deficits in abused and neglected preschoolers. Child Dev 1984;55:794–802.

107. Dubowitz H. Prevention of child maltreatment: what is known. Pediatrics 1989;83:570–577.

108. Showers J. The National Conference on Shaken Baby Syndrome. A Medical, Legal, and Prevention Challenge. Executive Summary. Alexandria, VA: National Association of Children's Hospitals and Related Institutions, 1997;28.

109. National Committee to Prevent Child Abuse. Help the Hurt Go Away [pamphlet]. South Deerfield, MA: National Committee to Prevent Child Abuse, 1990.

110. Helfer RE. A review of the literature on the prevention of child abuse and neglect. Child Abuse Negl 1982; 6:251–261.

111. Showers J. "Don't shake the baby": the effectiveness of a prevention program. Child Abuse Negl 1992; 16(1):11–18.

112. Smith SK. Child abuse and neglect: a diagnostic guide for the optometrist. J Am Optom Assoc 1988; 59(10):760–766.

113. Harley RD. Ocular manifestations of child abuse. J Pediatr Ophthalmol Strabismus 1980;17(1):5–13.

114. Kiffney GT. The eye of the "battered child." Arch Ophthalmol 1964;72:231–233.

115. Giangiacomo J, Barkett KJ. Ophthalmoscopic findings in occult child abuse. J Pediatr Ophthalmol Strabismus 1985;22(6):234–237.

116. Massicotte SJ, Folberg R, Torczynski E, et al. Vitreoretinal traction and perimacular retinal folds in the eyes of deliberately traumatized children. Ophthalmology 1991;98:1124–1127.

Appendix 18A

Resources for Information on Child Abuse

Organization	Description	Address	Contact Information
National Committee to Prevent Child Abuse (NCPCA)	Not-for-profit, volunteer-based organization committed to preventing child abuse through education, research, public awareness, and advocacy. Founded in 1972. Chapters in each state. Publishes a variety of materials on child abuse, abuse prevention, and parenting. Free catalog available.	332 S. Michigan Ave., Suite 1600 Chicago, IL 60604-4357 For orders: 200 State Rd. South Deerfield, MA 01373	(312) 663-3520

(800) 835-2671 |
National Clearing House on Child Abuse and Neglect Information	A clearinghouse for the National Center on Child Abuse and Neglect (NCCAN—federal agency under the U.S. Department of Health and Human Services) that provides information on research and programs related to child abuse and neglect.	PO Box 1182 Washington, DC 20013-1182	(800) 394-3366 (703) 385-7565 (fax) (703) 385-3206 E-mail: nccanch@calib.com Web site: http://www.calib. com/nccanch
Kidrights	For-profit publishing company. Free catalog available containing a variety of education materials on child abuse, child development, and parenting.	10100 Park Cedar Drive Charlotte, NC 28210	(800) 892-KIDS (fax) (704) 541-0113
SBS (Shaken Baby Syndrome) Prevention Plus	Catalog available that includes materials from "Never Shake a Baby" campaign and educational material for parents, professionals, and volunteers directed toward preventing child abuse.	649 Main St. Groveport, OH 43125	(800) 858-5222 (614) 836-8360 (fax) (614) 836-8359 E-mail: SBSPP@aol.com

Organization	Description	Address	Contact Information
American Humane Association	Provides public education, lobbying, and research to help prevent mistreatment of children.	63 Inverness Dr., E Englewood, CO 80112-5117	(303) 792-9900
National Center for Education in Maternal and Child Health (NCEMCH)	Funded through the Maternal and Child Health Bureau, this agency manages a database of projects funded by the bureau and collects information on maternal and child health.	2000 15th St., N, Suite 701 Arlington, VA 22201-2617	(703) 524-7802 (fax) (703) 524-9335 Web site: http://www.NCEMCH.org E-mail: info@NCEMCH.org
Child Welfare League of America Inc.	National federation of more than 800 agencies. The league and its affiliates work to improve the well-being of children and their families in the U.S. and Canada.	440 1st St., NW Washington, DC 20001-2085	(202) 638-2952 Web site: http://www.cwla.org

Appendix 18B
Referral Sources for Assistance

Organization	Description	Address	Contact Information
Childhelp USA/IOF Foresters National Child Abuse Hotline	Provides crisis counseling, child abuse reporting information, and information and referrals for every county in the United States.	1345 El Centro Ave. Hollywood, CA 90028	(800) 422-4453
Parents Anonymous (P.A.)	A self-help program for parents under stress and for abused children. Many local groups throughout the country; 32 in Texas.	675 West Foot Hill Blvd., Suite 220 Claremont, CA 91711 In Texas: 7801 N. Lamar, Suite F8 Austin, TX 78752	Outside Texas: (909) 621-6184 In Texas: (800) 554-2323
National Child Advocacy Center	Provides information, training, and technical assistance to those interested in child abuse, sexual abuse, and neglect.	200 Westside Square, Suite 700 Huntsville, AL 35801	(205) 543-6868
C. Henry Kempe National Center for the Prevention and Treatment of Child Abuse and Neglect	Provides information about neglect, evaluation, and treatment for families, and. consultation to professionals on cases	University of Colorado School of Medicine Pediatric Department 1205 Oneida Denver, CO 80220	(303) 321-3963

Chapter 19

Identification of Potential Learning Disabilities in Preschool Children

Jack E. Richman and Richard C. Laudon

During the past decade, optometry has evolved into more of a primary vision care profession through its expanded clinical education and training. The primary care optometrist is therefore often one of the first health care providers to have contact with children for eye and vision care services. This contact may serve as an entry point for the child into the complex array and variety of health care services. The primary care optometrist should pay attention to all aspects of child development, including general health, vision, and learning and behavioral development [1, 2].

The preschool years (3–5 years of age) are a critical period in the child's overall development. This period has significant impact on later levels of child development and is characterized by dramatic changes in growth and behavior. Children's language, vocabulary, and motor skills increase significantly during this time [3]. Some children may not develop at the normal rate or develop differently from other children in certain ways. In some of these children, these differences are obvious (e.g., deafness, visual or physical impairment) [4]. For others, the differences may be more subtle or seem insignificant to the casual observer. Certain subtle conditions, however, can place the preschool child at risk for later difficulties. Almost all health care providers who treat children encounter a variety of potential physical and behavioral problems that may contribute to academic and learning problems. Early detection of children likely to be at risk for later reading and learning problems is important;

however, many children with reading and learning problems are not detected or referred for diagnostic evaluations until they are well into the school-age years [5].

This chapter summarizes basic information the primary care optometrist should know about early identification and treatment of preschoolers at risk for reading and learning problems. It includes information about identification of factors that place a child at risk for developmental disabilities, screening procedures, early childhood care and education programs, and the role of the optometrist in this early identification and intervention process.

THE AT-RISK CHILD

Any interference with or delays in the normal process of development, especially during the critical preschool years, may place a child at risk for later problems. If these problems go unrecognized and untreated, permanent disabilities may result. When developmental delays or factors that interfere with development are detected, a child is considered to be at risk for later problems in health, behavior, and learning [6]. Difficulty in any aspect of the learning process may be due to a complex interaction between biological, sociocultural, and psychoeducational factors. Biological aspects of learning problems should be considered predisposing factors, whereas nonbiological aspects are classified as environmental causes [7].

Many biological factors have been suggested as potential links to childhood learning problems, including excessive maternal drug use of substances such as alcohol, heroin, cocaine, and tobacco; maternal malnutrition; premature birth; neonatal seizures; maternal infections; central nervous system trauma; and chronic neonatal infections.

Although these factors do not inevitably cause developmental problems, the health care provider should carefully monitor any child who is at risk due to the presence of any of these factors. The presence of additional risk factors should be determined by gathering more information about the child's home and sociocultural environment and, if warranted, by performing a direct assessment of that environment. Outcomes of exposure to risk factors characteristically vary from the full manifestation of a physical and learning problem, to a partial or mild appearance, to no detectable problem at all [8]. Children respond differently to the same risk factors, and these factors do not necessarily affect an individual child in an "all-or-none" fashion. Accurate prediction of a child's specific response to exposure to a risk factor is not really possible.

It is important to differentiate between identifying at-risk children and identifying children with current problems. Labeling a child or a situation as "at risk" is a clinician's projected judgment based on assessment of risk factors and their potential for causing future problems. In contrast, identification is the process by which a child, his or her environment, or both are assessed to determine the existence of a current problem. In either case, the focus should be on detecting a deficiency or developmental delay in its early stages through screening or more involved assessment procedures.

In theory, screening and determining a diagnosis are distinctly different processes, but it is not uncommon for results of screening to be thought of as an actual diagnosis [9]. For this reason, some tests lead to the labeling of children without a complete assessment being performed. The label may then be interpreted as a diagnosis and the diagnosis may lead to a recommended, but unnecessary, intervention [10]. The purpose of entry-level screening is to survey large groups of children to detect potential problems. Such screening procedures usually have lower reliability and validity than procedures designed for diagnostic classification and for generating specific prescriptions. At best, most screening procedures provide a preliminary indication that something may be wrong; at worst, the validity of entry-level screenings may be so low or insensitive that they do not identify children unless they exhibit obvious problems. To determine specific diagnoses and recommend appropriate interventions, assessment procedures with greater validity are essential.

The question of whether or not young children should ever be labeled as "at risk for academic failure" inevitably produces disagreement. Experts disagree about whether it is valid to consider a child to be "at risk" before he or she has been exposed to opportunities for demonstrating academic achievement. The possible disadvantages of such labeling have been discussed frequently in the literature. Labels may serve as self-fulfilling prophecies because they lower expectations of the child among parents and teachers [11], while children who internalize such labels may develop low self-concepts. Despite these disagreements, most parents and early childhood educators strongly support efforts to identify and intercede when deficiencies are seen during the earliest years of life. More and more individuals are hesitant, however, to endorse brief screening efforts because they are concerned about the negative effects of labeling and the potential for overlooking a child who may have significantly benefited from appropriate intervention [12, 13].

Regardless, any health care provider who encounters a preschool child with known risk factors or early signs of developmental delay should be aware of the fact that the child is at risk for later learning problems.

SCREENING PROCEDURES

The clinician should use multiple approaches to identify developmental delays and potential learning disabilities. The most time-consuming, yet most accurate methods use reliable, valid, standardized testing methods and procedures to measure development (e.g., the Bayley Scales of Infant Development) [14]. These instruments compare the scores of the individual being tested with normal levels for his or her age group. It is often impractical to use methods that require extensive time for testing—that is, more than 15–20 minutes—in a clinical office because of the time and complexity involved [15].

Developmental screening tools are a less time-consuming option than the more accurate complete assessment test batteries. These screening tools apply a standardized measure of development but use fewer items than the more sophisticated assessment tools. Developmental screening tests have been criticized, however [16]. Since screening tests can be superficial, developmental delays may be missed (under-referral) or may be indicated by the test when no real delay is present (over-referral). The Denver Developmental Screening Test (DDST), for example, is one of the most widely used screening tests, yet it may not detect delays that are subsequently identified, especially in the area of language skills [17]. It does not over-refer children because it tends to identify most children as normal, including children with language delays [18]. Developmental screening tests can still be time consuming. Although they have fewer items than the complete assessment and diagnostic batteries, they have to be presented more accurately. Since the screening tests have fewer items to conserve time, the items selected have to be administered more carefully to ensure accuracy and validity. This will require increased attention by the screener during the test and training in test application for the screener [19].

If the clinician does not have time to perform a developmental screening test, the third option is use of prescreening questionnaires. Parents can fill them out while they are waiting for their child's examination or complete them at home. This approach may be more cost effective and efficient than the use of screening instruments. Some of these systems have been shown to be valuable in identifying children with developmental delays when used under the correct conditions [20]. Prescreening questionnaires have several advantages. Parents are often excellent observers of their child's development and enjoy reporting their observations on a questionnaire. The completion of the prescreening questionnaires promotes parents' interests in developmental milestones and invites discussions about their child's development [21].

The final option for detecting developmental delays or risk factors is the use of surveillance. This option is being promoted by those critical of screening tests, which may be used without considering other information about the child and family. Surveillance is the art of being suspicious. The best way to increase the index of suspicion of a developmental delay in the child is to listen to parents' concerns, make observations about the child's behavior, and draw on multiple sources of information before identifying a child as being at risk for learning problems. This approach may be the least time consuming and theoretically is the most efficient method. However, this approach varies from practitioner to practitioner depending on individual clinical experience. According to Dworkin,

> Surveillance is a flexible, continuous process that is broader in scope than screening, whereby knowledgeable professionals perform skilled observations of children throughout all encounters during child health care.... It entails obtaining a relevant developmental history, making accurate and informative observations of children and eliciting and attending to parental concerns [22].

A child who does not seem to be developing appropriately based on what the clinician has seen in surveillance should be referred to or scheduled for a more comprehensive developmental assessment with specific clinicians who may address the area of concern. These may include such professionals as pediatricians, neurologists, speech-language pathologists, and occupational therapists. The following list contains examples of pointed questions that can be asked of the parents to aid in surveillance:

Do you have any concerns about your child's vision or hearing?
Did your child walk or talk later than you expected?
What recent changes have you seen in your child's development?
What kind of temperament did your child have as a baby?
What do you and your child enjoy doing together?
What are your child's favorite play activities?
What do you find most difficult about caring for your child now?

Surveillance examines more aspects of the child's development and environment than any single screening tool. It includes a developmental history, comments and observations during health and vision examinations, parent observations and concerns, and any other input from persons having contact with the child. Surveillance may also include reports on the child's performance in activities that have been recommended to encourage various aspects of cognitive and motor development. The information gained from screening tests and questionnaires may even be included. The overall

Table 19.1. Publishers for Developmental Screening Tests for Young Children

Name of Test	Publisher's Address
Developmental Indicators for Assessment of Learning-Revised (DIAL)	American Guidance Service Publishers Building Circle Pines, MN 55014
Early Screening Profile	See Developmental Indicators for Assessment of Learning-Revised (DIAL), above
Miller Assessment for Preschoolers	The Psychological Corporation 555 Academic Court San Antonio, TX 78204

success of surveillance as a technique varies depending on the practitioner's professional experience, knowledge, and acquired skills. Some clinicians may make excellent early referral and intervention decisions, whereas others take a "wait-and-see" approach based on similar information and only respond when it becomes obvious that the child has a significant developmental delay. Although parents may suspect a problem, they will frequently go along with the practitioner's advice. In some cases, precious time for early intervention may be lost. Surveillance has value, but its dependence on the practitioner skills and knowledge make its results highly variable. Its validity and reliability need to be examined through large-scale population-based studies.

Because all of the methods for identifying children at risk for reading and learning problems have both strengths and weaknesses, the practitioner may use several approaches to make a final decision regarding the developmental status of a child. The more options a practitioner has available to efficiently assess the developmental status of children, the more accurate his or her assessment will be.

In a review, Satz and Fletcher [12] discussed the need for earlier identification of learning disabled children and the problems related to this identification. They raised numerous concerns about the design of screening instruments, including their lack of longitudinal and outcome results. Continued expansion and development of instruments used for screening preschoolers is needed. Even if a very

sensitive screening instrument could be developed with excellent reliability, validity, and sensitivity, its results may not reflect all aspects of the developing child's strengths and weaknesses. It is ultimately up to the clinicians, educators, and parents to incorporate and apply these screening results in planning for the child's future needs.

Several developmental screening tests are individually administered and require at least 15–20 minutes to administer. The Denver II [17] is a revised version of the original DDST from the late 1960s. Despite the changes and improvements in the Denver II, it still has a number of serious limitations. Preacademic and academic skills are not assessed, which, as the authors themselves suggest, means that the test may not detect emerging or existing learning disabilities in children [18]. A wide range of other screening tools are available on the market, some of excellent and some of questionable quality. Tests that are standardized on a national basis and have reasonable sensitivity and specificity (i.e., how well they identified correctly children with developmental delays from those who did not) are the best. The three tests that meet these criteria are the Developmental Indicators for Assessment of Learning-Revised [23], the Miller Assessment for Preschoolers [24], and the Early Screening Profile [25]. For a list of these screening instruments and their publishers, see Table 19.1. All require 15–30 minutes to administer; are designed for children as young as 2 years of age; evaluate language, cognitive, and motor development; and incorporate parental observations and questionnaires. It is beyond the scope of this discussion to review and critique each assessment tool available. Several reviews address these issues in great detail [26–28].

ADMINISTERING SCREENING TESTS

The purpose of screening is to correctly identify as many at-risk children as possible; therefore, practical and efficient application of these procedures is essential. A multiperson approach that includes individuals who are trained and familiar with the screening instruments and cooperative and observant parents, teachers, and clinicians is required. To improve the validity and reliability of results, the examiner should become familiar with the child, have a language and interaction style appropriate for the child's background, and possess credentials and experience in understanding children and child development [29]. The less information gathered due to time constraints or an inexperienced or inadequately prepared screener, the less reliable and valid the final screening decision will be. The clinician needs to ensure that appropriate time for administration of screening tests is maintained.

REFERRAL

If a primary care optometrist determines that a young child may have developmental delays, he or she should refer the child to other professionals (e.g., pediatrician, occupational therapist, speech-language specialist) for further evaluation in addition to addressing any vision or ocular disorders. Preparing and informing the parents of the need for a referral and directing the referral to the appropriate sources are the two major steps in this process.

Parents are generally not pleased to learn that something may be "different" with their child. Even when they believe a problem may exist, they hope that someone will tell them that everything is fine and that their child will outgrow the problem. Unfortunately, many parents are told their child has a problem they did not know existed and the problem is explained in a way that the parents find difficult to understand. The key to this sensitive situation is the manner in which the practitioner presents his or her findings, observations, and concerns [30]. The practitioner should attempt to be sincere, honest, and use simple language. It is often helpful to integrate the parent's observations of the child with the results from any screening test. While explaining the results, attempt to demonstrate the test and what might be expected of a child of a similar age without a developmental delay. Initially, parents may be bewildered and deny that there is any problem. Give the parents time to react to recommendations and allow them the opportunity to ask questions. This may require another visit scheduled specifically to discuss this issue. It is important to understand the initial anxiety and possible emotions the parents are experiencing. By offering support as an advocate, they may feel they have a health care ally to assist in reviewing and discussing future decisions.

The next step, the actual referral, has been made easier by numerous federal laws, including the Education of the Handicapped Act (and its 1986 amendments) and the Individuals with Disabilities Act [31]. These laws require each state to develop and fund comprehensive programs for early-intervention services for infants, toddlers, and preschoolers with disabilities. When a state participates, it receives financial support for early intervention services. Each eligible child must include a multidisciplinary assessment; a written Individualized Family Service Plan developed by a multidisciplinary team and the child's parents; services designed to meet developmental needs, which may include special education, speech and language pathology, audiology, occupational therapy, physical therapy, psychological services, parent and family training and counseling services, transition services, medical services for diagnostic purposes, and health services necessary to enable the child to benefit from other early intervention services; case management services for every eligible child and his or her parents; qualified personnel to provide all services; a system for the establishment and maintenance of standards, certification, and licensing policies; and services provided at no cost to parents except when federal or state law provides for a system of payments by parents, including provision for a sliding-fee scale [32]. The actual process for early-intervention referrals varies from state to state. The simplest method for gaining access to the referral system and these services is through the special education services of the local school system, the state department of education, or the state department of public health. These agencies should provide the practitioner and the parents with eligibility criteria for services. The practitioner should become familiar with the intake process and clarify it for the parents. The child and family will go through an intake process with a service coordinator. This meeting often involves collecting basic information about the family and providing necessary information about the early intervention programs.

EFFICACY OF EARLY CHILDHOOD EDUCATION PROGRAMS

Early childhood care and education (ECCE) programs include early intervention, preschool education, and Head Start programs. Early intervention programs are designed for children of school age or younger who have or are at risk of developing a disabling condition or other special need that may affect their development. Early intervention programs provide services for both children and their families. These programs may be remedial or preventive in nature. Early intervention programs may be center based, home based, hospital based, or a combination [33].

The contribution of ECCE programs to children's development is an important public issue with critical implications for families, business, private philanthropy, and government. The extent to which ECCE programs produce long-term benefits in children's cognitive development, socialization, and academic success is a matter of some controversy.

After nearly 50 years of research, both quantitative and qualitative evidence has been found that early intervention increases the developmental and educational gains for the child, improves the functioning of the family, and reaps long-term benefits for society [33]. Early intervention has been shown to result in the child (1) needing fewer special education and other rehabilitative services later in life; (2) repeating grades less often; and (3) in some cases, being indistinguishable from nondisabled classmates years after intervention. Many studies and literature reviews report that intervention is more effective the earlier it occurs. A review [34] consisting of 36 studies of both model demonstration projects and large-scale public programs examined the long-term effects of these programs. The review carefully considers issues related to research design. It includes studies of preschool education, Head Start, child care, and home visiting programs and focuses primarily on the effects of program participation on children's cognitive development. The bulk of the evidence found that ECCE programs produced significant short-term effects on IQ during the early childhood years and sizable persistent benefits on the achievement, grade retention, special education, high school graduation, and socialization of children. In particular, the evidence of early intervention's ability to reduce grade retention and minimize use of special education services is very strong. However, not all programs produce these desired benefits, perhaps because of differences in quality and resource appropriations across the different programs. These studies indicate that early intervention therapy, language stimulation, and exposure to rich experiences at ages 3–4 years will potentially increase the achievement levels of children at risk for reading and learning difficulties.

ROLE OF THE OPTOMETRIST

Optometrists are often one of the first health care practitioners to care for young children. This opportunity places them in an excellent position, side by side with the pediatrician, to identify developmental delays in children. With knowledge about preschool screening and referral methods, supporting the parents, and working in conjunction with ECCE programs, the optometrist can potentially identify and advocate for children at risk for later reading and learning problems.

REFERENCES

1. Shonkoff JP, Dworkin PH, Leviton A. Primary approaches to developmental disabilities. Pediatrics 1979;64:506–514.
2. Hayman LL. Primary health care aspects of learning problems in young children. Topics Early Child Educ 1983;3(3):41-46.
3. Edwards CP. Normal Development in the Preschool Years. In EV Nuttall, I Romero, J Kalesnick (eds), Assessing and Screening Preschoolers. Psychological and Educational Dimensions. Boston: Allyn and Bacon, 1992;9–22.
4. Lifter K. Delays and Differences in the Development of Preschool Children. In EV Nuttall, I Romero, J Kalesnick (eds), Assessing and Screening Preschoolers. Psychological and Educational Dimensions. Boston: Allyn and Bacon, 1992;23–41.
5. Keogh BK, Daley SE. Early identification: one component of comprehensive services for at-risk children. Topics Early Child Educ 1983;3(3):7–16.
6. Adelman HS. Identifying learning problems at an early age: a critical appraisal. J Clin Child Psychol 1982;11: 255–261.
7. Peterson NL. Early Intervention for Handicapped and At-Risk Children: An Introduction to Early Childhood-Special Education. Denver: Love Publishing, 1987.
8. Nichols PL, Chen T. Minimal Brain Dysfunction: A Prospective Study. Hillsdale, NJ: Erlbaum, 1981
9. Meier JH. Screening, Assessment, and Intervention for Young Children at Developmental Risk. In N Hobbs (ed), Issues in the Classification of Children. San Francisco: Jossey-Bass, 1975.

10. Leigh JE. Early labeling of children: concerns and alternatives. Topics Early Child Educ 1983;3(3):7–16.

11. Foster G, Schmidt C, Sabatino D. Teacher expectations and the label "learning disabilities." J Learn Disabil 1976;9:58–61

12. Satz P, Fletcher JM. Early identification of learning disabled children: an old problem revisited. J Consult Clin Psychol 1988;56:824–829.

13. Lindsay GA, Wedell K. The early identification of educationally "at risk" children revisited. J Learn Disabil 1982;15:212–217.

14. Bayley N. Manual for the Bayley Scales of Infant Development. New York: The Psychological Corporation, 1969.

15. Romero I. Individual Assessment Procedures with Preschool Children. In EV Nuttall, I Romero, J Kalesnick (eds), Assessing and Screening Preschoolers. Psychological and Educational Dimensions. Boston: Allyn and Bacon, 1992;55–66.

16. Dworkin PW. Developmental screening—expecting the impossible? Pediatrics 1989;83:619–622.

17. Frankenburg WK, Dodds J, Archer P. The Denver II: a major revision and restandardization of the Denver Developmental Screening Test. Pediatrics 1992;89:91.

18. Meisels SJ. Can developmental screening tests identify children who are developmentally at risk? Pediatrics 1989;83:578–585.

19. Smith RD. The use of developmental screening tests by primary care pediatricians. J Pediatr 1986;93:524–527.

20. Eisert DC, Stumer RA, Mabe PA. Questionnaires in behavioral pediatrics: guidelines for selection and use. J Dev Behav Pediatr 1991;12:42–50.

21. Glascoe FP, Altemeier WA, MacLean WE. The importance of parents' concern about their child's development. Am J Dis Child 1989;143:955–958.

22. Dworkin PH. British and American recommendations for developmental monitoring: the role of surveillance. Pediatrics 1989;84:1,000–1,010.

23. Mardell-Czudnowski CD, Goldenberg DS. Developmental Indicators for the Assessment of Learning-Re-

vised. Circle Pines, MN: American Guidance Service, 1990.

24. Miller LJ. Miller Assessment for Preschoolers. San Antonio, TX: The Psychological Corporation, 1988.

25. Harrison PL, Kaufman AS, Kaufman NL, et al. Early Screening Profiles. Circle Pines, MN: American Guidance Service, 1990.

26. Glascoe FP. Developmental screening: rational, methods, and application. Inf Young Children 1991;4:1–10.

27. Cohn M. Screening Measures. In EV Nuttall, I Romero, J Kalesnick (eds), Assessing and Screening Preschoolers. Psychological and Educational Dimensions. Boston: Allyn and Bacon, 1992;83–98.

28. Miller LJ, Sprong TA. Psychometric and qualitative comparison of four preschool screening instruments. J Learn Disabil 1986;19:480–484.

29. Thurlow ML. Issues in the Screening of Preschool Children. In EV Nuttall, I Romero, J Kalesnick (eds), Assessing and Screening Preschoolers. Psychological and Educational Dimensions. Boston: Allyn and Bacon, 1992;67–82.

30. Solomon R. Pediatricians and early intervention: everything you need to know but are too busy to ask. Inf Young Children 1995;7(3):38–51.

31. Demers ST, Fiorello C, Langer KL. Legal and Ethical Issues in Preschool Assessment. In EV Nuttall, I Romero, J Kalesnick (eds), Assessing and Screening Preschoolers. Psychological and Educational Dimensions. Boston: Allyn and Bacon, 1992;43–54.

32. Zantal-Wiener, K. Preschool services for children with handicaps. ERIC Digest #450. ERIC Clearinghouse on Handicapped and Gifted Children. Reston, VA ED295394; 1995.

33. Smith, BJ. Does early intervention help? ERIC Digest #455. Revised. ERIC Clearinghouse on Handicapped and Gifted Children. Reston, VA ED295399; 1994.

34. Barnett SW. Long-term effects of early childhood programs on cognitive and school outcomes. Future Children 1995;5(3):1–19.

Index